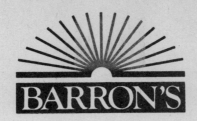

BARRON'S

HOW TO PREPARE FOR THE MEDICAL COLLEGE ADMISSION TEST

MCAT

SIXTH EDITION

by

Hugo R. Seibel, Ph.D.

Professor of Anatomy
Associate Dean of Medicine for Student Activities
School of Medicine and
School of Basic Health Sciences
Medical College of Virginia, Virginia Commonwealth University

and

Kenneth E. Guyer, Ph.D.

Associate Professor of Biochemistry
School of Medicine, Marshall University
Huntington, West Virginia

BARRON'S EDUCATIONAL SERIES, INC.
New York • London • Toronto • Sydney

All inquiries should be addressed to:
Barron's Educational Series, Inc.
250 Wireless Boulevard
Hauppauge, New York 11788

Library of Congress Catalog Card No. 89-17823

International Standard Book No. 0-8120-4288-3

Library of Congress Cataloging in Publication Data
Seibel, Hugo R.
    Barron's How to prepare for the Medical College Admission Test,
MCAT/by Hugo R. Seibel and Kenneth E. Guyer. —6th ed.
        p. cm.
    ISBN 0-8120-4288-3
    1. Medical colleges—United States—Entrance examinations—Study
guides.   I. Guyer, Kenneth E.   II. Title.   III. Title: How to
prepare for the Medical College Admission Test, MCAT.
    [DNLM: 1. Medicine—examination questions. W 18 S457b]
R838.5.S45   1990
610'.76—dc20
                                                89-17823
                                                CIP

PRINTED IN THE UNITED STATES OF AMERICA

0123   100   987654321

Contents

Preface

Can you prepare for the Medical College Admission Test (MCAT)? Some students are hesitant to utilize a book of this sort to assist in preparation for the medical college admission test, perhaps believing there is something dishonest about this method of preparation. Other students may believe that they can utilize this book or a similar one just before the test to prepare themselves.

In our estimation both of these viewpoints are incorrect. These practice materials should provide experience in timed tests of this type and point out areas of weakness for additional study in appropriate textbooks. By proper and careful preparation utilizing all possible modes, the individual is simply presenting his or her true potential for the study of medicine. For maximum benefit we would suggest that students begin their preparation two or three months before the examination. This will allow time to take some of the practice examinations, review the areas of weakness, and retake some of the practice examinations without having the pressure of time to produce undue frustration and a feeling of hopelessness.

Obtaining admission to medical school is a very difficult task today. We hope that, in preparing this volume, we have been able to offer you a greater chance of success. Good luck!

We wish to acknowledge the help we have received from many of our colleagues; a special thank you should be extended to H. Meetz; G. D. Meetz; J. Gregorek; J. D. Reynolds; W. M. Reams; C. Kirksey; R. J. Krieg; J. H. Johnson; S. S. Craig; J. D. Povlishock; W. Seibel; L. Crane; L. P. Gartner; L. M. Sawyer; G. J. Somori; W. J. McIntyre; J. Washburn; J. L. Poland; S. L. Quattropani; M. P. Golka; F. M. Bush; R. L. Salisbury; M. M. Sholley; G. Miller; C. H. Fowlkes; R. B. Brandt; P. L. Szabo; N. Whisner; J. Wood; J. P. Guyer; J. Kass; Lester Schlumpf; and Robert Lehrman. Particular gratitude is extended to Mrs. Marilyn P. Bertrand for her cheerful and spirited assistance and the typing of the manuscript. We are indebted to Mrs. Edith E. Seibel for her contributions and the proofreading of the book. Dr. Erwin E. Seibel deserves a special commendation since he contributed the bulk of the physics questions of this work.

Introduction

The MCAT was first administered to prospective medical students in the spring of 1977. It represents an attempt to evaluate (1) the student's knowledge and ability to solve problems in the areas of biology, chemistry, and physics, and (2) the student's skill in analysis of paragraphs, tabular material, graphs, etc. Separate scores will be reported for Biology, Chemistry, Physics, Science Problems (mixed scientific disciplines), Skills Analysis: Quantitative, and Skills Analysis: Reading. Since 1985, an essay topic has been administered on a trial basis as part of the MCAT. In 1991 the essay will become a permanent part of the exam.

It is expected that those taking the test will have the equivalent of one year of college study in each of the following scientific areas: biology, general and/or inorganic chemistry, organic chemistry, and physics. Although advanced study in one or more of these disciplines may give a better understanding of concepts, it is not intended that the questions will require a knowledge of concepts not taught in basic courses.

A mathematics background including one year of college mathematics should suffice for the science and quantitative skills questions; calculus is not required. Indeed, it has been suggested that high school courses including two years of algebra, use of trigonometric functions, memorization of sine and cosine of 0°, 90°, and 180°, facility in use of metric and English units and conversion from one set of units to another (when conversion factors are given); experimental error; statistics to include the concepts of arithmetic mean, range, variability, and significant figures; and vector addition and subtraction would represent adequate preparation in mathematics.

It is our suggestion that you begin preparation by studying the review sections of this book. Areas that are particularly difficult for you may require some review of your college texts. When you begin taking the practice tests, try to pace yourself to allow completion of each section within the allotted time. (If it is necessary to omit some questions because of time limitations, you may wish to go back after you have scored the test and try to answer them without the pressure of time.)

After taking your first practice test and correcting the answers, you should score your test as it will be done after the actual test. First count the number of correct answers in (1) Biology, (2) Chemistry, and (3) Physics. In each case this will represent the number of correct answers in that discipline in Science Knowledge and Science Problems.

The number of correct answers is the raw score and must then be converted into a 15-point scaled score *approximated by* the following tables. The approximation exists because raw score to scaled score tables may vary from test to test due to slight differences in degree of difficulty.

Biology		Chemistry		Physics	
Raw Score	Scaled Score	Raw Score	Scaled Score	Raw Score	Scaled Score
1–4	1	1–4	1	1–4	1
5–8	2	5–8	2	5–7	2
9–12	3	9–12	3	8–11	3
13–16	4	13–16	4	12–15	4
17–20	5	17–20	5	16–19	5
21–24	6	21–24	6	20–22	6
25–28	7	25–28	7	23–25	7
29–32	8	29–32	8	26–28	8
33–36	9	33–36	9	29–32	9
37–40	10	37–40	10	33–35	10
41–44	11	41–44	11	36–39	11
45–48	12	45–48	12	40–43	12
49–52	13	49–52	13	44–46	13
53–57	14	53–57	14	47–49	14
58–59	15	58–59	15	50–51	15

Although individual medical schools will vary with respect to the scores they require, a standard score of 11 or greater will probably be considered to be quite competitive. A standard score of 7 or less would indicate an area requiring substantial additional preparation. Before taking the next practice test, you should concentrate on areas of low score.

You will also be scoring Science Problems; Skills Analysis: Reading; and Skills Analysis: Quantitative. These will also be converted to standard scores as *approximated by* the tables below.

Science Problems		Skills Analysis Reading		Skills Analysis Quantitative	
Raw Score	Scaled Score	Raw Score	Scaled Score	Raw Score	Scaled Score
1–4	1	0–5	1	0–5	1
5–8	2	6–10	2	6–10	2
9–12	3	11–15	3	11–15	3
13–16	4	16–20	4	16–20	4
17–20	5	21–24	5	21–24	5
21–24	6	25–28	6	25–28	6
25–28	7	29–32	7	29–32	7
29–32	8	33–37	8	33–37	8
33–36	9	38–41	9	38–41	9
37–40	10	42–45	10	42–45	10
41–44	11	46–49	11	46–49	11
45–48	12	50–54	12	50–54	12
49–52	13	55–59	13	55–59	13
53–57	14	60–64	14	60–64	14
58–60	15	65–68	15	65–68	15

Before taking the next practice test, you should consider whether either of these latter three areas requires special attention. The Science Problems may be remediated by additional study and working problems. The two areas of Skills Analysis, however, may require a slightly different approach. Try going back over this part of the examination, reading carefully, and answering the questions again without a time limit. Read the paragraph again and try to determine why you missed certain questions. Be sure to use only the information in the paragraph. Then go on to additional practice examinations. One additional suggestion: Read the questions carefully before answering. Sometimes students answer the question they *expected* rather than the question that was asked. Try to avoid this pitfall.

If you are unable to read at the required rate and comprehension level, then your problem may be more serious. After studying the Reading Skills Analysis section of this book, you may want to review some reading selections from your Freshman English course.

As you progress through the other practice tests, you should develop facility in working faster to allow completion of each section. Although wild guessing is of no value, it is to your advantage to guess among a select number of answers if you have ruled out some answers.

Remember: we cannot hope to present everything you should have learned in years of study. We can only help you to identify areas of weakness, give some review of important concepts and provide experience and confidence in taking a test having the format of the Medical College Admission Test. We hope that this will allow you to reach your own potential on this test.

TIMETABLE FOR THE MCAT*

TOTAL TIME: Approximately 7 hours, plus 1 hour for lunch, 20 minutes for breaks

115 minutes	25B** 46C 44P	Science Knowledge (109 questions)	38 questions on biology 38 questions on chemistry 33 questions on physics
10 minutes	REST PERIOD		
78 minutes	Science Problems (60 questions)	21 questions on biology 21 questions on chemistry 18 questions on physics	
60 minutes	ESSAY		
60 minutes	LUNCH		
85 minutes	Skills Analysis: Reading (68 questions)		
10 minutes	REST PERIOD		
85 minutes	Skills Analysis: Quantitative (68 questions)		

* Format subject to change.   **Suggested Time for Each Discipline

SELF-SCORING CHARTS

Model Examination A	Total Possible	Raw Score	MCAT Score
Science Knowledge: + Science Problems			
Biology 38 + 21	59	+	
Chemistry 38 + 21	59	+	
Physics 33 + 18	51	+	
Science Problems	60		
Skills Analysis:			
Reading	68		
Quantitative	68		

Model Examination B	Total Possible	Raw Score	MCAT Score
Science Knowledge: + Science Problems			
Biology 38 + 21	59	+	
Chemistry 38 + 21	59	+	
Physics 33 + 18	51	+	
Science Problems	60		
Skills Analysis:			
Reading	68		
Quantitative	68		

Model Examination C		Total Possible	Raw Score	MCAT Score
Science Knowledge: + Science Problems				
Biology	38 + 21	59	+	
Chemistry	38 + 21	59	+	
Physics	33 + 18	51	+	
Science Problems		60		
Skills Analysis:				
Reading		68		
Quantitative		68		

Model Examination D		Total Possible	Raw Score	MCAT Score
Science Knowledge: + Science Problems				
Biology	38 + 21	59	+	
Chemistry	38 + 21	59	+	
Physics	33 + 18	51	+	
Science Problems		60		
Skills Analysis:				
Reading		68		
Quantitative		68		

Role of the MCAT

The MCAT in combination with college grades (overall and science GPA), types and quality of courses, letters of recommendation, extracurricular activities, major undergraduate institution attended, the interview, SAT, etc., is a screening device. The test is an objective measure and high scores will help an individual with average grades. Average or slightly lower MCAT scores probably do not significantly affect a superior college record. The literature points to a positive correlation between high MCAT scores (especially science subtests) and future success in the basic medical sciences (preclinical phase) and National Board of Medical Examiners Part I examination scores. The science knowledge tests in biology and chemistry and the science problems portions tend to have the highest correlations during the preclinical phase while the reading subtests retain their predictive value throughout.

TEST PREPARATION AND TEST-TAKING STRATEGIES COMPILED WITH THE HELP OF SUCCESSFUL MEDICAL STUDENTS

During the last 20 years, we have been involved in the training of approximately 5000 medical students; we have explored and discussed with them their test-taking strategies, since prospective medical students, and particularly students who are already in medical school, are probably the best, most efficient, and skillful test takers in the world. They must be good to survive and to cope with the volume of detailed material. To do this, they have learned to recognize key elements and have trained themselves to be hard and cold in their determination to accomplish the task.

Over the years, we have found some common attitudes and methods, which we would like to mention to you. We have met in group discussion with several of our present students, and they have helped us compile their test preparation and test-taking strategies, which they recommend highly.

Test Preparation

A. Key elements in preparation
    1. Study!
    2. Fine-tune your knowledge reservoir!
    3. Be ready—mentally and physically!

B. Review
    Most students did a preliminary review of the material they expected to master before they undertook intensive study. They stressed:
    1. During the time of intensive study, none of the material should appear new. A sense of familiarity with the material being studied usually avoids a feeling of cramming.
    2. Set aside regular time periods for this specific task; do not squeeze it in here and there! Regular time periods increase efficiency and delineate purpose.
    3. Skip superfluous material and adjust to repetitious material.
    4. If you detect major gaps in your knowledge, fill these in. Otherwise, they will bother you and distract you from your effort. *Remember*, it's easier to remember a story than to remember isolated facts.
    5. Study, if you can, in a chronological order! You learn the material this way, and you will feel more comfortable because of the sequence, and you will enhance your recall.
    6. During your studying, vary your attack as required.
        a. Read the material.
        b. Speak out the material.
        c. Write out the material.
        d. Sketch some of the material.
        e. Underline some of the material.
        f. Outline some of the material.
        g. Resort, if necessary, to mnemonic devices.
    7. Understand the material before you commit it to memory.
    8. Organize the material, and learn it in parts rather than in isolated, single details. Try to build a framework of facts.
    9. Note and focus in on similar ideas from different subject matters. Put them meaningfully together, and keep them in association. Integrate your material.

Taking the Examination

1. Get a good night's rest before the examination.
2. Do not change your eating habits if possible.
3. Go through your normal pattern of physical exercises and routines, and take the test in stride, as if it were part of the routine. It's another day's work.
4. Follow directions.
5. Proportion your time.
6. Do not become interested in your surroundings.
7. Do not keep "one eye" on the proctor and the other on your material.
8. Divorce yourself from everything, and let no disturbance influence your concentration.
9. Your eyes should be fixed on the printed page, and your only objective should be to accomplish your task efficiently, with speed and accuracy.
10. Remember that distractions can be internal as well as external; come to the examination having a positive attitude and a sense of pride and accomplishment.
11. Do not become impatient or discouraged if you cannot start at once effectively—most of us need a little warm-up period for our concentration to reach peak level.
12. Be interested in yourself! Self-interest leads to motivation to concentrate; remember, you are working for yourself and for your own future.
13. Do not get annoyed. If you do and your concentration lapses, let up and relax and regroup for a minute—take a quick break.
14. If your annoyance persists, try looking over the material you have successfully completed. Some people recover quickly and remotivate themselves by doing so.
15. Do not become discouraged by an "off-the-wall" question. Skip it and forget it and proceed with vigor. You are not alone.
16. Do not decrease speed because of fear that you might miss something.
17. If you should draw a temporary blank, besides reading, recite the question to yourself, or even write it out—this might help recall—you are utilizing all your senses.
18. Try to visualize the place in the book where this material appeared—this might lead you to relate facts and increase chances of recall. Sometimes, taking your mind completely off the subject might calm your nerves and restore your concentration.
19. Read the complete question before answering it. Check your answers to catch careless mistakes.
20. Do not read into or think too much about a question you feel you have answered correctly—you may arrive at implications not intended by the examiner, and you may more likely change your answer from right to wrong.
21. Do not rush too much: there is no prize for finishing early.

Do Your Best, and Good Luck!

David Cohen—Class of 1983, MCV
Nancy Armstrong—Class of 1983, MCV
Alan R. Swajkoski—Class of 1983, MCV
John M. Ogren—Class of 1983, MCV
Nancy Ensley—Class of 1984, MCV
Michael G. Waters—Class of 1985, MCV
Michael S. Glock—Class of 1985, MCV
Linda S. Beahm—Class of 1985, MCV
Martha A. Riggle—Class of 1985, MCV
Joan B. Weber—Class of 1986, MCV

A POSITIVE APPROACH TO ANSWERING QUESTIONS AND TO TEST TAKING

A positive, competitive approach and attitude are qualities of a successful individual. Hand in hand, however, goes a fund in knowledge. Nothing succeeds like knowledge of the subject matter for test taking. Indeed, the suggestions on test taking are all built on knowledge, which is strongly reinforced by your confidence, it, in turn, being supported by an understanding of the process involved in the successful answering of questions.

In this section, several specific questions will be selected from the Model Tests and will be examined not only for content but also for the process involved in the selection of the correct answer.

General Key Rules for Answering Questions

1. Are there specific disclaimers? *Best*, *all*, *none*, or some variety of negatives that separate the correct answer from the multiplicity of possible answers are the types of disclaimers to look for.

2. Are there specific qualifying words or topics that can be underlined? Sometimes these are the same as the disclaimers in item #1.

3. Are there similarities of choices in the answers? These similarities may allow elimination of choices.

4. Can some choices, such as the choice *all of the above*, be eliminated? Sometimes opposite choices help in the selection and in the narrowing down of the answers to one out of two possibilities.

5. If you can, sometimes a quick drawing or a formula will clarify the questions and initiate and aid in recall.

6. Remember, and keep in mind at all times, that all multiple-choice questions are really TRUE or FALSE decisions on a statement. Sometimes, in some cases, when in a quandary, they can best be answered by "I don't know" and "I'll proceed to the next question and not disturb my pace and concentration."

7. *Be positive!* If you have no good answers for several questions in a row, you positively *must forget them*. Do not dwell on failure, but have confidence in how much you know!

Application of Test-Taking Hints

We will use specific examples and apply our principles.

EXAMPLE: Model Examination B; Chemistry, Question 6

6. Glucose is NOT a (an)
   (A) aldose.
   (B) reducing sugar.
   (C) disaccharide.
   (D) sugar possessing optical activity.
   (E) monosaccharide.

ITEM 1:   Note the specific disclaimer *NOT*. This is an obvious and common one in test questions. You should *underline* this word.

ITEM 2:   Glucose is the topic of the question and should be *underlined*.

ITEM 3:   Similarity or dissimilarity of choices! There is a strong *dissimilarity* between choice (C): *di*saccharide and choice (E): *mono*saccharide. In fact, at this point, the answer is obvious to the knowledgeable individual. Since glucose is a *mono*saccharide, it cannot be a *di*saccharide; for the purpose of analyzation and this review, let us continue.

ITEM 4: Can choices be eliminated? Since both (C) and (E) cannot be true, *one* must be eliminated.

ITEM 5: A quick drawing to stimulate and help recall:

$$
\begin{array}{c}
\text{H} \qquad \text{O} \\
\diagdown \quad \diagup\!\!\diagup \\
\text{C} \\
| \\
\text{H}\!-\!\text{C}\!-\!\text{OH} \\
| \\
\text{etc.,} \\
| \\
\text{CH}_2\text{OH}
\end{array}
$$

ITEM 6: All multiple-choice questions are TRUE or FALSE statements!

For statement (A): "Glucose is NOT an aldose."

FACT: An aldose is an aldehyde carbohydrate. Look at the structure in item 5! This is indeed an aldehyde:

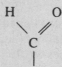

So, the choice is apparently true, but remember the disclaimer *NOT*. In this context, the answer for (A) is FALSE.

For statement (B): "Glucose is NOT a reducing sugar."

FACT: A reducing sugar is one that must be oxidized while reducing a metal ion ($Cu^{2+} \longrightarrow Cu^+$) (a gain of electrons is reduction). Remember the disclaimer *NOT*. In this context, the answer for (B) is FALSE.

For statement (C): "Glucose is NOT a disaccharide."

FACT: A disaccharide is a carbohydrate that may be hydrolyzed to a simpler carbohydrate. Carefully examine the sketch. Can this compound be hydrolyzed (split by water) into a smaller carbohydrate? Remember the disclaimer *NOT*. In this context, the answer for (C) is TRUE. During an examination with stress on speed and limited time, you would not wish to continue working on this question. Here, however, to continue the analysation of the process, please go on to the next statement.

For statement (D): "Glucose is NOT a sugar possessing optical activity."

FACT: An optically active compound requires an asymmetric carbon atom and no plane of symmetry. Examine the formula, and note carbon atom 2. Remember the disclaimer *NOT*. In this context, the answer for (D) is FALSE.

For statement (E): "Glucose is NOT a monosaccharide." Note the formula, and the opposite of choice (C). Remember the disclaimer *NOT*. In this context, the answer for (E) is FALSE.

In summary, we arrive at:

(A) FALSE
(B) FALSE
(C) TRUE
(D) FALSE
(E) FALSE

So, the answer is (C). Wow! That's easy if you know all the facts, but what if you don't? Suppose your array of answers was:

(A) FALSE
(B) I DON'T KNOW.
(C) TRUE
(D) FALSE
(E) FALSE

or a variation such as:

(A) I DON'T KNOW.
(B) I DON'T KNOW.
(C) TRUE
(D) I DON'T KNOW.
(E) I DON'T KNOW.

or:

(A) FALSE
(B) FALSE
(C) I DON'T KNOW.
(D) FALSE
(E) FALSE

The answer (C) is obvious in all three sets of answers above. However, what about:

(A) FALSE
(B) I DON'T KNOW.
(C) I DON'T KNOW.
(D) FALSE
(E) FALSE

Without additional information or a hunch or a gut feeling (which is a subliminal input), our advice would be to *let it go!* Pick one of the two, (B) or (C), and move on. You have a 50–50% chance of being right. The more "I don't know" answers for possible choices, the lower the probability of being right. So, for a particular examination, without additional information, decide to *always select* the first "I don't know" answer. This will cut through the random answer position on examinations. Remember that the answers on the key are randomly distributed. By adopting the above system, you put a degree of constancy into your pattern, and you don't float likewise. Your chances are drastically enhanced.

We will look at two more questions from the chemistry section of the first part of Model Examination B, using the same analytical techniques but in a less detailed way.

EXAMPLE: Model Examination B; Chemistry, Question 9

9. Alcohols have higher boiling points than do alkyl halides of the same chain lengths because
    (A) alcohols are more polar.
    (B) alcohols have higher molecular weights.
    (C) alcohols form ethers.
    (D) alcohols form intermolecular hydrogen bonds.
    (E) of all of the above.

KEY WORDS: Underline <u>Alcohols</u>, <u>higher boiling points</u>, <u>alkyl halides</u>, and <u>same chain lengths</u>.

(A) FALSE. Alkyl halides are more polar.
(E) "Of all of the above" can't be true if (A) is FALSE.
(B) FALSE. Halides have higher molecular weights than do alcohols.

(C) FALSE. The statement is true, but this is a chemical property not dealing with the physical property of a boiling point.

(D) TRUE. Compare CH_3OH to CH_3Cl

In summary, we arrive at:

(A)	FALSE
(B)	FALSE
(C)	FALSE
(D)	TRUE
(E)	FALSE

MCAT Science Review

The purpose of this section is to help the student review some key material quickly, to place some of his or her information in perspective and to help identify areas of weakness and strength. No attempt has been made to cover all of the material in the subject matter; but it is hoped that after the student has worked through the practice examinations and has studied the explanations to the questions, this section will amplify for him or her the highlights and essentials that are expected baseline knowledge for all educated people. A brief presentation such as this cannot cover all areas in sufficient depth. Some areas are omitted and others are presented only in a simplified manner. The individual who is well prepared will sometimes recognize compromises that must be made for the sake of brevity. This section should not be used as a substitute for a good general text in the areas but it should be used as a guide and in conjunction with a text so that the student may efficiently prepare for the MCAT. Again, we urge the student to begin preparation for the examination early and to be conscientious and thorough.

REVIEW OUTLINE

Biology

1. The Cell—Its Structure and Function
   A. Size
   B. Composition of Protoplasm
   C. Properties of the Cell and Protoplasm
   D. Components of a Typical Cell
   E. Cell Division—Mitosis
   F. Methods of Examining the Cell
   G. Eukaryotic vs. Prokaryotic Cell Structure

2. Classification of Living Organisms

3. Organization of the Human Body
   A. Organ System
   B. Four Basic Tissues

4. Skeletal System
   A. Axial Skeleton
   B. Appendicular Skeleton
   C. Characteristics of Bone
   D. Joints

5. Muscular System
   A. Classification
   B. Skeletal Muscles
   C. Muscle Attachment and Function
   D. Terms to Describe Movement
   E. Muscle Names
   F. Structural Organization of a Muscle Fiber
   G. Myofilaments
   H. Sarcoplasm

E. Carbohydrates
F. Lipids
G. Nucleotides and Nucleic Acids; Biosynthesis of Nucleic Acids and Proteins

Physics

1. Accelerated Motion
   A. Falling Objects—Gravity Acceleration
   B. Uniform Velocity
   C. Nonuniform Motion
   D. Uniform Deceleration
   E. Free Fall

2. Forces and Motion
   A. Forces and Acceleration
   B. Weight and Acceleration
   C. Negative Acceleration
   D. Resultant Forces
   E. Equilibrium States

3. Projectile Motion

4. Friction

5. Work and Power
   A. Work and Energy
   B. Power and Power Units

6. Energy
   A. Potential Energy
   B. Kinetic Energy

7. Momentum

8. Uniform Circular Motion
   A. Centripetal Acceleration
   B. Circular Motion
   C. Centripetal Force
   D. Centrifugal Force

9. Fluids at Rest
   A. Pressure
   B. Density
   C. Specific Gravity
   D. Buoyancy

10. Gravity

11. Temperature Calculations and Measurement

12. Heat
    A. Specific Heat
    B. Heat Lost = Heat Gained
    C. Heat of Vaporization

24. Mirrors
    A. Plane Mirrors
    B. Convex Mirrors
    C. Concave Mirrors

25. Lenses
    A. Concave Lenses
    B. Convex Lenses
    C. Combinations of Lenses

26. Composition of the Atom
    A. Subatomic Particles
    B. Isotopes
    C. Nuclear Reactions

27. Radioactivity
    A. Alpha Decay
    B. Beta Decay
    C. Half-life

28. Nuclear Energy
    A. Units of Measure
    B. Fusion Reactions
    C. Nuclear Fission

29. Photons
    A. Wave Property of Light
    B. Photon Energy
    C. Photoelectric Effect

30. Atomic Energy Levels
    A. Spectra
    B. Spectrum of Atomic Hydrogen

BIOLOGY

The Cell—Its Structure and Function

The cell is the basic unit of structure and function and basis of all life; all cells come from preexisting cells.

Size

Most cells are between 10 and 100μ (microns) in diameter. Measurements are made utilizing the following units:

$$1 \text{ cm} = 10 \text{ mm}$$
$$1 \text{ mm} = 1000\mu$$
$$1\mu = 10,000 \text{ Å (angstrom units)}$$

Average sizes of structures may be listed as follows:

cells about	10μ	(100,000 Å)
mitochondria about	1μ	(10,000 Å)
bacteria about	1μ	(10,000 Å)
viruses about	0.1μ	(1,000 Å)
macromolecules about	0.01μ	(100 Å)
molecules about	0.001μ	(10 Å)
hydrogen ion about	0.0001μ	(1 Å)

Resolution is commonly defined as the ability to discriminate two points and visualize them as two points, even though they are extremely close together. With the unaided eye these points might appear as one point, but the microscope can aid in resolving them as two. The resolution is dependent on the wavelength of the light source and can be calculated to be about one-half the wavelength. Examples of resolving power are:

human eye about 0.1 mm (100μ)
light microscope about 0.2μ (2000 Å)
electron microscope about 2–5 Å

Composition of Protoplasm

Protoplasm is made up mainly of proteins, carbohydrates, fats, salts and water; its average elemental composition is:

Oxygen 75+%
Carbon 10+%
Hydrogen 10%
Nitrogen 2+%
Sulfur about 0.2%
Phosphorus about 0.3%

Potassium about 0.3%
Chlorine about 0.1%
less than 0.1%—sodium
        calcium
        magnesium
        iron, etc.

Properties of the Cell and Protoplasm

1. Irritability
2. Conductivity
3. Respiration
4. Absorption
5. Secretion
6. Excretion
7. Growth
8. Reproduction
9. Metabolism

Components of a Typical Cell

Cells are commonly recognized as having two major compartments: *cytoplasm*—includes all components within the cell membrane but outside the nucleus, and *nucleoplasm*—includes everything within the nuclear membrane.

1. Cell Membrane: The cell membrane, or unit membrane, usually is about 75–100 Å thick; it is a trilaminar structure. As described by Danielli and Davson (1935), two protein layers sandwich a bimolecular lipid layer.

The cell membrane:

provides for a boundary resulting in a controlled environment.

is a relatively watertight barrier.

maintains a constant composition and environment resulting in homeostasis.

is semipermeable; only certain types of molecules are allowed to pass.

is composed mainly of proteins, lipids and carbohydrates; the major types of lipids found in nature are fats, phospholipids and steroids.

Structure. Electron microscopy suggests that the central region of the membrane consists of two layers of lipid molecules, mainly phospholipids and steroids. Each layer is thought to be one molecule thick. The phospholipid molecules are fairly long and have two functional poles: one exhibits lipid properties (it exhibits hydrophobic properties, repelling water); the other exhibits polar properties (it has a tendency to dissolve in water, and exhibits hydrophilic properties). The hydrophobic ends of both layers of lipid molecules associate with each other since they have affinity for one another. The hydrophilic portions face toward the protein layers; parts of proteins associate readily with water.

Electron microscopy substantiates that there is a light central layer surrounded by two denser layers. The two denser layers are thought to represent the proteins and hydrophilic portions of the lipid molecules while the light layer represents the hydrophobic portions of the lipid molecules.

Recent evidence, however, suggests that the arrangement of the protein molecules is far more complex. The protein molecules probably do not cover the entire surface but are arranged in definite, specialized, functional and structural packages throughout the entire membrane. Channels may exist where the lipid layers are interrupted and a continuous zone of hydrophilic molecules is present. This zone is thought to be occupied by a pore. A pore is only a few angstrom (Å) units in diameter and allows for the passage of water, inorganic ions and very small molecules.

Membranes vary and are highly specialized. All membranes, however, are made up of the same basic molecules and possess similar characteristics. The particular amount and arrangement of proteins, lipids and carbohydrates at the cell surface, however, impart specific properties. It is at these specific sites that different molecules are processed.

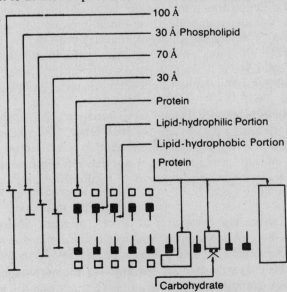

100 Å
30 Å Phospholipid
70 Å
30 Å
Protein
Lipid-hydrophilic Portion
Lipid-hydrophobic Portion
Protein
Carbohydrate

Composite representation of a lipoprotein membrane

Activities. As pointed out before, the plasma membrane is semi-permeable. It controls the passage of materials into and out of the cell. The movement of materials into and out of the cell is called *transport*.

There are two types of transport—passive, or transport that does not require the cell's energy, and active, which does require energy expenditure.

There are two types of passive transport—diffusion and osmosis.

In *diffusion* molecules pass from an area of higher concentration to that of lower concentration until the concentrations are equal on both sides of the membrane. Diffusion, in other words, follows the concentration gradient.

Osmosis is the movement of water across the semi-permeable membrane. Water will pass into a more concentrated solution and this passage of water will equalize the concentration of dissolved substances on each side of the membrane so that equilibrium is theoretically achieved.

Equilibrium implies an equal number of molecules of all dissolved material per unit volume on each side of the membrane compartment; the same applies to the concentration of each individual diffusable component.

Gases pass through the cell membrane with ease. Water and small molecules pass more readily than large molecules and lipid soluble materials enter the cell easier than nonlipid-soluble substances.

Active transport requires the cell to expend energy to allow materials to pass through the membrane. (Also called uphill transport, energy dependent transport can operate against concentration gradients.)

Electrical charge has also to be considered. The inside of the cell is usually electrically negative in comparison to the outside environment.

In active transport, materials enter the cell in membrane-bound vesicles, formed by the membrane. This process is known collectively as *endocytosis*. When it involves solid material we speak of *phagocytosis*; liquid material enters via *pinocytosis*. The process of expulsion of material is known as *exocytosis*.

Special Sites. To amplify the complexities of the cell membrane some general statements are in order at this point.

Cells must be held together and specialized structures are required. Adjacent cell membranes interdigitate and intercellular cement is utilized.

A *desmosome* is a specialized area of connection between adjacent cellular membranes (macula adherens).

A *terminal bar* is a dense area surrounding the apical cellular surface. It includes the tight junction (zona occludens) and the loose junction (zona adherens).

Layers of material (probably mucopolysaccharide) secreted by the cell are found on the surface of the cell. The most prominent layer is the *basement membrane*, or *basal lamina*. The thick cellulose cell wall of plants falls within the above category. These structures are boundaries and must be traversed by material entering and leaving the cell.

2.   **Intercellular Space:** Cells are usually separated by a space of about 100–200 Å. Only at specialized contact points do cells appose each other. The space is filled mainly by a matrix of proteins and polysaccharides which function in cementing cells to one another. Some cells possess special extracellular polysaccharide substances: cartilage is rich in chondroitin sulfate; joints have large amounts of hyaluronic acid; and cell walls of plants are composed largely of cellulose.

3. **Cytoplasmic Matrix:** The cytoplasm of a cell appears homogeneous, translucent, and structureless; the homogeneous mass, which is also called cell-sap or hyaloplasm, contains inorganic substances and organic compounds of varying molecular sizes. The more peripheral layer of this matrix is also known as ectoplasm (plasmagel). It appears more rigid and seems to lack granules completely.

4. **Cellular Inclusions:** These may be composed of proteins, fats, carbohydrates, granules, pigments, and crystals.

a. *Secretion granules (products of cell activity)*. These are usually membrane-bound products that await extrusion by the cell (exocrine secretion into ducts or endocrine secretion into the extracellular space and capillaries). Release of secretory product from the cells is via exocytosis. Under the general term endocytosis (taking into the cell), are the more specific terms, pinocytosis (taking in of fluid) and phagocytosis (taking in of solids).

b. *Lipid droplets*. These are globular accumulations synthesized by the cell. During periods of need they may serve as a source of energy.

c. *Glycogen granules*. These are small spherical units synthesized by the cell. They serve as storage reservoirs of carbohydrates.

d. *Pigment granules*. These may be of two types: endogenous pigments derived from cell metabolism or exogenous pigments taken in by the cell. Hemosiderin is an example of an exogenous pigment, while the lipochromes and the melanins are endogenous in nature.

e. *Vacuoles*. Under this general term may be classified any membrane-bound globular structure.

f. *Plastids*. The plastids are composed of leucoplasts, chromoplasts and chloroplasts. Leucoplasts resemble chloroplasts but have no chlorophyll; they manufacture starch, oil and protein. Chromoplasts possess pigments and are responsible for the color of flower petals. Chloroplasts possess chlorophyll, which is capable of capturing light energy to produce glucose from CO_2 and H_2O.

5. **Mitochondria:** Mitochondria are the best known of the cellular organelles. They had been described during the 19th century, notably by Kollicker and Fleming. Altman, using Janus green, was able to stain them in 1890. Structurally, the mitochondrion is composed of an outer trilaminar membrane and an inner trilaminar membrane; the inner one forms folds which are known as *cristae*. The space between the two membranes is about 6–10 nm wide.

Mitochondria as a whole and specifically the cristae vary greatly in size, shape and number not only in different cells but also in the same cell depending on its functional state. Mitochondria are present in greater numbers in cells exhibiting high levels of activity and having more energy requirements. Muscle and glandular tissues fall in the above category.

DNA has been found in the mitochondria of animals and the chloroplasts of plants. Mitochondria are capable of division and are not generated *de novo*.

Granules have been observed in the mitochondrial matrix. Their identity is in question, however; some believe that they might be reservoirs of calcium and other divalent ions. Phosphate is taken up with Ca^{2+} and calcium phosphate deposits might be the end result.

Mitochondria are the biochemical powerplants of cells. They recover energy from foodstuffs (via Krebs cycle, or citric acid cycle; tricarboxylic acid cycle and the respiratory chain) and convert it via phosphorylation into adenosine triphosphate (ATP). In this manner they produce the energy necessary for the metabolic processes.

Enzymes. The organization of enzymes and coenzymes (especially enzymes involved in oxidative phosphorylation) in the cristae appears to be highly specific facilitating an orderly and proper sequence of reactions.

Enzymes concerned with the Krebs cycle are presumed to be either free in the mitochondrial matrix (internal medium) or loosely bound to the membranes since they are readily recovered when mitochondria are disrupted. The electron transport components involved in respiratory activity and the oxidative phosphorylation systems are presumed to be tightly bound to the inner membranous system. Electron transport and oxidative phosphorylation seem to be coupled.

Enzymes then are associated with the outer membrane, the inner membrane, the space between the outer and inner membranes, and the matrix.

DNA and Protein Synthesis. Most extranuclear DNA, if not all, can be found in mitochondria (and in plants, in the chloroplast). There is evidence that proteins are synthesized in mitochondria under the direction of mitochondrial DNA. In biochemical preparations of mitochondria the synthesizing enzymes necessary for RNA and proteins have been isolated. However, there also is considerable documentation that the code for the enzymes involved in oxidative phosphorylation originates in nuclear DNA. Therefore, it must be assumed that mitochondrial DNA is involved only in the partial coding of the proteins manufactured in the organelle.

Krebs Cycle. Mitochondria are involved in the Krebs or citric acid cycle in which organic acids are oxidized to CO_2. In each successive step oxidation of a single carbon of the chain takes place and each reaction requires a different enzyme. The Krebs cycle reactions are further described under the topic "Carbohydrates" on page 133.

The ATP produced is a small molecule and can diffuse out of the mitochondrion into the cytoplasm and participate in the *endothermic* reactions of the cell.

6. Chloroplast: For completeness sake, let us examine the homologue of the mitochondria in plants—namely, the chloroplasts. Joseph Priestley discovered photosynthesis in 1771. In 1888 Haberlandt associated chloroplasts directly with oxygen production. Just as cellular respiration takes place in the mitochondria, photosynthesis occurs in chloroplasts. Composition of chloroplasts: 56% protein, 35% lipid, 8% chlorophyll.

Chloroplasts are somewhat larger and exhibit more variability than mitochondria. They are bounded by two membranes and possess an amorphous ground substance, or *stroma,* throughout which rows of parallel membranes called *grana* are distributed. These membranes house the photosynthetic machinery.

Photosynthesis. In photosynthesis light energy (photons) is absorbed by chlorophyll in the chloroplasts and utilized in the production of sugars from water and atmospheric carbon dioxide.

The process (light dependent reaction) may be outlined as follows:

$$CO_2 + H_2O \xrightarrow[\text{radiant energy}]{\text{green plants}} (CH_2O)_n + O_2 + H_2O$$
$$\text{sugars \&}$$
$$\text{starches}$$

or

$$6CO_2 + 12H_2O + \text{light} \xrightarrow{\text{chlorophyll}} 6O_2 + C_6H_{12}O_6 + 6H_2O$$

The oxygen produced is returned to the air. The sugars are used by mitochondria and the energy produced joins the high energy bonds of ATP. Chloroplasts can also produce ATP independently. Broadly speaking the photosynthetic process, due to its production of water, carbohydrates and oxygen, sustains all higher forms of life. Once the sugar has been produced no distinction can be made in the biochemical processes of plants and animals.

As implied before, photosynthesis is a two reaction process: one is dependent on light while the other is known as the dark reaction. They may be summarized as follows:

Light-dependent reaction
    results in production of ATP (adenosinetriphosphate) from ADP (adenosinediphosphate) via phosphorylation
    results in formation of reduced NADP from NADP (nicotinamide adenine dinucleotide phosphate)
    results in release of oxygen from water
    results in ATP production

Dark reaction
    results in carbohydrates from carbon dioxide
    utilizes the ATP and reduced NADP from the light reaction

As in the mitochondrion the sequence of reactions dictates a high degree of molecular organization. During fractionation studies most of the enzymes of the dark reaction can be isolated in the supernatant. The enzymes of the light reaction are associated with the membranous structures. In general terms one can speculate that while carbohydrate synthesis occurs in the stroma, the production of ATP, reduced NADP and O_2 is associated with membranes.

7. **Endoplasmic Reticulum** (ER): This cellular organelle had not been observed with the ordinary light microscope; it was first described using phase microscopy by Porter, Claude and Fallam in 1945. In general terms it is an extensive network of interconnecting channels. The endoplasmic reticular membranes are unit membranes (trilaminar). When ribosomes line the outer surface, it is designated as *rough endoplasmic reticulum* (RER). The primary form of this organelle is the rough variety. The smooth is derived from the rough due to the loss of ribosomes. The amount of each depends on the cell type and the cellular activity.

The RER (rough endoplasmic reticulum) is the synthetic machinery of the cell (messenger RNA influences that machinery, but itself is manufactured in the nucleus). It is mainly concerned with protein synthesis. Smooth endoplasmic reticulum (SER) is mainly concerned with lipid or fat synthesis. In the liver, SER probably plays a significant role in the detoxification of potentially harmful substances.

Ribosomes (probably in the form of polysomes; a group of ribosomes, like rosettes) are located on the external surface of ER. The rough endoplasmic reticulum is highly developed in protein-secreting cells such as found in the pancreas. Autoradiographic methods have revealed that labeled amino acids first appear on the RER (polysomes); then in the cisternae of the ER, where the material is processed and transported; later in the Golgi complex, where it is chemically modified and condensed; then in secretion granules (in the case of pancreas, zymogen granules), which move towards the cell surface (secretory pole); and finally in the extracellular space (via exocytosis) as a released secretory granule.

The movement of the material from the ribosomal area on the membrane into the ER seems to require no special energy or transport enzymes. Evidence is available for transport by the ER of: lipoproteins, lysosomal hydrolases, peroxisomal enzymes, albumin, and a variety of other molecules.

The isolated microsome cell fraction contains enzymes involved in the synthesis of: phospholipids, steroids, and triglycerides.

Both RER and SER can function in lipid synthesis; however, usually we assign prominence of the RER to protein-secreting cells and to the SER to steroid-secreting cells. The steroid hormone-producing cells of the adrenal and testis are rich in SER. The SER (sarcoplasmic reticulum) is extremely extensive and specialized in cardiac and smooth muscle. It encases the myofibrils and functions in the release and sequestering of calcium ions needed during contraction. It is obvious that the membranes are very dynamic systems and are extremely adaptable to the demands and needs of the cell.

8. **The Golgi Complex:** This structure was well known to light microscopists and was first described by Camillo Golgi in 1898.

All eukaryotic cells, except for the red blood cell, possess a Golgi apparatus; in plants the sacs of the Golgi complex are referred to as *dictyosomes*. The Golgi apparatus is composed of numerous and diverse channels of cisternae (flattened sacs) and interspersed vesicles and granules; it is a very heterogeneous cellular organelle. It is located usually near one pole of the nucleus and in close relation to the centriole.

Generally speaking, the Golgi complex is prominent in glandular cells and is thought to function in the production, concentration, packaging, and transportation of secretory material. Important enzyme systems are associated with the membranes (flattened cisternae or round vesicles or sacs) of the Golgi complex. It is thought that substances manufactured by the endoplasmic reticulum are transferred to the Golgi cisternae, processed there, and then stored or released by the cell. The Golgi elaborates polysaccharide moieties.

The functions of the Golgi apparatus are highly diverse and complex. During the early period of elucidating the processes of this organelle a condensing role was ascribed; it has now been shown that not only does condensing of products take place but also certain factors, such as carbohydrate moieties, are contributed and added to glycoproteins. Sulfation is also carried out.

Recently, utilizing cell fractions containing Golgi material, high concentrations of glycosyl transferase were detected; these enzymes catalyze the polymerization of sugars into polysaccharides and also attach sugars to glycoproteins. Evidence shows phosphatase, thiamine pyrophosphatase (TPPase) and nucleoside diphosphatase (NDPase) activity in the Golgi zone.

As pointed out in a previous section, when radioactive tracers (tritium labelled amino acids) are utilized, they appear first over ribosomes, then in the ER, and later the protein is found in or near the Golgi complex. However, when tritium labelled sugars are employed they first make their appearance in the Golgi. This fact has fostered the idea that the Golgi complex is the site of synthesis of secretory polysaccharides.

The associations, interrelationships, and interactions of the various membranous components of the organelle are not completely elucidated. However, a certain amount of association and transformation is evidenced. The peripheral sacs of the Golgi are probably related to the endoplasmic reticulum; the central ones, however, seem to be different. The products that come from the Golgi apparatus are very complex in nature and exhibit mixtures of proteins and polysaccharides, or lipids and proteins in a variety of concentrations. Concentration or condensing is thought to be accomplished by the extrusion of water.

Lysosomes (organelles containing hydrolytic enzymes) have been linked to the Golgi membranes. Vesicles containing acid phosphatase have been shown to originate from the Golgi zone. The presence in the Golgi (a good marker) of galactosyltransferase activity which is absent from other membranes might help shed light on the complex functions.

In summary one can link the Golgi complex to:

secretion,
membrane biogenesis,
lysosome formation,
membrane recycling,
hormone modulation.

Secretory proteins undergo modifications such as: glycosylation, sulfation, proteolytic processing, and condensing and concentrating.

Lysosome: The term lysosome, denoting a membrane-bound lytic particle or body, was introduced in 1955 by Christain DeDuve. Lysosomes were described as containing proteolytic enzymes (hydrolases).

Lysosomes contain acid phosphatase and other hydrolytic enzymes. These enzymes are enclosed by a membrane and are released when needed into the cell or into phagocytic vesicles. The enzymes found in lysosomes are probably manufactured by the endoplasmic reticulum and Golgi apparatus. The membrane surrounding these enzymes confines these potentially lethal chemicals so that they can perform their functions without harming the cell. The enzymes not only digest material which the cells ingest but also function in the debridement of the cell, a process known as *autophagy.* Prominent examples of cells with conspicuous lysosomes are the granulocytic leucocytes and macrophages; these specific lysosomes are also known as *bacteriocidal lysosomes.* Acid phosphatase activity is the most widely used enzyme marker and so far over fifty hydrolases have been identified.

Related to the lysosome is the *phagosome.* The phagosome, as the lysosome, is membrane bound; it is a structure in which phagocytized bacteria or other substances that enter the cell are transported. Lysosomes come in contact and fuse with phagosomes and in this fashion a *secondary lysosome,* or *phagolysosome,* is created.

Where all lysosomes are produced is still in question. Most lysosomal enzymes, however, are produced first by ribosomes, then processed by the endoplasmic reticulum, shipped from there either to lysosomes directly or processed further via the Golgi membranes to finally enter the lysosomal pool.

Lysosomal enzymes have the capacity to hydrolyze all classes of macromolecules. A generalized list of substrates acted upon by respective enzymes is given below:

Lipids by lipases and phospholipases;
Proteins by proteases;
Polysaccharides by glycosidases;
Nucleic acids by nucleases;
Phosphates (organic-linked) by phosphatases;
Sulphates (organic-linked) by sulfatases.

9. Peroxisomes: Peroxisomes are found in virtually all mammalian cell types and probably arise from swellings of the endoplasmic reticulum. These structures are often smaller than lysosomes. The enzymes they possess are active in the production of hydrogen peroxide (urate oxidase, D-amino acid oxidase, α-hydroxyacid oxidase), and one functions in destroying hydrogen peroxide (catalase). Other oxidases have been proposed also. The peroxisomes function in purine catabolism and in the degradation of nucleic acids.

10. Nucleus: The nucleus was first described by Robert Brown in 1831. The nucleus is surrounded by a double layer of the typical trilaminar membrane which is pierced by small pores. The pores measure about 50–80 nm in diameter. The pores allow and serve in the interchange of nuclear and cytoplasmic material. For example, messenger RNA can pass into the cytoplasm to elicit its effect. The outer membrane of the nuclear envelope (exposed to cytoplasm) has ribonucleoprotein particles (ribosomes) attached to it and may also be continuous with the RER. The inner membrane (exposed to nuclear content) lacks ribosomes.

Approximate composition of the nucleus:

80% protein,
15% DNA (deoxyribonucleic acid),
5% RNA (ribonucleic acid),
3% lipid.

Functions: Simply speaking, the nucleus controls the metabolic aspects of the cell and is responsible for its structural integrity, function, survival and the passage of the hereditary material to the next generation. The nucleus is necessary for: life, growth, differentiation, and reproduction.

DNA Structure. DNA—deoxyribonucleic acid—is a nucleic acid. A nucleic acid is a polymer of nucleotides. The combination of a *purine* or *pyrimidine* base, a sugar, and phosphoric acid is called a *nucleotide*. *Deoxyribose* is the sugar in DNA; ribose is the other nucleic acid, ribonucleic acid, or RNA.

DNA molecules are composed of two nucleotide strands coiled together in a double helix. Watson and Crick (1953) proposed a double helix model of DNA. The two strands consist of sugar-phosphate backbones which are connected by pairs of bases. The DNA molecule may be illustrated as follows:

Single chain

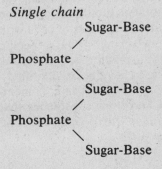

Double chain

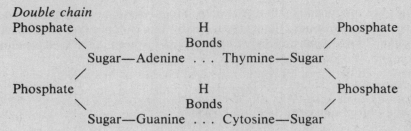

Phosphate   H   Phosphate
Bonds
Sugar—Adenine . . . Thymine—Sugar
Phosphate   H   Phosphate
Bonds
Sugar—Guanine . . . Cytosine—Sugar

Each strand is a chain of nucleotides. All DNA nucleotides consist of a 5-carbon sugar (deoxyribose) with a phosphate group attached at one end and a nitrogen-containing ring compound (the base) at the other. The nitrogenous bases are: adenine and guanine (*purines*) and thymine, cytosine, and uracil (*pyrimidines*). In DNA they pair specifically in the following manner:

adenine and thymine
guanine and cytosine

In RNA they pair as follows:

adenine and uracil
guanine and cytosine

The paired bases are held together chiefly by hydrogen bonds. The strands complement each other since the base sequence present on one determines the base sequence of the other. Duplication of this material involves the splitting of the unions between purines and pyrimidines; each nucleotide then acquires a new complementary nucleotide and the phosphate and pentose moieties are then joined enzymatically and the duplication process has taken place.

The phosphate groups of DNA are negatively charged. Basic dyes (hematoxylin, Feulgen stain) which are positively charged stain the DNA and RNA since positive and negative charges attract each other. The regions that attract a basic stain are referred to as *basophilic*.

DNA Functions. One of the premier functions of DNA is the production of RNA. Most RNA is produced in the nucleus. DNA and RNA are similar. They are both nucleotide chains; however, RNA differs in the following manner:

RNA is single stranded (certain viruses are exceptions)
the 5-carbon sugar in RNA is ribose

CHARACTERISTICS OF DNA AND RNA

DNA	RNA
double stranded sugar—deoxyribose base—thymine	single stranded (mainly) sugar—ribose base—uracil

DNA determines and acts as a template for RNA synthesis. With the help of a transcription enzyme (RNA polymerase) a complementary RNA strand is produced. The base pairings are as follows:

DNA	*RNA*
T-thymine	A-adenine
C-cytosine	G-guanine

Once RNA has been manufactured in the nucleus it moves fairly quickly into the cytoplasm.

Messenger RNA (mRNA) from the nucleus brings the coded message for protein synthesis to ribosomal RNA (rRNA). Ribosomal RNA imparts the message to *transfer RNA* (tRNA), which carries the specific amino acids coded for to the ribosomes, where protein synthesis is carried out.

Chromatin. The survival of the cell, organism, and species depends upon the chromatin material in the nucleus. Chromatin is DNA combined with protein, and stains with basic dyes. During the interphase of the cell cycle some chromosomes are visualized as tight coils and are referred to as *heterochromatin.* Heterochromatin is metabolically quite inactive and appears more electron dense. When chromosomes are active in the synthetic process, they are loosely coiled and one speaks in terms of *euchromatin,* which is more granular in appearance.

11. Ribosomes and Polysomes: Ribosomes may be free or attached to the membranes of the endoplasmic reticulum, which is then designated as rough ER. Ribosomes are the sites of protein synthesis in the cell. If ribosomes appear in clusters (rosettes) in the cytoplasm, they are commonly termed *polyribosomes* or *polysomes.*

Ribosomes are dense structures measuring about 15–25 nm in diameter. Both ribosomes attached to the endoplasmic reticulum and the free ones in the cytoplasm, form polyribosomes and perform identical functions.

Ribosomes possess RNA known as ribosomal RNA (rRNA) and both rRNA and messenger RNA (mRNA) are produced on DNA templates in the nucleus. Ribosomal RNA is very large in comparison to transfer RNA (tRNA), while the size of mRNA varies greatly.

Even though protein synthesis was discussed earlier, a brief repeat is in order since a form of RNA is an intricate part of every step. Amino acids are attached in the cytoplasm to tRNA, which consists of specific base triplets. The tRNA bonds to complimentary base triplets on the mRNA (formed on a DNA template in the nucleus). Therefore, specific base pairing and the nucleotide sequence of the mRNA determines the position of the tRNA sequence and thus the amino acid sequence. Amino acids are linked and form a polypeptide chain which eventually is released from the RNA. Transfer RNA and mRNA interaction form the ribosome mRNA complex and accomplish the synthesis of proteins.

As said earlier, ribosomes are complexed into polyribosomes; the number of ribosomes in a polyribosome seems to vary from 10 to 20. The importance of the polyribosome complex seems to lie in the fact that as amino acid sequences are laid down on the ribosome-mRNA complex in several areas, multiple chains of polypeptides are probably synthesized simultaneously on the polysomes using the same mRNA molecules.

12. Microtubules: These structures are usually associated with centrioles and basal bodies. They are also present in the cytoplasm of various cells, in particular the axons of neurons. Microtubules apparently function in the maintenance of the structural integrity (shape and rigidity) of the cell. Transport of material and movement of cilia and flagella are also ascribed to these organelles.

The microtubules are generally found to be 20–30 nm in diameter; their length is considerable. They are not membrane limited but their walls seem to be composed of regular units when observed in cross section. About a dozen units are seen and are thought to be composed of proteins called *tubulins.*

13. Microfilaments: These structures are prominent in the microvilli of the absorptive cells of the intestines. They have been shown to be associated with the regions of the terminal web and the desmosome. Their diameter is usually 5–8 nm, and they are observed in groups of various sizes and distributions. They seem to work in conjunction with microtubules and function in maintaining the cytoskeletal configuration of the cell and in cellular movements.

14. Centrioles, Cilia and Flagella: The centrioles are self-reproducing organelles that play an important role in the separation of the chromosomes during mitosis. Before division of the cell the centriole splits into two and the daughter centrioles migrate to opposite sides of the nucleus. They form the center of the *spindle* and *aster* configuration during cell division; from the centriole the microtubules of the spindle radiate. Electron microscopy reveals that centrioles are composed of a peripheral cylinder which consists of 9 parallel sets of tubules in a triplet pattern. The triplets are embedded in an amorphous matrix.

Organelles almost identical in structure to the centriole are the basal bodies of cilia and flagella. A *basal body* is present at the base of each cilium and flagellum and it has the 9 + 0 configuration of the centriole. The centriole and basal bodies may, therefore, be closely related. Basal bodies control the structural makeup of cilia and flagella.

The structure and function of cilia and flagella are similar. They, like the centriole, have nine (9) sets of tubules arranged in a peripheral cylinder; the sets, however, are doublets, not triplets. And unlike centrioles, cilia and flagella have an additional pair of central tubules. Therefore we can summarize the arrangement in centrioles as 9 + 0, and in cilia and flagella as 9 + 2.

There are usually two centrioles per cell (diplosome); many cilia per cell and usually only one flagellum. The two centrioles are usually arranged perpendicular to each other. Centrioles have no specific relationship or association with a membrane, but cilia and flagella are in a sense bounded by an extension of the cell membrane. Cilia and flagella participate in active movements. Cilia beat in unison and move liquid and particles on the surface of cells (ciliated epithelium of respiratory tract) while flagella move the whole cell or organism.

The nitrogenous bases can be listed as adenine, guanine, thymine, cytosine, and uracil. They pair in the following manner in DNA:

(1.) adenine and thymine
(2.) guanine and cytosine

There are four nitrogenous bases in RNA: adenine pairs with uracil and cytosine pairs with guanine.

The Watson and Crick model clearly illustrates the above pairings. Duplication of this material involves the splitting of the unions between purines and pyrimidines; each nucleotide then acquires a new complementary nucleotide and the phosphate and pentose moieties are then joined enzymatically and the duplication process has taken place.

RNA of the nucleolus provides the vehicle for the coded messages of the nuclear DNA to reach the machinery of the cell. Ribosomal RNA and RNA of the nucleolus are quite similar; ribosomal RNA probably is derived from RNA of the nucleolus. Messenger RNA from the nucleus brings the coded message for protein synthesis to ribosomal RNA. Ribosomal RNA imparts the message to transfer RNA, which carries the specific amino acids to the ribosomes, and protein synthesis is carried out.

Cell Division-Mitosis

For purposes of convenience, mitosis is divided into prophase, metaphase, anaphase, and telophase; the process, however, is a continuous one. The major events during the phases are:

1. Prophase: Chromosomes become distinct and nucleolus (nucleoli) disappear(s); centriole(s) and asters and spindle appear; nuclear membrane disappears.

2. Metaphase: Chromosomes move to the equator of the cell and duplicate.

3. Anaphase: The two chromatids split apart and start migration toward the poles of the spindle; the spindle loses its definition.

4. Telophase: Chromosomes lengthen and become less distinct; nucleoli reappear. The next period of growth and rest is known as *interphase*.

5. Interphase: Cell growth; protein synthesis; DNA synthesis; chromosome duplication.

Methods of Examining the Cell

1. Histological Methods:

a. *Microscopy*. Microscopes are usually classified according to the type of energy source. Besides the straight light microscope and the electron microscope, the researcher utilizes polarization, phase contrast, interference, ultraviolet, and X-ray microscopes.

b. *Stains*. Dyes are used in solution to stain generally the nucleus and/or cytoplasm, or specifically, particular cell components. Dyes in general are neutral salts having both acidic and basic radicals. A basic dye exhibits its coloring property because of the basic radical it possesses. Structures stained by it are designated as basophilic—the nucleus, for example. An acidic dye exhibits its staining property because of the acidic radical. Structures delineated by it are acidophilic—the cytoplasm, for example.

Examples of stains routinely employed:

1) Hematoxylin, a common histologic stain, stains nuclei blue;
2) The common histological stain eosin (H&E) and other acidic dyes, such as picric acid, stain the general cytoplasm;
3) Iron hematoxylin, which stains chromosomes, mitochondria, Golgi complex, and contractile elements of muscle cells black or dark blue;
4) Carmine, which stains nuclei red-purple;
5) Basic aniline dyes, such as toluidine blue, azure A and methylene blue, which stain mucopolysaccharides metachromatically;
6) Mallory's connective tissue (CT) stain, which stains collagen fibers bright blue, nuclei red or orange, and various cell components blue, red, orange or purple;
7) Reticular fibers, which are argyrophilic, are stained brown by silver impregnation methods.

2. Histochemical Methods: Tissues are composed of various chemicals such as proteins, carbohydrates, lipids, inorganic salts and miscellaneous substances, and various tests are used to detect these chemicals.

Examples:

1) Proteins (with tyrosine)—yellow color;
2) Enzymes—various tests for phosphatases, lipases, oxidases, esterases, and dehydrogenases;
3) Carbohydrates—glycogen by periodic acid Schiff (PAS) test results in a magenta or purple color; glycoproteins give a positive PAS magenta color. Basal laminae and reticular fibers are strongly PAS positive;
4) Lipids—Sudan dyes or osmic acid;
5) Nucleic acids—Feulgen reaction is specific for DNA, but not for RNA, which can be detected by ribonuclease. Both DNA and RNA are basophilic (because they are both acids).

3. Fixation: The fixative must modify the cell to resist further treatments and also to make further treatments possible. Fixatives may be classified as either coagulant or non-coagulant. Examples of each are:

1) *coagulant:* methanol, ethanol, acetone, nitric acid, hydrochloric acid, picric acid, trichloroacetic acid and mercuric chloride.
2) *non-coagulant:* formaldehyde, glutaraldehyde, osmium tetroxide, potassium dichromate, acetic acid, and potassium permanganate.

Fixatives can also be subclassified into two categories. The following are examples:

1) *additive:* osmium tetroxide, formaldehyde, and glutaraldehyde.
2) *non-additive:* methanol, ethanol, and acetone.

4. Method of Preparation

1) *Fixation:* a piece of tissue is placed in a killing (preservative) solution; processes of the cell are stopped as close to normal as possible;

2) *Dehydration:* water is usually removed from the tissues by passing it through a series of increasing strengths of alcohol solutions;

3) *Embedding:* embedding places the tissues in a solid medium;

4) *Sectioning:* tissue is cut into 5 microns or 5000 nm for light, and about 60 nm for electron microscopic evaluation;

5) *Staining:* dyes for light microscopy and heavy metals for electron microscopy enhance visualization.

Eukaryotic vs. Prokaryotic Cell Structure

Eukaryotes: All higher animals and plants, as well as protozoa, are eukaryotes, and their cells possess the following characteristics:

A nucleus surrounded by a nuclear membrane (nucleolemma)

Discrete chromosomes that are present in the nucleus and undergo reduplication.

DNA (deoxyribonucleic acid) that stores the vital information for the functioning of the cell.

DNA synthesis as the mode of duplication. Mitosis separates chromosomes which have already duplicated.

Cellular metabolites such as protein, RNA, vacuoles, ribosomes, and mitochondria in the cytoplasm.

Cilia and flagella that possess the basic structure of two inner fibrils surrounded by nine outer ones. (Flagella of eukaryotic and prokaryotic organisms are structurally different.)

In addition, most eukaryotic cells are surrounded by a lipoprotein cell membrane; some also possess a cell wall (plants).

Prokaryotes: Bacteria (and blue-green algae) are the organisms which make up this important category. They possess the following characteristics:

1) The nucleus or nucleoid consists mostly of DNA and is never enveloped by a nuclear membrane. DNA is visualized as fine fibrils and is not organized into chromosomes. Mitosis does not occur.

2) In the cytoplasm vacuoles and mitochondria are absent. Many of the reactions that take place in the mitochondrion of the eukaryotic cell are carried out by the prokaryotic cell membrane.

3) Cytoplasmic granules which store carbohydrates, lipids, or volutin (polymetaphosphate) are present.

4) Ribosomes are present.

5) A cell membrane surrounds the cytoplasm; however, unlike the eukaryotic cell membrane, it lacks sterols and is made up only of phospholipid and protein.

6) The cell membrane is a highly synthetic structure: it contains the respiratory enzymatic machinery; is the site of DNA attachment; and serves in the control of permeability.

7) A cell wall giving integrity to the organism is present. In some cells constituents such as endotoxins play a role in disease. (Cell wall structure determines susceptibility to the attack by chemotherapeutic agents.)

8) A polysaccharide-polypeptide capsule is laid down outside the cell wall. This material may play a vital role in the virulence of a pathogenic bacteria since it can interfere with the ability of the host's leukocytes to phagocytize the bacteria. The capsular material of each bacterial strain is unique.

9) Flagella, if present, have a structure different from that of eukaryotes. Each flagellum consists of a single fibril (not the typical 11 axial fibrils), which originates from a basal granule of the cytoplasmic membrane.

10) They may produce spores (endospores) which are thick-walled and protect them during unfavorable conditions. Spores exhibit greater resistance to heat, drying, freezing, chemical agents and radiation than their vegetative counterparts. Spores possess the compound dipicolinic acid; the calcium salt of this acid plays a role in resistance to heat (the higher the calcium dipicolinate concentration, the more heat resistant).

Reproduction and Genetics in Eukaryotes and Prokaryotes: Genetic stability in eukaryotes and prokaryotes is comparable. Frequency of mutations is the same. Eukaryotes introduce changes via sexual reproduction (combination of gametes). They also reproduce asexually using various methods. Sexual reproduction *per se* does not occur in prokaryotes. However, three very effective processes do result in the mixing of genetic material. They are:

a. *Transformation*. DNA released from a donor cell into a medium is taken up and incorporated by a recipient cell; it results in the replacement of part of the cell's genetic material.

b. *Conjugation*. Genetic material is transferred from one bacterium to another via a conjugation bridge.

c. *Transduction*. Genetic material is transferred from one bacterium to another via a bacteriophage (a bacterial virus).

Classification of Living Organisms

Taxonomy is the classification of living organisms based on characteristics and ancestry. Two *kingdoms*—animal and plant—are easily distinguished. In general, members of the former consume food and are mobile while those of the latter are stationary and produce their own nutrients.

Several systems have evolved to classify the great variety of living organisms. One such system divides living things into five kingdoms based on (1) the presence (eukaryotic) or absence (prokaryotic) of membrane-bound nuclei in the cells; (2) the number of cells forming the organism, and (3) the mechanism for nutrition. This five-kingdom classification system is shown in the following table.

FIVE-KINGDOM CLASSIFICATION SYSTEM		
Kingdom	**Characteristics**	**Examples**
Monera	unicellular without organized nuclei; absorb or produce their own nutrients	bacteria, blue-green algae
Protista	unicellular with membrane-bound nuclei; ingest, absorb or produce nutrients via photosynthesis	protozoans, algae
Fungi	multicellular with membrane-bound nuclei; absorb nutrients	mushrooms, molds
Plants	multicellular with membrane-bound nuclei and a cell wall; possess chlorophyll and undergo photosynthesis	flowering plants and trees; evergreens
Animals	multicellular with membrane-bound nuclei; ingest nutrients	mammals, birds, amphibians, fish, reptiles, insects, crustaceans, etc.

These kingdoms can be divided into three main groups based on the mode of nutrition—photosynthetic organisms (plants and algae), organisms which absorb their nutrients (bacteria and fungi), and organisms which engulf or ingest their nutrients (protozoa and animals).

Each kingdom is further divided into phyla (sing. phylum), which are subdivided as follows: phyla → into classes → into families → into genera → into species. Each of these groups may be divided into 6 additional subgroups.

All living organisms are given a scientific name using the combination of genus and species. Under this binomial naming system, the scientific name for a human is *Homo sapiens*. To illustrate the classification system a demonstration of how one classifies a human is given below:

CLASSIFICATION OF THE HUMAN

Classification Group		Distinguishing Features
Kingdom	Animalia	Consume food and are mobile.
Phylum	Chordata	Notochord, hollow nervous system (neural tube) dorsally positioned, gill slits in pharyngeal wall, heart ventral to digestive system.
Subphylum	Vertebrata	Segmental vertebral column.
Class	Mammalia	Mammary glands for nourishment of young; hair or fur; warm-blooded; diaphragm.
Order	Primates	Large cerebral hemispheres; opposable digits; nails; highly developed sense of sight—eyes directed forward; teeth specialized for different functions.
Family	Hominidae	Walk with two limbs (bipedal locomotion); binocular color vision.
Genus	Homo	Ability to speak and most highly developed and largest brain.
Species	sapiens	Large skull, high forehead, reduced size of brow (supraorbital) ridges, prominent chin; decreased amount of body hair.

Organization of the Human Body

A multicellular organism is composed of millions of cells organized into functional units (organs and systems) which are formed by various groups of similar cells (tissues) working together. These cells are embedded in intercellular substances and tissue fluids. A *tissue* consists of a group of cells performing a similar function. Four basic tissues compose the human (mammalian) body: epithelium, connective tissue, muscle and nerve tissues. The four basic tissues may be organized to form functional units known as *organs*. Each organ has a definite function which results from the combined functions of the various tissue components. Several organs which function together as a unit for a specified purpose make up an organ *system*. The animal *organism* is composed of several interrelated organ systems. The human body is composed of the systems listed in the following table.

Organ Systems

The human body is composed of the systems listed in the following table.

ORGAN SYSTEMS IN THE HUMAN

System	Functions
Muscular	Produces motion of body parts and viscera.
Skeletal	Supports the body, protects organs and produces blood cells.
Circulatory	Transports nutrients, wastes, gases (oxygen and carbon dioxide), hormones, blood cells throughout body; also protects body against foreign organisms.
Nervous	Responds to internal and external stimuli; regulates and coordinates body activities and movements.
Integumentary	Limits and protects the body as a whole; prevents excess loss of water and functions in regulating body temperature.
Digestive	Enzymatically breaks down food materials into usable and absorbable nutrients.
Respiratory	Functions in the exchange of gases (oxygen and carbon dioxide).
Urinary	Removes body wastes from blood stream and helps regulate homeostasis of internal environment.
Reproductive	Perpetuates the living organism by the production of sex cells (gametes) and future offsprings.
Endocrine	Regulates body growth and function via hormones.

Four Basic Tissues

1. Muscle Tissue: Muscle tissue is contractile in nature and functions to move the skeletal system and body viscera.

TYPES OF MUSCLE

Type	Characteristics	Location
Skeletal	striated, voluntary	skeletal muscles of the body
Smooth	non-striated, involuntary	walls of digestive tract and blood vessels, uterus, urinary bladder
Cardiac	striated, involuntary	heart

2. Nervous Tissue: Nervous tissue is composed of cells (*neurons*) that respond to external and internal stimuli and have the capability to transmit a message (*impulse*) from one area of the body to another. This tissue thus induces a response of distant muscles or glands, as well as regulating body processes such as respiration, circulation, and digestion. Nervous tissue composes the central (brain and spinal cord) and peripheral (peripheral nerves, ganglia and receptors) nervous systems and the special sensory receptors (eye, ear, taste buds and olfactory region).

3. Epithelial Tissue: Epithelial tissue covers the external surfaces of the body and lines the internal tubes and cavities. It also forms the glands of the body. Characteristics of epithelial tissue (epithelium) are that it

  (1) has compactly aggregated cells;
  (2) has limited intercellular spaces and substance;
  (3) is avascular (no blood vessels);
  (4) lies on a connective tissue layer—the basal lamina;
  (5) has cells that form sheets and are polarized;
  (6) is derived from all three germ layers.

TYPES OF EPITHELIUM

Classification	Location(s)	Function(s)
Simple squamous epithelium	Endothelium of blood and lymphatic vessels; Bowman's capsule and thin loop of Henle in kidney; mesothelium lining pericardial, peritoneal and pleural body cavities; lung alveoli; smallest excretory ducts of glands.	Lubrication of body cavities (permits free movement of organs); pinocytotic transport across cells.
Stratified squamous keratinized epithelium	Epidermis of skin.	Prevents loss of water and protection.
Stratified squamous nonkeratinized epithelium (moist)	Mucosa of oral cavity, esophagus, anal canal; vagina; cornea of eye and part of conjunctiva.	Secretion; protection; prevents loss of water.
Simple cuboidal epithelium	Kidney tubules; choroid plexus; thyroid gland; rete testis; surface of ovary.	Secretion; absorption; lines surface.
Stratified cuboidal epithelium	Ducts of sweat glands; developing follicles of ovary.	Secretion; protection.
Simple columnar epithelium	Cells lining lumen of digestive tract (stomach to rectum); gall bladder; many glands (secretory units and ducts); uterus; uterine tube (ciliated).	Secretion; absorption; protection; lubrication.
Pseudostratified columnar epithelium	Lines lumen of respiratory tract (nasal cavity, trachea and bronchi) (ciliated); ducts of epididymis (stereocilia); ductus deferens; male urethra.	Secretion; protection; facilitates transport of substances on surface of cells.
Stratified columnar epithelium	Male urethra; conjunctiva.	Protection.
Transitional epithelium	Urinary tract (renal calyces and pelvis, ureter and urinary bladder).	Protection.

Epithelial cells may also have specializations at the cell surface. For example,

microvilli—fingerlike projections of plasma membranes. Mainly located at luminal surfaces of absorptive cells (brush border of proximal convoluted tubules and striated border of intestinal epithelium).

cilia—motile organelles extending into the luman consisting of specifically arranged microtubules. Mainly located in respiratory epithelium and part of female reproductive tract.

flagella—similar to cilia. Primary examples are human spermatozoa.

stereocilia—are actually very elongated microvilli.

4. Connective Tissue: Connective tissue is the packing and supporting material of the body tissues and organs. It develops from mesoderm (mesenchyme). All connective tissues consist of three distinct components: ground substance, cells and fibers.

a. *Ground substance*. Ground substance is located between the cells and fibers, both of which are embedded in it. It forms an amorphous intercellar material. In the fresh state, it appears as a transparent and homogeneous gel. It acts as a route for the passage of nutrients and wastes to and from the cells within or adjacent to the connective tissue. The ground substance is composed of mucopolysaccharides (*glycosaminoglycans*), proteins, lipids and water. The primary glycosaminoglycans found in the ground substance are chondroitin sulfate and hyaluronic acid, the latter present in greater quantity.

b. *Fibers*. The fiber components of connective tissue add support and strength. Three types of fibers are present: *collagenous, elastic* and *reticular*.

Collagen fibers (white fibers) are the most numerous fiber type and are present in all types of connective tissue in varying amounts. Collagen bundles are strong and resist stretching. They are found in structures such as tendons, ligaments, aponeuroses and fascia, which are subjected to pull or stretching activities.

Elastic fibers (yellow fibers) are refractile fibers which are thinner (0.2 to 1 μm diameter) than collagen fibers. They are extremely elastic and are located in structures with a degree of elasticity, such as the walls of blood vessels (elastic arteries), true vocal cords and trachea.

Reticular fibers are thinner (0.2 to 1 μm diameter) than collagenous fibers. They are arranged in an intermeshing network (reticulum) which supports the organ. Reticular fibers are inelastic. They are found in the walls of blood vessels, lymphoid tissues (spleen and lymph nodes), red bone marrow, basal laminae and glands (liver and kidney).

c. *Cells*. The *cells* of connective tissue are primarily attached and non-motile (*fixed cells*), but some have the ability to move (*wandering or free cells*). The typical cells found in connective tissue are:

Fibroblasts constitute the largest number of cells present in connective tissue. In an actively secreting state, they are flattened stellate-shaped cells with an oval nucleus and basophilic cytoplasm due to the numerous rough endoplasmic reticulum. In the inactive state, they appear as elongated spindles with a more basophilic oval or elongated nucleus. In this state, they are referred to as *fibrocytes*. The latter are the main cellular constituents of connective tissue structures such as tendons and ligaments. Only the nuclei of fibrocytes are observed between the fibers since the cytoplasm is indistinct. The terms fibrocyte and fibroblast are often used interchangeably.

Mesenchymal cells are undifferentiated connective tissue cells which have the potential to differentiate into other types of connective tissue cells. They are primarily found in embryonic and fetal tissues; some are thought to be present in the adult abutting the walls of capillaries. They are smaller than fibroblasts and are stellate in shape. They are capable of moving by extending their cell processes into the gel-like ground substance.

Macrophages (histiocytes) may be fixed or free. Free macrophages may wander through the connective tissue by extending their cell processes. Fixed macrophages are very numerous in loose connective tissue. They are polymorphic in shape and contain an oval nucleus. They have the ability to engulf extracellular material (foreign matter or necrotic cells). Macrophages are difficult to distinguish except when they are actively phagocytosing material and thus contain many vacuoles.

Adipocytes (fat cells) are found in most connective tissue, either singly or in groups. If the connective tissue layer is primarily composed of fat cells, it is referred to as adipose tissue. An adipocyte is a round, large cell with a distinct, dense nucleus usually located at the periphery of the cytoplasm. The majority of the cytoplasmic (cell) volume is taken up by a large lipid droplet. Due to the clear appearing cytoplasm and dark nucleus at one pole, the cell has a signet ring appearance. Fat cells do not undergo mitosis.

Mast cells are ovoid cells with small round nuclei. The cytoplasm contains numerous coarse basophilic granules which also stain metachromatically and are soluble in water. The mast cell granules are composed of *histamine* and an anticoagulant known as *heparin*. Histamine dilates blood vessels and increases the permeability of capillaries, thus increasing interstitial fluid. Mast cells take part in the allergic response of the body. Mast cells are found in most connective tissue and are numerous in the respiratory tract and near small blood vessels.

Plasma cells have a characteristic eccentric nucleus which contains chromatin arranged in a definite pattern near the nuclear envelope. This pattern gives a ''cartwheel or spoke wheel'' appearance. The juxtanuclear cytoplasm appears clear and less basophilic due to the Golgi complex located in this area. Plasma cells are found in the lamina propria of the gastrointestinal tract. They function in protecting the body against bacterial invasion by secreting antibodies (immunoglobulins—IgG) into the circulating blood.

Reticular cells are star-shaped cells which join via their processes to form a cellular network. They are found abutting reticular fibers in certain glands and lymphoid tissues.

Pericytes are located in the adventitia of blood vessels. They are believed to be multipotential cells which may differentiate into various connective tissue cells as well as into smooth muscle cells.

White blood cells or leukocytes. Certain white blood cells migrate out of the blood into the extracellular ground substance. The main leukocytes found in the connective tissue are lymphocytes, monocytes, eosinophils, basophils and neutrophils. The leukocytes in connective tissue are similar in structure and function to those in the blood. The agranular leukocytes migrate in large numbers under normal conditions. Lymphocytes accumulate in areas in response to chronic inflammation. Neutrophils also migrate in large numbers into the interstitium during an inflammatory response. Eosinophils occur in areas involved in allergic reactions, such as the respiratory tract.

Skeletal System

The skeletal system of vertebrates is an *endoskeleton*—that is, it is within the body— as compared to an *exoskeleton* characteristic of arthropods. The human skeletal system provides:

(1) support
(2) protection of vital organs
(3) sites for muscle attachment
(4) storage site of body calcium and phosphates
(5) sites for blood cell formation

The *human skeleton* consists of bone and cartilage. The bones form the main rigid structure of the skeleton. The human skeleton consists of about 206 bones, some of which are fused while others are joined together at sites which permit various degrees of movement. The sites of junction, or articulation, whether movable or immovable, are known as *joints*.

The human skeleton is divided into an *axial skeleton* and an *appendicular skeleton*.

Axial Skeleton

The axial skeleton consists of 80 bones forming the trunk (spine and thorax) and skull.

Vertebral Column: The main trunk of the body is supported by the spine, or vertebral column, which is composed of 26 bones, some of which are formed by the fusion of a few bones. The vertebral column from superior to inferior consists of 7 cervical (neck), 12 thoracic and 5 lumbar vertebrae, as well as a sacrum, formed by fusion of 5 sacral vertebrae, and a coccyx, formed by fusion of 4 coccygeal vertebrae. Each vertebra consists of a body anteriorly and an arched posterior region circumscribing an inner central canal, the *vertebral canal*, which extends from the foramen magnum at the base of the skull through the sacrum. The vertebral column functions to support the trunk of the body and to protect the spinal cord located in the vertebral canal. The vertebrae of the cervical, thoracic and lumbar regions are separated from each other by round fibro-cartilaginous articular discs known as *intervertebral discs*. The entire vertebral column is held together by ligaments.

Ribs and Sternum: The axial skeleton also contains 12 pairs of *ribs* attached posteriorly to the thoracic vertebrae and anteriorly either directly or via cartilage to the *sternum* (breastbone). The ribs and sternum form the *thoracic cage*, which protects the heart and lungs. Seven pairs of ribs articulate with the sternum (*fixed ribs*) directly, and three do so via cartilage; the two most inferior pairs do not attach anteriorly and are referred to as *floating ribs*.

Skull: The *skull* consists of 22 bones fused together to form a rigid structure which houses and protects organs such as the brain, auditory apparatus and eyes. The bones of the skull form the *face* and *cranium* (brain case) and consist of 6 single bones (*occipital, frontal, ethmoid, sphenoid, vomer* and *mandible*) and 8 paired bones (*parietal, temporal, maxillary, palatine, zygomatic, lacrimal, inferior concha* and *nasal*). The *lower jaw* or *mandible* is the only movable bone of the skull (head); it articulates with the temporal bones.

Other Parts: Other bones considered part of the axial skeleton are the *middle ear bones* (*ossicles*) and the small U-shaped *hyoid bone* that is suspended in a portion of the neck by muscles and ligaments.

Appendicular Skeleton

The *appendicular skeleton* forms the major internal support of the appendages—the *upper* and *lower extremities* (limbs).

Pectoral Girdle and Upper Extremities: The arms are attached to and suspended from the axial skeleton via the *shoulder* (*pectoral*) *girdle*. The latter is composed of two *clavicles* (*collarbones*) and two *scapulae* (*shoulder blades*). The clavicles articulate with the sternum; the two *sternoclavicular joints* are the only sites of articulation between the trunk and upper extremity.

Each upper limb from distal to proximal (closest to the body) consists of hand, wrist, forearm and arm (upper arm). The *hand* consists of 5 *digits* (fingers) and 5 *metacarpal* bones. Each digit is comprised of three bones known as *phalanges*, except the thumb which has only two bones. The *wrist* consists of eight *carpal* bones which articulate with metacarpals. The *forearm* consists of two bones, the *ulna* on the side of the fifth digit (little finger) and the *radius* on the thumb side. The articulation between radius and ulna at the wrist permits rotation of the radius over the ulna during pronation (palm facing backward) and supination (palm turned forward). The ulna articulates at the elbow joint with the *humerus* creating a hinge joint and movement of the arm. The humerus, in turn, is connected to the shoulder girdle at the *glenoid cavity* of the scapula.

Pelvic Girdle and Lower Extremities: The lower *extremities*, or legs, are attached to the axial skeleton via the *pelvic* or *hip girdle*. Each of the two coxal, or *hip*, *bones* comprising the pelvic girdle is formed by the fusion of three bones—*ilium, pubis* and *ischium*. The coxal bones attach the lower limbs to the trunk by articulating with the sacrum.

From distal to proximal the lower limb consists of foot, ankle, shank and thigh. The *foot* consists of 5 digits (*toes*) and 5 *metatarsals*. The digits contain 3 *phalanges* each, except for the big toe, which has two. The *ankle* is formed by 7 *tarsal* bones. The shank region is supported by two bones, the *tibia* and *fibula*. The tibia is larger, is located medially, forms the shin, and articulates at the knee joint with the *femur* (*thigh bone*). The knee joint is protected anteriorly by the kneecap, or *patella*. The femur articulates with the *acetabular fossa* of the coxal bone.

THE HUMAN SKELETAL SYSTEM	
Part of the Skeleton	**Number of Bones**
Axial Skeleton	**80**
Skull	22
Ossicles (malleus, incus and stapes)	6
Vertebral column	26
Ribs	24
Sternum	1
Hyoid	1
Appendicular Skeleton	**126**
Upper extremities	64
Lower extremities	62

Characteristics of Bone

Bone is a specialized type of connective tissue consisting of cells (*osteocytes*) embedded in a calcified matrix which gives bone its characteristic hard and rigid nature. Bones are encased by a *periosteum*, a connective tissue sheath. All bone has a central marrow cavity. *Bone marrow* fills the marrow cavity or smaller marrow spaces, depending on the type of bone.

Types of Bone: There are two types of bone in the skeleton: *compact bone* and *spongy* (cancellous) bone.

Compact Bone. Compact bone lies within the periosteum, forms the outer region of bones, and appears dense due to its compact organization. The living osteocytes and calcified matrix are arranged in layers, or *lamellae*. Lamellae may be circularly arranged surrounding a central canal, the *Haversian canal*, which contains small blood vessels. This unit of a Haversian canal circumscribed by Haversian lamellae is known as an *Haversian system*, or *osteon*. Osteons are oriented along the longitudinal axis of the bone and communicate with each other, the periosteum, and the marrow cavity via oblique or transverse canals known as *Volkmann's canals*. Blood vessels enter and leave and are distributed throughout bone via the Haversian and Volkmann's canals. Irregular lamellae structures, the *interstitial lamellae*, are present between the Haversian systems. They are remnants of resorbed lamellar systems resulting from the remodelling of bone. The inner (next to marrow cavity) and outer (next to periosteum) limits of compact bone are formed by lamellar structures, the *inner* (*endosteal*) and *outer* (*periosteal*) *circumferential lamellae*, respectively. The Haversian systems are the major component of compact bone and lie between these two circumferential lamellae. The marrow cavity and Haversian canals are lined by *endosteum*, a thin layer of connective tissue. Both the endosteum and periosteum contain *osteogenic cells*, which can transform into bone-forming cells, or *osteoblasts*.

Spongy bone. Spongy bone consists of *bars*, *spicules* or *trabeculae*, which form a lattice meshwork. Spongy bone is found at the ends of long bones and the inner layer of flat, irregular and short bones. The trabeculae consist of osteocytes embedded in calcified matrix, which in definitive bone has a lamellar nature. The spaces between the trabeculae contain bone marrow.

Bone Cells: The cells of bone are osteocytes, osteoblasts, and osteoclasts. *Osteocytes* are found singly in *lacunae* (spaces) within the calcified matrix and communicate with each other via small canals in the bone known as *canaliculi.* The latter contain osteocyte cell processes. The osteocytes in compact and spongy bone are similar in structure and function.

Osteoblasts are cells which form bone matrix, surrounding themselves with it, and thus are transformed into osteocytes. They arise from undifferentiated cells, such as mesenchymal cells. They are cuboidal cells which line the trabeculae of immature or developing spongy bone.

Osteoclasts are cells found during bone development and remodelling. They are multinucleated cells lying in cavities, *Howship's lacunae,* on the surface of the bone tissue being resorbed. Osteoclasts remove the existing calcified matrix releasing the inorganic or organic components.

Bone Matrix: *Matrix* of compact and spongy bone consists of collagenous fibers and ground substance which constitute the organic component of bone. Matrix also consists of inorganic material which is about 65% of the dry weight of bone. Approximately 85% of the inorganic component consists of calcium phosphate in a crystalline form (hydroxyapatite crystals). Glycoproteins are the main components of the ground substance.

MAJOR TYPES OF HUMAN BONES

Type of Bone	Characteristics	Examples
Long bones	Width less than length.	Humerus, radius, ulna, femur, tibia.
Short bones	Length and width close to equal in size.	Carpal and tarsal bones.
Flat bones	Thin flat shape.	Scapulae, ribs, sternum, bones of cranium (occipital, frontal, parietal).
Irregular bones	Multifaceted shape.	Vertebrae, sphenoid, ethmoid.
Sesamoid	Small bones located in tendons of muscles.	—

Joints

The bones of the skeleton articulate with each other at *joints,* which are variable in structure and function. Some joints are immovable, such as the *sutures* between the bones of the cranium. Others are *slightly movable joints*; examples are the *intervertebral joints* and the *pubic symphysis* (joint between the two pubic bones of the coxal bones). These contain fibrocartilage plates separating the articulating bones and have a slight gliding motion. The most common joints are *freely movable joints*. They are also referred to as *synovial joints* since their joint capsules are lined by a serous *synovial membrane* which produces a lubricating fluid—*synovial fluid*—between the articulating bones. The *capsule* is a fibrous connective tissue sheath which encases the joint. Another feature of synovial joints is that a thin layer of *hyaline cartilage* lines the articular surfaces of the abutting bones. The synovial joints can be classified according to the type of motion permitted by the structure of the joint.

TYPES OF JOINTS

Joint Type	Characteristic	Example
Ball and socket	Permits all types of movement (abduction, adduction, flexion, extension, circumduction); it is considered a universal joint.	Hip and shoulder joints.
Hinge (ginglymus)	Permits motion in one plane only.	Elbow and knee, interphalangeal joints.
Rotating or pivot	Rotation is only motion permitted.	Radius and ulna, atlas and axis (first and second cervical vertebrae).
Plane or gliding	Permits sliding motion.	Between tarsal bones and carpal bones.
Condylar (condyloid)	Permits motion in two planes which are at right angles to each other (rotation is not possible).	Metacarpo-phalangeal joints, temporomandibular.

Adjacent bones at a joint are connected by fibrous connective tissue bands known as *ligaments*. They are strong bands which support the joint and may also act to limit the degree of motion occurring at a joint.

Muscular System

Classification

A muscle cell not only has the ability to propagate an action potential along its cell membrane, as does a nerve cell, but also has the internal machinery to give it the unique ability to contract.

Most muscles in the body can be classified as striated muscles in reference to the fact that when observed under a light microscope the muscular tissue has light and dark bands or striations running across it. Although both skeletal and cardiac muscles are striated and therefore have similar structural organizations, they do possess some characteristic functional differences. Skeletal muscle contraction, for example, is made up of the contraction of many motor units. A motor unit consists of a single motor neuron coming from the spinal cord of the central nervous system and all the muscle fibers which it innervates (a few to 2000).

In contrast to skeletal muscle, cardiac muscle is a functional syncytium. This means that although anatomically it consists of individual cells the entire mass normally responds as a unit and all of the cells contract together. In addition, cardiac muscle has the property of automaticity which means that the heart initiates its own contraction without the need for motor nerves. Motor nerves may alter this inherent rhythm but the resource for initiating the contraction lies within the special cardiac cells called pacemaker cells. Here an action potential is initiated and spreads to the other cardiac cells.

Non-striated muscle consists of multi-unit and unitary (visceral) smooth muscle. Visceral smooth muscle has many of the properties of cardiac muscle. To some extent it acts as a functional syncytium e.g., areas of intestinal smooth muscle will contract as a unit. Smooth muscle is part of the urinary bladder, uterus, spleen, gallbladder, and numerous other internal organs. It is also the muscle of blood vessels, respiratory tracts, and the iris of the eye.

The basic contractile mechanism is probably the same in all muscle types although the structural organization of smooth muscle is very different from that of striated muscle. We will concentrate on skeletal muscle, knowing that what we discuss can be applied to cardiac muscle and to some extent to smooth muscle.

Skeletal Muscles

In order for the human being to carry out the many intricate movements that must be performed, approximately 650 skeletal muscles of various lengths, shapes, and strength play a part. Each muscle consists of many muscle cells or fibers held together and surrounded by connective tissue that gives functional integrity to the system. Three definite units are commonly referred to:

(1) endomysium—connective tissue layer enveloping a single fiber;
(2) perimysium—connective tissue layer enveloping a bundle of fibers;
(3) epimysium—connective tissue layer enveloping the entire muscle.

Muscle Attachment and Function

For coordinated movement to take place, the muscle must attach to either bone or cartilage or, as in the case of the muscles of facial expression, to skin. The portion of a muscle attaching to bone is the tendon. A muscle has two extremities, its origin and its insertion; the origin is the relatively fixed attachment site, while the insertion is the end attached to a structure that will be moved when the muscle contracts. A pair of muscles usually control the movement of a joint; they are opposing or antagonistic muscles. For example, a flexor muscle is opposed by an extensor.

Terms to Describe Movement

Flexion is bending, most often ventrally to decrease the angle between two parts of the body; it is usually an action at an articulation or joint.

Extension is straightening, or increasing the angle between two parts of the body; a stretching out or making the flexed part straight.

Abduction is a movement away from the midsagittal plane (midline); to abduct is to move laterally.

Adduction is a movement toward the midsagittal plane (midline); to adduct is to move medially and bring a part back to the mid-axis.

Circumduction is a circular movement at a ball and socket (shoulder or hip) joint, utilizing the movements of flexion, extension, abduction, and adduction.

Rotation is a movement of a part of the body around its long axis.

Examples: a. The atlas (1st cervical vertebra) rotates on the axis (2nd cervical vertebra).
b. The thigh may be rotated medially or internally; it may also be rotated laterally or externally.

Supination refers only to the movement of the radius around the ulna. In supination the palm of the hand is oriented anteriorly; turning the palm dorsally puts it into pronation. The body on its back is in the supine position.

Pronation refers to the palm of the hand being oriented posteriorly. The body on its belly is the prone position.

Inversion refers only to the lower extremity, specifically the ankle joint. When the foot (plantar surface) is turned inward, so that the sole is pointing and directed toward the midline of the body and is parallel with the median plane, we speak of inversion. Its opposite is eversion.

Eversion refers to the foot (plantar surface) being turned outward so that the sole is pointing laterally.

Opposition is one of the most critical movements in humans; it allows us to have pulp-to-pulp opposition, which gives us the great dexterity of our hands. In this movement the thumb pad is brought to a finger pad. A median nerve injury negates this action.

Muscle Names

The names of some muscles may appear strange; the naming, however, is based essentially on anatomical position, function, shape, or other feature. Here are some examples:

1. **Position and Location:**

   a. Pectoralis major and minor — pectoral region of thorax; the major is larger

   b. Temporalis — temporal region of head

   c. Infra- and supraspinatus — below and above spine of scapula

   d. External and internal intercostals — refers to their location in the intercostal spaces

2. **Principal Action:**

   a. pronators (e.g., pronator quadratus) and supinators — pronator refers to palm down and supinator to palm up; quadratus refers to the shape

   b. Flexors and extensors (e.g., flexor and extensor digitorum) — flexors and extensors of digits

   c. Levator scapulae — elevator of the scapula (shoulder)

3. **Shape:**

   a. Trapezius — trapezoid in shape

   b. Rhomboid major and minor — rhomboid in shape

4. **Number of Divisions (Heads) and Position:**

   a. Biceps brachii — two-headed muscle in anterior brachium (arm)

   b. Triceps brachii — three-headed muscle in posterior brachium (arm)

5. **Size, Length, and Shape:**

   a. Flexor pollicis longus and brevis — long and short flexors of the thumb

   b. Rhomboid major and minor — major is larger in size; rhomboid in shape.

6. Attachment Sites:

a. Sternocleidomastoid   extends from sternum and clavicle (cleido) to mastoid process

b. Sternohyoid   extends from sternum to hyoid bone

Structural Organization of a Muscle Fiber

A muscle fiber is a single muscle cell. If we look at a section of a fiber we see that it is complete with a cell membrane called the sarcolemma and has several nuclei located just under the sarcolemma—it is multinucleated. Each fiber is composed of numerous cylindrical fibrils running the entire length of the fiber.

The fibril exhibits light and dark bands—the "I" and "A" bands respectively. The "I" band is bisected by the "Z" line and the "A" band by the "M" line. There is a somewhat lighter band within the "A" band that is called the "H" band. An even lighter area in the middle of the "H" zone on either side of the "M" line is called the "pseudo-H" band.

These striations are produced by the arrangement within the fibril of myofilaments which make up the contractile machinery. A sarcomere, the area between two "Z" bands, is the functional unit of muscle; it is the region between two "Z" lines and consists of an "A" band and half of two abutting "I" bands. Refer to the illustration of the relaxed myofibril (page 35) for the positions of these lines and bands.

Myofilaments

1. The thick and thin myofilaments form the contractile machinery of muscle and are made up of proteins. Approximately 54% of all the contractile proteins (by weight) is myosin. The thick myofilament is composed of many myosin molecules oriented tail-end to tail-end at the center with myosin molecules staggered from the center to the myofilament tip.

2. The second major contractile protein is actin. Actin is a globular protein. The thin myofilament contains two chains of F-actin arranged in a twisted fashion. This configuration gives the thin myofilament a certain periodicity. Associated with the thin myofilament along its entire length is the globular protein troponin. The presence of troponin along with tropomyosin-B inhibits myosin-actin interaction—it represses actomyosin formation. Calcium ions released following an action potential in the fiber membrane and T-tubules bind with troponin. Calcium-troponin binding removes the inhibition of actomyosin formation.

Sarcoplasm

The sarcoplasm (cytoplasm of the muscle cell) contains Golgi complexes near the nuclei. Mitochondria are found between the myofibrils and just below the sarcolemma. The myofibrils are surrounded by smooth endoplasmic reticulum (*sarcoplasmic reticulum*) composed of a longitudinally arranged tubular network (*sarcotubules*). This network is continuous with dilated sacs, *terminal cisternae*, which lie transversely across the fiber near the center of the "I" band. Near this same point the sarcolemma invaginates into the sarcoplasm, forming a tubular channel called the T (*transverse*) *tubule*, which branches and extends among the myofibrils. A branch of the T system is interposed between the two terminal cisternae at the junction between any two sarcomeres (directly over the "Z" line). The complex (terminal cistern–T tubule–terminal cistern) formed at this position is known as a *triad*. The T tubules function to bring a wave of depolarization of the sarcolemma into the fiber and thus into intimate relationship with the terminal cisternae. The sarcoplasmic reticulum concentrates calcium ions (Ca^{2+}) within its lumen, but depolarization of the T-tubule membrane induces the nearby terminal cisternae of the sarcoplasmic reticulum to release this Ca^{2+} into the sarcoplasm among the myofilaments. The Ca^{2+} becomes associated with the troponin of the thin myofilament, bringing about contraction as discussed below.

Excitation

Contraction in a skeletal muscle is triggered by the generation of an action potential in the muscle membrane. Each motor neuron upon entering a skeletal muscle loses its myelin sheath and divides into branches with each branch innervating a single muscle fiber, forming a *neuromuscular junction*. Each fiber normally has one neuromuscular junction which is located near the center of the fiber. A *motor unit* consists of a single motor neuron and all the muscle fibers innervated by it. The *motor end plate* is the specialized part of the muscle fiber's membrane lying under the neuron.

The impulse arriving at the end of the motor neuron causes liberation of *acetylcholine* from vesicles in the neuron terminal. The acetylcholine acts at specific sites normally found only on the motor end plate section of the fiber membrane and increases the permeability of the motor end plate. The resulting Na^+ influx produces a depolarizing potential called the end-plate potential. This in turn depolarizes adjacent areas of the fiber membrane, triggering an action potential which is propagated in both directions from the central neuromuscular junction toward the fiber ends. Normally the magnitude of the end-plate potential is sufficient to discharge the muscle membrane, so that each impulse in the nerve ending produces a response in the muscle. The acetylcholine is rapidly destroyed by the enzyme *acetylcholinesterase* which is found in high concentrations at the neuromuscular junction.

Contraction

According to the sliding filament theory (Huxley) the sarcomere response to excitation involves the sliding of thin and thick myofilaments past one another making and breaking chemical bonds with each other as they go. Neither the thick nor thin myofilaments change in length. If we could imagine observing this contraction under a light microscope we would see the narrowing of the "H" and "I" bands during contraction while the width of the "A" band would remain constant.

The word *contraction* refers to those processes which are manifested externally by either a *shortening* of a muscle or by *tension development* in a muscle. If the muscle length is held constant, the contraction is referred to as an *isometric contraction*. In an isometric contraction the passive tension remains constant with the *active tension* being added to it to produce the *total tension* of the muscle.

If the muscle shortens during contraction, it is called an *isotonic contraction* and the total tension remains constant.

Muscle Twitch

A muscle's response to a single maximal stimulus is a *muscle twitch*. The beginning of muscular activity is signalled by the record of the *electrical activity* in the sarcolemma. The *latent period* is the delay between imposition of the stimulus and the development of tension.

Tetanus

When a volley of stimuli is applied to a muscle, each succeeding stimulus may arrive before the muscle can completely relax from the contraction caused by the preceding stimulus. The result is *summation*, an increased strength of contraction. If the frequency of stimulation is very fast, individual contractions fuse and the muscle smoothly and fully contracts. This is a *tetanus*.

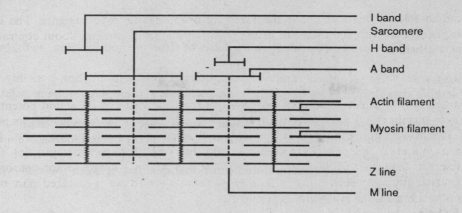

Relaxed Myofibril

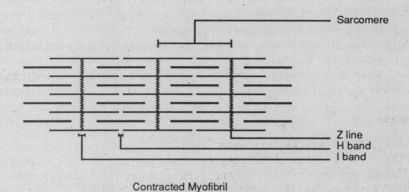

Contracted Myofibril

SCHEMATIC OF SKELETAL (STRIATED) MUSCLE

Energy Sources

In any phenomenon including muscular contraction the energy input to the system and the energy output from the system are equal. Let us consider first the energy sources for muscular contraction. The immediate energy source for contraction is ATP which can be hydrolyzed by actomyosin to give ADP, P_1, and the energy which is in some way associated with cross-bridge motion.

The ultimate source of this ATP is the ATP produced by the intermediary metabolism of carbohydrates and lipids. Skeletal muscle has the biochemical machinery to utilize both. With mild exercise oxygen availability after an initial period of adjustment is sufficient so that the aerobic pathways for ATP production can keep pace with the ATP utilization during the exercise—a new equilibrium is reached. During short-term, violent exertion, however, aerobic energy production cannot keep pace with energy utilization and even during the onset of mild exercise aerobic energy production initially lags behind energy utilization. Yet the ATP concentration remains constant. The reason is that there are stores of CP (creatine phosphate) in muscles and ATP levels can be maintained at the expense of CP levels. In these cases of insufficient oxygen availability ("oxygen debt") anaerobic pathways can produce enough additional ATP to permit those short-term bursts of exercise but lactic acid is generated. This incomplete oxidation produces substantially less energy than the complete aerobic oxidation to carbon dioxide and water.

Types of Muscle Fibers

Skeletal muscle fibers can be described, on the bases of structure and function, as follows:

1. *White (fast) fibers*—contract rapidly; fatigue quickly; energy production is mainly via anaerobic glycolysis; contain relatively few mitochondria; examples are the muscles of the eye.
2. *Red (slow) fibers*—contract slowly; fatigue slowly; energy production mainly via oxidative phosphorylation (aerobic); contain relatively many mitochondria; examples are postural muscles.
3. *Intermediate fibers*—have structural and functional qualities between those of white and of red fibers.

Circulatory System

Functions

The circulatory system serves:

(1) to conduct nutrients and oxygen to the tissues;

(2) to remove waste materials by transporting nitrogenous compounds to the kidneys and carbon dioxide to the lungs;

(3) to transport chemical messengers (hormones) to target organs and modulate and integrate the internal milieu of the body;

(4) to transport agents which serve the body in allergic, immune, and infectious responses;

(5) to initiate clotting and thereby prevent blood loss;

(6) to maintain body temperature;

(7) to produce, carry and contain blood;

(8) to transfer body reserves, specifically mineral salts, to areas of need.

General Components and Structure

The circulatory system consists of the heart, blood vessels, blood and lymphatics. It is a network of tubular structures through which blood travels to and from all the parts of the body. In vertebrates this is a completely closed circuit system, as William Harvey (1628) demonstrated. The heart is a modified, specialized, powerful pumping blood vessel. Arteries, eventually becoming arterioles, conduct blood to capillaries (essentially endothelial tubes), and venules, eventually becoming veins, return blood from the capillary bed to the heart. (Malpighi [1661] demonstrated the capillary system.) The system is lined entirely by endothelium. Fluids (mostly water) which leave capillaries return as lymph to the blood stream via lymphatic channels. The spleen, liver, and bone marrow function in the formation, destruction and replacement of blood cells.

Systemic arteries orginating from the left side of the heart (via the aorta) distribute oxygenated and nutrient-rich blood to the body. The systemic venous system returns deoxygenated blood to the heart. The pulmonary arterial circuit delivers this blood from the right side of the heart to the lungs and the pulmonary venous component returns oxygenated blood to the left side of the heart. Arteries travel away from the heart; veins come to it.

Course of Circulation

Systemic Route:

a. *Arterial system.* Blood is delivered by the pulmonary veins (two from each lung) to the left atrium, passes through the bicuspid (mitral) valve into the left ventricle and then is pumped into the ascending aorta; backflow here is prevented by the aortic semilunar valves. The aortic arch toward the right side gives rise to the brachiocephalic (innominate) artery which divides into the right subclavian and right common carotid arteries. Next arising from the arch is the common carotid artery, then the left subclavian artery; these two arise independently from the arch. In general the carotids split into external and internal carotids which supply the head and neck and brain. The subclavians supply the upper limbs. As the subclavian arteries pass the first rib they are renamed axillary arteries. When the axillary arteries leave the axilla (armpit) and enter the arm (brachium) they are called brachial arteries. Below the elbow these main trunk lines divide into ulnar and radial arteries, which supply the forearm and eventually form a set of arterial arches in the hand which give rise to common and proper digital arteries. The descending (dorsal) aorta continues along the posterior aspect of the thorax giving rise to the segmental intercostal arteries. After passage "through" (behind) the diaphragm it is called the abdominal aorta. Branches are:

inferior phrenic arteries to the diaphragm and adrenal gland,
middle suprarenal (adrenal) artery to the adrenal,
celiac artery to the stomach, part of duodenum, liver, and spleen,
superior mesenteric artery to the small intestines, the cecum, ascending, and transverse colon
renal arteries to the kidneys and adrenals,
ovarian and testicular arteries to the respective gonads,
inferior mesenteric artery to the descending and sigmoid colon, and to the superior portion of the rectum,
lumbar segmental arteries to the abdominal wall.

At the pelvic rim the abdominal aorta divides into the right and left common iliac arteries. These divide into the internal iliacs, which supply the pelvic organs, and the external iliacs, which supply the lower limb.

As the external iliac artery passes below the inguinal ligament into the thigh, its name changes to femoral artery. In the region posterior to the knee joint the artery is known as the popliteal artery; it divides into an anterior tibial artery to the anterior leg, a posterior tibial artery to the posterior leg, and a peroneal artery to the lateral aspects of the leg. The anterior and posterior tibial arteries eventually give rise to metatarsal and digital arteries for the supply of the dorsal and plantar aspects, respectively, of the foot.

b. *Venous system.* Veins are frequently multiple and variations are common. They return blood originating in the capillaries of peripheral and distal body parts to the heart. Tributaries converge and eventually all the blood of the body except that from the lungs and heart itself reaches the right atrium via the superior and inferior venae cavae.

The superior vena cava is formed in the following manner. The internal jugular veins, from the brain and deep face and neck, and the external jugular veins, from the superficial face and neck, join the subclavian veins, which receive the drainage of the upper limb and form right and left brachiocephalic (innominate) veins. The two brachiocephalic veins join to form the superior vena cava. Also joining the superior vena cava is the azygous system of veins, which drains the chest wall.

The inferior vena cava has the following origin. Femoral veins, from the lower limb, become in the abdominal cavity the external iliac veins, which receive the internal iliac veins from the pelvis and form the common iliac veins. The common iliac veins join to form the inferior vena cava. The inferior vena cava receives the renal veins, veins from the body wall, the right gonadal vein and the hepatic veins, from the liver, before passing through the diaphragm into the thorax to enter the right atrium of the heart.

Hepatic Portal System: Blood draining the alimentary tract (intestines), pancreas, spleen and gall bladder does not return directly to the systemic circulation, but is relayed by the hepatic portal system of veins to and through the liver. In the liver, absorbed foodstuffs and wastes are processed. After processing, the liver returns the blood via hepatic veins to the inferior vena cava and from there to the heart.

Pulmonary Circuit: Blood is oxygenated and depleted of metabolic products such as carbon dioxide in the lungs. The pathway is as follows:

(1) Deoxygenated blood arrives in the right atrium and passes through the tricuspid valve into the right ventricle.

(2) It leaves the right ventricle via the pulmonary (trunk) artery and passes to the lungs; backflow is prevented by the pulmonary semilunar valves.

(3) In the capillary network of the lung, blood is oxygenated. It then leaves the lung via two pulmonary veins each from the right and left lung and passes to the left atrium.

(4) Blood passes through the bicuspid valve into the left ventricle and from there is expelled to the rest of the body via the ascending aorta; backflow is prevented by the aortic semilunar valves.

Lymphatic Drainage: A network of lymphatic capillaries permeates the body tissues. Lymph is a fluid similar in composition to blood plasma, and tissue fluids not reabsorbed into blood capillaries are transported via the lymphatic system eventually to join the venous system at the junction of the left internal jugular and subclavian veins. Like veins, lymphatics possess valves. Interposed along the course of some lymph vessels are lymph nodes. These nodes filter lymph and add lymphocytes to the circulation. Lymph nodes possess an outer cortex and an inner medulla. Lymphoid follicles are present in the cortex; irregular cords of lymphocytes make up the medulla.

The Heart

The heart is a highly specialized blood vessel which pumps 72 times per minute and propels about 4,000 gallons (about 15,000 liters) of blood daily to the tissues. It is composed of:

endocardium (lining coat; epithelium)
myocardium (middle coat; cardiac muscle)
epicardium (external coat or visceral layer of pericardium; epithelium and mostly connective tissue)
impulse conducting system

Mammals possess modified cardiac muscle fibers specialized for conduction (Purkinje system). The heart has an automatic rhythmic beat. Cardiac (autonomic) nerves exert an influence on heartbeat but serve only to change the force and frequency of the contractions in accordance with the physiologic needs of the organism.

Cardiac Nerves: Modification of the intrinsic rhythmicity of the heart muscle is produced by cardiac nerves of the sympathetic and parasympathetic nervous system. Stimulation of the sympathetic system increases the rate and force of the heartbeat and dilates the coronary arteries. Stimulation of the parasympathetic (vagus nerve) reduces the rate and force of the heartbeat and constricts the coronary circulation. Visceral afferent (sensory) fibers from the heart end almost wholly in the first four segments of the thoracic spinal cord.

Cardiac Cycle: Alternating contraction and relaxation is repeated about 75 times per minute; the duration of one cycle is about 0.8 second. Three phases succeed one another during the cycle:

(a) atrial systole: 0.1 second,
(b) ventricular systole; 0.3 second
(c) diastole: 0.4 second

The actual period of rest for each chamber is 0.7 second for the atria and 0.5 second for the ventricles, so, in spite of its activity, the heart is at rest longer than at work.

Blood

Blood is composed of cells (corpuscles) and a liquid intercellular ground substance called plasma. The average blood volume is 5 or 6 liters (7% of body weight). Plasma constitutes about 55% of blood volume, cellular elements about 45%.

Plasma: Over 90% of plasma is water; the balance is made up of plasma proteins and dissolved electrolytes, hormones, antibodies, nutrients, and waste products. Plasma is isotonic (0.85% sodium chloride). Plasma plays a vital role in respiration, circulation, coagulation, temperature regulation, buffer activities and overall fluid balance. The plasma proteins (albumin, globulin and fibrinogen) are responsible for the viscosity of blood, carry immune material and control osmotic pressure. Fibrinogen, in bleeding, is transformed into fibrin and helps form a clot. Plasma defibrinated by clotting is known as *blood serum*.

Blood Cells: There are two types of blood cells: red blood cells (RBC), or erythrocytes, and white blood cells (WBC), or leukocytes. Cell fragments called blood platelets are also present in mammalian blood.

a. *Erythrocytes—RBC*. These cells are biconcave discs about 7.7 microns in diameter. Mature cells lack a nucleus. The normal RBC hematocrit is about 36–45. The normal RBC counts are $5.2 \times 10^6/mm^3$ in males and $4.5 \times 10^6/mm^3$ in females. *Hemoglobin*, a complex molecule of iron and protein, is present in the cell. Red blood cells carry oxygen (in the form of oxyhemoglobin) from the lungs to the tissues and transport carbon dioxide from the tissues to the lungs. The membranes of the RBC carry Rh antigen and blood group antigens. Red blood cells have a life span of about 3 months. They are removed from the circulation by the spleen and replaced by new red blood cells formed in bone marrow. In the breakdown of hemoglobin, bilirubin is excreted and iron is retained.

b. *Leukocytes—WBC*. These cells differ from red blood cells by having nuclei and by exhibiting ameboid movement. A normal count of WBC in circulating blood is about 5–$9 \times 10^3/mm^3$. WBC contain phosphatases, liberate proteolytic enzymes, and function mainly in phagocytosis, proteolysis and antibody formation. An increase in the number of leukocytes is called *leukocytosis*, a decrease *leukopenia*.

There are two main types of leukocytes: nongranular and granular.

Non- or Agranular Leukocytes

1. *Lymphocytes* make up between 20 and 25% of total leukocytes and are seldom phagocytic. They originate from lymphoid tissue and bone marrow, function in immunologic responses and the detoxification of noxious substances; and are prevalent at sites of chronic inflammation. Some live several years.

2. *Monocytes* make up between 3 and 8% of total WBC. They are sometimes phagocytic and help in debridement.

Granular (possess abundant, specific granules) Leukocytes

1. *Neutrophils* make up about 65–75% of leukocytes. They are twice as large as a RBC and have a lobulated nucleus. They are the most active and phagocytic, providing the first line of defense against invading organisms. Dead neutrophils become *pus*.

2. *Eosinophils* make up about 2–5% WBC. They possess large red acidophilic granules and a bilobed nucleus. Large numbers are found at sites of parasitic infections and allergic reactions (specifically, in the respiratory and digestive tracts). Eosinophils function in the destruction of antigen-antibody complexes.

3. *Basophils* make up 0.5% or less of the total white blood cell count. They are rarely phagocytic. Basophils contain large quantities of basophilic granules. They are involved in immune phenomena, and produce heparin, which prevents the clotting of blood.

c. *Blood platelets*. These cytoplasmic structures are not true cells but are cell fragments characteristic of mammalian blood. (In lower vertebrates, cells called thrombocytes have a function similar to platelets.) Blood platelets average about three microns in diameter. About 250–350,000/mm^3 are normally present. These structures arise by the fragmentation of cytoplasmic processes of giant bone marrow cells. Platelets agglutinate and adhere to regions of injured vessels; they plug wounds of blood vessels. They help physically in clotting and form thromboplastin (thrombokinase), an integral chemical component of clot formation.

Blood Clotting: Platelets contribute thromboplastin (thrombokinase), an enzymatically active substance. Thromboplastin interacts with calcium ions and prothrombin (a plasma protein). Prothrombin is an inactive precursor of the catalyst thrombin. In the presence of these components prothrombin is converted to thrombin. Subsequently thrombin reacts with the plasma protein fibrinogen, forming fibrin. Fibrin is an insoluble, coagulated protein which clots. A clot also contains blood cells. Diagrammatically we can represent clotting reactions as follows:

$$\text{platelets} \longrightarrow \text{thromboplastin}$$
$$\downarrow$$
$$\text{prothrombin} + Ca^{2+} \longrightarrow \text{thrombin}$$
$$\downarrow$$
$$\text{fibrinogen} \longrightarrow \text{fibrin}.$$

Anticoagulants. An anticoagulant is a substance that prevents or retards coagulation of blood. Examples are: *heparin,* an acid mucopolysaccharide which occurs most abundantly in the liver; *aspirin* (acetylsalicylic acid), which also acts as an analgesic, antipyretic, antirheumatic compound; and the drug *Dicumarol,* a tradename for bihydroxycoumarin.

Blood Pressure: Blood pressure is usually measured by placing a sphygmomanometer cuff around the arm compressing the brachial artery and vein. Maximum blood pressure is obtained during ventricular contraction (systole) and minimum blood pressure indicates ventricular rest (diastole). The normal blood pressure listed for a young adult is 120 systolic and 80 diastolic (mm Hg).

Respiratory System

The respiratory system is composed of a conduit for air and an air-blood interface for gaseous exchange in the alveoli of the lungs. The function of the lung is to facilitate movement of oxygen from the air into the pulmonary circulation and the movement of carbon dioxide from the body out. This is accomplished by simple diffusion from an area of high concentration to one of a low partial pressure.

The conducting passages of the respiratory system can be listed as:

1) external (anterior) nares
2) nasal cavity with conchae, meatuses and sinuses
3) internal (posterior) nares
4) nasopharynx
5) oropharynx (communicates with oral cavity and mouth anteriorly)
6) laryngeal pharynx
7) larynx (possesses false and true vocal cords)
8) trachea
9) primary (left and right) bronchi
10) secondary (three named ones per lung—one per lobe) bronchi
11) tertiary bronchi
12) respiratory bronchioles
13) alveolar ducts
14) alveolar sacs
15) alveoli

The tracheobronchial tree (anatomic dead space) consists of about 16 generations of branches, while the respiratory unit is made up of an additional seven generations of respiratory bronchioles, alveolar ducts, and alveolar sacs for a total of 23 generations. The last seven are functional in gas exchange. (The upper parts of the respiratory system function in the removal of inhaled particles.)

Removal of Inhaled Particles

Large particles are filtered by hairs and mucous material in the nose and respiratory tract. Air is also warmed and humidified. Mucus is continually moved by cilia towards the throat and expelled by swallowing, expectoration or through the nose. No cilia are present in alveoli; macrophages and leukocytes debride this area. Material so gathered is removed via the lymphatic system.

Pulmonary Ventilation

Respiration refers to the gaseous exchanges which occur between the body as a whole and the environment. It entails:

1) ventilation of the lungs
2) gas exchange between lungs and blood
3) transport of gases in the blood
4) gas exchange between blood and interstitial fluids of the body

Ventilation must be adequate in environments ranging from sea level to high altitude and under degrees of physical activities ranging from sleep to exertion.

Respiratory minute ventilation is the amount of air which one inspires or expires each minute. It is equal to the amount of air inspired with each breath (the *tidal volume*) times the frequency (the number of breaths per minute). Normally with each breath we inspire about 500 ml and breathe at a rate of 12 breaths per minute. The resting respiratory minute ventilation under these conditions is 6 l/min. During severe exercise, the respiratory minute ventilation may reach 80 to 100 l/min; this is an indication of the practical upper limit of our respiratory system. Thus a 15-fold increase in ventilation is possible, indicating that the respiratory system has considerable reserve.

Inspiration and Expiration

During inspiration the thoracic cavity expands, its volume increases and air rushes into the respiratory tract due to the creation of negative pressure; the musculature involved is the diaphragm (innervated by the phrenic nerve) and the external intercostal muscles (innervated by intercostal nerves). During its contraction the diaphragm descends as much as 7 cm; the external intercostal muscles raise the rib cage. Relaxation of these muscles, the stabilization of the thoracic cage by the internal intercostals, contraction of the abdominal musculature, plus the elasticity of the lung, return the organ to the pre-inspiratory resting phase. A normal breath involves a volume of about 500 ml. Normal expiration is passive and involves no great muscular contraction. When ventilation exceeds about 40 l/min, expiratory (abdominal) muscles come into play to speed up expiration. By contracting, they push on contents of the abdominal cavity which then push the diaphragm upward, forcing air out of the lungs.

Positive and Negative Pressure Breathing

Gases flow from regions of higher pressure to those of lower pressure. Thus, when the gas pressure in the alveoli is equal to that of the surrounding atmosphere, no movement of gas occurs. For inspiration to occur, the alveolar gas pressure must be less than the atmospheric pressure. There are two ways in which this pressure difference can be produced. The first is by positive pressure breathing as is the case when using a resuscitator. Here the pressure at the nose and mouth (the atmospheric pressure) is made greater than the alveolar gas pressure. The second method is by negative pressure breathing as is the case when using the iron lung. Here the alveolar gas pressure is lowered below atmospheric pressure.

Normal breathing is a form of negative pressure breathing. If we plot intra-alveolar pressure (intrapulmonary pressure) during inspiration and expiration, we see that enlarging the thorax and lungs enables the alveolar gas to expand until its pressure drops below that of the surrounding atmosphere and the inflow of gas then occurs. For expiration to occur, the alveolar gas pressure must be made greater than the atmospheric pressure. This is produced by the natural recoil of the lungs, during which time the alveolar gas is compressed until its pressure is above atmospheric pressure. Gas then flows out of the lungs. Resistance to respiration arises due to the elastic fibers of the lung itself and the surface tension phenomena (forces) present at any liquid-air interface.

Since the inner surface of the lung is lined with a fluid (surfactant, which has a low surface tension), surface tension forces play a role. As a result of this surface tension the alveolus will tend to collapse unless opposed by the inflating pressure. The amount of pressure needed to oppose surface tension and maintain inflation is determined by the Law of Laplace:

$$p = \frac{2T}{\text{radius}}$$

where p = the inflation pressure, T = surface tension forces, and radius means the radius of the alveoli.

With a plasmalike liquid lining the lungs (constant surface tension), as the radius decreases (deflation) the distending pressure increases. Also, smaller alveoli would require a greater distending force than the larger alveoli.

The density of the surfactant molecules at the liquid-air interface is such that at high lung-volumes there are few surfactant molecules per unit of area and the surface tension is relatively high (like plasma). As deflation occurs, the surfactant molecules become more concentrated at the liquid air interface, and surface tension becomes relatively low (like surfactant). Thus, during deflation, the alveolar radius is decreasing tending to increase the needed distending pressure, but the surface tension is becoming less, which tends to decrease the required distending pressure. The lung, therefore, has alveoli which will not collapse until very low pressures are reached (because the surface tension is low), and can have small and large alveoli existing side by side (because the surface tension is area dependent).

Absence of the ability to produce surfactant is a key element in hyaline membrane disease. Infants afflicted die of respiratory distress because their lungs collapse with each breath due to the high surface tension. Extreme muscular efforts are required for reinflation and respiration is very labored in these cases.

Neuronal Control and Integration of Breathing

Normal spontaneous breathing is under control of motor neurons (primarily the phrenic nerves) which innervate the respiratory muscles. Brain impulses regulate and modulate the process. Voluntary activity originates in the cerebral cortex, automatic (autonomic) control rests in the pons and medulla of the brain.

The respiratory center, located in the medulla, has an inspiratory and an expiratory portion. The ventral portion produces forced and deep inspiration; the dorsal portion produces expiration.

Rhythmicity is spontaneous (12–15 times/minute) but is modulated by centers in the pons and medulla and by input from afferent vagal (stretch) receptors located in the lung. Stretching of the lung during inspiration reflexly limits the inspiratory drive.

Smooth muscle in the walls of the airways is innervated by parasympathetic and sympathetic nerves. Parasympathetic stimulation causes bronchoconstriction and an increase in airway resistance. Sympathetic stimulation produces relaxation. (Therefore, during an asthmatic attack it is helpful to inhale an aerosol containing a sympathomimetic drug, a drug that mimics the action of stimulating the sympathetic nervous system.)

Gas Exchange in the Alveoli

Abutting the alveoli (about 150 million/lung) is a large capillary bed providing an enormous diffusion area (about 90 m^2) with an extremely thin barrier (about 5000 Å) for gaseous exchange. Gas exchange takes place only in the alveoli and not in the tracheobronchial tree; the nonfunctional space (anatomic dead space) volume comprises about 150 ml. The alveolar portion, known as the respiratory zone, has a volume of about 2,000 ml. The diffusion pathway for alveolar gas may be listed as:

1) surfactant (lowers surface tension)
2) alveolar epithelium
3) interstitium (fused basement membranes)
4) capillary endothelium (epithelium)
5) plasma
6) red blood cell

Oxygen Transport

Oxygen is transported mainly in the form of oxyhemoglobin. Normal hemoglobin (Hb) values are, respectively, 14 g/100 ml for women and 16 g/100 ml for men. Blood then contains an average of 15 g hemoglobin/100 ml blood; each gram of hemoglobin can combine with 1.39 ml of oxygen. Fully oxygenated blood can be calculated thus:

$$(15 \text{ g Hb}/100 \text{ ml blood}) \times (1.39 \text{ ml O}_2/\text{g Hb})$$

to contain 21 ml O_2/ml blood. This is known as the *oxygen capacity* of blood.

If the concentration of oxygen against the PO_2 is plotted, a sigmoid shaped curve, also called the *oxygen dissociation curve,* is obtained.

Four factors affect the affinity of hemoglobin for oxygen:

1) pH
2) temperature
3) concentration of 2,3-diphosphoglycerate (DPG)
4) carbon dioxide

A decrease in pH, an increase in temperature or an increase in DPG will facilitate the release of oxygen in the tissue capillaries.

Actively metabolizing tissues have a higher temperature and produce metabolic acids (e.g., lactic acid) and carbonic acid via the reaction of released carbon dioxide and water. An increase in CO_2 and a decrease in affinity of hemoglobin for oxygen with a decrease in pH and an increase in carbamino Hb is called the *Bohr effect*. Most of the oxygen released is due to the decrease in PO_2 in the interstitial fluid but an extra amount is released due to these factors. Chronic hypoxia increases the amount of DPG and thus facilitates oxygen release by this mechanism.

Carbon Dioxide Transport

While some carbon dioxide remains in plasma, most diffuses into red blood cells. Here, it can be (1) transported in physical solution, (2) bound to the amino groups of hemoglobin as carbamino hemoglobin, or, most importantly, (3) converted to bicarbonate ions via its interaction with water to form carbonic acid, which almost completely dissociates into bicarbonate and hydrogen ions. This reaction occurs rapidly in red blood cells because the cells contain the enzyme carbonic anhydrase, which catalyzes the reaction.

The carbon dioxide in plasma can also be transported (1) in physical solution, (2) bound to the amino groups of plasma proteins (although the amount carried as carbamino compounds in plasma is small compared to the amount carried in red blood cells as carbamino hemoglobin), or (3) as bicarbonate ions. Few bicarbonate ions are produced in the plasma, however, since there is no carbonic anhydrase in plasma.

Bicarbonate ions produced in the red blood cells diffuse into the plasma because of the concentration gradient. However, the red blood cell membrane is not very permeable to cations so no positively charged ion can accompany the bicarbonate ions into the plasma. The result is that the inside of the red blood cell is slightly positive and so attracts negatively charged chloride ions from the plasma. This exchange of chloride for bicarbonate is referred to as the *chloride shift*. Thus, although bicarbonate is produced in red blood cells it is transported in plasma.

The hydrogen ions produced are buffered to a great extent by hemoglobin. The fact that reduced hemoglobin holds hydrogen ions more strongly than oxyhemoglobin means that as oxygen is released to tissues hydrogen ions generated by the addition of carbon dioxide can be taken up by the deoxygenated (reduced) hemoglobin. Slightly more hydrogen ions are produced than can be handled by the reduced hemoglobin produced. Thus, the pH of venous blood is slightly lower than that of arterial blood.

Since deoxygenated hemoglobin forms carbamino compounds much more readily than oxygenated hemoglobin does, venous blood can handle more CO_2 than can arterial blood.

The changes in the quantity of oxygen and carbon dioxide in the lungs are as indicated:

	Inspired Air, %	Expired Air, %	Change, %
Oxygen	20.96	16.02	4.94 loss
Carbon dioxide	0.04	4.48	4.44 gain

The carbon dioxide resulting from cellular metabolic activity diffuses into the blood since it is less concentrated there; here it then either combines with hemoglobin or is converted into carbonic acid:

$$CO_2 + H_2O \longrightarrow H_2CO_3$$

The carbonic acid reacts with sodium in the plasma to form sodium bicarbonate:

$$H_2CO_3 + Na^+ \longrightarrow NaHCO_3 + H^+$$

or it can react with potassium in the hemoglobin to form potassium bicarbonate:

$$H_2CO_3 + K^+ \longrightarrow KHCO_3 + H^+$$

In the lungs the carbon dioxide is dissociated from the bicarbonate and hemoglobin and diffuses into alveolar space air for exchange.

Chemical Regulation of Respiration

Chemical stimulants of physiological importance that affect respiration are:

1) increased arterial PCO_2 (hypercapnia),
2) decreased arterial PO_2 (hypoxia),
3) an increased arterial hydrogen-ion concentration (acidosis).

Arterial $[H^+]$ and PO_2 are monitored by carotid and aortic bodies which contain nerve endings that are sensitive to arterial pH and PO_2. The carotid bodies lie near the carotid sinus at the bifurcation of the common carotid arteries and send impulses through fibers of the glossopharyngeal nerves. The aortic bodies lie near the arch of the aorta; their neural fibers are part of the vagus nerves.

Increases in arterial PCO_2 are also sensed to some extent by these peripheral chemoreceptors (carotid and aortic bodies) but, more importantly, by a central chemosensitive area on the surface of the medulla overlying the medullary respiratory center. This central chemosensitive area, bathed in cerebrospinal fluid (CSF), is sensitive to changes in $[H^+]$ in the CSF. Although hydrogen ions poorly penetrate the blood-brain barrier which separates arterial blood and CSF, carbon dioxide can rapidly diffuse between the two fluids. Thus, arterial PCO_2 and CSF PCO_2 equilibrate. Once in the CSF, carbon dioxide reacts with water to form carbonic acid, which dissociates into bicarbonate and hydrogen ions. The central chemosensitive area is sensitive to the pH changes thus produced. In a similar manner (but of less importance) arterial PCO_2 alters arterial pH, which is best detected by the carotid and aortic bodies.

Oxygen lack stimulates ventilation solely by its effect on the peripheral chemoreceptors, but alveolar PO_2 must fall to low levels (50–60 mm Hg) before ventilation begins to increase. However, some chemoreceptor discharge is present at normal oxygen tensions. Hypercapnia, which often accompanies hypoxia, will potentiate sensitivity of peripheral chemoreceptors to hypoxia. Hypoxia is the stimulus for increased ventilation observed at high altitudes.

Acidosis stimulates ventilation mainly via peripheral chemoreceptors. Arterial $[H^+]$ may also effect the central chemosensitive area but its influence there is slow in onset and much less pronounced. Hyperventilation driven by acidosis will ''blow off'' CO_2 and generate alkalosis in the CSF, which tends to depress ventilation. The results of these opposing forces is a lesser increase in ventilation than would occur with a constant arterial PCO_2. The effects of acidosis and either hypoxia or hypercapnia are additive with no complicated potentiation occurring.

Ventilation is much more sensitive to hypercapnia than to either hypoxia or acidosis. Changes in ventilation produced by hypercapnia are only slightly altered when the peripheral chemoreceptors are denervated, indicating the importance of the central chemosensitive area in monitoring CO_2. Hypoxia potentiates this CO_2 sensitivity.

Urinary System

The urinary system helps maintain homeostasis of the body by excreting wastes and regulating the content of the blood. It consists of two kidneys, two ureters, a urinary bladder and a urethra. Kidneys produce the excretory product; three tubular structures serve as a passageway for the excretory material (urine) to reach the outside of the body.

Structure of the Kidney

The kidney is a bean-shaped organ encased by a fibrous capsule and embedded within a fatty connective tissue and perirenal fascia. The kidney lies deep to the *peritoneum* (i.e., retroperitoneal) which lines the abdomino-pelvic cavity. It is approximately 10 centimeters long, 5 centimeters wide and 3 centimeters thick. Its medial aspect, which is indented or concave, is known as the *renal hilus* (*hilum*); it is the location for the renal arteries and veins as well as for the renal pelvis. The hilus leads into a cavity, the *renal sinus,* within the kidney which contains fat, blood vessels, nerves, calyces and renal pelvis.

The internal aspect of the kidney when bissected in a medial to lateral plane presents two zones, an outer *cortex* and an inner *medulla*. The medulla is adjacent to the renal sinus. The cortex is redder in appearance and has fine striations known as *medullary rays*. These striations are due to medullary structures (collecting tubules) extending into the cortex. The medulla consists of triangular (pyramidal) structures, *the renal pyramids,* separated by columns of cortical material known as *renal columns*. The bases of the renal pyramids face the cortex while the apices or *papillae* extend into the *minor calyces*.

The kidney is divided into functional *lobes,* each defined as one renal pyramid, its abutting cortex and part of the two adjacent renal columns. There are about 6 to 18 lobes. A *lobule* of a kidney is considered to be a medullary ray and the adjacent nephrons draining into the collecting ducts forming the ray.

The functional unit of the kidney is the *uriniferous tubule,* which consists of a *nephron* and a *collecting tubule* (duct) within the kidney. There are 1 to 3 million per kidney. The individual nephron is considered by many as the functional unit and the collecting tubule as a separate entity being part of the internal excretory pathway for urine.

Nephron: The nephron is a tubular structure about 30 to 40 millimeters long and lined by epithelium. It functions in producing an ultrafiltrate and then reabsorbing material from and excreting substances into the filtrate resulting in an excretory product. It consists of several morphologically and physiologically different sections forming a continuous tubular unit. The regions of a nephron sequentially are: Bowman's capsule, proximal convoluted tubule, loop of Henle, and distal convoluted tubule. The latter is continuous with the collecting tubule (excretory duct) draining it. The loop of Henle extends into the medullary pyramid while the other three regions are found entirely in the cortex.

Nephrons vary in their level or position in the cortex with some, the *cortical nephrons*, being at the periphery of the cortex, and others, the *juxtamedullary nephrons*, abutting the medulla. These vary in that the size of the renal corpuscle and the length of the loop of Henle are larger in the juxtamedullary nephrons.

Bowman's capsule is an invaginated blind sac lined by a simple squamous epithelium. The latter forms two layers, the *visceral* and *parietal layers*, continuous with each other at the capsule's vascular pole, as well as separated by a cavity, *Bowman's space*. The visceral layer of Bowman's capsule is intimately related with the capillary network, known as the *glomerulus*, located between an *afferent and an efferent arteriole*. The Bowman's capsule forms a unit with the glomerulus referred to as the *renal corpuscle (corpuscle of Malpighi)*. The proximal and distal convoluted tubules are located adjacent to their renal corpuscle. The region of the capsule where the arterioles enter and exit is the *vascular pole*, while the *urinary pole* is located where Bowman's space is continuous with the proximal convoluted tubule. The visceral layer consists of specialized star-shaped epithelial cells, the *podocytes*, abutting the endothelium of the tuft of capillaries.

The lumen of the capillary and Bowman's space are separated by the *filtration membrane or barrier,* which consists of fenestrated endothelium; *basement membrane*, between endothelium and podocyte; and *filtration-slit membranes,* between the podocyte processes known as *pedicels* (end feet) abutting the basement membrane. The ultrafiltrate formed enters the capsular space and then passes into the proximal convoluted tubule which is lined by a low columnar or cuboidal epithelium.

The loop of Henle consists of the following three sequential regions:

(1) descending thick limb (straight portion of proximal tubule)
(2) thin limb, forming a loop which connects descending and ascending thin limbs; lined by simple squamous epithelium
(3) ascending thick limb (straight portion of distal tubule).

Collecting Tubules: The route for the filtrate and excretory product is from Bowman's space through the proximal convoluted tubule, descending thick and thin limbs of the loop of Henle, ascending thin and thick limbs, distal convoluted tubule and then into the collecting tubule. The latter unite and form 10–25 larger collecting ducts (papillary ducts of Bellini) which extend into the renal pyramids and terminate at the papillae.

The urine passes from the ends of these large collecting ducts into funnel-shaped collecting vessels, the *minor calyces,* into which the papillae extend. The 7 to 18 minor calyces empty into 2 to 3 *major calyces,* which are larger funnels that terminate in the *renal pelvis*. The renal pelvis is the terminal collecting site for urine in the kidney and is continuous with the ureter at the hilum of the kidney.

Tubular Passageways

The *ureter* is a long muscular tube which connects the renal pelvis to the urinary bladder. It passes inferiorly on the posterior abdominal wall, enters the pelvis by crossing the pelvic inlet, and then pierces the wall of the urinary bladder at its posterior-lateral aspect. The smooth muscles which are part of the bladder and surround the oblique path of the ureter through the wall act as a sphincter of the ureter.

The *urinary bladder* is located in the pelvis superior and posterior to the pubic bone, anterior to the uterus in the female, anterior to the rectum in the male. The bladder consists of a thick wall composed of three intermeshing smooth muscle layers known as *detrusor muscles*. The bladder functions to store urine as well as to expel it. The excretory pathways and the bladder are lined by the urinary type of the epithelium known as transitional epithelium.

The *urethra* is a fibromuscular tube that transmits urine to the outside of the body. It is continuous inferiorly with the urinary bladder. It traverses the prostate gland and then exits the pelvic cavity by passing through the pelvic floor (urogenital diaphragm) and terminates at the external urethral orifice of the penis or in the vestibule of the female.

The male urethra (20 centimeters in length) is longer than the female urethra (2–6 centimeters) and consists of three parts: the *prostatic, membranous* and *spongy urethrae*. The spongy urethra is within the corpus spongiosum of the penis which forms the glans penis.

Functions of the Kidney and Uriniferous Tubules

The kidney, during production of urine,

a) excretes the waste products of metabolism;
b) maintains the fluid volume of the extracellular regions of the body;
c) excretes foreign materials from the body;
d) regulates the type and concentration of salts retained in the body (maintain electrolyte balance);
e) regulates the total body water;
f) regulates the acid-base balance of the body.

The physiological processes occurring during the production of urine are

a) *filtration*—the production of an ultrafiltrate of plasma within Bowman's space;
b) *reabsorption*—the selective removal of material from the ultrafiltrate as it passes through the tubular nephron and the return of these substances into peritubular capillaries;
c) *secretion*—the cells forming the nephron actively secrete material into the filtrate;
d) *passive diffusion*—diffusion of fluids along the osmotic gradient.

Filtration: Filtration occurs at the renal corpuscles through the filtration barrier, which permits the passage of water and various solutes from the capillary lumen into Bowman's space but retains cells and large proteins. The ultrafiltrate produced (125 ml/min) enters the capsular space to be transported through and modified by the remaining portions of the nephron. Approximately 170–180 liters of ultrafiltrate are produced in 24 hours; this results in about 1 to 2 liters of urine per day. The production of the ultrafiltrate results from:

a) the filtration pressure (about 25 mm Hg), which is the differential between hydrostatic pressure within the glomerular capillaries (about 75 mm Hg) and total pressure resulting from osmotic pressure (30 mm Hg) and the intratubular pressure in Bowman's space and nephron (20 mm Hg). The resulting filtration pressure forces substances from the blood through the filtration barrier and into the nephron;
b) blockage of proteins larger than 70,000 molecular weight by the filtration membrane.

The ultrafiltrate is similar to plasma and isotonic to blood. It is composed of amino acids, urea, uric acid, salts, creatinine, glucose and small amounts of albumin.

Reabsorption: The isotonic ultrafiltrate enters the proximal convoluted tubules which are lined by cuboidal or low columnar epithelium with numerous apical microvilli (brush border). Filtrate volume is decreased by approximately 80% as it passes through the proximal convoluted tubule (PCT) through reabsorption of substances from the tubule lumen into interstitial spaces and then peritubular capillaries. Major resorption of substances from the ultrafiltrate occurs, therefore, in the PCT and results in:

a) the active reabsorption of all the glucose;
b) the active reabsorption of 85% of the sodium chloride;

c) the passive diffusion, due to the osmotic gradient, of 85% of the water from the filtrate;

d) the active transport of all amino acids, ascorbic acid and proteins. (Protein is broken down to amino acids in phagolysosomes following pinocytosis at the apical microvillar border.)

Secretion: The cells of the proximal convoluted tubule also secrete creatinine into the tubular lumen, as well as materials foreign to the body, such as phenol red, antibiotics and various radiopaque dyes. The amount of a substance reabsorbed is controlled; what is not resorbed from the tubule lumen is excreted. (In diabetes, glucose concentration in the blood and thus the ultrafiltrate is high; not all glucose is resorbed, and the remainder or excess is excreted in the urine.)

Passive Diffusion: The loop of Henle functions by setting up the mechanism (countercurrent multiplier system) in the renal medulla for the production of *hypertonic urine*. The descending limb of the loop is permeable to water, Na^+ and Cl^-. These materials pass through the walls according to osmotic gradients. Water diffuses out of the tubule lumen into the more concentrated (hypertonic) interstitial tissue of the renal pyramids; Na^+ and Cl^- diffuse passively into the tubule.

The ascending limb of the loop differs in that its wall is impermeable to water. Therefore, water remains in the tubule. Also, chloride ions are actively reabsorbed and pumped into the interstitium surrounding the loop of Henle, as well as into the collecting ducts passing through the medullary pyramid. Sodium ions are thought to diffuse passively out of the tubules in conjunction with the Cl^-. This decrease in sodium chloride concentration of the filtrate results in a hypotonic filtrate at the distal end of the loop of Henle as it enters the distal convoluted tubule. The flow of the sodium chloride out of the tubule also increases its concentration in the surrounding interstitial tissue, which thus becomes hypertonic. This hypertonic interstitium is essential for production of hypertonic urine as the filtrate passes through the collecting ducts of the renal pyramid.

Hormonal Control of More Secretion and Resorption

The simple cuboidal epithelium lining the distal convoluted tubule may also increase the Na^+ concentration in the interstitium by reabsorbing Na^+. At the same time potassium ions (K^+) are excreted into the tubular lumen. The latter processes are regulated by *aldosterone*, a hormone produced by the adrenal cortex. The distal convoluted tubules also participate in maintaining the acid-base balance of the blood by adding hydrogen and ammonium ions into the filtrate.

The permeability of water through the walls of the distal convoluted tubules and collecting tubules is regulated by the *antidiuretic hormone* (ADH) secreted by the posterior lobe of the pituitary gland (neurohypophysis). The presence of this hormone makes these tubules more permeable to water. Since the interstitium of the renal pyramids is more highly concentrated (hypertonic) than the filtrate, water exits the collecting tubules and passes into the interstitium. This process continues along the length of the collecting ducts and results in concentrating the urine which therefore is *hypertonic*. The amount of water resorbed is regulated by ADH production. For example, an increase in ADH increases resorption of water resulting in a more hypertonic urine, while a decrease in ADH decreases resorption resulting in the excretion of more water and therefore, a diluted or hypotonic urine. Diuretic drugs counteract the action of ADH, causing less water resorption and increased urine volume. The osmotic gradient in the renal pyramids is also maintained by the *vasa recta* adjacent to the collecting tubules due to flow of water and Na^+ into and out of the vessel lumen. This establishes a countercurrent exchange system between the arterioles and venulae rectae.

Integumentary (Skin) System

The skin and the specialized organs derived from the skin (hairs, nails and glands) form the integumentary system.

Skin

The skin lines the external surface of the body. It is continuous with the mucous membranes of (1) the respiratory pathways via the nose; (2) the digestive tract via the mouth and anus; and (3) the genitourinary system via urethra and/or vagina.

Functions: The skin functions by surfacing the body and thus protecting it from dehydration as well as from damage by the elements in the external environment. The skin also helps maintain normal body activities. The skin

(1)   Protects the body against dehydration. The skin is impermeable to water which, therefore, prevents loss of body fluids. This property permits humans, as well as other animals, to live in a non-fluid environment such as land.

(2)   Protects the body against abrasive forces. The ability to withstand frictional forces also allows humans to walk and perform manipulatory skills with the hands.

(3)   Protects the body against damage from toxic chemicals and extreme heat.

(4)   Protects the body from the harmful effects of ultraviolet rays. This is primarily the function of the melanin pigment secreted by the melanocytes in the epidermis.

(5)   Acts as a barrier to infectious organisms invading the body.

(6)   Takes part in regulating the temperature of the body. The degree of heat loss or retention is regulated by neurovascular processes. The body is cooled by the evaporation of water (sweat) from its surface.

(7)   Functions to excrete body wastes and fluids via the production of sweat by the sweat glands.

(8)   Acts as a primary sense organ of the body for general somatic sensations, such as touch, pressure, heat, cold and pain.

(9)   Plays a role in the production of vitamin D through the action of ultraviolet light. The latter transforms vitamin D precursors (7-dehydrocholesterol) found in the skin into vitamin D.

Structure: Skin consists of the *epidermis* and *dermis* (*corium*). Deep to the dermis and therefore, the skin, is the *hypodermis,* which is also known as the *subcutaneous* or superficial connective tissue of the body. The latter comprises loose connective tissue with various amounts of adipose cells (tissue).

Epidermis: The epidermis is derived from the ectoderm and is composed of a keratinized stratified squamous epithelium. The epidermis varies in thickness depending on the function of the specific region of the body. Its thickness is used to differentiate two types of skin—thick and thin.

Thick skin denotes skin with a thicker epidermis which contains more cell layers when compared to *thin skin*. The epidermis ranges in thickness from 0.07 millimeter to 1.4 milimeters. Skin itself (both epidermis and dermis) ranges from 0.5 millimeter to greater than 4 millimeters. The epidermis, similar to other epithelial layers, is avascular and lies on a basal lamina (basement membrane). The latter separates it from the underlying dermis to which the basal layer of epidermal cells is anchored.

The epidermis consists of specific cell layers which differ in their morphology and function. The layers of the epidermis of thick skin (sole of foot and palm) from the basal lamina (dermis) to the free surface are:

1.   stratum basale or germinativum
2.   stratum spinosum
3.   stratum granulosum
4.   stratum lucidum
5.   stratum corneum

The combined layers of the strata basale and spinosum are also referred to as the *stratum malpighi* or *malpighian layer.*

In thin skin the stratum lucidum is absent and the stratum granulosum often appears as a discontinuous layer. The strata spinosum and corneum are always present as distinct layers but are thinner than in thick skin.

The layers of skin represent the different stages through which the epidermal cells (keratinocytes) pass as they undergo the process of keratinization from their origin in the stratum basale to their sloughing off as dead keratinized cells at the free surface.

The five layers of thick skin are characterized as follows:

1. Stratum basale
    a) Simple cuboidal to columnar epithelial cell layer resting on the basal lamina.
    b) Cells with the ability to divide (mitosis) and thus give rise to cells which migrate into the overlying stratum spinosum. This continuous process replenishes the keratinized epithelial cells which are shed from the surface.
    c) *Melanocytes,* which synthesize the brown pigment, *melanin,* in the form of pigment granules (*melanosomes*). Melanocytes have long cell processes which extend among the cells of the strata basale and spinosum. Via these processes they release and transfer melanosomes to the cells of the stratum malpighi. Increased exposure to UV light stimulates an increase in the secretion and release of melanosomes by the melanocytes, which results in the darkening of the skin (tanning). Dark color skin results from melanin, from carotene, a yellowish pigment, and from the degree of vascularity of the area, which adds a reddish-blue tint.

2. Stratum spinosum—consists of several layers of polygonal (polyhedral) cells which adhere to each other via desmosomes.

3. Stratum granulosum
    a) Consists of 3 to 5 layers of flat epithelial cells with pycnotic nuclei.
    b) Has a granular appearance due to the accumulation of irregular granules, the *keratohyalin granules,* within the cytoplasm. The granules are basophilic and are not encased by a membrane. The keratohyalin granules are associated with the numerous tonofilaments; both are involved in the production of keratin.
    c) The cells also contain *membrane-coating granules* (lamellated granules) composed of mucopolysaccharides and phospholipids. The latter are secreted into the intercellular regions surrounding the cells of the stratum granulosum. This intercellular matrix appears to block the passage of substances through the epidermis.
    d) The keratinocytes die in this stratum.

4. Stratum lucidum
    a) It is a homogeneous translucent layer separating the strata granulosum and corneum in thick skin.
    b) Consists of 3 to 5 layers of flat, elongated cells whose organelles and nuclei are indistinct or absent.

5. Stratum corneum
    a) Composed of layers of compressed, flat, cornified (keratinized) cells which lack nuclei and organelles. These scalelike cells are often referred to as *horny cells.*
    b) The most superficial horny cells slough off or desquamate constantly.

Dermis: The *corium,* or dermis, is the connective tissue layer between the epidermis and hypodermis. Depending on the region, its thickness may range between 0.5 millimeters to 4 millimeters. The border between these two strata is irregular in contour. This is caused by the irregular pattern of the surface of the dermis, to which the epidermis conforms. In a section perpendicular to the skin's surface, the dermis is seen to project into folds of the epidermis. These connective tissue projections are known as *dermal ridges* (*or papillae*); the epidermal regions between these ridges are the *epidermal or interpapillary pegs* (*ridges*). The dermal ridges are more numerous in thick skin (palm and soles), where greater abrasive forces occur. Since the epidermis follows the contour of the skin, the irregular contour of the dermis is projected onto the surface of the skin as ridges and grooves. The orientation and patterns of these surface grooves differ according to the skin region. They are very evident in the palm and fingers. The pattern is also extremely specific for each individual as is illustrated by the use of fingerprints to identify a person. These fingerprints, therefore, are actually the impressions of the grooves on the surface of the skin which represent the contour of the dermo-epidermal junction.

The dermis consists of two strata, the *papillary* and *reticular* layers.

Papillary layer. The *papillary layer* abuts the epidermis and forms the dermal ridges (papillae). It is thinner than the reticular layer and is composed of loose connective tissue. It consists of fine collagen, reticular, and elastic fibers associated with typical connective tissue cells (mainly fibroblasts and macrophages). The region abutting the basal cell layer is organized into a basement membrane. The processes of the basal cells anchor in the fibers of the membrane. The dermal ridges have extensive capillary networks. The epidermis is nourished by the diffusion of nutrients from this vascular bed. The papillary layer also contains encapsulated sensory receptors.

Reticular layer. The *reticular layer* is thicker and is composed of dense irregular connective tissue. The collagen and elastic fibers are thicker and coarser and form an interlacing network. Most fibers are primarily oriented parallel to the surface forming lines of skin tension called *Langer's lines*, which are important for surgical incisions. Capillaries are sparse. A rich nerve supply as well as encapsulated receptors are present in this layer. The reticular layer is the location of epidermal derivatives such as sweat and sebaceous glands and hair follicles. It also contains smooth muscles (arrector pili) associated with hair follicles and skeletal muscles in the head and neck (muscles of facial expression).

Glands

Glands are specialized organs derived from skin. There are two basic types: sebaceous and sweat.

Sebaceous Glands: Sebaceous glands are *simple branched alveolar* (*acinar*) *glands* with a *holocrine* mode of secretion. They are found in all areas of the body except the palms and soles. The excretory ducts of several glands open into the necks of a hair follicle.

The cells of the gland differentiate and become progressively larger as they accumulate lipid droplets in their cytoplasm. The cells eventually rupture releasing their lipid content and cell remnants into the lumen. The latter comprise the oily secretion of the sebaceous glands called *sebum,* which helps protect the skin from becoming extremely dry.

Sweat Glands: Sweat is a watery fluid containing ammonia, urea, uric acid and sodium chloride. The production of sweat is important for the excretion of some body wastes and the regulation of body temperature and is under nervous system control.

There are two types of sweat glands: eccrine and apocrine.

Eccrine Sweat Glands: The *eccrine sweat glands* are simple, coiled tubular glands with a merocrine mode of secretion. These glands are the ones that are typically considered when discussing sweat glands. Up to three million are found distributed all over the body in humans, except at the margin of the lip, glans penis, and ear drums. The largest number occur in the thick skin of the palms and soles. The *secretory tubular* unit is very coiled and is located in the reticular layer of the dermis near the hypodermis.

Apocrine Sweat Glands: The *apocrine sweat glands* are very large glands which are thought to have a merocrine mode of secretion. They occur mainly in the hypodermis of the axilla, areola of breast, labia majora and scrotum. They are branched tubular glands whose secretory tubule is very dilated. Their secretory product is more viscous. The excretory ducts open into the hair follicles above the openings of this sweat gland.

The *ceruminous glands* of the external auditory canals, which secrete wax, and the *glands of Moll,* in the eyelid margin, are also considered to be apocrine sweat glands.

Hair

Hairs are long, filamentous keratinized structures derived from the epidermis of skin. The process of keratinization is similar to that in skin since cells divide, differentiate, and move toward the surface and become keratinized. Hairs are found covering the whole body except palms, soles, sides of fingers and toes, glans and prepuce of penis, clitoris and labia minor.

Structure: A hair consists of a *shaft*, which extends above the skin surface, and a *root*, which lies within the skin. The root is encased by a tubular *hair follicle* composed of epidermal and dermal cell layers. At its deeper end, the follicle dilates and forms an invaginated *hair bulb* which is continuous with the root. The invaginated portion of the hair bulb contains a connective tissue papilla, the *dermal papilla*, which has a rich blood supply.

Hairs consist of three concentrically oriented epidermal layers, the *medulla, cortex* and *cuticle*. The *medulla* forms the center of the hair and consists of two or three layers of cuboidal cells found only in coarse hair; these cornified cells contain soft keratin. The medulla is encased by the *cortex*, which constitutes the largest part of the hair. It consists of several layers of keratinized cells which contain numerous filaments embedded in an amorphous matrix. The latter form the *hard keratin* found in these compactly arranged spindle-shaped cells. Melanin granules are found in the cells of the cortex giving hair its coloration. Air in the intercellular region of these cells also affects the pigmentation of hairs. The *cuticle* surrounds the cortex and consists of a single layer of transparent, enucleated cells which form keratinized scales.

Hair Follicle: The *hair follicle* consists of two sheaths, the *epithelial root sheath* and the *connective tissue root sheath*. The epidermally derived epithelial root sheath abuts the cuticle and is subdivided into the *inner epithelial root sheath* and the *outer (external) epithelial root sheath*. The *inner epithelial root sheath* extends from hair bulb to the level of the excretory duct of the sebaceous glands. It comprises three layers: (1) the *cuticle root sheath*, abutting the cuticle; (2) *Huxley's layer*; and (3) *Henle's layer*, adjacent to the outer epithelial root sheath. These layers are composed of keratinized cells containing soft keratin. The cells of the inner epithelial root sheath arise from the *hair matrix* in the hair bulb and migrate upward from it.

The *outer epithelial root sheath* is continuous with the epidermis of the skin. Close to the hair bulb the outer epithelial root sheath consists of a simple cuboidal layer similar to the stratum germinativum.

The *connective tissue root sheath* (or *dermal root sheath*) is derived from the dermis and consists of three layers: (1) the *glassy membrane*, the innermost layer which is a non-cellular translucent membrane that corresponds to the basal lamina deep to the epidermis; (2) the *middle layer*, similar to the papillary layer of the dermis, and consisting of fine connective tissue fibers arranged in a circular pattern; and (3) the *outer layer*, similar to the reticular layer and consisting of longitudinally arranged coarse collagen fibers.

Hair Growth: Growth of a hair depends on the viability of the epidermal cells of the hair matrix which lie adjacent to the dermal papilla in the hair bulb. The matrix cells abutting the dermal papilla proliferate and give rise to cells which move upward to become part of the specific layers of the hair root and the inner epithelial root sheath. The hair matrix, therefore, functions similarly to the malpighian layer of the epidermis since it gives rise to cells which become cornified as they move toward the surface. Due to this upward movement of the cells arising from the hair matrix, the hair (root and shaft) grows outward. Hairs do not grow continuously but have specific growth and rest periods which vary according to the area of the body. Hair growth is influenced by growth hormone and the sex hormones.

Hair Musculature: Hairs are oriented at a slight angle to the skin surface and are associated with *arrector pili muscles*. These smooth muscle bundles extend from the dermal root sheath to a dermal papilla. Contraction results in the standing up of the hairs and raising of the skin surrounding the hair. This produces what is referred to as *gooseflesh* or *goose pimples*.

Nails

Nails are translucent plates of keratinized epithelial cells on the dorsal surface of distal phalanges of fingers and toes. The nail plate consists of a *body* and *root*, formed by compact layers of cornified epithelial cells similar to the stratum corneum. The *nail body* is the main portion of the plate lying on the *nail bed*, which is an epidermal layer consisting primarily of the malpighian cell layer. The proximal end of the body is continuous with the *nail root* at the *lunula*. The lunula is the crescentric whitish region at the proximal part of the nail.

Deep to the root and continuous with the proximal end of the nail bed is the *nail matrix*. The latter is a thickened stratum malpighi which gives rise to new cells that migrate upward and become keratinized. The matrix, therefore, functions in producing cornified cells composed of hard keratin which are added to the proximal end of the nail plate (root). This process increases the length of the nail. Nails increase in length at about 0.5 millimeters per week.

The *cuticle*, or *eponychium*, is a fold of the stratum corneum which extends over the surface of the nail body in the area of the lunula.

A similar fold, the *hyponychium*, occurs deep to the distal free margin of the nail plate. The hyponychium is actually a thickening of the stratum corneum of the skin where the nail bed and epidermis of the skin are continuous.

Digestive System and Nutrition

Nutrition

The environment must supply its organisms with adequate nutrients via the food supply. Organisms require the basic elements making up protoplasm, the enzymes that catalyze and control the metabolic activity, and vitamins and hormones that have profound effects on the overall function of the system. Elements that are needed in very small quantities are called trace elements. No organism is independent of the environment, but on nutritional self-sufficiency we can classify organisms into autotrophs and heterotrophs. Heterotrophs include all animals; autotrophs include all those that carry out photosynthesis and can manufacture organic constituents from inorganic material. Although all organisms require intake of nutrients, we shall confine this discussion to nutrition and digestion in higher animals (particularly humans).

Unit for Measuring Value of Foods: The kilocalorie (kcal) is the unit of heat used in measuring the value of foods for producing heat and energy in the human body. It is equivalent to the amount of heat that is required to raise the temperature of one kilogram of water one degree Celsius. The kilocalorie is $1000 \times$ calorie, the amount of heat required to raise the temperature of one gram of water $1°C$.

Proteins: Few free amino acids are available in the diet. Amino acid intake is primarily in the form of proteins (high molecular weight heteropolymers of amino acids). Amino acids are necessary for the production and maintenance of protoplasm. Certain amino acids are denoted as essential in all higher animals; these are: L-leucine; L-methionine; L-phenylalanine; L-valine; L-lysine; L-isoleucine; L-threonine and L-tryptophan. In the rat, however, all of the above eight plus histidine and arginine are essential. Among the nonessential amino acids (synthesized by the organism) are glycine, alanine, serine, cystine, tyrosine, and proline. Not all proteins have a complete complement of all amino acids; therefore, dietary intake must be adjusted to meet the needs of the organism.

Carbohydrates: Of primary importance in human nutrition are the monosaccharides, disaccharides, and polysaccharides. Monosaccharides ordinarily are simple 5- or 6-carbon sugars; they cannot be broken down into smaller units. Common examples are glucose and fructose.

Disaccharides are formed by the union of two 6-carbon monosaccharides and thus contain 12 carbons; they can be broken down by hydrolysis into their component hexose sugars. Common examples are sucrose (containing glucose and fructose) and lactose (containing glucose and galactose). Polysaccharides are large molecules formed by the union of many monosaccharides; they can be broken down into their respective monosaccharides. Common examples are glucose polymers, starch, and glycogen.

Fats: Fats may be grouped into simple lipids, compound lipids, and lipids derived from simple and compound lipids by hydrolysis. Fat are composed of three fatty acid molecules joined to a molecule of glycerol. Simple lipids are esters of fatty acids with various alcohols. Waxes possess alcohols other than glycerol. Cholesterol esters are a combination of fatty acids and sterol alcohols such as cholesterol. Compound lipids are composed of esters of fatty acids and glycerol; they also incorporate other chemical groups. Derived lipids are obtained by hydrolysis of simple and compound lipids and can be grouped into free fatty acids, alcohols, and sterol alcohols. Fatty acids may be either saturated or unsaturated. The unsaturated fatty acids may contain cis or trans double bonds, but cis double bonds are more common.

Vitamins: Vitamins are organic substances which are needed in minute quantities; vitamins often play a role as part of an enzyme system. Vitamins are used up in the metabolic activities and must be constantly replaced; the organism, however, is not capable of synthesizing a vitamin (at least in sufficient quantities) and must obtain it from the outside. Autotrophs have no requirement like heterotrophs for vitamins. Deficiency of a vitamin reduces the metabolic efficiency of the process which depends on it and symptoms arise for the deficiency diseases. Most deficiency diseases in the young will lead to stunting. Vitamins can be grouped into fat-soluble and water-soluble substances.

Fat-soluble Vitamins:

1. *Vitamin A.* This vitamin is formed from the carotenoid provitamins (yellow pigments of most vegetables and fruits). Deficiency in man causes poor dark vision adaptation, conjunctivitis and keratinization of the cornea.

2. *Vitamin D.* This vitamin does not occur naturally and is manufactured in the animal body by the utilization of ultraviolet light. Deficiency in humans mainly affects calcification of bones and teeth; in the child, rickets and in the adult, osteomalacia are consequences. The vitamin enhances the absorption of calcium and phosphorus from the intestinal tract.

3. *Vitamin E.* This vitamin is essential for normal reproduction in a variety of animals. Deficiency causes non-motility of sperm (sterility) and general loss of sexual instincts in the male. In the female, while conception and early embryological development are not impaired, about halfway through the pregnancy the fetus will abort. In the human the need for this vitamin is unclear.

4. *Vitamin K.* This vitamin is necessary for the production of prothrombin and thus for normal blood clotting to occur. Deficiency causes abnormally long clotting times and hemorrhage.

Water-soluble Vitamins:

1. *Thiamine (Vitamin B_1).* This vitamin is essential for the proper functioning of the nervous system; it is an antagonist to acetylcholine. Deficiency will result in beriberi in humans and polyneuritis in birds.

2. *Riboflavin (Vitamin B_2).* Riboflavin functions in the conversion of tryptophan to nicotinic acid. No recognized disease is associated with a deficiency. General problems with vision, skin, coordination and growth do occur.

3. *Niacin (Nicotinic acid).* Niacin is the functional group of the coenzymes NAD and NADP. Deficiency results in blacktongue in canines and pellagra in humans. Dermatitis and neurological lesions are manifestations of pellagra. As noted above, tryptophan may be converted to nicotinic acid.

Minerals: Minerals are also utilized by the tissues of the body. Among the most common ones found on the label of a bottle of vitamin and mineral supplements are calcium, phosphorus, potassium, sodium, magnesium, chlorine, manganese, iodine, iron, zinc, copper, cobalt, bromine and fluorine. Except in unusual circumstances, of course, these will be in the normal diet and need not be taken in pills.

The Digestive System

Regionalization of the Embryonic Gut:

1)   Foregut (supplied mainly by celiac artery): pharynx, esophagus, stomach, and cranial portion of duodenum from which the primordia of the liver, gall bladder and pancreas arise.

2)   Midgut (supplied by superior mesenteric artery): caudal duodenum, jejunum, ileum, and ascending colon and 2/3 of transverse colon including the appendages cecum and vermiform appendix.

3)   Hindgut (supplied by inferior mesenteric artery): distal third of transverse colon, descending colon, sigmoid colon, and rectum.

Parts of the Adult Digestive Tract: The parts of the human intestinal tract may be listed in the following order: oral cavity (receives salivary gland secretions); oral and laryngeal pharynx; esophagus; cardiac sphincter; stomach; pyloric sphincter; duodenum (receives bile and pancreatic secretions); jejunum (absorption of nutrients); ileum (absorption of nutrients); cecum; ascending colon (water absorption); transverse colon; descending colon; sigmoid colon; rectum; and anal sphincter.

The Oral Cavity. The oral cavity is divided into:

a)   Vestibule: the area between cheek and teeth.
b)   The Lip: composed of a core of skeletal muscle and covered externally by skin.
c)   The Cheek: structure similar to the lip.
d)   Oral Cavity Proper: area from teeth to fauces.
e)   The Tongue: composed primarily of a core of skeletal muscle and glands and covered by a mucous membrane. The anterior 2/3 of the upper (oral) portion is separated from the posterior 1/3 (pharyngeal) portion by the sulcus terminalis.

Three types of lingual papillae appear as surface projections:

a)   Circumvallate papillae, located along the sulcus terminalis and possessing taste buds;
b)   Filiform papillae, the most numerous;
c)   Fungiform papillae, relatively few but possessing taste buds.

f)   The Teeth: two sets occurring during lifetime. In childhood, there are 20 temporary primary (deciduous) teeth present; this dentition lacks premolars (bicuspids) and has only two instead of three pairs of molars (tricuspids) in each jaw. After about the age of six, the primary dentition is replaced by a set of 32 symmetrically arranged permanent (succedaneous) teeth. Each jaw contains beginning at the front: 2 central incisors, 2 lateral incisors, 2 cuspids, 4 premolars (bicuspids), and 6 molars (tricuspids).

The basic parts of a tooth are:

a)   crown—above gum margin;
b)   root—1 to 3 cm below gum margin;
c)   alveolus—root socket in jaw bone;
d)   neck—junction of root and crown;

e) periodontal membrane—attaches the root to the alveolar wall;

f) pulp chamber—extends from crown into root canals;

g) apical foramen—canal opening at the tip of root;

h) dental pulp—soft core of loosely arranged connective tissue occupying the chamber and containing blood vessels and nerves to teeth;

i) tooth wall with dentin, which borders pulp; enamel, which covers the crown and thins at the neck; and cementum, which encrusts the root and thins at the neck.

g) Salivary Glands: There are 3 pairs of major salivary glands.

1) Parotid (largest gland)—located in relation to the mandibular ramus below and anterior to the ear. It is a compound tubulo-alveolar, serous gland of the merocrine type. Connective tissue divides the gland into lobes and lobules. The major duct (Stenson's) opens into the vestibule of the oral cavity opposite the second upper (maxillary) molar.

2) Submandibular (intermediate in size)—located in relationship to the mylohyoid muscle, medial and inferior to the mandible. It is a tubulo-alveolar, merocrine gland (mixed-mucus and serous). The major duct (Wharton's) opens on the anterolateral margin of the frenulum of the tongue.

3) Sublingual (smallest gland)—a collection of glands located under the mucous membrane of the floor of the mouth. It is a tubulo-alveolar merocrine gland with mostly mucous acini. The major duct (Bartholin's) empties on the side of the frenulum of the tongue, having joined the submandibular duct.

Tubular Digestive Tract. The adult tubular digestive tract has a general structural plan of mucosa, submucosa, muscular tunic and adventitia.

1) Mucosa
   a) moist surface epithelium
   b) connective tissue (lamina propria)
   c) thin muscular layer (muscularis mucosae)
   d) villi (evaginations of the mucosa)
2) Submucosa
   a) connective tissue
   b) plexi of nerves and ganglion cells termed Meissner's plexus
   c) some areas may contain glands
   d) rich in blood vessels
3) Muscular tunic
   a) inner circular smooth muscle layer
   b) outer longitudinal smooth muscle layer
   c) Auerbach's myenteric plexus—between the two muscle layers is located a parasympathetic plexus of nerves associated with numerous ganglion cells
4) Adventitia
   a) connective tissue containing blood vessels, nerves and lymphatics
   b) peritoneal covering (mesothelium) known as a serosa, located in some regions

Esophagus (about 10–12 inches). The upper ⅓ of the esophagus features skeletal muscle (voluntary), the middle ⅓ both skeletal and smooth (involuntary) muscle, the lower ⅓ as the rest of the digestive tract only smooth muscle.

The Stomach. The stomach is highly vascular, contains gastric glands, and has smooth muscle fibers extending around the glands. There are two types of gastric glands: cardiac and fundic.

1) Cardiac glands secrete mucus
2) Fundic glands:
   a) mucous and epithelial cells—secrete mucus; this mucus protects against autodigestion and neutralizes acid to a small degree.

b) parietal or oxyntic cells—secrete hydrochloric acid (HCl). Acid (pH below 5.5) is necessary to convert pepsinogen into pepsin; at pH 2, this reaction is almost instantaneous. Parietal cells secrete acid under the influence of the hormone gastrin (probably of greatest importance); parasympathetic mediation via acetylcholine; histamine; and the presence of foodstuffs, such as peptides and amino acids.

c) chief (zymogenic) cells—secrete pepsinogen, the precursor of pepsin (proteolytic enzyme). These cells also secrete and release the hormone gastrin, and some are also implicated in the production of rennin and gastric intrinsic (anti-pernicious anemia) factor.

d) argentaffin cells—thought to secrete serotonin, a vasoconstrictor substance.

Small Intestine. The small intestine has 3 major regions:

1) Duodenum (10 inches)
2) Jejunum (8.5 feet)
3) Ileum (12.5 feet)

The small intestine has mucosal surface modifications:

a) Villi (projections of mucosa)—covered by simple columnar epithelium and having a core of connective tissue; they are broad in the duodenum, fingerlike in the ileum. In the core of the villus (in the connective tissue layer called the lamina propria) are found lymphocytes, eosinophils, plasma cells, macrophages, capillaries and *lacteals* (lymphatic capillaries).

b) Microvilli—present on columnar absorptive cells covering villi and lining crypts; we speak in terms of a striated border.

Large Intestine (cecum, ascending, transverse and descending colon)

Colon and Rectum

The Major Digestive Glands

Pancreas: The pancreas has both an exocrine and endocrine secretory function. Two excretory ducts are usually present and enter the second part of the duodenum. Exocrine glandular elements are arranged in acini. Acinar cells have a basal zone which is basophilic and an apical zone with zymogen granules which are the precursors of the enzymes in pancreatic juice—namely trypsin, chymotrypsin, amylase, and lipase. Acinar cells secrete:

(1) trypsinogen, which will be converted into trypsin.
(2) chymotrypsinogen, which will be converted into chymotrypsin.
(3) procarboxypeptidase, which will be converted into carboxypeptidase.

The above reactions are autocatalyzed (trypsinogen-trypsin). Trypsin, chymotrypsin and carboxypeptidase attack proteins and polypeptides and eventually render amino acids which can be absorbed.

Pancreatic lipase, amylase and proteases are controlled by the presence of foodstuffs and hormones. As acid chyme enters the duodenum from the stomach, secretin is released and fluid and bicarbonate are secreted.

Pancreatic juice:

1) neutralizes the acid chyme in the duodenum
2) provides enzymes for the digestion of proteins, carbohydrates and fats.

Islets of Langerhans are the endocrine portion of the pancreas. The endocrine cell aggregations are interspersed irregularly among the acini. Three cell types can be identified:

1) A, or alpha, cells, which are presumed to form glucagon.

2) B, or beta, cells which are more numerous than A cells and produce insulin.

3) D, or delta, cells; their significance is uncertain but they might represent multipotent resting cells.

Liver: The liver has the following functions:

a) Removal of bile pigments from blood which are excreted in bile.
b) Storage of glycogen.
c) Conversion of fats, and perhaps proteins, to carbohydrates (*gluconeog enesis*).
d) Maintenance of the constancy of blood glucose level.
e) Deamination of amino acid with urea as a by-product.
f) Metabolism of fat and storage in the liver.
g) Synthesis of plasma proteins such as fibrinogen, prothrombin, and albumin.
h) Storage of essential vitamins (A, D, B_2, B_3, B_4, B_{12}, and K).
i) Embryonic hemopoietic (blood cell forming) organ.

Gallbladder: *Bile,* which is secreted continuously by the hepatocytes, is collected and transported via the hepatic ducts and cystic duct into the gallbladder, where it is stored and concentrated. When demand exists bile is released and flows into the cystic duct which connects with the common bile duct (formed by union of common hepatic and cystic ducts), which empties into the second part of the duodenum.

General Functional Schema of the Digestive Tube (ingestion, digestion, egestion)

Oral Cavity:

a) Receives food and perceives taste, odor, texture and temperature.
b) Grinds foodstuffs to facilitate the action of enzymes.
c) Adds enzymes, mucus and moisture and shapes the bolus for the process of swallowing.

Pharynx and Esophagus: The oral and laryngeal pharynx, and the esophagus are essentially conduits for food to reach the stomach.

Stomach: Food is received, stored and churned; digestive juices are added; and the digestive process started in the mouth is continued. Intrinsic factor (anti-pernicious anemia factor) is secreted.

Small Intestines: Digestion is completed and most absorption takes place in jejunum and ileum.

Large Intestines:

a) Water and electrolytes are reabsorbed to preserve that delicate balance in the body.
b) Food is propelled along for elimination (egestion).

Intestinal Motility

Intestinal motility facilitates:

1) the mixing of food with secretions and enzymes
2) the contact of foodstuffs with the intestinal mucosa
3) propulsion along the tube (peristalsis).

This process is controlled by the nervous system, hormonal secretions, and intestinal distension and similar phenomena.

Epinephrine (from the adrenal) inhibits contraction; serotonin (from the small intestines) stimulates contractions.

Innervation of the Intestinal Tract

The nerves supplying the intestinal tract affect smooth muscle, glands, endocrine tissue and control motility and secretion. Motility or *peristalsis* is a wave of compression (contraction) that is followed by a regional relaxation. The gut musculature (smooth) is controlled by the autonomic nervous system.

Sympathetic Innervation: Effects of sympathetic innervation are:

a)   some excitation of salivary secretion
b)   a decrease of motility and secretion in the stomach and small intestines due mainly to the vasoconstrictive action
c)   an inhibition of muscular contraction and intrinsic ganglion cell activity due to the release of the neurotransmitters epinephrine and norepinephrine

Parasympathetic Innervation: Effects of the parasympathetic innervation are:

a)   stimulation of motility and secretion via its supply of the intrinsic plexi and the release of the neurotransmitter acetylcholine
b)   release of gastrin

Summary of Digestive Juices

Saliva: Saliva is protective and digestive. In this manner, it

a)   dissolves food and passes it over the taste buds
b)   lubricates food
c)   starts starch digestion (contains -amylase which breaks down 1,4-glycosidic bonds of glucose molecules as in starch)
d)   contains antibacterial enzymes (lysozymes)

Saliva is composed of

a)   water
b)   electrolytes
c)   enzymes (chiefly ptyalin, or salivary amylase)
d)   mucin
e)   glycoproteins
f)   blood group proteins
g)   gamma globulins

Ptyalin. Ptyalin (salivary amylase), produced chiefly by the parotid, submandibular, and sublingual salivary glands, functions in the breakdown of starch into molecules of the disaccharide maltose.

Gastric Juices: Gastric juice is composed of

a)   water
b)   hydrochloric acid (HCl)
c)   inorganic salts
d)   mucus
e)   enzymes (pepsin, rennin, and lipase)

About 2 or 3 liters of gastric juices are secreted within a 24-hour period. Food usually remains in the stomach for 3 or 4 hours. The pH of gastric juice usually varies from about 0.9 to 1.5. This acidity allows pepsin to act and inhibits ptyalin (salivary amylase).

Pepsin, a proteinase of gastric juice, is derived from its precursor pepsinogen, which is secreted by the chief cells of the gastric mucosa. Pepsin acts upon protein substrates, breaking them down to amino acids, proteoses, and peptones.

Rennin. Rennin is secreted by the stomach. This enzyme splits some peptide bonds in casein to produce a calcium-precipitable paracasein.

Mucus. Mucus is composed of proteins, glycoproteins, polysaccharides, intrinsic factor, plasma proteins, and blood group substances.

Intrinsic factor. Intrinsic factor, produced by the parietal cells of the stomach, is a mucoprotein. It binds to vitamin B_{12} and "protects" it until it is absorbed in the ileum and then transported actively into the circulation.

Pancreatic Juice: Pancreatic juice contains proteolytic, lipolytic, and amylolytic enzymes.

Pancreatic amylase. Pancreatic amylase is an enzyme which hydrolyzes starch to maltose.

Steapsin. Steapsin, or pancreatic lipase, facilitates the digestion of fats.

Trypsinogen. Trypsinogen is secreted by the pancreas and converted by enterokinase to the active enzyme *trypsin*. Trypsin's substrates are proteins but specifically it further disintegrates proteoses and peptones.

Chymotrypsinogen. Chymotrypsinogen is the precursor in pancreatic juice of the enzyme *chymotrypsin*. Trypsin is active in this conversion. Chymotrypsin acts with trypsin to hydrolyze proteins and protein products to polypeptides and amino acids.

Bile: Bile is secreted by the liver, stored and concentrated in the gall bladder, and poured into the duodenum. It primarily contains bile salts (such as cholic acid, chenodeoxycholic acid, deoxycholic acid and lithocholic acid), cholesterol phospholipids (lecithins), pigments (bilirubin), mucin and sodium, potassium, calcium and other elements. It aids in the emulsification, digestion, and absorption of fat. It also contributes to the alkalinization of the intestinal contents.

Lacteals are found in the villi of the small intestines; they are part of the lymphatic system and function to take up chyle containing fat in lipoproteins.

Hormones of the Digestive Tract

Endocrine cells of the gut originate from the neural crest. Hormones of the gastrointestinal tract are produced by the mucosa of the stomach (gastrin) and by the small intestines (secretin and cholecystokinin). These gastrointestinal hormones are polypeptides which affect:

1) water balance;
2) electrolyte balance;
3) enzyme secretions;
4) motility;
5) digestion;
6) absorption;
7) growth; and
8) hormonal release.

The general stimuli for their release are:

1) nervous activity;
2) physical extension;
3) chemical stimuli.

Specific stimuli for the three key hormones are:

1) Gastrin—distension, vagal stimulation, and presence of proteins and amino acids.
2) Secretin—acid chyme (hydrogen ion) released when the pH falls below 4.5.
3) Cholecystokinin—presence of proteins and amino acids and of monoglycerides, fatty acids.

Primary actions are as follows:

1) Gastrin
   a) stimulates gastric acid and pepsinogen secretion,

b) increases the distension of the stomach and gastric motility.
2) Secretin
   a) stimulates the pancreas to secrete pancreatic fluid and bicarbonate
   b) stimulates biliary fluid secretion and bicarbonate
   c) potentiates the enzymatic response to cholecystokinin
   d) slows gastric motility and emptying
   e) stimulates pepsinogen secretion and
   f) inhibits gastrin release.
3) Cholecystokinin
   a) stimulates pancreatic enzyme secretion
   b) increases the pancreatic bicarbonate response to secretin
   c) increases the distensibility of the stomach and inhibits gastric emptying
   d) induces gallbladder contractions and emptying.

General Digestion of the Major Food Groups

Carbohydrates: Starch digestion begins in the oral cavity under the influence of α-amylase and ends in the small intestines after exposure to pancreatic amylase. Products resulting from the above processes are further hydrolyzed by enzymes associated with the microvilli of the intestinal cells. For example: (1) maltase acts on maltose and maltotriose to yield glucose units; (2) sucrase acts on sucrose to produce glucose and fructose; (3) lactase breaks down lactose to yield monosaccharide subunits.

Proteins: Digestion begins in the stomach by the action of pepsin, which has a specificity for peptide bonds; it is inactivated by pancreatic juice. When products are transferred from the stomach to the duodenum, this stimulus results in the release of cholecystokinin (CCK) which is responsible for the release of pancreatic proteolytic enzymes such as: (1) endo- and exopeptidases, (2) trypsin, (3) chymotrypsin, (4) elastase.

Fats: In the stomach fat products are acted upon by pepsin; when the products are released into the duodenum, cholecystokinin stimulates the pancreas to secrete lipases and the gallbladder to release its contents, which emulsify fat droplets resulting in the formation of micelles. The absorption is completed in the jejunum.

Nervous System

The nervous system is usually divided into: a) central nervous system (brain and spinal cord) and b) peripheral nervous system (peripheral nerves and ganglia). The peripheral nervous system is divided into a somatic system and visceral (autonomic) system.

Nervous Tissue

Nervous tissue consists of neurons (nerve cells and their processes) and supportive elements. Neuroglia in the central nervous system and Schwann cells in the peripheral nervous system are the supportive elements.

The Neuron

The neuron is a cellular element and, as a highly specialized cell, it carries out the function of nervous transmission. The neuron is like many other cells within the body in that it consists of a nucleus with an associated nucleolus and a cytoplasm which is rich in organelles, the most prominent of which are the rough-surfaced endoplasmic reticulum (Nissl substance), mitochondria, and the Golgi apparatus. In addition to the above characteristics, it should be noted that neurons possess numerous cytoplasmic processes or appendages. In almost all of the many varieties of neurons, there are two kinds of processes: the *dendrites* and the *axon*.

The Dendrites:
1. are direct extensions of the cytoplasm.
2. are generally multiple.

3. provide an increased surface area, the dendritic zone, to allow for synaptic interaction.

The Axon:

1. There is only one per neuron.

2. This process arises from a conical elevation of cytoplasm which is devoid of rough-surfaced endoplasmic reticulum (Nissl) and this area is called the *axon hillock*.

3. It is usually thinner and longer than the dendrites of the same neuron.

4. It may be surrounded by a *myelin sheath* which is produced by the *oligodendrocytes* in the CNS and by the *Schwann cells* in the PNS. Discontinuities in this myelin sheath occur at intervals known as the *nodes of Ranvier*. Though many axons are myelinated and are referred to as myelinated nerve fibers, numerous others possess no myelin ensheathment and thus are referred to as unmyelinated nerve fibers.

5. At its ending, the axon transmits impulses: a. to other neurons—the site of this impulse transmission being called a *synapse*; and, b. to effector cells such as muscle fibers or gland cells. This junction with skeletal muscle fibers constitutes a *motor end plate*.

The Action Potential: An impulse traveling along a neuron is an electrical phenomenon initiated by a temporary change in the permeability of the neuron's cell membrane. To understand this change, one must first examine the condition of a resting, or unstimulated, neuron. The membrane possesses specific sites for the active transport of sodium ions (Na^+) and potassium ions (K^+). At these sites, sodium is transported out of the cell, and potassium is transported inward. Both ions tend to return to their original positions through pores, but Na^+ ions are less successful than are K^+ ions. Thus, the unstimulated neuron accumulates a larger concentration of positive ions (both Na^+ and K^+) outside its membrane than in its cytoplasm. A voltmeter would measure this difference as about 70 millivolts, with the inside of the neuron being negative; this is called the *resting potential* or *membrane potential*.

A sufficient stimulus—whether it be mechanical, chemical, or electrical—causes a radical but temporary change in the permeability of the affected membrane region. The membrane possesses specific channels that can allow sodium to pass, and others for potassium; in a resting membrane both are closed. A stimulus causes the sodium channel to open, and accumulated sodium ions outside the membrane rush into the interior by diffusion. Their number is sufficient to reverse the interior charge, making it about 40 millivolts positive. This change, in turn, causes the potassium channels to open, allowing a loss of potassium ions from the cytoplasm. Thus, the initial gain of interior positive ions (Na^+) is countered by a loss of positive ions (K^+), and the cytoplasm once again is negatively charged. The charge reversal, from negative to positive to negative, occurs within only a few milliseconds. The phenomenon is termed an *action potential*.

Immediately after an action potential, the sodium and potassium channels close again, and the two types of ions are pumped back to their original sites. During this refractory period of several milliseconds, an additional stimulus will not lead to another action potential.

Initiation of the action potential at any point of a neuron's membrane acts as a stimulus to the adjacent membrane material; therefore, the effect is of an action potential flowing along the membrane. The result is the "message" that moves quickly over the length of a motor neuron's axon. It is also the message that flows along and into a muscle fiber that has been stimulated by events at a motor end plate, because the membrane of a muscle fiber can act like that of a neuron.

The Synapse: The synapse is the site of contact between two neurons; it may be, and most commonly is, between an axon and a dendrite; however, contacts between an axon and the cell body and between axons and axons have also been observed. A typical synapse seen between an axon and dendrite (axodendritic synapse) has the following properties:

1. As the axon terminal reaches the synaptic site, it forms a bulbous head called a *bouton*. This bouton, which constitutes the presynaptic element of the synapse, contains numerous mitochondria and specialized vesicles, the synaptic vesicles, which contain the various neurotransmitters (acetylcholine is the primary one).

2. The dendrite, which constitutes the postsynaptic element of the synapse, is separated from the bouton by a cleft which varies in width from 150 to 200 Å.

3. This axo-dendritic synapse is *not* a site where cytoplasmic continuity is established between the axon and the dendrite, as both the pre- and postsynaptic elements are separated by a cleft. However, via the process of synaptic vesicle release, this axo-dendritic synapse establishes a functional (chemical) continuity across the expanse of the cleft.

Classification of Neurons

Multipolar Neurons: Most abundant; somatic and visceral motor, and associational.

Unipolar Neurons: Somatic and visceral *sensory* neurons; cell bodies are located in cranial sensory and dorsal root ganglia; peripheral process goes out to receptor and central process travels into the central nervous system.

Bipolar Neurons: Special *sensory* neurons; cell bodies are located in special sense organs; i.e., eye (retina), ear (spiral and vestibular ganglia), and nose (olfactory epithelium).

Groups of Neurons

Nucleus: cluster of nerve cell bodies *within* the central nervous system.

Ganglion: cluster of nerve cells bodies *outside* the central nervous system.

Cortex: layered arrangement of nerve cells bodies on the surface of the cerebrum and cerebellum (gray matter).

Supportive Elements

Neuroglia—Supportive Elements of the Central Nervous System: Neuroglia, the supportive elements of the central nervous system, are of several types.

1. Astrocytes. Astrocytes are fibrous and protoplasmic; their perivascular feet end on capillaries. They are located between capillary (or pia matter) and neurons and are implicated in the blood-brain barrier. Eighty percent of brain capillary surfaces are covered by perivascular end feet of astrocytes.
2. Oligodendrocytes. Oligodendrocytes function in the myelinization of central nervous system axons.
3. Microglia. Microglia are of questionable origin and role; they may be macrophages of the central nervous system.

Supportive Elements of the Peripheral Nervous System:

1. Schwann (neurolemmal) Cells. These are involved in the myelinization of peripheral nervous system axons.
2. Satellite Cells. These cells surround nerve cell bodies in the ganglia (e.g., dorsal root ganglia) of the peripheral nervous system.

The Central Nervous System

The central nervous system is made up of the brain and the spinal cord.

Spinal Cord: Before one can appreciate the organization of the cerebral mass and brain stem, it is necessary to understand the basic structural organization found throughout the extent of the spinal cord.

Cross Section View. If one were to examine a cross section through any level of the spinal cord, the following would be seen:

1.   A centrally located H-shaped mass which contains the cell bodies of neurons. This H-shaped mass is divided into dorsal and ventral columns, or *horns*. Cell bodies responsible for sensory phenomena are located in the dorsal horns, cell bodies for motor phenomena in the ventral horns. This H-shaped mass is collectively referred to as the *gray matter*.

2.   Peripheral to this H-shaped mass, *white matter,* made up primarily of myelinated nerve fibers.

3.   Entering the spinal cord at the apex of the dorsal horn, or column, the dorsal root of the spinal nerve. The cell bodies of these fibers are unipolar and are located in the dorsal root ganglion. The ventral root exits from the ventral horn of the gray matter. The cell bodies of these fibers are multipolar and located in the ventral horn.

4.   White matter divided into three masses of fibers known as *funiculi*. These three funiculi are:

    a)   the dorsal funiculus, located between the dorsal midline and the dorsal root,

    b)   the lateral funiculus, located between the dorsal and ventral roots,

    c)   the ventral funiculus, located between the ventral root and the ventral midline.

Within each funiculus are found bundles of fibers (axons) called *tracts*. The fibers within a specific tract have a common origin, termination, and function and either descend or ascend in the cord.

5.   An orderly arrangement of gray and white matter that remains constant throughout the spinal cord, varying only in relative mass.

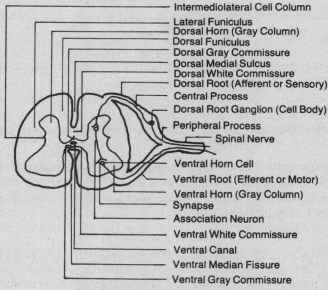

- Intermediolateral Cell Column
- Lateral Funiculus
- Dorsal Horn (Gray Column)
- Dorsal Funiculus
- Dorsal Gray Commissure
- Dorsal Medial Sulcus
- Dorsal White Commissure
- Dorsal Root (Afferent or Sensory)
- Central Process
- Dorsal Root Ganglion (Cell Body)
- Peripheral Process
- Spinal Nerve
- Ventral Horn Cell
- Ventral Root (Efferent or Motor)
- Ventral Horn (Gray Column)
- Synapse
- Association Neuron
- Ventral White Commissure
- Ventral Canal
- Ventral Median Fissure
- Ventral Gray Commissure

Transverse section of spinal cord

Gross Anatomy and Relationships. The spinal cord viewed as a whole also has the following characteristics:

1.   It is cylindrical, about 1/2 inch in diameter and 18 inches in length, and has *cervical* and *lumbar enlargements* due to the involvement of these cord levels with the innervation of the upper and lower limbs.

2.   It runs within the bony *vertebral canal* but is shorter than the canal since vertebral column growth exceeds cord growth. The spinal cord ends at vertebral level L_1–L_2 (Lumbar 1–2).

3.   It is protected not only by the bony vertebral column but also by three connective tissue sheaths known collectively as the *meninges* (dura mater, arachnoid membrane and

pia mater). *Cerebrospinal fluid* is in the subarachnoid space (between arachnoid and pia) and bathes the cord and cushions it from shock.

4.   There are 31 pairs of *spinal nerves* that are connected to the cord by *dorsal* and *ventral roots*: 8 *cervical*, 12 *thoracic*, 5 *lumbar*, 5 *sacral* and 1 *coccygeal*.

5.   The spinal nerves exit from the vertebral canal through *intervertebral foramina*.

6.   It is beause the cord ends at vertebral level L_2 that *lumbar punctures* (spinal taps) can be done safely below that level. (Nerve roots arise from the cord and extend below this level to exit at the specific vertebral level. These roots are collectively called *cauda equina* and are deflected away from the needle and therefore are not damaged.)

The Brain: The brain is divided into three parts: the cerebrum (two cerebral hemispheres), the brain stem, and the cerebellum. The brain stem is, in turn, divided into the medulla, pons, midbrain, and diencephalon. Important facts about the structure and functions of each of the parts is given below.

Cerebrum. The cerebrum consists of two hemispheres that are joined by a broad band of commissural fibers, the *corpus callosum*. Eminences on the surface are known as *gyri* and the furrows as *sulci* or *fissures*.

Each cerebral hemisphere is divided into five lobes:

1.   *frontal*—contains the major motor areas (motor speech area).
2.   *parietal*—is concerned with sensory impressions such as touch, pressure, and pain.
3.   *occipital*—is concerned with vision.
4.   *temporal*—is concerned with hearing.
5.   *insula*—is found deep within the Sylvian fissure.

The cerebrum is the seat of intelligence, consciousness and rational behavior and possesses areas for speech and writing.

Medulla Oblongata. The medulla oblongata is structurally derived from the myelencephalon and is continuous with the spinal cord at the *foramen magnum* and extends to the caudal portion of the pons. The medulla controls movement of eyelids (in blinking), sneezing, coughing, chewing, swallowing, and vomiting, and contains centers for the autonomic control of respiration (breathing), heartbeat (rate and force), contractility of blood vessels, visceral movement (gastric juice production and peristalsis), and glandular secretion (salivation).

Pons. The pons is essentially a crossing and relay station for nerve tracts. It is a conduit through which the cerebral cortex communicates with the cerebellum. It contains the motor nuclei that exert control over facial expression and mastication, and it possesses cell bodies that control lacrimation and salivation, and it serves as a relay station of tactile sensation for the facial system.

Midbrain. The midbrain serves as a relay center for auditory and optic phenomena. It houses the oculomotor nucleus, which controls extraocular movements, and exerts autonomic control over pupillary constriction and the process of accommodation.

Diencephalon. The diencephalon is itself divided into the thalamus and the hypothalamus.

Thalamus.

1.   Maintains the internal environment of the organism.
2.   Processes all sensory input except olfactation.
3.   Maintains a subconscious sense of comfort.
4.   Serves as the main relay station between the cerebrum and the rest of the nervous system.
5.   Serves in the integration of motor activities via its relay activity between the basal ganglia, the cerebellum and the cerebral cortex.

Hypothalamus. The hypothalamus regulates body temperature, osmotic balance, blood pressure, and sleep.

Cerebellum. The cerebellum is derived from the metencephalon. It integrates unconscious proprioceptive impulses, integrates and modulates vestibular functions and body equilibrium. The cerebellum is also responsible for muscular synergy of the body; it coordinates the smooth, accurate and orderly sequences of muscular contraction and movement. Without cerebellar influence muscle activity is disorganized and crude. There is, however, no conscious perception.

The Peripheral Nervous System

The peripheral nervous system is made up of a somatic portion and an autonomic portion.

Somatic Peripheral Nervous System: The somatic portion of the peripheral nervous system is made up of cranial nerves and spinal nerves.

Cranial Nerves. The cranial nerves are those peripheral nerves which leave the brain. It is customary to subdivide the cranial nerves into twelve pairs and to number and name these pairs as follows:

I.	Olfactory nerve	VII.	Facial nerve
II.	Optic nerve	VIII.	Vestibulocochlear (auditory) nerve
III.	Oculomotor nerve	IX.	Glossopharyngeal nerve
IV.	Trochlear nerve	X.	Vagus nerve
V.	Trigeminal nerve	XI.	Spinal accessory nerve
VI.	Abducens nerve	XII.	Hypoglossal nerve

No.	Nerve	General Components	Peripheral Termination and Modality Supplied	Damage to Nerve Results in
I	Olfactory	Sensory	Nasal mucosa—olfaction	Anosmia; Parosmia
II	Optic	Sensory	Rods and cones of retina—vision	Visual field defects
III	Oculomotor	Motor	Superior, inferior and medial rectus muscles and inferior oblique muscle—rotate eyeball	Strabismus or squint—deviation of the eyeball; Diplopia—double vision
		Motor	To a muscle which constricts pupil	Dilated pupil; Loss of light reflexes
			To ciliary muscle whose contraction thickens lens	Loss of accommodation
IV	Trochlear	Motor	Superior oblique muscle—rotates eyeball	Strabismus and diplopia
V	Trigeminal	Motor	Muscles of mastication—mastication	Paralysis of the muscles of mastication
		Sensory	Skin of face and mucosa of mouth and nose—supplies sensation	Loss of sensation over the distribution of V; Loss of reflex; Tic douloureux—pain over the distribution of V

No.	Nerve	General Components	Peripheral Termination and Modality Supplied	Damage to Nerve Results in
VI	Abducens	Motor	Lateral rectus muscle—moves eyeball laterally	Loss of the ability to abduct eyeball
VII	Facial	Motor	Muscles of facial expression	Facial paralysis (Bell's palsy); Expressionless face with a drooping mouth
		Sensory	Taste buds on the anterior ⅔ of the tongue	Loss of taste on the anterior ⅔ of the tongue
VIII	Vestibulocochlear	Sensory (Vestibular portion)	Cristae of semicircular canals—provides for equilibrium	Vertigo, nystagmus and nausea
		Sensory (Cochlear portion)	Hair cells in the organ of Corti—provides for hearing	Deafness
IX	Glossopharyngeal	Motor	Parotid gland—provides for glandular secretion	Loss of secretion
		Sensory	Taste buds in the posterior ⅓ of the tongue	Loss of taste in the posterior ⅓ of the tongue
		Sensory	Epiglottis, root of tongue, soft palate	Loss of gag reflex
X	Vagus	Motor	Palate and pharyngeal constrictors and intrinsic muscles of larynx	Aphonia and dysphonia
		Motor	Via the cardiac and pulmonary ganglia to the cardiac muscle and to the smooth muscle and the glands of the pulmonary and gastrointestinal systems—provides for autonomic regulation of the above named organs	Autonomic disturbances
XI	Spinal Accessory	Motor	Trapezius and sternomastoid muscles	Difficulty in rotating head or raising chin
XII	Hypoglossal	Motor	Muscles of the tongue	Paralysis of tongue

Spinal Nerves. Thirty-one pairs of spinal nerves are connected to the spinal cord. Like any nerve, a spinal nerve is composed of nerve fibers (axons and their sheaths) coursing together outside the central nervous system. Spinal nerves are surrounded by well-organized, protective connective tissue sheaths, i.e., endoneurium, perineurium and epineurium.

Spinal nerves contain both sensory and motor fibers.

a) Sensory:
   1) from receptors in skin and skeletal muscle (G.S.A.—general somatic afferent)
   2) from receptors in smooth muscle in walls of organs and blood vessels (G.V.A.—general visceral afferent).

b)   Motor:
   1)   to skeletal muscle (G.S.E.—general somatic efferent)
   2)   autonomic fibers to smooth muscle, cardiac muscle, and glands (G.V.E.—general visceral efferent).

Sensory Pathway. A typical sensory pathway contains three neurons in a chain from the receptor on the surface of the body to consciousness in the cerebral cortex (Primary: 1°, Secondary: 2°, and Tertiary: 3° neurons).

   1° neuron: has its unipolar cell body in the dorsal root ganglion; its peripheral process goes out to the receptor through the spinal nerve; its central process follows the dorsal root and synapses in the C.N.S. with a second order (2°) neuron.
   2° neuron: has its cell body in the central nervous system; those cell bodies concerned with pain and temperature are found within the spinal cord; those concerned with touch and pressure are localized in the medulla of the brain. The axon of this 2° neuron then crosses the midline and ascends to the thalamus, where it synapses with a third order (3°) neuron.
   3° neuron: has its cell body in the thalamus; its axon ascends to the cerebral cortex.

Voluntary Motor Pathway. A typical voluntary motor pathway contains two neurons from the cerebral cortex to the effector organ in skeletal muscle.

   Neuron 1: (upper motor neuron) has its cell body in the cerebral cortex; its axon descends, crosses in the medulla and terminates in relation to lower motor neurons found in the ventral horn.
   Neuron 2: (lower motor neuron) has its cell body in the ventral horn of the spinal cord; its axon (efferent fiber) leaves the spinal cord through the ventral root and follows the spinal nerve to the skeletal muscle, where it terminates as a motor end plate.

Autonomic Nervous System: The autonomic nervous system innervates all smooth muscle, cardiac muscle, and glands. The autonomic nervous system is divided into a sympathetic (flight and fight) component and parasympathetic (maintains homeostasis) component. The autonomic nervous system exerts important influences on the intrinsic eye musculature, skin glands, the cardiovascular, gastrointestinal, respiratory, endocrine, and reproductive systems.

   Fear, rage, pain, and the like evoke sympathetic activity that mobilizes the resources of the body. Gastrointestinal activity is curtailed; heart rate and blood pressure increase and coronary arteries and bronchioles dilate.

Reflex Arc

   The typical pathway of a reflex may be outlined as follows: sensory receptor on dendrite of dorsal root ganglion cell ——→ ganglion cell ——→ axon of cell ——→ dorsal root ——→ dorsal horn of spinal cord ——→ either directly to motor cell in ventral horn or via internuncial (association) neuron to ventral horn motor cell ——→ axon via ventral root ——→ spinal nerve ——→ effector organ (e.g., muscle).

Organs of Special Sense

The Eye

The visual system is made up of the eye and complex nerve pathways for interpretation by the cerebral cortex and subcortical centers for the purpose of:

   1)   Refraction of light rays and the focusing thereof on the retina for the production of an image;
   2)   Conversion of light rays into a nervous impulse;
   3)   Transmission to visual centers of the brain for interpretation.

The visual system is composed of the following structures: eyelids, tearing apparatus (lacrimal gland), extrinsic muscles, and the eyeball and optic nerve. We will concentrate on the eyeball and optic nerve.

Eyeball and Optic Nerve: The eye is nearly spherical and about 2.5 cm in diameter. The eyeball is composed of three coats—namely, an outer fibrous layer, a middle, vascular and pigmented layer, and an inner or retinal layer—and the refractive elements—the cornea, the aqueous humor, the lens and the vitreous humor.

Two clinical problems concerned with the size of the eyeball must be identified:

a) *myopia* (near-sightedness)—In this condition the eyeball is longer than normal and light rays come to focus in front of the retina.

b) *hyperopia* (far-sightedness)—In this condition the eyeball is shorter than normal and light rays come to focus in back of the retina.

Outer Layer. The outer fibrous tunic is the opaque *sclera* (white of the eye), which anteriorly becomes the transparent, non-vascular *cornea*. The sclera maintains the shape of the eye and gives attachment to the external ("extrinsic") ocular muscles. The cornea is composed of five layers and is one of the refractive elements.

Middle Layer. The middle vascular and pigmented tunic is the *choroid,* which anteriorly becomes the *ciliary body* and the *contractile iris*. The ciliary body, attached to the *lens* via the suspensory ligaments, aids in focusing light rays on the retina. Contraction of the ciliary muscles mediated by the parasympathetic portion (Edinger-Westphal nucleus) of the oculomotor nerve decreases the tension on the suspensory ligaments, allowing the lens to increase in thickness. The *pupil* is the central opening of the iris; its size is regulated by the amount of light present. Two smooth muscles regulate the opening; the constrictor, or sphincter pupillae, is innervated by the parasympathetic system (oculomotor nerve) and reduces the size of the pupil, while the dilator, or dilator pupillae, receives its innervation from the sympathetic system and enlarges the diameter of the pupil.

Inner Layer. The innermost tunic, the retinal layer, consists of ten layers of cells and fibers. Three layers are of neuronal importance:

a) rod and cone layer; here light energy is transformed into chemical and electrical energy;

b) bipolar cells, which allow for internal nerve impulse transmission;

c) ganglion cells which give rise to the *optic nerve*.

There are about 120 million rods and 6 million cones present per eye. The rods contain rhodopsin, or visual purple, which converts photons (basic unit of light) into chemical and then into electrical energy. Rhodopsin is formed from vitamin A; a deficiency of vitamin A may result in night blindness. Rods are very sensitive and function in dim light but yield no color discrimination. Cones contain iodopsin: they are concerned with bright light vision, visual acuity (scotopic vision) and color perception.

Bipolar cells make contact with many rods and cones to receive their impulses which they in turn transmit to the ganglion cells whose axons give rise to the optic nerve. It is estimated that the one million ganglion cells receive information from approximately 130 million rod and cone receptors.

The area at which optic nerve fibers exit is called the *optic disc* or *blind spot*. No photoreception takes place there but the central artery and vein of the retina may be observed there.

Directly in line (visual axis) with the center of the cornea is the *macula lutea*. This area exhibits a high concentration of cones; the center, known as the *fovea centralis,* is the area of most acute vision. The image formed on the retina is inverted; this is inverted again—corrected—by the brain.

The Ear

The ear, which is located in the temporal bone, essentially serves in a dual capacity. It is an auditory organ for the sense of hearing (40–20,000 cycles/second) and a vestibular organ monitoring the effects of gravity and position of the head. Hearing utilizes the cochlear mechanism; vestibular functions are modulated by the utricle, saccule and the three semicircular canals.

Irritative lesions to the vestibular system may result in nystagmus, vertigo, nausea, incoordination or any other disorders of equilibrium or posture.

The auditory functions of the ear are:

1) reception and conduction of sound waves,
2) amplification of the waves,
3) transduction of the waves into nerve impulses,
4) transmission of the impulse to conscious centers.

The vestibular functions of the ear are:

1) reception of stimuli and response to movements of the head and gravitational influences on the head,
2) nerve transmission to higher centers for reflex and postural adjustments to maintain equilibrium.

The ear is commonly divided into the external ear, the middle ear, and the inner ear.

The External Ear: The auricle, or pinna, is composed of skin molded on a complex elastic cartilage; it serves to gather and funnel sound waves into the external auditory meatus (canal), which terminates at the tympanic membrane, or eardrum. In the skin of the meatus are located fine hairs and large sebaceous glands. Coiled, tubular ceruminous glands are also present; they discharge a brownish secretion which in conjunction with the sebaceous products and desquamated cells produce a waxy product known as cerumen.

The Middle Ear: The middle ear is a cavity continuous superiorly with the mastoid air cells and inferiorly, via the auditory (Eustachian) tube, with the nasopharynx. The auditory tube is ordinarily open and serves to equalize the internal and external pressures on the eardrum. Within the cavity are located three ossicles. From external (eardrum) to internal (oval window), they are respectively the malleus (hammer), the incus (anvil), and the stapes (stirrup). These small bones function in transduction: they translate the displacement of the tympanic membrane, produced by sound waves, into mechanical energy.

On the medial wall of the middle ear are the vestibular window (oval) and the cochlear window (round). The vestibular window houses the base of the stapes; the cochlear window is closed by a membrane. Movement of the eardrum sets up vibrations of the stapes in the oval window; these are transmitted to perilymph in the scala vestibuli (bony labyrinth). The movement is transferred to the endolymph in the cochlear duct (membranous labyrinth) and from there to perilymph in the scala tympani and then is dissipated through the movement of the membrane in the round window. Sound vibrations may be transmitted by surrounding bone in case of middle ear disease (deafness); therefore, the outer and middle ear are not absolutely essential for hearing.

The Inner Ear: The internal ear, located in the petrous portion of the temporal bone, consists of a complex series of fluid (endolymph)-filled sacs, the membranous labyrinth, housed within bony cavities (bony labyrinth), which are filled by perilymph. The interconnecting membranous channels serve static and kinetic senses (vestibular) as well as hearing (auditory).

The vestibular apparatus comprises: three semicircular canals, utricle, and saccule.

The auditory mechanism is housed in the cochlear duct. Both senses are transmitted by the stato-acoustic nerve (cranial nerve VIII) to the brain. This nerve is also named "vestibulocochlear nerve"; in the past it has been called the "auditory nerve."

The Cochlea. The cochlear duct is a helical tube of about 2½ turns housed in its bony labyrinth. The duct separates the bony tube into two channels, the scala tympani and scala vestibuli. At the apex the scala tympani and scala vestibuli communicate; this point is termed the helicotrema. The scala vestibuli begins at the oval window and the scala tympani terminates at the round window.

Pulsations are set up in the perilymph of the scala vestibuli by movements of the stapes at the oval window. They are propagated either via the helicotrema directly to the scala tympani or may pass through the vestibular membrane, activate movement in the endolymph of the cochlear duct, and then pass via the basilar membrane into the perilymph of the scala tympani. The pulsations stimulate the receptor (hair) cells located on the basilar membrane and elicit the phenomenon of hearing. Movements of the endolymph, varying with the volume and pitch of the sound waves are registered in specific regions of the organ of Corti. The cochlear division of the stato-acoustic nerve transmits the information to the medulla, then to the midbrain, the thalamus, and, finally, interpretation takes place in the cerebrum.

The Vestibular Apparatus. Head movements are perceived by the three semicircular canals, attached at right angles to the utricle. Displacement of the head causes endolymph to elicit a response in the sensory hair cells of the crista. Position with respect to gravity is monitored by movement of otoliths (calcium carbonate crystals) on the sensory hair cells, in the macula of the utricle and sacculus. The vestibular division of the stato-acoustic nerve (CN VIII) relays the information to the medulla, then to the cerebellum, where muscle coordination is elicited.

Semicircular Canals. There are three canals. Each possesses an ampulla with a modified, sensory epithelium (crista ampullaris) which is associated with neuronal reception. Each crista is stimulated by movements occurring in the plane of its specific canal. Rotational movement leads to a compensatory response of the eyes, head and limbs.

Utricle. The sensory epithelium is located in a region known as the macula. Gelatinous material in which are embedded crystals (otoliths) cover the hair cells. Any change in position of the head in space and any linear acceleration will result in pressure from the crystals on the hair cells and a compensatory reaction such as righting of the body and eye coordination.

Saccule. The morphology of the saccule is similar to that of the utricle. The saccule responds to vibrational stimuli.

The Olfactory System

The olfactory system may be visualized as a highly specialized mucous membrane located in the roof of each nasal cavity. Four primary odors—fragrant, acid, burnt and rancid—are perceived. Olfactory stimulation is caused by gaseous and odiferous substances in solution. Olfactory sero-mucous glands secrete a watery fluid continuously. This allows for reception of dissolved substances and also lessens retention and lingering of stimulation. The receptive cells, bipolar ganglion cells, end in bulbous knobs that possess about 10 olfactory hairs; these serve as the sensory receptors. The sense of smell is subject to fatigue; no structural differences are correlated with discrimination of different kinds of odors. Reception follows this route:

Bipolar cells of olfactory epithelium → Olfactory bulb → Olfactory tract (cranial nerve I) → Olfactory stria → Olfactory cortex.

The Gustatory System

In higher vertebrates the sense of taste is generally restricted to the oral cavity (tongue and epiglottic region). Taste buds are located in vallate, foliate and fungiform papillae. The receptors in the taste bud are neuroepithelial cells. Substances must be in solution and the four modalities of taste—sweet, sour, salt and bitter are specific and regionalized.

Sweetness is localized mainly on the tip of the tongue, sour and salt mainly on the central areas and bitter on the back of the tongue.

Endocrine System

Two systems modulate, integrate, and control the activities of the body; they are the nervous and endocrine systems. The response in nervous control is rapid while control via the endocrine system is fairly slow and longer lasting. The endocrine glands are ductless and secrete their products, called hormones, into the capillaries (bloodstream). Hormones are substances that are secreted into the bloodstream and travel to their target organs to elicit their effects. The product of the target organ may also feed back upon the organ that stimulated its activity and production and thus manipulate its cycle of function. It may shut off the supply of stimulating hormone; this activity is called a negative feedback. The controlling mechanism can be thought of as a neuro-endocrine-somatic tissue relationship, or the brain affecting the pituitary gland, which in turn affects the target organs, which then elicit their effect upon the body tissues and cells. Hormones cannot be classified into one chemical class; they are, however, all organic substances and may be proteins, peptides, amino acids (or amino acid derivatives), and steroids, or prostaglandins (derivatives of essential fatty acids). Generally the glands which produce protein hormones embryologically originate from the alimentary tract; they are the anterior pituitary, thyroid, parathyroids, and pancreas. Glands which produce steroid products are derived from the celomic mesothelium and are the testes, ovaries, and adrenal cortex. Glands whose products are small molecular weight amines arise from cells of nervous tissue derivation and are the neurohypophysis and the adrenal medulla.

It is the purpose of this chapter to give the student a brief description of each endocrine organ, its products, and the results of hypo- and hypersecretion.

The Pituitary Gland (Hypophysis)

The pituitary gland is commonly divided into an anterior and a posterior lobe according to origin. The anterior lobe (adenohypophysis) originates from the oral epithelium of the roof of the mouth in the embryo (Rathke's pouch) while the posterior lobe (neurohypophysis) is a downgrowth of the floor of the brain (in relation to the third ventricle and the hypothalamic areas).

Three cell types are found in the anterior lobe: chromophobes 50%; acidophils 40%; basophils 10%. Chromophobes are considered to be resting cells.

Hormones Secreted by Acidophils (Alpha Cells):
1. *Somatotropic hormone (STH)*
    a. Stimulates general body growth
    b. Hypersecretion—before ossification is complete, giantism
               —after ossification is complete, acromegaly
    c. Hyposecretion—dwarfism
2. *Lactogenic hormone* or luteotrophic hormone (LTH) or prolactin
    a. Promotes growth of breast which was already stimulated by estrogen and progesterone, especially during the last trimester of pregnancy
    b. Promotes and maintains lactation
    c. Helps in the maintenance of the corpus luteum
    d. Promotes maternal instinct

Hormones Secreted by Basophils (Beta and Delta Cells):
1. *Beta cells*
    a. Thyroid stimulating hormone (TSH)
        (1.) Stimulates the thyroid gland to produce its hormones T_3 (triiodothyronine) and T_4 (tetraiodothyronine or thyroxin)

(2.) Modulates the iodide trapping mechanisms

(3.) Hypersecretion—goiter, exophthalmos

(4.) Hyposecretion—diminished thyroid function and lethargy

  b. Adrenocorticotropic hormone (ACTH)

(1.) Stimulates the adrenal cortex to produce glucocorticoids (cortisol, etc.)

(2.) Does *not* stimulate mineralocorticoid activity (aldosterone production)

(3.) Affects production of adrenal androgens

  c. Melanocyte stimulating hormone (MSH) or intermedin

(1.) Function poorly understood in humans

(2.) This hormone causes the dispersion of pigment in the chromatophores of the skin of cold-blooded vertebrates and a darkening of the skin results; the action of MSH allows for quick changes in the skin color in response to changes in the external environment.

  2. *Delta cells*

    a. Luteinizing hormone (LH) in female
Interstitial cell stimulating hormone (ICSH) in male

(1.) In the female this hormone is necessary for preovulatory development of the ovarian follicle, ovulation, and formation of the corpus luteum.

(2.) In the female it modulates the production of estrogen and progesterone.

(3.) In the male this hormone stimulates the interstitial cells of the testes, which results in a secretion of testicular androgens.

    b. Follicle stimulating hormone (FSH)

(1.) In the female this hormone stimulates the growth of the ovarian follicle.

(2.) In the male FSH stimulates the testes to produce sperm (spermatogenesis).

Hormones of the Neurohypophysis:

The posterior lobe or neurohypophysis develops from the floor of the third ventricle of the brain. The function of this portion of the pituitary gland is to store and release the hormones oxytocin (produced by the paraventricular nucleus of the hypothalamus) and vasopressin or antidiuretic hormone (ADH, produced by the supraoptic nucleus of the hypothalamus).

  1. *Oxytocin*

    a. Stimulates the contraction of the smooth muscle of the uterus and may play some role in the initiation of labor

    b. Stimulates the ejection of milk by affecting the myoepithelial cells of the breast tissue (mammary gland)

  2. *Vasopressin; antidiuretic hormone (ADH)*

    a. Acts upon the renal tubules to aid water resorption and thereby restricts diuresis; a lack of hormone results in the condition known as diabetes insipidus (the production of large volumes of dilute urine).

The Pituitary Portal System: In humans the pituitary gland receives its blood supply via the right and left superior and the right and left inferior pituitary arteries from the internal carotid artery system. These vessels supply the hypothalamic areas, the pituitary stalk, and the posterior lobe. The anterior lobe, however, receives no arterial blood supply. The entire blood supply to the anterior lobe is derived from the pituitary portal veins. These veins arise from the capillary network of the median eminence and the infundibular stem. The vascular tufts of the primary capillary system are in close relationship with the nerve endings of the hypothalamo-hypophyseal tract. It is hypothesized that upon excitation these nerve fibers liberate their secretory products into this system, which then, via the portal veins, transports these neurosecretory products to the sinusoids of the anterior lobe. It is in this manner that the activity of the anterior lobe is governed by the hypothalamic areas.

The Thyroid Gland

The thyroid gland is derived from the pharynx (the foramen cecum of the tongue). Its structural unit is the follicle; the follicle is composed of a unit of epithelial cells that surround a colloid space. Colloid is located extracellularly and contains thyroglobulin. The function of the thyroid gland is to produce colloidal material which contains the thyroid hormones (T_3—triiodothyronine and T_4—thyroxin) which affect the rate of metabolism of all the tissues of the body.

The iodides consumed in our food and water are absorbed and carried to the iodide pool in the extracellular fluid via the circulatory system. Five basic events can be identified in thyroid hormone production: a. trapping iodide; b. oxidation of iodide to organic iodine; c. synthesis of hormone; d. storage of hormone as the thyroglobulin moiety in the follicle; and e. release of the hormone into the circulation. TSH from the anterior pituitary influences greatly the trapping mechanism; thiocyanates block this mechanism while thiouracil blocks the oxidation and synthetic steps. These compounds are classified as antithyroid agents.

The production of the hormone thyrocalcitonin has been implicated with the parafollicular cells of the thyroid gland. This hormone is an antagonist of parathyroid hormone and its functions are to lower the serum calcium level and to enhance the deposition of calcium in bone.

Action of Thyroid Hormone:

1. *Controls the rate of metabolism.*

2. *Controls the growth, maturation, and differentiation of the organism.*

3. *Influences nervous system activity.*

Problems Associated with Thyroid Function:

1. *Cretinism.* Congenital failure of proper development of the thyroid gland. The cretin is a dwarf physically and mentally.

2. *Myxedema.* Acquired thyroid deficiency in the adult. This deficiency can be of two types:

    a. Thyroid deficiency due to thyroidectomy, neoplasms, thyroiditis, and so forth.

    b. A pituitary deficiency in the secretion of TSH.

The thyroid in these cases appears atrophic, hard, and fibrous. The clinical picture is the presentation of a patient who is fairly heavy, phlegmatic, and devoid of expression; his skin is rough and dry and sensitive to cold. The patient is sluggish mentally and physically. Laboratory tests would show a low basal metabolic rate, low protein bound iodine, and a high serum cholesterol level.

3. *Goiter.* Any enlargement of the gland not due to neoplasm or inflammatory disease. Endemic goiters are due to lack of intake of iodine caused by deficiency in the soil and water. This results in increased TSH production, thyroid compensatory hypertrophy, and eventual exhaustion of the gland.

4. *Hyperthyroidism.* Increased activity by the organ. The patient exhibits loss of weight, nervousness, irritability, increased metabolic rate, rapid heart rate, sweating, and so forth. Exophthalmos, a protrusion of the eyeballs, is exhibited and thought to be due to an increased production of TSH. Hyperthyroidism may be an adjunct to the development of a goiter or may arise *de novo*.

The Parathyroid Glands

There are usually four parathyroid glands which are embedded in the thyroid gland. The parathyroid glands produce parathyroid hormone, which governs the metabolism of calcium and phosphorus. The parathyroids are essential to life; their removal results in cramps, convulsions, tremors, and eventually death due to tetany. The condition is due to the increased irritability of the muscular and nervous system caused by the decrease of calcium levels in the blood and body fluids. The activity of the parathyroids depends on the level of ionized calcium in the serum.

Problems Associated with Parathyroid Function:

1. *Hypoparathyroidism.* This condition results in a decrease of urinary excretion of phosphorus and its concomitant rise in the serum; this results in a shift in the calcium-phosphorus serum levels and a decline in calcium resorption from bone. The fall in serum calcium will produce tetany. Low serum levels of calcium may also be influenced by deficient intake of calcium, deficiency of vitamin D in the diet, problems with intestinal absorption or increased demand for calcium during pregnancy.

2. *Hyperparathyroidism.* Tumor is the most frequent cause of this condition. In this condition urinary phosphorus excretion is elevated and serum levels are decreased. Calcium resorption from bone is increased and serum levels rise. The glomerular filtrate is saturated and stones may form. Secondary renal disease may occur.

The Pancreas

The pancreas is both an endocrine and exocrine gland. The endocrine portion to be discussed is located in the islets of Langerhans. The function of the islets of Langerhans is to produce insulin by the beta cells and glucagon by the alpha cells. A deficiency of insulin production results in the disease known as diabetes mellitus (elevated blood sugar level). The beta cells do not seem to depend upon any outside trophic influences and the primary physiologic stimulus for insulin production seems to be the level of the blood sugar.

Insulin promotes the removal of glucose from the blood and also the conversion of glucose to glycogen in muscle and liver. It increases the rate of oxidation of glucose in the tissues, the conversion of carbohydrates into fats, the mobilization of fatty acids from adipose tissue, and the rate of protein synthesis.

Glucagon is the glycogenolytic hormone produced by the alpha cells of the pancreas; its principal action is to stimulate the conversion of glycogen to glucose by the liver. Glucagon also increases the peripheral utilization of glucose; therefore, it should not be referred to as simply the antagonist of insulin. Its secretion is controlled by the concentration of blood glucose and blood insulin level. If insulin levels rise and blood glucose levels drop, glucagon secretion increases.

The Adrenal Glands

The adrenal is composed of a cortex and a medulla. The cortex is derived from mesoderm of the Wolffian ridge in conjunction with the sex glands, while the medulla is of ectodermal, neural crest origin in conjunction with the anlage of the sympathetic nerve cells. In fetal life the adrenal is composed almost completely of cortex, but after birth the entire fetal cortex rapidly degenerates and is replaced by the adult cortex and medulla. The cortex, which produces the mineralocorticoids and glucocorticoids, is divided into three zones: a. the most peripheral zona glomerulosa; b. the intermediate zona fasciculata; and c. the zona reticularis bordering the medulla. The function of the adrenal cortex is to produce the sex hormones: androgens, estrogens, and progesterone, and the corticosteroids: glucocorticoids and mineralocorticoids.

The zona glomerulosa is rich in lipids, especially cholesterol, from which the mineralocorticoids are formed. Aldosterone is the most powerful mineralocorticoid. Mineralocorticoids function in the retention of water, sodium, and chloride, and increase urinary loss of potassium and phosphorus by action on the renal tubules. This regulation of the electrolytes is essential to life. No pituitary control is present.

The zona fasciculata and reticularis are the sources of the glucocorticoids; i.e., 17-hydroxycorticosteroids. Corticosterone (hydroxycorticosterone), cortisone (compound E), and hydrocortisone (cortisol or compound F) are the most widely known compounds.

The levels of these hormones are increased by ACTH; they are gluconeogenic in nature. They convert amino acids into sugar instead of protein and in this way increase blood sugar and liver glycogen levels. Cortisone—in addition to influencing protein, carbohydrate, and fat metabolism— a. affects the permeability of cell membranes; b. interferes with the antigen-antibody response by inhibiting antibody formation; and c. suppresses the inflammatory response. Cortisone, however, only relieves the symptoms of disease without influencing the cause.

The zona reticularis is responsible for the production of the sex hormones or 17-keto-steroids. The action of these hormones is no different from the action of the estrogens, androgens, and progesterone (the regular sex hormones produced by the testes and ovaries); i.e., they masculinize the body and increase the synthesis of amino acids and protein from nitrogen; they favor the retention of nitrogen, phosphorus, potassium, sodium, and chloride. ACTH has some control of these hormones.

Problems Associated with Adrenal Cortex Function:

1. *Hypofunction or chronic adrenal insufficiency.* Addison's disease. This condition is due to inadequate amounts of steroid hormones. Deficiency of glucocorticoids makes the patient easily susceptible to stress; deficiency or mineralocorticoids leads to a fall in serum sodium and rise in serum potassium. These patients lack proper resistance to infection and are easily dehydrated. Patients exhibit general languor and debility, a very weak heart, irritability of the stomach, and a peculiar change in skin color due to the deposition of melanin; this feature is highly characteristic.

2. *Hyperadrenalism*
   a. Overfunction of zona glomerulosa—aldosteronism (Conn's syndrome).
   b. Overfunction of zona fasciculata—(Cushing's syndrome).
   c. Overfunction of zona reticularis—adrenal virilism (Adreno-genital syndrome).

Primary Aldosteronism—Conn's Syndrome:
Characterized by:
1. Periodic severe muscular weakness or paralysis.
2. Intermittent tetany and paresthesia.
3. Hypertension.
4. Renal disfunction.

Cushing's Syndrome:
Characterized by:
1. Painful adiposity of face, neck, and trunk (full moon face).
2. Excess hair growth in the female and preadolescent males.
3. Peculiar body striations.
4. Sexual dystrophy.
5. Muscular weakness and atrophy.
6. Hypertension.

Adrenal Virilism—Adrenogenital Syndrome:
Characterized by:
1. Excess hair growth.
2. Virilism.
3. Excessive muscularity.

The adrenal medulla is intimately connected with the nervous system and develops from the neural crest. The cells of the adrenal medulla are modified ganglion cells and receive stimulation from the preganglionic fibers whose cell bodies are located in the intermediolateral cell columns of the spinal cord in the thoraco-lumbar segments dealing with the sympathetic outflow of the autonomic nervous system. Sectioning of the splanchnic nerves to the adrenal medulla will result in cessation of secretion, while stimulation of these nerves enhances secretion markedly. The function of the adrenal medulla is to secrete adrenalin (epinephrine) and nor-adrenalin (nor-epinephrine).

In general these hormones help the body in frightful and stressful situations. They affect the vascular system, the heart, respiration, carbohydrate metabolism, the pupillary dilators, the intestines, and uterine musculature.

A clinical picture of nor-adrenalism during which these pressor amines are produced in excess will show: a. hypertension; b. headache; c. palpitation; d. dyspnea; e. weakness; and f. chest and/or abdominal pain, etc.

The Testes

The testes function in the production of sperm and also contain interstitial cells, which produce the male sex hormone testosterone. Testosterone promotes and maintains the development of the male accessory genital organs (prostate and seminal vesicles) and secondary sex characteristics, i.e., beard growth, hair growth (pubic, axilla, trunk and limbs), and scrotal growth. It maintains spermatogenesis, is responsible for the deepening of the voice, the greater muscular development of men, sex urge, and acne at puberty. It also exerts an influence upon nitrogen, electrolyte and water balance within the system. Both males and females produce estrogens and androgens; it is the ratio of the two which determines male and female characteristics.

General Functional Schema of Both Sexes

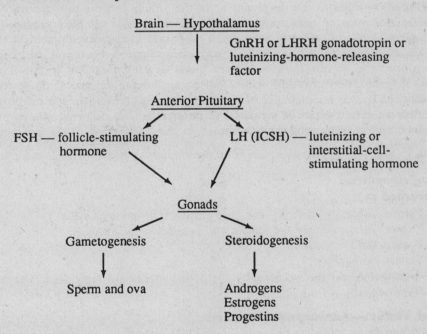

Brain — Hypothalamus

GnRH or LHRH gonadotropin or luteinizing-hormone-releasing factor

Anterior Pituitary

FSH — follicle-stimulating hormone

LH (ICSH) — luteinizing or interstitial-cell-stimulating hormone

Gonads

Gametogenesis

Steroidogenesis

Sperm and ova

Androgens
Estrogens
Progestins

Steroidogenesis is similar in the ovary and the testis; the difference is in the predominance and quantity of the secretions. The androgen testosterone is the predominant secretion of the testis, while in the ovary the estrogen estradiol and the progestin progesterone predominate.

Actions of LH and FSH in the Male: These hormones act on the testis to promote:

1) androgen secretion,
2) spermatogenesis.

Hormonal Control of Spermatogenesis:

1. Pituitary secretions regulate spermatogenic activities.
2. Interstitial-cell-stimulating hormone (ICSH) affects seminiferous tubules via androgen secretion.
3. FSH affects maturation of spermatids.
4. FSH and GH maintain spermatogenesis.

Androgenic and Anabolic Actions of Testosterone:

1. Maintenance of spermatogenesis.
2. Maintenance of structure and function of the sex accessory organs.
3. Promotion of secondary sex characteristics (size of genitalia, voice, glandular secretions, muscle development, and hair distribution),
4. Normal development and body growth.
5. Psychological balance.
6. Suppression of LH via feedback mechanism.

The Ovaries

Like the testes, the ovaries are endocrine glands; they have three functions: a. they produce the female gamete (ovum); b. they produce estrogens, which function in the preparation for fertilization of the egg and in the production of secondary female sex characteristics; and c. they produce progesterone, which prepares the uterus for implantation. FSH from the pituitary initiates the development of the follicle and the production of estrogen; when the level of estrogen rises above a certain point, it shuts off FSH production, ovulation occurs, and LH and prolactin production take over in the development of the corpus luteum, which secretes progesterone. This hormone prepares the uterus for implantation of the fertilized egg; it promotes mammary gland development and prohibits additional ovulation. If fertilization does not occur, the corpus luteum regresses, progesterone production falls, and since maintenance of the lining of the uterus depends on progesterone, menstruation is the next phase of the cycle. If fertilization has occurred, the corpus luteum is maintained and secretes progesterone almost to the termination of the pregnancy.

Ovarian Cycle: It occurs from menarche to menopause, is typically 28 days long, and can be divided into two phases:

1) follicular or estrogenic,
2) luteal or progestational.

Menstrual Cycle

The ovarian cycle and the menstrual cycle of the uterus are integrated. The menstrual cycle can be divided into four phases:

1) menstrual phase (days 1–5);
2) proliferative or follicular phase (days 6–13), followed by ovulation (day 14);
3) secretory or luteal phase (days 15–25);
4) ischemic phase (days 26–28).

Uterine Changes during the Menstrual Cycle: Menses (days 1–5) involves the sloughing off of necrotic endometrium, blood, and uterine fluid, which is discharged as menstrual flow. During the proliferative phase (days 6–13) the primary hormonal stimulus is estrogen from the follicle, which promotes proliferation of uterine epithelium and glandular tissue. Ovulation generally occurs on day 14 of the cycle. During the postovulatory phase (days 15–25) the uterus is under the combined effects of estrogen and progesterone from the corpus luteum. This hormonal milieu promotes increased vascularity, further development of glands, their increased secretory activity (including glycogen accumulation), hypertrophy, and fluid accumulation. These changes prepare the uterus for implantation of a fertilized ovum, should fertilization occur. If fertilization does not occur, the corpus luteum begins to regress after day 25, leading ultimately to the onset of menses.

Hormonal Control of the Menstrual Cycle: The suppressed (and even declining) plasma gonadotropin (FSH and LH) levels during the follicular phase are due to the negative-feedback inhibitory effects of estrogen being secreted from developing follicles. The small, abrupt rise in plasma estrogen is believed to trigger the ovulatory LH surge (by suspension of negative feedback or by positive feedback). During the luteal phase negative-feedback suppression is reestablished, but in this period feedback is due to the combined effects of estrogen and progesterone. Luteal failure occurs at about 26 days. It results in an abrupt withdrawal of estrogen and progesterone and hence in a release of feedback inhibition, which accounts for the rise in FSH and LH at the beginning of a new cycle.

Female Contraception

Female oral contraceptives represent combinations of synthetic progestational compounds (19-nortestosterone derivatives such as norgestrol and norethindrone) with synthetic estrogen. The original rationale behind the pill was that the synthetic progestin in the presence of estrogen would block the ovulatory LH surge. The progestins are effective because they also cause the cervical mucus to produce an environment (like that in the luteal phase) hostile to sperm.

The Placenta

While the placenta is mainly concerned with support and nourishment of the developing embryo, it secretes estrogens, progesterone, and chorionic gonadotropin. Excess chorionic gonadotropin (similar to luteinizing hormone) is excreted in the urine and is the basis of most pregnancy tests. The estrogen production by the placenta inhibits FSH production and in this manner inhibits follicle development during pregnancy.

The Pineal

The pineal organ is a diencephalic outgrowth. It has been linked to photoperiodism and seasonal breeding; experimental evidence now suggests that it produces an antigonadotropic substance. How the pineal influences the reproductive organs remains to be established.

The Prostaglandins

Prostaglandins (PGs) are hormonelike substances; they play a role in cellular metabolism. Their function, unlike that of hormones, is limited to immediate areas; in this respect they may be labeled as tissue hormones. These substances, which are derivatives of prostanoic acid, are C_{20} fatty acids containing a five-membered ring; they are found in almost every type of human and animal tissue and elicit a multitude of effects. Prostaglandins exert control over processes such as reproduction, inflammation, nerve impulse transmission, blood pressure and blood clotting, smooth muscle activity, and hormone secretion.

Major Actions of the Prostaglandins:

1. Lower blood pressure.
2. Modulate smooth muscle activity.
3. Inhibit the release of glycerol and fatty acid from adipose tissue.
4. Decrease nervous system excitability.
5. Modulate uterine smooth muscle.

6. Induce labor.
7. Modulate the bronchial tree.
8. Suppress gastric secretions.
9. Amplify pain response.
10. Stimulate renin secretion.
11. Modulate platelet aggregation.
12. Shrink swollen nasal passages.
13. Increase intraocular pressure.
14. Mediate inflammation.
15. Stimulate steroid production.
16. Promote sodium excretion.
17. Potentiate the pain-producing action of bradykinin.
18. Modulate norepinephrine release.

The Small Intestine

Food materials stimulate the secretion of certain hormones by the gastrointestinal mucosa and they may be summarized as follows:

1. Secretin: from duodenal mucosa—stimulates pancreatic juice secretion which is low in enzymatic content.

2. Pancreozymin: from duodenal mucosa—stimulates pancreatic juice secretion rich in enzymes.

3. Cholecystokinin: from duodenal mucosa—stimulates the contraction and emptying of the gall bladder.

4. Enterogastrone: from duodenal mucosa—inhibits motility and depresses the acid secretion by the stomach.

5. Gastrin: from pyloric region of stomach—enhances acid secretion by the stomach.

Reproductive System

Reproductive Organs

Male: Seminiferous tubules of the testis, epididymis, vas deferens, seminal vesicles, prostate, prostatic urethra, membranous urethra, penile urethra, glans penis.

Female: Ovaries, oviduct, uterus, vagina; the breasts (accessory organs).

Hormonal Control

For a detailed discussion of the hormonal interactions concerning the reproductive system, the reader is referred to the section dealing with the endocrine system. However, the cyclic activity of the female organism is briefly summarized since it is of the utmost importance and quite difficult.

The reproductive cycle is under hormonal regulation; gonadotropic hormones of the pituitary (anterior lobe) stimulate the ovaries to produce a mature egg. The pituitary and ovaries have a reciprocal effect upon each other. FSH (follicle stimulating hormone) from the pituitary elicits estrogen production from the developing follicle. When estrogen concentration reaches a certain blood level, it inhibits FSH production. At that time the egg is discharged and the cells lining the follicle come under the influence of another gonadotropin, LH (luteinizing hormone), which influences the development of the corpus luteum. The corpus luteum produces the hormone progesterone, which influences the wall of the uterus in preparation for implantation. As the concentration of progesterone rises, LH production is checked. If fertilization has occurred, the production of FSH is curtailed throughout the period of gestation through the production of estrogen by the placenta and ovary. If fertilization does not occur, the cycle begins anew.

Gametogenesis and Meiosis

The production of gametes, or sex cells—egg and sperm, is known as gametogenesis. Since an individual possesses an equal amount of genetic material from both parents and the same number of chromosomes as either parent, a reduction to one half that number must be accomplished in the development of the egg and sperm. Eggs and sperms are haploid; and a fertilized egg (zygote) possesses the diploid number of the parent again. The reduction occurs during meiosis.

The process of meiosis is best demonstrated in the following manner:

Haploid gametes; either sperm (spermatids) or egg (ova).

$$\underline{1,2} + \underline{1a, 2a}$$

The above unite in fertilization (form zygote) and the diploid adult somatic and primary germ cells are formed.

$$\downarrow$$
$$\underline{1, 1a, 2, 2a}$$

Primary germ cell in the adult undergoes spermatogenesis (male) or oogenesis (female); the result eventually will be haploid cells.

Tetrad formation

$$\downarrow$$
$$\underline{1, 1, 1a, 1a, 2, 2, 2a, 2a}$$

The first meiotic or reduction division occurs next, and results in the following:

$$\underline{1, 1a, 2, 2a} \qquad + \qquad \underline{1, 1a, 2, 2a}$$

Meiosis II occurs now and four haploid cells are produced.

$$\underline{1, 2} \quad \underline{1a, 2a} \qquad \downarrow \qquad \underline{1, 2} \quad \underline{1a, 2a}$$

Even though we have not indicated it, random assortment does take place during the process and chromosome combinations other than those illustrated are possible. In the human male four functional cells (sperms) are produced while in the human female one functional cell (egg) and three polar bodies are produced. This is the general gamut of the process of meiosis.

Mature Gametes

Types of Eggs: Isolecithal eggs are primitive and have a small amount of yolk that is distributed equally; examples are sea urchin eggs and amphioxus eggs. Telolecithal eggs have a large amount of yolk concentrated at one pole (lower or vegetal pole); examples are fish, amphibia, reptile, and bird eggs. Centrolecithal eggs show a concentration of yolk in their center; insect eggs are the prime example.

Semen: Semen is a fluid secreted by the male accessory sex glands, namely, the prostate, seminal vesicles, and bulbo-urethral glands. Fructose is added by the prostate, as are acid phosphatase, citric acid, calcium, and fibrinolysin. The seminal vesicles add phosphoryl-choline. The vas deferens is just a tube through which sperm are transported from the testes to the urethra. Between 3 and 4 ml of semen comprise one ejaculation, which contains between 300 and 400 million sperm cells.

Chromosomes: Forty-four autosomal chromosomes are present in every diploid cell of the human body. Mature gametes, however, are haploid. The total chromosome number of the human being is 46 (male 44 plus X and Y; female 44 plus X and X).

Other Modes of Reproduction

Budding, as in hydra, involves the multiplication of cells in one region of the organism and the organization of these cells into a new individual.

Binary fission or **mitosis** is a division of a cell into two equal parts and in this respect two new organisms (cells).

Parthenogenesis involves a mechanism in which a single cell is set apart for the purpose of reproduction. This cell has the capability to develop into a new organism.

A **hermaphrodite** possesses both male and female reproductive tissue.

Development

Fertilization

The development of a new organism starts with fertilization, the process during which the male and female gametes unite in the *ampulla* of the oviduct (Fallopian tube). The *diploid* (2N) number of chromosomes is achieved in this fusion. The egg (oocyte) is transported from the ovary down the oviduct by the *ciliary* movement and *peristaltic* action of the tube. Sperm pass quite rapidly from the vagina into the uterus, and then into the oviduct; they are propelled by the contractions of the musculature of the uterus and the oviduct and by the tail motion of the sperm itself.

Before fertilization can occur the spermatozoa must undergo *capacitation*, a process during which some of the protective coating of the head is removed. An *acrosome reaction* also occurs; during this process enzymes which are necessary to penetrate the protective barrier of the oocyte are released.

Of the approximately 350 million sperm deposited in a single ejaculation only about 350 reach the egg. Only one is necessary for fertilization but the others, it is thought, help in the dispersal of *corona radiata* cells (a circle, or "crown," of ovarian nurse cells that accompany the egg to this point) by release of enzymes such as hyaluronidase.

After passing through the corona radiata, the fertilizing sperm touches the *zona pellucida,* a protective membrane surrounding the oocyte. The zona reaction then takes place; this prevents multiple sperm penetration. The sperm next touches the inner oocyte cell membrane and fusion of both membranes occurs. Upon entrance of the sperm, the secondary oocyte completes its second maturation division. The nucleus of the now mature ovum is known as the *female pronucleus*. When the male and female pronuclei come in contact, their nuclear membranes vanish, and the chromosomes intermingle. Fertilization is now complete, and the fertilized egg is known as a *zygote*.

Fertilization therefore consists of:

a) penetration of the corona radiata barrier,
b) penetration of the zona pellucida,
c) penetration of the oocyte membrane.

Fertilization results in:

a) restoration of diploid number of chromosomes and variation of species,
b) determination of sex,
c) initiation of cleavage.

Cleavage

About 30 hours after fertilization, the zygote reaches the two-cell stage. Mitotic divisions rapidly increase the number of cells at this time; these small cells are termed *blastomeres* and the developing organism (now a solid ball) is called the *morula*. At approximately the 16-cell stage the zygote consists of centrally located cells, the *inner cell mass*, and a covering layer, the *outer cell mass*. The inner cell mass gives rise to the embryo proper, while the outer cell mass forms the *trophoblast*, which becomes the fetal component of the *placenta*. (In some species, cleavage of an ovum may occur without fertilization; the process is referred to as *parthenogenesis*.)

Blastocyst Formation

As the morula reaches the uterine cavity, fluid starts to accumulate internally between the inner cell mass and the outer cell mass and eventually forms a single cavity, the *blastocele*. The zygote is then referred to as the *blastocyst*. The inner cell mass (at this point located at one pole) now assumes the name *embryoblast*, and the outer cell mass, or *trophoblast*, at this time forms the epithelial wall of the *blastocyst*. By two weeks of gestation, the developing zygote has passed through the morula and blastocyst stages and has begun the implantation process by which it invades the uterine tissue to establish contact with the maternal circulation.

Implantation in the Uterus

Endometrium (uterine mucosa, an epithelium) lines the uterus; *myometrium* forms the thick, middle muscular layer; and *perimetrium* covers the outside of the organ. When the blastocyst arrives the *uterine mucosa* is in the *secretory* or *progestational* phase. Uterine arteries are dilated, glands are enlarged, mucin and glycogen are being produced and the tissue resembles a sponge. Implantation usually occurs either along the anterior or posterior wall of the uterus.

Second Week (Bilaminar Germ Disc Formation)

As the blastocyst embeds the trophoblast differentiates into an inner *cytotrophoblast* and an outer *syncytiotrophoblast* layer. Syncytiotrophoblastic processes invade the endometrial epithelium and stroma. *Lacunae* (spaces) soon appear in the syncytiotrophoblast and fill with maternal blood and secretions; this nutritive material, called *embryotroph*, reaches the embryoblast by diffusion (a primitive uteroplacental circulation). The embryoblast differentiates into *endoderm* and *ectoderm* (two of the three primary germ layers) which form a flat disc known as the *bilaminar germ disc*. Between the cytotrophoblast and ectoderm layer the *amniotic cavity* develops, while beneath the ectoderm, the single layer of endoderm proliferates to form the definitive *yolk sac*. As development proceeds, the extra-embryonic coelom, the cavity between the embryoblast and the trophoblast, expands and the large *chorionic cavity* is formed. Within the chorionic sac, the embryo and its amnion and yolk sac are suspended. Extraembryonic mesoderm lines this cavity and covers the embryoblast, thus connecting it to the trophoblast. As soon as blood vessels develop this connecting stalk will become the *umbilical cord*.

Highlighting this period is the development of the *primitive streak* on the surface of the ectoderm facing the amniotic cavity. The primitive streak functions as the *blastopore* during gastrulation. The cephalic end of this streak is known as the *primitive node*. During gastrulation, mesoderm cells segregate from the ectoderm layer and migrate between the ectoderm and endoderm by way of the primitive streak. In this manner the third primary germ layer, the *mesoderm* is formed between the ectoderm and endoderm except at the prochordal plate (buccopharyngeal membrane) and cloacal membrane.

The *allantois* appears as an outpocketing in the caudal end of the primitive gut around day 16. It stores excretory products in lower forms; it remains rudimentary in humans but plays a vital role as a source of vascular stem cells. During this period, formation of the *somites* from *mesoderm* and formation of the *central nervous system* from *ectoderm* begins. Mesoderm also gives rise to the blood vessels which eventually connect the placenta and the embryo.

Second Month (Germ Layer Differentiation)

During this period the main organ systems become established and external body features such as limb buds, face, ear, nose and eyes become apparent.

Ectodermal Derivatives:

1. The *central and peripheral nervous system,* which develops in conjunction with the notochord. The notochord develops from the notochordal process and establishes a primitive axis for the embryo. (The nucleus pulposus of the intervertebral disc in the adult is the remnant of the notochord.) The established *neural plate* (composed of neuroectoderm above the notochord) forms a neural groove by differential growth and eventually becomes a *neural tube* giving rise to *brain vesicles* and the central canal of the *spinal cord. Neural crest cells,* intermediate in position between the neural tube and surface ectoderm, develop into *dorsal root* and *cranial sensory* ganglia and their associated neurons.

2. *Placodes.* Many complex sensory structures begin their development as placodes, which are simple, localized ectodermal thickenings which invaginate into the underlying tissues and there differentiate into their definitive structures.

a) An *otic placode* forms the *otic pit* and the *otic vesicle* giving rise eventually to organs of hearing and equilibrium.

b) A *lens placode* under induction of the *optic vesicle* gives rise to the lens of the eye.

c) A *nasal placode* gives rise to the *olfactory epithelium* of the nose.

3. The *epidermis,* including hair and nails, and subcutaneous connective tissue.

4. *Mammary glands,* the *pituitary gland* and the *enamel of the teeth.*

Mesodermal Derivatives: The sheet of mesoderm first gives rise to *paraxial mesoderm* (it will become the future paired *somites*), second to the *intermediate mesoderm* (it will become the future excretory units) and third to the *lateral plate* mesoderm (it will split into *somatic* and *splanchnic* (visceral) layers) which will line the intraembryonic *coelomic cavity.*

a. *Somite Differentiation.* Somites are individual blocks of paraxial mesoderm arranged as paired chains along the length of the notochord and neural tube. Each somite will form bone, muscle, and dermis for a specific body segment. At the beginning 4 occipital, 8 cervical, 12 thoracic, 5 lumbar, 5 sacral and 8–10 coccygeal pairs of somites are present; the first occipital and the last 5–7 coccygeal disappear at a later stage. Each somite is organized into a sclerotome, a myotome, and a dermatome.

1. *Sclerotome.* This is formed by *mesenchyme,* or primitive connective tissue, which is multipotent and differentiates into:

a) *fibroblasts,* which give rise to reticular, collagenous and elastic fibers of connective tissue;

b) *chondroblasts,* which give rise to cartilage;

c) *osteoblasts,* which give rise to bone of the vertebral column.

2. *Myotome.* Each myotome gives rise to the skeletal musculature of its segment.

3. *Dermatome.* Cells of this nature give rise to the dermis (skin) and subcutaneous tissue under the skin.

b. *Intermediate Mesoderm Differentiation.* Cells in the cervical and thoracic region will give rise to *nephrotomes;* more caudally located cells form the *nephrogenic cord.* These will become the excretory units of the urinary system.

c. *Lateral Plate Mesoderm*

1. *Somatic.* These cells form the lining of the intraembryonic coelomic cavity and give rise to the non-segmental skeletal muscle of both wall and serous membranes which will eventually line the pericardial, pleural and peritoneal cavities of the adult.

2. *Splanchnic.* These cells differentiate into *angioblasts,* which will give rise to blood cells and the cardiovascular and lymphatic systems. True blood formation starts in the second month and occurs in the liver, spleen, bone marrow and lymph nodes.

Other Mesoderm Derivatives. Besides the structures described, mesoderm also gives rise to the gonads and their ducts, the cortex of the adrenal glands, and the spleen. It is also the source of the smooth muscle of the viscera.

Endodermal Derivatives: This germ layer provides:

1) the epithelial lining of the gastrointestinal system
2) the epithelial lining of the respiratory system
3) the parenchyma of the tonsil, thymus, thyroid, parathyroid, liver and pancreas
4) the epithelial lining of the urinary bladder and urinary tract
5) the epithelial lining of the auditory (Eustachian) tube and the tympanic cavity (middle ear).

At eight weeks the fetus stage has been reached and the dramatic changes leading to organ formation have taken place. The embryonic period now enters a phase of remarkable growth until the *conceptus* is ready for delivery.

Fetal Membranes and Placenta

The fetal membranes are the: amnion, yolk sac, allantois, and chorion. While these membranes originate from the zygote only the *yolk sac* and *allantois* contribute to embryonic structures.

The Amnion: The amniotic cavity is filled with fluid derived from the maternal circulation and from excretory products of the fetus. Amniotic fluid is swallowed by the fetus and taken up by the gastrointestinal system. The embryo, suspended by the umbilical cord, floats in the amniotic fluid. Amniotic fluid:

1) serves as a cushion and absorbs jolts,
2) allows the fetus to move,
3) helps in temperature regulation,
4) separates the amnion from the embryo,
5) provides a hydrostatic wedge during birth.

The Yolk Sac: The yolk sac is formed in the chorionic cavity and is connected to the umbilical cord. No yolk storage takes place in the human. However, the yolk sac plays a role in:

1) nutrient transfer before placental circulation is established,
2) blood development,
3) formation (endodermal component) of the gut,
4) formation (epithelial component) of the respiratory system,
5) formation of the germ cells (spermatogonia and oogonia).

The Allantois: This structure serves in the following manner:

1) it contributes to blood formation,
2) the allantoic blood vessels become the umbilical arteries and vein,
3) via the urachus the bladder is connected to the umbilicus.

The Placenta:

Structure. The placenta is composed of two parts:

1) the maternal part, derived from the endometrial decidua basalis,
2) the fetal part, derived from the chorionic villi.

Decidua. The decidua is the functional layer of the endometrium during pregnancy. Three zones are differentiated:

1) decidua basalis—this is the part deep to the conceptus, which forms the maternal placenta,

2) decidua capsularis—this is the part superficial to the conceptus and closest to the uterine cavity,

3) decidua parietalis—this is the term applied to the remaining portion of the uterine mucosa.

Chorionic Component. Originally the entire chorionic sac is covered by villi; however, around week eight, the villi not associated with the decidua basalis start to degenerate. The villi in relation to the decidua basalis increase in number and size and become the functional fetal portion of the placenta. The maternal and fetal components form an intimate anatomical and functional unit.

Function. Deoxygenated blood is carried from the fetus via the umbilical arteries to the placenta (villi). No mixing of maternal and fetal blood occurs. Exchange takes place over the endothelial barrier of the fetal vessels. Oxygenated blood passes into fetal placental veins, which form the umbilical vein, which supplies the fetus.

The main functions of the placenta are:

1) exchange of metabolic and gaseous products,
2) synthesis of glycogen, cholesterol and fatty acids,
3) synthesis of hormones,
4) transmission of antibodies

Fetal and Neonatal Circulation

The cardiovascular system is designed to meet the needs of the fetus and at birth quickly to adapt to the demands of a new circuit and environment.

Fetal Circulation: Placenta → umbilical vein → ductus venosus of liver (half of the blood bypasses in this manner the hepatic circulation) → inferior vena cava → right atrium → foramen ovale, between right and left atria (blood bypasses the pulmonary circuit) → left atrium → left ventricle → ascending aorta → descending aorta → two umbilical arteries → placenta.

Blood that enters the right ventricle from the right atrium leaves via the pulmonary artery but bypasses the pulmonary circuit by passing through the ductus arteriosus, which connects the pulmonary artery to the aortic arch. In this manner blood reaches the aorta.

Changes at Birth: Due to a cessation of placental blood flow and the activation of the respiratory system because of pressure on the thoracic cavity and the replacement of amniotic fluid by air in the bronchial tree, certain changes are necessary:

1) ductus arteriosus closes due to muscular constriction of its wall,
2) blood flow through the lungs increases and results in a rise of pressure in the left atrium,
3) right atrial pressure drops due to cessation of placental circulation,
4) the above pressure differentials result in the closing of the foramen ovale and complete pulmonary circulation is established,
5) the umbilical arteries close
6) the umbilical vein and ductus venosus close.

Adult Derivatives

	Fetal structure	Adult structure
1)	umbilical vein	→ ligamentum teres
2)	ductus venosus	→ ligamentum venosuum
3)	umbilical arteries	→ a) superior vesicle arteries
		b) medial umbilical ligaments
4)	foramen ovale	→ fossa ovalis
5)	ductus arteriosus	→ ligamentum arteriosum

Multiple Pregnancy

Twinning: Twinning occurs in about 1% of normal births; about 2/3 are of the *dizygotic* (fraternal) twin type. The frequency of dizygotic twins increases with the age of the mother and is influenced by heredity. (No age correlation exists as far as *monozygotic* [identical] twins are concerned.) If a first pregnancy results in twins, subsequent twinning is about 3 to 5 times greater than in the normal population. The *genotype* of the mother seems to be the key determining factor in the frequency of twin births.

Monozygotic Twins (Identical Twins). A single ovum and sperm are involved. The zygote usually splits by the blastocyst stage of development. These embryos have a common placenta and chorionic cavity but possess separate amniotic cavities. These individuals have the same sex and blood groups, and a strong resemblance in external features. (Their phenotypes and genotypes are identical.)

Dizygotic Twins (Fraternal Twins). Two separate oocytes and two separate sperms are involved. Both zygotes are totally different genetically. They may or may not be of the same sex. These zygotes implant independently and develop their own placenta and membranes. (Fraternal twins are not identical in phenotype or genotype. They are no more similar than any other non-twin siblings.)

Triplets: Triplets occur once in about 8,000 pregnancies. They may result from:

1) one zygote and therefore be identical,
2) two zygotes, and therefore give rise to one set of identical twins and one independent infant,
3) three zygotes and result in three independent individuals.

Types of multiple births higher than triplets are rare but similar combinations do occur.

Genetics

Chromosomes within the nucleus of the cells are the source of DNA (deoxyribonucleic acid), the inheritable material; chromosomes contain specific units called genes which are arranged in linear order on the chromosomes. Genes are paired elements, held together in a specific linkage arrangement. One member of each pair of genes separates during germ cell production; therefore, each germ cell contains only one set. An allele is one of a pair of genes that occupies the same locus on homologous chromosomes. Genotype refers to the genetic make-up of the organism. The genotype is expressed via phenotypic characteristics that are visible and observable under normal circumstances.

Mendel is responsible for the discovery of several intriguing phenomena:

1. He showed that each member of a pair of genes will be found in a different gamete; they were contributed to that individual by his parents and underwent no change such as blending while they were associated. This is Mendel's first law (law of segregation) which affirms that *allelomorphs segregate*.

2. Mendel also documented that the distribution of members of one pair has absolutely no bearing on the distribution of another pair. For example, if an individual possesses one pair of alleles Y and y, and another pair Z and z, the individual will produce approximately equal numbers of gametes of the four possible chance combinations of one member from each pair (YZ; Yz; yZ; yz). This law is known as independent assortment; the law does not apply to linked genes but only to genes located on different chromosomes. Independent behavior of chromosomes during meiosis is essential.

Mendel also showed that certain characteristics mask other traits; this phenomenon is known as dominance.

Genetic phenomena are best explained and demonstrated by problem solving, and it will be attempted in this manner.

Mendelian Characteristics

Dominance: Dominance is expressed in terms of a pair of alleles. A gene which produces and expresses the same characteristic whether it is present alone (in the heterozygous state matched to a gene not possessing the same trait) or with a gene possessing the same trait (in the homozygous state) is said to be dominant to the allele with which it is paired. The allele which is ineffective in the expression of its trait in the heterozygote is said to be recessive to the dominant. Let us illustrate with the following example.

The trait of green eyes did not occur in the F_1 (offspring from parents) but made its appearance in the F_2 (offspring of F_1 or offspring of offspring from the parents) generation. We are dealing with a recessive trait that is being masked by a dominant one. AA (brown eyes) bred with aa (green eyes) results in all F_1, Aa (genotypically heterozygous but phenotypically A; all brown eyes). Breeding of the offspring Aa with Aa results in 1 AA 2 Aa 1aa genotype and 3:1 phenotype. The above demonstrates a one factor cross.

Let us now demonstrate several typical two-factor crosses:

1. Crossing of two types of organisms yields the classical 9:3:3:1 ratio. The cross would be considered an expression of phenotypic ratio.

The example calls for a cross between individuals possessing a genetic makeup of RrSs $\times$ RrSs. Construct the Punnett square below and see the results in a 9:3:3:1 phenotypic ratio.

	RS	Rs	rS	rs
RS	RRSS	RRSs	RrSS	RrSs
Rs	RRSs	RRss	RrSs	Rrss
rS	RrSS	RrSs	rrSS	rrSs
rs	RrSs	Rrss	rrSs	rrss

R__S__ or RS = 9
R__ss or Rss = 3
rrS__ or rrS = 3
rrSS or rrss = 1

2. In rabbits, rough coat is dominant over smooth coat. Brown is dominant over grey fur color. A rough, brown male is mated to a couple of smooth, grey females. The offspring are counted as: 18 rough, brown; 21 rough, grey; 16 smooth, brown; 24 smooth, grey. If this male had been mated to a female of his own genotype, what proportion of the offspring would have exhibited rough, grey coats? The answer is 3 out of 16 and is obtained in the following manner.

Basic genetic knowledge is applied.

rough = (dominant)
smooth = (recessive)
brown = (dominant)
grey = (recessive)

The male is crossed to several smooth grey females; they had to be homozygous recessive genotype. Since all four combinations appeared, we can assume that the male was genotypically heterozygous even though he appeared phenotypically dominant. If first we crossed this heterozygous male RrBb $\times$ rrbb, the result would be RrBb; Rrbb; rrBb; rrbb; in other words the four combinations given. Now let us cross the RrBb male $\times$ RrBb female; the following combinations would have to be considered in both male and female: RB; Rb; rB; rb. If these are crossed, we find 3 out of 16 possess rough grey coats (namely RRbb; Rrbb and Rrbb).

Incomplete Dominance: Seeds from a self-pollinated gold flowering plant produce 56 charcoal, 130 gold and 61 beige flowering plants. The plant is heterozygous with incomplete dominance of its traits.

The phenomenon illustrated here is incomplete dominance (blending of two traits). Let us assume:

charcoal	C	
beige	B	
gold		BC

Cross: → BC × BC

Result:
1 BB (beige)
2 BC (gold)
1 CC (charcoal)

Backcross: A backcross consists of crossing a dominant phenotype with a pure homozygous recessive. In this manner a breeder can determine if the phenotype is heterozygous or homozygous. The backcross is used, therefore, to determine if a line is genotypically pure.

Probability Ratios: Genetic ratios are probability ratios. If, for example, we mate (B = black dominant; b = grey recessive) two heterozygous black squirrels (Bb) and 4 offspring are produced, the ratio of 3 black and 1 grey should be probable. However, what are the chances of all black and all grey litters?

Many crosses of heterozygous (Bb) animals will result in a fairly close 3:1 ratio. We, therefore, can see that we have 3 chances out of 4 to produce an individual exhibiting the dominant trait, and 1 chance out of 4 to show the recessive trait.

Therefore, to produce black squirrels (BB or Bb, 3 out of 4) we multiply ¾ × ¾ × ¾ × ¾ = 81/256; to produce grey squirrels (bb, 1 out of 4) we multiply ¼ × ¼ × ¼ × ¼ = 1/256.

Polygenic Traits

In morning glories, genes C and P are necessary for pink flowers. In the absence of either (ccP__ or C__pp) or both (ccpp) of these genes, the flowers are blue. What will be the result of the following crosses as far as flower color of the offspring and proportion of the offspring are concerned? Cross a. Ccpp × ccPp = 1 pink : 3 blue; b. ccpp × CcPp = 1 pink : 3 blue.

In essence the expression of pink requires C__ P__, and all others will be blue. The offspring may be Cc or cc with equal probability (i.e., 50%); the same is true for Pp and pp (50%). If the chance of C__ is 0.5 and the chance of P__ is 0.5, then the chance of C__ P__ is 0.5 × 0.5 = 0.25. Thus, 1/4 will be pink and 3/4 will be blue.

Sex Determination: A male carries an XY and a female an XX complement of chromosomes. If a male embryo were to result, the sperm that fertilizes an egg would have to possess a Y chromosome.

Sex-Linked Traits: Both sexes carry a complete complement of sex-linked genes. A female, however, with the XX arrangement will only exhibit a recessive gene if it has received it from both parents (a rare event if we are dealing with an uncommon gene of the population) while in the male with the XY arrangement the recessive gene cannot be masked since there is no partner X chromosome and, therefore, a larger number of recessive genes are expressed (examples are hemophilia and color blindness). A man receives his X chromosome from his mother and passes it on to his daughters not his sons. His daughters in this respect are the carriers of his sex-linked traits and their sons will be the affected ones. Let us illustrate with an example. The normal czarinas of Russia produced sons suffering from hemophilia, a disease that is caused by a sex-linked recessive gene, h. The more dominant gene, H, produces normal blood clotting. Genotypically, these women must have carried Hh (X_H and

X_h). A daughter, depending on the father ($X_H Y$ or $X_h Y$), could have carried $X_H X_h$ or $X_H X_H$ while a son could have been born with either an $X_H Y$ or an $X_h Y$ (hemophilic) chromosomal complement.

Another way of expressing a sex-linked or, strictly speaking, sex-limited phenomenon is shown in the example below.

A cattle breeder has in his herd a y-linked trait which produces white stockings. A calf sired by a white-stockinged bull is born. The breeder determines that the chances of white stockings by this inheritance are 50%. If the calf born had been a female, the chances of exhibiting the trait (or serving as a carrier) were zero. The explanation is that the male may contribute gametes containing either X or Y chromosomes, but the female can contribute only gametes containing X chromosomes. If the X chromosome is contributed by the male, an unaffected female offspring will result; if the Y chromosome is contributed by the male, an affected male offspring will result. These two possibilities are of equal probability (i.e., 50%). If the sex of the offspring is known, there is no doubt about whether it has the trait. All males (100%) and no females (0%) would have the trait. Females could not even be carriers for a Y-linked trait.

Mutation: A mutation may be thought of as a sudden change in the genetic makeup of the organism. It may be beneficial or harmful. It may occur spontaneously or may be experimentally produced with chemicals, X-rays, cosmic rays, and so forth. It may or may not be passed on to the next generation because, for example, it may be lethal or otherwise preclude reproduction.

Blood Types: The ABO blood grouping system is explained on the basis of a single triallelic system with genes A, B, and O operating at a single genetic locus. Phenotypic and genotypic characteristics may be expressed as follows:

Phenotype	Genotype
A	A/A; A/O
B	B/B; B/O
O	O/O
AB	A/B

The A and B genes appear to be codominant; they are dominant over O, which is recessive.

As can be seen from the above table, there are four major blood types and the explanation as to universal donor and recipient is based on the following:

Type	Agglutinogens on Cells	Agglutinins in Serum and Plasma
AB—can receive A, B, AB or O (universal recipient)	A, B	none
A —can receive A, O	A	anti b
B —can receive B, O	B	anti a
O —can receive only O, but can give to all; therefore, O is the universal donor	O	anti ab

Rh Factor: Rhesus (Rh) agglutinogen is present in humans and is represented by a dominant gene R. The agglutinogen of an Rh positive fetus passes across the placenta, enters the maternal blood stream, and elicits the production of an agglutinin (antibody) by the mother. The agglutinin passes into the circulation of the fetus and if present in sufficient concentration can produce agglutination, at times fatal to the developing fetus.

Mode of Inheritance of Some Common Human Traits: Among the human traits inherited as single-gene dominants are:

a) brachydactyly (short digits),
b) white forelock in the hair,
c) blue sclera (white of the eye),
d) Rh-positive blood.

Among the traits inherited as recessives:

a) albinism (lack of skin pigment),
b) alkaptonuria (urine turns black).

Sex-linked traits:

a) hemophilia,
b) colorblindness.

Crossing-Over: During the process of meiosis a recombination of genetic material is possible. One way this is effected is through crossing over. In crossing-over, comparable portions of chromatids are exchanged. Since crossing-over is more the rule than the exception, we shall illustrate it with two diagrams. These portions may differ in alleles but they do carry the same gene sites (loci) and control the same specific trait, as, for example, eye color.

Let us start with one pair of homologous chromosomes:

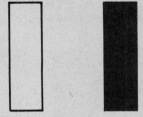

As illustrated, replication results during the first part of meiosis in four chromatids:

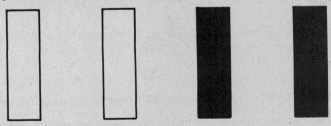

Of the four chromatids, two may exchange materials in a process known as crossing-over:

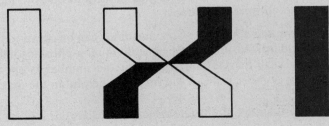

The configuration shown by the central two chromosomes is termed a chiasma, the region where crossing-over occurs. After separation in the second reduction division of meiosis, the resulting chromatids include two recombinants, having new combinations of genetic material.

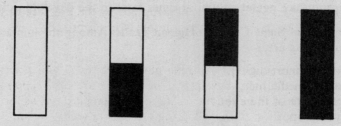

We shall next illustrate crossover using two specific genes.

Parents

$$
\begin{array}{ccc}
| & & | \\
A & & a \\
| & + & | \\
B & & b \\
| & & |
\end{array}
$$

Two gametes unite and form a new hybrid individual (F_1).

F_1

$$
\begin{array}{cc}
| & | \\
A & a \\
| & | \\
B & b \\
| & |
\end{array}
$$

Without crossover these four gametes are produced:

$$
\begin{array}{cccc}
| & | & | & | \\
A & A & a & a \\
| & | & | & | \\
B & B & b & b \\
| & | & | & |
\end{array}
$$

With crossing-over these four gametes are produced,

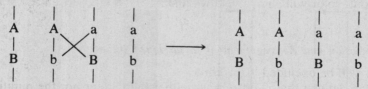

and the result is two new types of gametes with new combinations of genes.

Crossing-over may occur anywhere along the chromosome; however, the recombination frequency is higher for genes separated by a greater distance than those that are close together. Crossing-over has provided the investigator with the tool to measure distances between genes and make chromosome maps.

Abnormalities in Chromosome Number: Chromosomes can be identified in somatic cells and a *karyotype,* a standardized display of an individual's chromosomes, can be constructed. Chromosomes vary in size and shape but the number is species specific. In humans the chromosome number is 46. A karyotype is helpful in the diagnosis of genetic abnormalities.

In humans some abnormalities of chromosome number are:

Down's syndrome (formerly called mongolism) This phenomenon is most often characterized by three, instead of two, chromosomes 21 in group G; a total number of 47 chromosomes are present in these individuals.

Turner's syndrome Females possess only one X chromosome (not the normal female XX). Total number of chromosomes present is 45.

Klinefelter's syndrome This syndrome is characterized by the presence of two X chromosomes and a Y, which results in 47 chromosomes being present.

Epistasis (or Gene Interaction): In morning glories, genes C and P are necessary for pink flowers. In the absence of either (*ccP__* or *C__pp*) or both (*ccpp*) of these genes, the flowers are blue. What will be the result of the following crosses as far as flower color of the offspring and proportion of the offspring are concerned?

$$Ccpp \times ccPp = 1 \text{ pink}:3 \text{ blue};$$

$$ccpp \times CcPp = 1 \text{ pink}:3 \text{ blue}$$

In essence the expression of pink requires $C\_\_P\_\_$, and all others will be blue. In this example, the epistasis is of the complementary interaction type. The offspring may be Cc or cc with equal probability (i.e., 50%); the same is true for Pp and pp (50%). If the chance of $C\_\_$ is 0.5 and the chance of $P\_\_$ is 0.5, then the chance of $C\_\_P\_\_$ is $0.5 \times 0.5 = 0.25$. Thus, 1/4 will be pink and 3/4 will be blue.

Polygenic Traits: Certain conditions are determined by genes at several loci. Each of the genes involved has a small effect which may be additive. Expression of this kind of trait is usually very sensitive to environmental influences.

Lethal Genes: Certain genes are lethal in the homozygous condition and cause the demise of the organism. An example is yellow coat in mice. If two hybrid yellow mice are mated the typical 1:2:1 genotypic ratio results—namely, 1/4 homozygous dominant (yellow dead embryos), 1/2 hybrid (yellow mice), and 1/4 homozygous recessive (wild type or agouti mice), but the phenotypic ratio among the live born mice is 2 yellow: 1 gray.

Modifying Genes: These genes affect the performance of other genes but apparently exhibit no trait of their own. If, for instance, in mice the gene for black hair is present, the gene for agouti color will elicit a yellow banding. When it is absent there is no effect.

Paternity Exclusion and Reassignment of Misassigned Infants

1) Paternity will be excluded if the child
   a) Has an antigen that is present in neither the mother nor the putative father;
   b) Does not have an antigen that the putative father has and would have had to give to his progeny (for example, a type O child and a type AB putative father).

2) Correct reassignment of infants misassigned to parents in a hospital is often achieved by looking for any of the following kinds of incompatibilities between the infants and the couples and then assigning each infant to the couple with which only compatibilites exist:
   a) The child has an antigen present in neither spouse;
   b) The child lacks one or more antigens that either or both spouses would have had to give him/her.

3) Increased probability of exclusion of a falsely accused male or of correct parental reassignment of misassigned infants results if several kinds of blood groups, HLA, and some of the following kinds of other genetically determined proteins are also included in the studies: hemoglobins, serum proteins, red cell enzymes, and several other enzymes.

The Animal Kingdom

Distribution of Living Organisms

Every living organism has a distinct yet interactive role, a place, and a mode of life, which are determined by that individual's structure and physiological makeup. The earth represents diverse *habitats* (places where one lives), which are characterized by conditions such as temperature, moisture, soil conditions, terrain, pressure, chemical cycles (gases and minerals), sunlight, seasonal variations, and others; organisms (species) must adapt and adjust their *life cycles* to the *climate* they live in. No species lives in a vacuum and is entirely independent; all are part of an integrated, systematically functioning, living (dynamic) *community* that includes many varieties of plants, animals, viruses, etc.

Although many populations of different species live together as a *community*, and although *turnover* is continuous, automatic, and self-adjusting, the result is an internally balanced community; there is a remarkable numerically steady state that is determined essentially by food supply, reproduction, and protection of the bonds of interdependency of community members.

Six factors are important to any habitat.

1. *Temperature* controls the speed of every reaction; raising the temperature by 10°C doubles the speed. While there exists a large range of temperature, most life exists in a narrow range; species have limits, and most are destroyed by excess at either end of the scale. Warm-blooded organisms (mammals and birds) possess internal regulation of body temperature, whereas cold-blooded animals (fishes, reptiles, amphibians, and invertebrates) do not and their function is directly related to their external environment. The oceans represent a fairly stable environment, and marine organisms are less prone to seasonal variations. Many land animals have adapted to seasonal changes by migration or hibernation.

2. *Moisture* (water) is critical to the existence of life since it is a solvent (minerals used by plants), a constituent of tissues, and the medium in which many species live and breed. The water cycle (evaporation, cloud formation, precipitation, drainage, and soil percolation) is dynamic and continuous (between sea, land, and air) and affects every particle of the universe. Also, water prevents rapid temperature fluctuations, a critical element in homeostasis.

3. *Soil conditions* are a crucial factor. The chemical makeup of the soil determines the presence or type of plants and, in some cases, the animals of the region. Texture and porosity play a role in moisture content, pH, and the presence or abscence of burrowing animals. Slope affects drainage, while exposure to sunlight modulates absorption of heat.

4. *Pressure* varies with elevation (atmospheric pressure reflected in barometric reading) and with depth (water pressure: 15 pounds/10 meters equals one atmosphere of pressure). Availability of oxygen decreases with increasing altitude and depth. People living at high altitudes have higher red blood cell (erythrocyte) counts to compensate.

5. *Chemical interchange* occurs continuously in all habitats. Here are three good examples:

   a. Oxygen derived from air and water serves the oxidative machinery of life; after usage it returns to the life cycle in the form of carbon dioxide or, combined with hydrogen, as water. Carbon dioxide is used in the process of photosynthesis; some of the oxygen released is utilized by plants in respiration, but most is returned to the environment.

   b. Nitrogen is utilized directly by nitrogen-fixing bacteria to produce plant proteins; after utilization by animals these become animal proteins, and their eventual metabolic fate results in nitrogeneous wastes. These wastes are converted by bacteria into nitrites and ammonia with release of nitrogen into the atmosphere; the nitrites are converted into nitrates, which again are utilized to make plant proteins.

   c. Carbon is the backbone of protoplasm; it is derived from carbon dioxide (via photosynthesis) and synthesized into carbohydrates, which, together with proteins and fats, comprise the tissues of all plants and animals. Metabolism returns carbon for recycling as carbon dioxide.

6. *Sunlight* provides all the energy utilized by most living organisms. Energy is transformed from one type to another, but it is neither created nor destroyed. Lavoisier (1743–1794) showed that processes of organisms conform to the First Law of Thermodynamics—namely, the total amount of energy in a system is constant but is capable of transformation. Radiation from the sun includes heat, visible light, and ultraviolet radiation. Solar radiation, especially of the longer wavelengths, controls most climatic variations because of the effects of soil heating, water evaporation, and air expansion. Light controls the photoperiod responsible for the flowering of plants and the migration of animals.

Interrelationships of Animals

Competition for food, shelter, and mates is considerable; some organisms (termites, bees), however, have developed a coorperative society based on distinct roles (workers, protectors, reproducers, nurses, etc.). Plants (producers—autotrophs) commonly compete for sunlight (energy), minerals, and water. The passing of energy from one organism to another constitutes the *food chain* or pyramid; the small (more abundant) are eaten by the large (fewer in number). Plants are eaten by *herbivores* (primary consumers); these in turn are eaten by *carnivores* (secondary consumers); and as larger carnivores eat smaller ones the energy is passed along the chain. As the energy is transferred through the predator chain, the total declines progressively, and successive members are usually larger in size but fewer in number. Organisms eaten by a predator are called *prey*; an organism that consumes its own species is considered a *cannibal*, and one that devours dead material is a *scavenger*.

Factors such as disease control the number of organisms in the food chain; organisms such as viruses, rickettsias, bacteria, protozoans, parasitic worms, and arthropods which by themselves are populations also control the populations on/in which they live. The *parasite* obtains its food from its host, generally harming the host. *Ectoparasites* (lice) live *on* the host, while *endoparasites* (trichina worm) live *in* the host (gut or tissues). Some parasites such as the tick are intermediate hosts, as demonstrated in the transmission of Rocky Mountain spotted fever. Parasites that may destroy the host are called *pathogenic*, and are a considerable element in the regulation and control of the host population. All viruses are parasitic, and bacteria that lack photosynthetic abilities (are saprotrophic) are also parasitic.

The long-term relationship of two organisms of different species is commonly referred to as *symbiosis*. When one gains without harming the other, we speak of *commensalism* (barnacles on whales and epiphytes—plants—that grow on another host plant); in *mutualism* both parties are benefited (the flagellate in the termite digests the wood the termite eats, and the tick bird on the rhinoceros eats ticks, and cleans and warns the larger animal of danger).

Saprophytism is the obtaining of food from dead or decaying material (bacteria of decay and filamentous fungi are examples); the saprophytes essentially function to release chemicals back to the food chain. Without their role many essential elements would soon be unavailable, and the balance of energy transfer and transformation would be disturbed.

As previously emphasized, no organism can be successful in isolation since every specialized being depends on others for some product or process. The smallest congregation of like organisms is the *family*; a larger number comprises a *population*. The key element of a population is the fact that its members interbreed with one another; all populations are composed of *species*. Reproductive barriers exist between species. Speciation has many causes, such as separation by differences in climate, mountain ranges, rivers, or just distance. Only inheritable variations (e.g., skin color) controlled by genes are transmitted to new generations; acquired ones (e.g., muscle build) die with the individual. Individual variations of the members of a species are denoted as *polymorphism*, while the differences due only to sex are referred to as dimorphism.

All organisms live together in a dynamic state under the influence of environmental (chemical and physical) factors; not all are friendly since natural enemies exist for every species (they consume one another or compete for the same food source). Protective adaptation helps in survival. Many organisms blend well into their surroundings (polar bears are white), so that they are hard to see; some organisms such as the flounder can adapt readily to several backgrounds, and others (insects are good examples) mimic their surroundings (butterflies look like flowers and leaves).

Population Dynamics

According to their mode of mobility, organisms are classified as *free-living* (the organism gets around by itself) or *sessile* (it is fixed to another structure). Among both groups there are *solitary* (independent) individuals and others that live in colonies (groups).

All organisms of one species that live in a definable area comprise a population that has distinct organizational features.

As part of the group dynamics of a population, certain factors must be considered:

1) *population density* — the number of organisms in a unit of area,
2) *birth rate* — the number of new organisms per unit of time,
3) *mortality rate* — the number of organisms dying per unit of time,
4) *reproductive or biotic potential* — the potential of a population to increase its numbers under optimal conditions.

Populations are usually considered in terms of the number per unit occupying a given area. As mentioned before, the number of larger organisms is considerably smaller. *Biotic potential* (maximum rate of increase) is continuously checked by *environmental resistance* (competition, disease, inclement climate, etc.). When a population settles in a new area, growth at first is slow (lack of mates), then increases rapidly (exponentially), and finally levels off as an equilibrium is reached because of limits of food supply, the settling of suitable habitats, and the increase of parasites and predators. Usually, as a population increases the environmental resistance, which initially was low, also increases as a result of population density.

A dynamic community of different plants and animals (interdependent) evolves to form an *ecosystem* with the physical environment. No situation is permanent; and while some changes occur rapidly, most are due to a sequential *succession* (lake–pond–swamp–grassland). No one species is present in every corner of the world; geography (geographical range) and environment (ecological range) are key elements. Physical (land and water), climatic (temperature and moisture), and biological (food and predators) barriers are limiting factors to the spread of populations.

Each species requires certain minimal elements for growth and reproduction; this fact led Liebig in 1840 to formulate the "law of the minimum," which states that the rate of growth of an organism is limited by the factor present in the scarcest amount. Too much of a certain factor, according to Shelford (1913), can be just as limiting since the well being of a species is determined by its *range of tolerance*. Organisms are usually more sensitive during development and early and late in life. The range varies greatly from factor to factor. *Stenothermic* organisms can tolerate only slight variations in temperature, while *eurythermic* organisms are able to survive a wide range.

Major Environments – Habitats

1. Water:

a. *Salt Water*. Over 70 percent of the earth is covered by salt water, and the environment, while varying widely overall, is quite stable in a specific region in regard to temperature (a range of 35°C), gas composition, and salinity (30–37 parts of salt per thousand). Ocean currents affect movements of marine organisms and the adjacent regional climate. Tidal fluctuations affect organisms in the shore region. Depth varies, pressure increases with depth, while light decreases with depth (about a 600-ft limit).

b. *Fresh Water*. Freshwater bodies are scattered in their distribution, have less volume and depth, and exhibit great variability in temperature, gas composition, mineral content, light penetration, and mobility. Organisms living in fresh water, because of its low salinity (low osmotic pressure), have had to develop organs for effectively regulating the osmotic pressure. Unlike oceans, freshwater bodies are subject to periodic drying, changing flow rates, and high turbidity.

2. Land or Terrestrial Habitat:

The greatest variability is present on land, when one considers minerals, topography, temperature, water content, air movement, and light. Temperature and moisture vary tremendously with the seasons, altitude, latitude, and with topography. Soil and air temperatures vary as much as 120°C.

Learning, Conditioning, Rhythms

1. Learning:

Many definitions of learning exist, but the process of learning, simply defined, is a change in the behavior of an organism based on some experience or practice. Many organisms have been very successful without much learning; their inborn patterns or instincts allow them to compete for food, find shelter, mate, and live out their life spans. Familiar examples of instinctive behavior are spiders spinning webs (specific patterns), birds building nests and migrating and returning, and fish returning to spawning grounds thousands of miles away. More complex, but still instinctive, are societies of bees and ants where a definite division of labor exists. Humans, on the other hand, while high in the evolutionary scale, must learn from their interaction with the environment and use that knowledge to succeed; for many years a human child is quite dependent, while most animals from day 1 are quite independent. Changes in behavior are often hard to assess but might include:

(a) a new pattern of the organism, and

(b) a change in the response to a stimulus not previously exhibited.

2. Conditioning:

Many of our actions seem automatic, and in most instances we cannot attribute definite reasons for them. These behaviors (responses) may be learned even though we have no recollection of the learning process. On the other hand, many actions are unlearned reflexes. An example of the latter is the fact that the autonomic nervous system (sympathetic and parasympathetic) allows an organism to adapt to certain phenomena. When we walk into bright sunlight the sphincter pupillae contracts, but if we enter a dark area the dilator opens the pupillary opening; the sphincter is under parasympathetic, and the dilator under sympathetic, control. For close vision (reading) convergence and change in the shape of the lens allow the eye to accommodate. Salivary secretion (parotid, submandibular, and sublingual glands) and tearing by the lacrimal gland of the eye are other superb examples of these homeostatic reflexes. Fright produces an increase in heart rate, blood pressure, and metabolic states to prepare an organism to cope; all this takes place at the subconscious level.

Classical Conditioning. Some actions, however, can be learned by a process called *classical conditioning*, that is, learning to associate two previously linked phenomena. First reported by Pavlov in 1927, it is exemplified by the responses of dogs to the introduction of food. When a dog sees or smells food, it is stimulated to begin a reflexive behavior—secretion of saliva. Pavlov restrained dogs in a harness and then simply used an auditory stimulus such as a bell. When the bell was rung, the dog did not secrete saliva. When food alone was provided, the expected salivary secretion occurred. If, thereafter, the two stimuli—bell and food—were presented for some time simultaneously, salivary secretion occurred. After many trials, the bell alone elicited the salivary response; the dog had learned to react to a different stimulus via conditioning. In 1920 Watson showed the same reaction in an 11-month-old baby, who was conditioned by a loud noise and the presentation of a furry object to eventually be frightened by fur alone. Many of the results of conditioning can be reversed through reconditioning the organism to a different association.

Pavlov identified five components of classical conditioning:

1) unconditioned stimulus—the food; it automatically stimulates salivation;
2) conditioned stimulus—the bell; it is neutral at the beginning but eventually effective and undistinguishable;
3) reinforcement—the pairing of two stimuli;
4) unconditioned response—salivation—the automatic response by the parasympathetic division of the autonomic nervous system;
5) conditioned response—the bell—the response as a result of learning by the central nervous system; the unconditioned and conditioned stimuli function as one.

Five other aspects of conditioning should be mentioned.

1. Extinction. The conditioned response can be reversed. Pavlov showed that, after an animal was conditioned, if for some time thereafter only the bell was rung without food being offered, the flow of saliva started to decrease and eventually stopped.
2. Spontaneous Recovery. In this set of experiments, Pavlov let a response achieve extinction and then gave the animal a long rest from the experimental protocol. After this rest the bell was rung and the response reappeared. This spontaneous recovery may explain phenomena we all experience, such as fears or preferences for certain things for which we have no conscious basis.
3. Stimulus Generalization. In these experiments, Pavlov was able to show that somewhat different but basically similar stimuli (e.g., different tones of music) may evoke the same response and effect. The more similar the new stimulus is to the familiar one, the stronger the response usually will be.
4. Stimulus Discrimination. In another set of experiments, food was offered to animals only at the sound of a specific bell, and salivation was elicited only when that particular bell was rung. The animal did not salivate at the ringing of a different bell; it had learned to discriminate between different stimuli.
5. Onset of Neurotic Behavior. In 1927 Pavlov also observed that, after an animal had learned stimulus discrimination and then the difference between the two stimuli was decreased to the point where the animal could not recognize it, the animal's behavior become unpredictable and aberrant.

In general, conditioning is best accomplished when a short interval between stimuli is used and when positive phenomena are elicited or are the end result. Conditioning is also enhanced when the stimulus is truly different (strong and novel) from many of the background stimuli.

Operant Conditioning. The results described above are due chiefly to the influence of the learning process on autonomic reflexes. However, other forms of behavior are also of consequence in reactions to stimuli. When, for instance, a cat is introduced into a new environment, the animal will react by exploring and marking its territory. In this case, the organism itself is acting on the environment, and the activity is referred to as *operant behavior*. Learning can modify these actions, as Skinner demonstrated in the 1930s with the help of a box and a food bar to reward the animal for a certain action.

In 1938 Skinner observed that a rat placed in a box explored actively and even pressed a bar that released a pellet of food. At first the animal did not make an association but soon learned to connect the pressing of the food lever with the dispensing of food and a reward for the action of pressing. The key element in this situation is that reinforced operant behavior is repeated (the lever is pressed frequently), while nonreinforced activities are quickly abandoned. Extinction, spontaneous recovery, and stimulus generalization and discrimination are also part of operant behavior.

Instrumental Conditioning (Operant) and the Law of Effect. In 1898 Thorndike addressed similar issues and found that, when cats were placed in a box and had to learn to open the door in order to obtain food, the reward enhanced their conditioning. The law of effect essentially states that, when a stimulus is followed by a reward, the response is strong, consistent, and likely to be repeated by the experimental subject.

Certain factors called *reinforcers* have been identified by psychological researchers:

1. Primary—in animals, food and water.
2. Secondary—love and affection, shown, for example, by petting.
3. Immediate—a reward given upon accomplishing a feat produces the most efficient learning.
4. Constant—repeated (short-interval) stimuli result in very efficient and rapid learning.
5. Partial—extinction is less apt to occur if there is at least partial reinforcement.

Operant Escape—Escape Learning. When an animal is exposed to an unpleasant stimulus (shock), it will quickly learn to leave the environment to avoid the experience.

Operant Avoidance—Active Avoidance Learning. If an animal is conditioned to a warning signal (bell) and knows that a shock will follow, it will heed the warning and rapidly leave the hostile environment.

Aversive Conditioning. In this experimental setup the unconditioned stimulus is offensive and is of negative value to the organism. In this case the organism (e.g., after a shock is administered) not only exhibits a specific response such as muscular twitching but also develops a generalized "fear reaction," which results in modification of heart rate, respiratory activity, sweating, etc.

Primary Activities. Many activities occur as the organism goes through life, but some very organized ones are limited to early development. Human beings are fairly helpless, but other animals (e.g., rats) on day 1 can perform highly complex motor patterns independently. Two classical phenomena of rat behavior will serve as examples:

1. Suckling. Suckling involves some very complicated sensory input aspects, helps meet the nutritional needs of the organism, is an effective reinforcing activity leading to other skills, and provides thermal support and transport for the young. In order for suckling to occur, the mother's nipple must be coated by amniotic fluid, saliva, or both; the pup *in utero* swallows and excretes amniotic fluid during the last trimester and it is that familiarity with the substances that directs the pup's first act of suckling. Also, since the mother licks the pups and the nipples (milkline), saliva is a behavioral stimulus. The key factor in this primary activity is that it is the animal's previous exposure to the stimulus that leads it to react to it (it has had gustatory and olfactory clues). Thereafter, however, the pup's saliva becomes the stimulus. Ability of the pup to adapt to its new environment is categorized as developmental plasticity.

2. Huddling. This activity is undertaken by neonates and is beneficial in temperature regulation, which results in less energy expenditure by the young (a homeostatic response). Huddling is not a self-serving mechanism; it benefits the whole brood. An animal starting at the periphery will eventually end up in the center, and so on; the

shifting of places helps the group to survive and to adapt to and identify with littermates. Young animals that know their littermates will find their nest readily.

Conditioning and Biofeedback. Biofeedback manipulation is an attempt by the physician to let the individual know what his/her spontaneous functions—heart rate, blood pressure, respiratory activity, skin and internal body temperature, brain waves, peristaltic activity, muscular activity—are at a particular time and circumstance. Patients learn, for example, to recognize when their muscles are tense and may with conditioning be able to relax them to avoid spasms or relieve tension; in the same way vascular headaches may perhaps be avoided. In these procedures patients learn to manipulate and control nonconscious processes. Although results have been mixed, this arena has excited the imagination of researchers and is undergoing active analysis.

3. Rhythms—Biological Clocks: Interest has mainly focused on rhythms that appear in close approximation with natural periodicities such as day-night cycles; tidal rhythms; monthly, seasonal and annual phenomena; circadian rhythms (about 24 hours); and circa-tidal rhythms (12-hour cycles in marine organisms).

Rhythms are present from the cellular to the tissue–organ–system–organismal level, and from unicellular organisms to humans. Circadian rhythms persist even when the cues for the cycle are deleted. When cues are controlled, cycles are extremely constant and exact, but in the wild they tend to vary slightly. There is considerable evidence that endogenous and autonomic, genetically controlled mechanisms account for the persistence of rhythms.

Most living things, both animals and plants, show a circadian rhythm of activity and rest. It is well documented that humans perform differently on physiological and psychological tests at different periods of the day and night. Local time is not a critical factor, as has been well established by shift workers who work at night and sleep during the day; the shift worker's temperature is falling during the daytime, while in the rest of the population, which is working, temperatures are rising. The shift worker at the same time exhibits low levels of adrenal steroids, while in the rest of the population levels are high. These are relevant examples that the body's biological clock adjusts to the mechanical clock of society.

Characteristics of Rhythms. Rhythms are usually described in terms of four characteristics.

1) *Period*—the number of times required to complete the cycle; it is the time between peaks.
2) *Frequency*—the number of times that a peculiar event, such as sleeping occurs.
3) *Phase*—time location when a specific event occurs in a particular organism; the highs and lows of a substance are phase phenomena. Adrenal corticosteroid levels in day and night workers can be described as 180 degrees out of phase;
4) *Amplitude*—the extent (amount) of change that takes place (e.g., body temperature varies as much as 2° during one cycle).

Factors that Affect Rhythms. Among the commonly cited factors that influence rhythms are these six:

1) geomagnetic fields,
2) cosmic rays,
3) electric fields,
4) X-rays,
5) light and darkness,
6) atmospheric pressure.

Cycles can be disrupted by many factors; commonly cited ones are shift work, jet travel, and space flight.

Importance of Rhythms. As a consquence of our daily circadian rhythms we have a susceptibility or a resistance to drugs, stress, allergy, pain, infection, and many other factors. The responsiveness to different regimens, doses, and procedures have ramifications in therapeutic plans. The outcome of surgical procedures and the effect of anesthetic agents certainly are influenced by rhythms and the time they were performed and administered, respectively. Pain tolerance, for instance, shifts according to the time of day (more pain is experienced at night). What is just an annoyance at one time in the cycle is fatal at another point. Births and deaths mainly occur at night and in the early morning. Ulcers, allergies, and psychoses are more prevalent in the spring. Arctic hysteria is a winter phenomenon. In humans, deaths from arteriosclerotic disease peak in January and suicides in May.

To illustrate the importance of rhythms in every activity, here is a partial list of the factors they influence:

1. Body and skin temperature
2. Blood pressure
3. Pulse rate
4. Respiration
5. Blood sugar levels and glucose tolerance
6. Hemoglobin levels
7. Protein utilization and amino acid levels
8. Production and breakdown of ATP
9. Adrenal hormone levels
10. Urinary production, volume, and rate and urinary electrolytes
11. Mitosis
12. Enzyme activities
13. EEG rhythms
14. Stamina and physical vigor
15. Emotional state
16. Metabolic rate
17. Pancreatic enzymatic activity and insulin production

Evolution

The cornerstone of evolution is the fact that species arise from preexisting species.

Key People and Concepts

Aristotle (384–322 B.C.) philosophized that living organisms represent a succession and progression of more suitable forms, rather than random creations.

Redi (1626–1898) showed by experiment that organisms do not arise spontaneously from nonliving material; he demonstrated that maggots did not appear in meat unless the meat was exposed to flies, which laid thier eggs on it.

Spallanzani (1729–1799) repeated Redi's work and showed that no life appeared in solutions first boiled and then protected from air.

Lamarck (1744–1829) believed that simple animals and plants are spontaneously generated but that lineage presents a series of evolutionary forms and that there can be independent branching and development. However, his incorrect ideas of inherited characteristics and of use and disuse of parts overshadowed his correct ideas that individual variations are retained because of adaptive value and that these variations lead to the emergence of different species suited for particular environments.

John Ray (1627–1705) was the first to attempt to define a species and to point out the difference between constant and incidental features of organisms.

Louis Pasteur (1822–1895) showed that life cannot arise in a medium from which all living things are excluded.

Charles Darwin (1809–1882) and *Alfred Russel Wallace* (1823–1913) documented the fact that natural processes can bring about a gradual development of new types.

Alfred Russel Wallace sent a manuscript to Darwin that dealt with the tendency of organisms to depart from the original type. Wallace had observed the same things as Darwin had on his voyage on the *Beagle*, and Darwin, being the scholar and gentleman he was, forwarded Wallace's article for publication and included a short article on his own observations. The failure of the articles to arouse much interest gave Darwin the impetus to proceed with his own work, and in 1859 he published his *Origin of Species by Natural Selection*. He argued two main premises:

1. No two members of a species are exactly alike even if they have the same parents.
2. Some variations are advantages, giving the organism the chance to branch out into new environments and to enlarge its numbers, while others are detrimental and diminish its chances of survival.

These premises lead to the conclusion that a population is likely to change in the relative frequency of its various characteristics (i.e., it *evolves*), because of the *natural selection* of some characteristics over others. The environment was cited as a major cause of natural selection, because it weeds out organisms with unfavorable characteristics and strengthens those with favorable variations.

As one can gather, the modern theory of evolution is not the work of a single individual, but it was Darwin, via his careful documentation and voluminous writings, who marshaled the evidence.

Process of Evolution

The basis of evolution is the inheritable genetic material; the forces (natural selection) can be demonstrated by the principles of Mendelian population genetics. Free reproduction within a population results in the shuffling and reshuffling of the genetic pool. As two populations (sister populations) interbreed, the total genetic material of a species continues to be shuffled, and one can readily see that inheritable features may arise by sexual recombination or by mutation. The individuals whose genes are passed on to the next generation with greater frequency will be those whose genes give them the ability to produce many viable offspring, because of their favorable ability to survive, to mate, to produce gametes, and to have the offspring survive to their own age of reproduction. It is via this mode that a genetically favorable trait is spread and a change that starts in one individual is distributed to the whole population. Generally, many such changes occur before a new species evolves; evolution is a very slow process. Thus, this basic process of evolution consists of:

1) The appearance of an inheritable trait by sexual recombination or mutation, and
2) the spreading of this trait via reproduction to successive generations.

In 1906 De Vries proposed that mutations (sudden changes in the genetic material) were largely responsible for many evolutionary features exhibited, since they are transmitted to future generations. Radiation (cosmic and other), mutagens (chemicals), and temperature probably cause most mutations. Most are unfavorable; advantageous ones, however, survive if occurring in gametes and are often utilized by humans (short-legged sheep that cannot jump fences readily and many varieties of flowers are good examples).

Adaptive Radiation

In speciation one ancestor species gives rise to several descendant species, and as the process continues the new type in turn becomes a potential ancestor for many lines; it can be likened to a tree trunk and its branches and branches of branches. This is not a ladder effect since many presently living species had a common ancestor and simply represent contemporary specimens of adaptive radiation.

Extinction

Obviously, not all the branches reach the top, and for many reasons not always clearly understood certain species became extinct. Lack of adaptation to the constantly changing environment and competition (basically for food) between two different species in the same location are the dominant factors controlling the fine balance between survival and extinction.

When a common ancestor gives rise to several descendent lines that, although closely related, have adapted in different ways and developed dissimilar characteristics in response to diverse states, one speaks of evolutionary *divergence*. On the other hand, when unrelated groups adapt to the same environment and a common set of features is developed, even though there is no common ancestry, the process is termed *convergence*. Even though similarities are developed, however, there is never identity.

Analogy and Homology

In unrelated organisms, structures performing similar functions have developed; if function is the only unifying element these structures are said to be *analogous* (examples are the wing of a bird and the wing of a bee).

If body parts exhibit similar structure but their functions are diverse, one suspects a common ancestry and speaks of *homology* (the wing of a bird and the upper extremity of a human have a common bone pattern). When a structure becomes nonfunctional, as the appendix has in humans, it is termed *vestigial*.

This association of structure and function led to the biogenetic law, which states, "Ontogeny repeats phylogeny"; in other words, as an individual develops it passes through the developmental stages of the larger group to which it belongs. For example, embryos of land vertebrates possess rudiments of gills at one state. However, the embryonic stages are far from perfect recapitulations of ancestors' evolutionary history.

CHEMISTRY

General Chemistry

The Atom

John Dalton's theories—still accepted

    a. An element is composed of atoms. All atoms of an element possess the same chemical properties.

    b. Atoms of different elements have different properties.

    c. During a chemical reaction (nuclear reactions excepted, of course) atoms and elements are not created nor do they disappear.

    d. Atoms of more than one element may react to form compounds. In a pure compound the number of atoms of each element is constant.

Components of the Atom

  1. **Nucleus:** The nucleus—found at the center of an atom—contains neutrons and protons.

    a. Neutrons—no charge—mass of about 1 dalton

    b. Protons—charge of +1—mass of about 1 dalton. Number of protons in an atom determines the atomic number and the identity of the element.

2. **Electrons:** Electrons—charge of -1—mass of about 0.0005 dalton. Number of electrons circling the nucleus is equal to the number of protons in the nucleus.

Placement of Electrons—Energy Levels

1. **Quantum numbers:**

   a. Principal quantum number, n, determines the shell. It may be 1, 2, 3, 4, etc., in increasing distance from the nucleus and increasing energy. The K shell has a principal quantum number of 1.

   b. Angular momentum quantum number, l, determines the subshell. $l = 0, 1, 2, \ldots, (n - 1)$.

   c. Magnetic quantum number, m_l, determines the orbital: $m_l = l, l - 1, \ldots, 0, \ldots, 1 - l, -l$. The energies are virtually identical.

   d. Spin quantum number, m_s, describes the spin of an electron. Allowed values are $+\frac{1}{2}$ and $-\frac{1}{2}$.

2. **Pauli exclusion principle:** No two electrons in an atom may have exactly the same quantum number (i.e., all four).

3. **Total number of electrons in a shell:** The total number of electrons in a shell is $2n^2$.

4. **Order of filling orbitals:** Orbitals are filled from lower to higher energy levels. They may be designated in shorthand form. For example, the following oxygen atom may be designated as $1s^2 2s^2 2p^4$. Within the $2p$ orbitals, it is possible for an electron to be in $2p_x$, $2p_y$, or $2p_z$. Hund's rule states that one electron of parallel spin will go into each of these until each has one electron; additional electrons of antiparallel spin will then be added as necessary until all are filled.

$$
\begin{array}{cccccc}
 & & & & \overline{} & \\
 & & & & 2p & \\
1s & 2s & & 2p_x & 2p_y & 2p_z \\
\text{Oxygen } (\uparrow\downarrow) & (\uparrow\downarrow) & & (\uparrow\downarrow) & (\uparrow) & (\uparrow) \\
\end{array}
$$

5. **The excited state:** The situation described above is that of the ground state. By input of energy it is possible to raise electrons to higher energy levels. When electrons drop back from these higher energy levels (excited state) to the levels required by the ground state, there is emission of radiation (emission spectrum).

Periodic Table

The Periodic Table arranges the elements from left to right in order of increasing atomic number. The Periodic Law states that: The properties of the elements are periodic functions of their atomic numbers.

1. **Groups:** Vertical columns are called groups. All elements in the same group have the same number of valence electrons and, therefore, related chemical properties. For example, Group IA elements have only one electron in their outermost principal energy level. They tend to lose this electron readily to form $+1$ ions. Group VIIA elements have seven valence electrons. They tend to gain one electron to form -1 ions. At the extreme right of the table is the group known as the noble gases. These elements have complete outer shells and are essentially non-reactive. Properties of elements in other groups are now known to be related to placement of their electrons.

2. **Periods:** Horizontal rows of the table are called periods. Elements in the same period have the same number of principal energy levels. From left to right across a period, many properties exhibit periodicity (change with changes in atomic structure). For example, from left to right, atomic radii and metallic characteristics decrease while ionization energy and electronegativity increase.

Gases

1. Ideal gas law: Although early laws were formulated by Boyle, by Charles, and by Gay-Lussac to explain parts of the interrelationships between temperature, pressure, and volume of a gas, one simple formula sums it up:

$$\frac{P_1 V_1}{T_1} = \frac{P_2 V_2}{T_2} = nR$$

where P = pressure in atmospheres or torr
V = volume
T = absolute temperature in convenient units
n = moles of the gas
R = universal gas constant in appropriate units

Real gas behavior deviates from the ideal gas law at low temperature and high pressure.

2. Partial pressures:

$$P_T = P_1 + P_2 + \cdots + P_n$$

(i.e., the total pressure of a mixture of gases is equal to the sum of the partial pressures)

3. Diffusion—Graham's Law: Rate of diffusion is inversely proportional to the square root of the molecular weight.

$$\frac{v_1}{v_2} = \sqrt{\frac{m_2}{m_1}}$$

where v = velocity
m = molecular weight

Thus, a gas of twice the molecular weight will diffuse 0.71 as fast.

Liquids and Solids

Ideal gases are assumed to have negligible intermolecular interactions. Within a homologous series of organic compounds, the boiling point increases with increasing molecular weight. The same relationship may be seen within the halogens.

There are, however, forces in some compounds that cause them to be liquids or even solids at temperatures at which their molecular weights would suggest that they should be gases.

1. Dipole forces: In certain asymmetrical molecules the electrons become unevenly distributed between regions, and there results a partial positive charge in one region (and a partial negative charge in another). Molecules become arranged so that there is electrostatic attraction between adjacent molecules.

2. Hydrogen bonds: Hydrogen in one molecule may bond to oxygen, nitrogen, or fluorine in another molecule. The energy required to break this bond is about 10 kcal.

3. London-van der Waals dispersion forces: These forces involve interaction between molecules on the basis of their polarizability. They may be important in nonpolar compounds.

4. Ionic forces: Oppositely charged ions exhibit coulombic attraction.

Phase Changes

1. Nature of the solid, liquid, and gaseous phases:
where A is melting or fusion
B is freezing
C is vaporization or boiling
D is condensation

$$\text{Solid} \underset{B}{\overset{A}{\rightleftharpoons}} \text{Liquid} \underset{D}{\overset{C}{\rightleftharpoons}} \text{Gas}$$

2. **Energy of phase transition:**
   a. The energy involved in conversion from the solid to the liquid phase is H_f.
   b. The energy involved in conversion from the liquid to the gaseous phase is H_v.
   c. All molecules in one phase do not have the same energy—there is a range. A liquid at a temperature below its boiling point is subject to some of its molecules being vaporized by virtue of the fact that some molecules are sufficiently energetic to be converted into the gaseous state. The temperature of the liquid, however, is a measure of the average kinetic energy.

3. **Phase diagram:** The phase diagram allows the visualization of possible phases at particular temperatures and pressures.

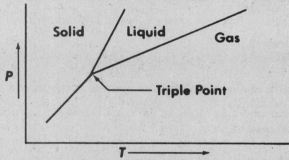

Note that the lines between phases in the phase diagram represent those conditions of pressure and temperature at which the phases indicated on the two sides of the lines may coexist. The point of intersection of the three lines is designated as *the triple point*; at this temperature and pressure all three phases may coexist.

Chemical Compounds

1. **Percent Weight and Empirical Formula:** Chemical compounds are pure substances that may be broken into two or more elements. A molecule is the smallest unit of a compound that still retains the properties of the compound; an atom is the smallest unit of an element.

A particular chemical compound will always have the same percentage composition by weight. Considering the compound iron (III) oxide, it is found to consist of:

$$Fe = 69.94\%$$

$$O = 30.06\%$$

Since it is agreed that a molecule of a compound is made up of whole atoms of elements, we will try to find the lowest multiple(s) of whole numbers. We may do this in two steps:

(1) Divide each percentage by the atomic weight of that element. .

$$Fe = \frac{69.94}{55.85} = 1.252$$

$$O = \frac{30.06}{16.00} = 1.879$$

(2) Convert these numbers to the lowest whole multiple(s).

$$\frac{1.879}{1.252} = 1.501$$

This would indicate 1.5 atoms of oxygen for each atom of iron. Since it is agreed that whole atoms are involved, the simplest formula would be Fe_2O_3. This is known as the empirical formula.

2. Molecular Formula: In some cases, however, the molecular weight of a compound does not agree with its empirical formula. (This is often true of organic compounds and sometimes true of inorganic ones.) The organic compound glucose may be used as an example. Its elemental composition would give an empirical formula of CH_2O. From molecular weight determination, however, we can show that the molecular formula is $C_6H_{12}O_6$.

3. Mole and Avogadro's Number: If the molecular weight is known, we may weigh that many grams of the compound and we will have a mole. A mole of any compound contains 6.023×10^{23} molecules of that compound. This is known as Avogadro's number.

Balanced Chemical Equations

Chemical equations may be written in unbalanced or balanced form.

1. Inorganic Chemistry:

$$H_2 + O_2 \rightarrow H_2O$$

This equation tells us that diatomic molecules of hydrogen and oxygen react to form water. Inspection indicates, however, that there are 2 atoms of oxygen on the left side but there is only 1 atom of oxygen on the right side. This does not agree with what we know about conservation of matter.

We could increase the atoms of oxygen on the right side by placing the coefficient 2 before H_2O, thus indicating 2 molecules of H_2O. This unbalances the hydrogen, however, with 2 atoms of hydrogen on the left and 4 on the right. We can correct this by placing the coefficient 2 before the H_2:

$$2H_2 + O_2 \rightarrow 2H_2O$$

Inspection indicates that there are now 4 atoms of hydrogen on each side and 2 atoms of oxygen on each side.

This is now a balanced equation. The coefficients tell us that 2 diatomic molecules of hydrogen will react with 1 diatomic molecule of oxygen to form 2 molecules of water. Since the same number of molecules (i.e., Avogadro's number) are required for a mole of any material, we can also say that 2 moles of hydrogen react with 1 mole of oxygen to produce 2 moles of water.

2. Organic Chemistry: The equation

$$C_3H_8 + O_2 \rightarrow CO_2 + H_2O$$

is not balanced. Since there are 3 atoms of carbon on the left and 1 atom on the right, we need to multiply carbon dioxide by 3. Similarly, we need to multiply water by 4 to balance the hydrogen. Then, however, there will be too few oxygens on the left. We need to multiply O_2 by 5. Our balanced equation is then:

$$C_3H_8 + 5O_2 \rightarrow 3CO_2 + 4H_2O$$

Check to see that this equation is balanced. It tells us that 1 mole of propane reacts with 5 moles of oxygen to produce 3 moles of carbon dioxide and 4 moles of water.

Solutions

1. Concentration units:
  a. Molarity
      moles/liter = grams/molecular weight/liters of solution
  b. Molality = moles of solute/kilograms of solvent
  c. Normality = equivalents of solute/liters of solution
  d. Equivalents = grams/equivalent weight

2. **Colligative properties:** Based on the number of dissolved particles, without regard to their nature.

  a. Boiling point elevation

   Boiling point elevation $= K_b m$

   where K_b is a constant for the specific solvent and $m =$ molality of solute.

Note, however, that a 1 molal solution of NaCl would have twice the calculated effect since it would be 1 molal each in Na^+ and Cl^- (i.e., 2 molal total).

  b. Freezing point depression

   Freezing point depression $= K_f m$

   where K_f is a constant for the specific solvent and $m =$ molality of solute particles (see comment above regarding ionizable solutes).

  c. Osmotic pressure. When an aqueous solution is placed on one side of a semi-permeable membrane and pure water on the other side, there is net movement of water across the membrane. The applied pressure required to produce a net movement of zero is called the osmotic pressure.

$$\pi V = nRT$$

where $\pi =$ osmotic pressure
  $V =$ volume
  $n =$ moles of particles in solution
  R is the universal gas constant
  T is the temperature, kelvin units (K)

3. **Solubility:** A comparatively insoluble inorganic compound in water is in equilibrium with its soluble ions.

$$Al(OH)_3 \downarrow \rightleftharpoons Al^{3+} + 3OH^-$$

The solubility product constant is K_{sp}.

$$K_{sp} = 5 \times 10^{-33} = [Al^{3+}][OH^-]^3$$

Thus, in the specific case of $Al(OH)_3$, if the product of the molar concentration of OH^- raised to the third power and Al^{3+} exceeds 5×10^{-33}, precipitation will occur.

Acids and Bases, pH, and Buffers

1. **Acids:**

  a. Bronsted-Lowry acid—a material that donates a proton:

$$HCl + H_2O \longrightarrow H_3O^+ + Cl^-$$
  (acid)

  b. Lewis acid—a material that accepts an electron pair

2. **Base:**

  a. Brönsted-Lowry base—a material that accepts a proton:

$$H_3O^+ + NaOH \rightleftharpoons 2H_2O + Na^+$$
  (base)

  b. Lewis base—a material that donates an electron pair

3. **Strength of acids and bases:**

  a. Strong acids and bases. A strong acid or base is assumed to be completely ionized. Therefore the concentration of acid is equal to the concentration of hydrogen ions (or hydronium ions).

$$HCl + H_2O \longrightarrow H_3O^+ + Cl^- \quad or \quad HCl \longrightarrow H^+ + Cl^-$$

    b. **Weak acids and bases**

        (1) $HF \rightleftharpoons H^+ + F^-$

$$K_a = \frac{[H^+][F^-]}{[HF]} = 7 \times 10^{-4} \text{ (in this specific case)}$$

Consider a $1M$ solution of HF for example:

$[H^+] = [F^-]$

So, $K_a[HF] = [H^+][F^-] = [H^+]^2$

and $[H^+] = \sqrt{K_a[HF]} = \sqrt{7 \times 10^{-4}} = 2.6 \times 10^{-2}$

In this example HF is called a conjugate acid, capable of releasing a proton. F^- is called a conjugate base, capable of combining with a proton.

        (2) **Bases**

$NH_3 + H_2O \rightleftharpoons NH_4^+ + OH^-$

$K_b[NH_3] = [NH_4^+][OH^-]$

$K_b = 1.8 \times 10^{-5}$ for this particular base.

Computation similar to that for acid would allow one to determine the $[OH^-]$ for a 1 molar NH_3 solution. H_2O is not included in the equilibrium expression.

4. **pH, pOH, and pK_w:**

    a. $pH = -\log[H^+]$

       The pH of pure water is 7.

    b. $pOH = -\log[OH^-]$

       The pOH of pure water is 7.

    c. $pK_w = pH + pOH = 14$

    d. **Changes in pH and hydrogen ions.** Remember that pH is a logarithmic scale. A decrease of one unit in pH (e.g., from 7 to 6) indicates an increase in hydrogen ions by a factor of 10.

5. **Solutions of salts:**

    a. A solution of the salt of a strong acid and a strong base is highly ionized and neutral.

    b. A solution of the salt of a strong acid and a weak base is acidic.

    c. A solution of the salt of a weak acid and a strong base is basic.

6. **Buffers:** A buffer is a solution containing a weak acid or a weak base *and* a salt of that weak acid or weak base.

    a. The ionization of a weak acid, HA, may be shown as

$$HA \rightleftharpoons H^+ + A^-$$

    b. The ionization constant is defined as

$$K_a = \frac{[H^+][A^-]}{[HA]}$$

    c. The negative logarithm of K_a is defined as pK_a. It is then possible to define a useful relationship called the Henderson-Hasselbalch equation:

$$pH = pK_a + \log \frac{[\text{conjugate base}]}{[\text{conjugate acid}]}$$

In the example we have already considered, of course, A^- would be the conjugate base and HA would be the conjugate acid in the buffer pair.

Although the conjugate acid is weakly ionized, it is assumed that the salt that produces the conjugate base is strongly ionized. Thus, the mixture of 500 ml each of $0.1M$ acetic acid and $0.1M$ sodium acetate would produce 1 liter of a solution that contains $0.05M$ acetic acid and $0.05M$ acetate ion. The Henderson-Hasselbalch equation would provide us with

$$pH = pK_a + \log \frac{(0.05)}{(0.05)} = pK_a + \log 1 = pK_a$$

Thus, a mixture of equal concentrations of the conjugate base and the conjugate acid will produce a pH equal to the pK_a. From a practical standpoint it is usually considered that a buffer system is useful in the restraint of changes of pH only over the range of $pK_a \pm 1$ pH unit.

7. **Volumetric calculations with acids and bases:**
   a.   Molarity = grams acid or base/molecular weight/liters
   b.   Normality = grams acid or base/equivalent weight/liters

For a monoprotic acid such as HCl, the normality equals the molarity. For a diprotic acid such as H_2SO_4, the normality is twice the molarity.

   c.   Number of equivalents in neutralization:

$$L_{acid} \times N_{acid} = L_{base} \times N_{base} = \text{number of equivalents}$$

   d.   Neutralizations may be done using the experimental technique of titration.

Electrochemistry

The electrolytic cell uses the flow of electrical current to cause a chemical reaction to occur. This type of chemical reaction is an oxidation-reduction (otherwise known as redox). In the electrolysis of molten NaCl, there is production of both Na and Cl_2. The half reactions involved are:

$$Na^+ + e^- \rightarrow Na^0 \qquad \text{(reduction)}$$
$$2Cl^- \rightarrow Cl_2^0 + 2e^- \quad \text{(oxidation)}$$

In balancing these half reactions, we must first balance one half reaction against the other to obtain the same number of electrons in each:

$$2[Na^+ + e^- \rightarrow Na^0] = 2Na^+ + 2e^- \rightarrow 2Na^0$$
$$1[2Cl^- \rightarrow Cl_2^0 + 2e^-] = 2Cl^- \rightarrow Cl_2^0 + 2e^-$$

When these balanced half reactions are added together, the electrons drop out to give a balanced equation for the net reaction:

$$2Na^+ + 2Cl^- \rightarrow 2Na^0 + Cl_2^0$$

or

$$2NaCl \rightarrow 2Na^0 + Cl_2^0$$

Thermodynamics

1. **Laws:**
   a.   *First law.* Energy can neither be created nor destroyed.
   b.   *Second law.* The spontaneous flow of heat is always unidirectional from the higher to the lower temperature.
   c.   *Third law.* The entropy of all pure crystalline solids may be taken as zero at the absolute zero of temperature.

2. **Change in enthalpy:** The change in enthalpy is ΔH. A negative ΔH for a reaction indicates that the products have a lower heat content than the reactants; therefore, heat is evolved. Since enthalpy is independent of the route of a reaction, it is possible to algebraically add reactions.

$$Pb(s) + O_2(g) \longrightarrow PbO_2(s) \qquad \Delta H = -66.1$$
$$2H_2O(g) \longrightarrow 2H_2(g) + O_2(g) \qquad \Delta H = +115.6$$

Sum $\quad Pb(s) + 2H_2O(g) \longrightarrow PbO_2(s) + 2H_2(g) \qquad \Delta H = +49.5$

In this example the overall reaction input of heat would be required.

3. Change in entropy: The change in entropy is ΔS. Entropy may be described as the degree of disorder of a system. It is also seen as unrecoverable energy. Without the addition of energy to a system, entropy increases to a maximum.

4. Changes in Gibbs free energy: Changes in Gibbs free energy are ΔG. Some of the energy of a reaction is unavailable for useful work. The term ΔG indicates the energy that is available for useful work.

$$\Delta G = \Delta H - T \Delta S$$

where $T =$ absolute temperature, K°

A negative ΔG indicates a spontaneous reaction. A positive ΔG indicates a reaction that would be spontaneous in the reverse direction. When $\Delta G = 0$, the system is at equilibrium.

Rate Processes in Chemical Reactions

1. Rate-Controlling Step: Although we sometimes write an equation in a simple way such as

$$A + B \rightarrow X + Z$$

it is not always so simple. There may be many intermediates in the process. For example, a product C could be formed, and then converted to D, etc. Somewhere along such a series of steps there would be a slowest or rate-controlling step. In spite of the other series of reactions, as the name implies, this step would control or determine the rate of the overall reaction.

2. Activation Energy, Catalysts, Enzymes: Although a reaction is thermodynamically favorable, it will often require a certain activation energy.

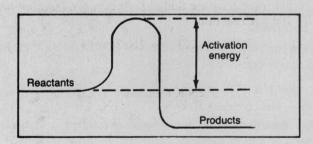

A catalyst or an enzyme (essentially a biological catalyst) may substantially increase the rate of a reaction by decreasing the activation energy that is required.

3. Equilibrium Constant: Consider a reversible reaction:

$$A + B \rightleftharpoons C + D$$

We may calculate an *equilibrium constant*:

$$K_{eq} = \frac{[C][D]}{[A][B]}$$

4. Le Chatelier's Principle: Le Chatelier's principle states that when a system is at equilibrium, it will shift to relieve any stress placed upon it. Thus, in the above example, addition of more C to the system would bring about the consumption of D and the production of more A and B (without changing the equilibrium constant).

General Principles

Characteristics of Mixtures and Compounds

Mixture	Compound
1. Physical union	Chemical union
2. No new substances are formed	New substances are formed
3. Can be separated by physical means	Can be separated by chemical means
4. Elements form no definite proportions	Elements form definite proportions

Reactions

1. Single Replacement Reaction: In a single replacement reaction a more active element reacts with a compound to replace a less active one. A new element and a new compound are the result.

Examples: $Fe + CuSO_4 \longrightarrow FeSO_4 + Cu$
$Zn + CuSO_4 \longrightarrow ZnSO_4 + Cu$

2. Double Replacement Reaction: Double replacement reactions involve a double exchange; compounds react chemically to form two new compounds.

Examples: $NaCl + AgNO_3 \longrightarrow NaNO_3 + AgCl$
$HCl + NaOH \longrightarrow NaCl + H_2O$

In the first example a precipitate $(AgCl)$ is formed and in the second example a weakly ionized compound (H_2O) is formed. In the other cases (e.g., $NaCl + KNO_3$) a double replacement reaction could be written, but the equilibrium would involve all possible combinations of cations and anions since neither a precipitate, nor a gas, nor a weakly ionized compound is formed.

3. Synthesis Reaction: In a synthesis reaction two or more elements or compounds can unite to form a single compound.

Examples: $Fe + S \xrightarrow{\Delta} FeS$
$CO_2 + H_2O \longrightarrow H_2CO_3$

4. Decomposition Reaction: In a decomposition reaction a compound is broken down into simpler compounds or into its elements.

Examples: $2KClO_3 \longrightarrow 2KCl + 3O_2$
$2HgO \longrightarrow 2Hg + O_2$

Role of Enzymes in a Reaction

Consider the following reaction:

$$A + B + C \xrightarrow{\text{E (enzyme)}} ABCE \longrightarrow D + F + E$$
$$1 \qquad\qquad 2 \qquad\qquad 3 \qquad 4 \quad 2$$

Substrate(s) or reactant(s) (1) react(s) with the enzyme (2) to form an enzyme–subtrate complex (3). This complex breaks down into product(s) (4), and free enzyme (2) ready for the formation of a new enzyme–substrate complex is available again.

An enzyme speeds up the rate of the reaction but is not used up itself in the reaction.

Temperature Conversion Factors

On the Celsius scale (°C) the freezing point of water is 0°, and the boiling point is 100°. On the Fahrenheit scale (°F) they are respectively 32° and 212°.

The absolute Kelvin scale lists as absolute zero a temperature of −273°C, and therefore the Kelvin and Celsius scales differ only in the choice of point zero. Kelvin temperature is, therefore, 273 plus the Celsius temperature. Let us illustrate and work two examples:

1. 104°F is what temperature on the Kelvin scale? The answer is 313 K and is obtained in the following manner:

First we must convert Fahrenheit to Celsius by using the following formulas:

$$\text{Celsius equals } \frac{5}{9} \times (\text{Fahrenheit} - 32)$$

$$\text{Fahrenheit equals } \frac{9}{5}\ C + 32$$

$$\text{Celsius} = \frac{5}{9} \times (104 - 32)$$

$$C = \frac{5}{9} \times 72$$

$$C = 40°$$

Now we take 273°, add 40°, and obtain a Kelvin temperature of 313 K.

2. 45°C will equal how many degrees F?

We utilize the conversion factors:

$$F = \frac{9}{5}\ C + 32$$

or

$$C = \frac{5}{9}(F - 32)$$

$$F = \frac{9}{5}(45) + 32$$

$$F = 81 + 32$$

$$F = 113°$$

Formulas and Laws

1. **Specific Gravity:** Specific gravity is usually expressed as the weight of an object in air divided by the loss of weight when weighed in water.

Example: A ball of steel weighs 300 grams in air and 250 grams when submerged in water; its specific gravity is 6.

$$\text{Specific Gravity} = \frac{\text{Weight in Air}}{\text{Loss of Weight}}$$

$$\text{Specific Gravity} = \frac{300}{50} = 6$$

2. **Density:** Density is expressed as $\dfrac{M \text{ (mass)}}{V \text{ (volume)}}$

Example: A piece of iron 60 inches long, 12 inches wide and 2 inches high has a mass of 2000 lb. The density of this piece is 1.39 lb./in.^{3} and was obtained as follows:

$$D = \frac{M}{V} = \frac{2000 \text{ lb.}}{60 \text{ in.} \times 12 \text{ in.} \times 2 \text{ in.}}$$

$$D = \frac{2000 \text{ lb.}}{1440 \text{ in.}^3} = 1.39 \text{ lb./in.}^3$$

Organic Chemistry

It is not possible to present a course in organic chemistry in the limited space we have allotted. All we can hope to do is to help you review some of the high points.

General Considerations

1. **Definition:** Organic chemistry is the chemistry of compounds of carbon. Historically, it has been the study of chemical compounds from living or dead organisms. Until 1828, it was believed that these compounds could not be synthesized from "inorganic" compounds outside living organisms. This theory was first breached by Friedrich Wöhler in 1828; he was successful in synthesizing urea from the inorganic compound, ammonium cyanate.

2. **Bonds:** In general, the bonds in the stable organic compounds are covalent bonds, formed by the sharing of electrons between atoms. If the electrons are shared unequally between two atoms, the bond is said to be a polar bond (e.g., C—Br or C—O).

Such a polar bond is a dipole, and the molecule possesses a dipole moment. The dipole moment is calculated by multiplying the charge by the distance of separation. Thus methane (CH_4) has a dipole moment of zero. By comparison, CH_3Cl has a dipole moment of 1.87.

3. **Electronic Configuration of the Carbon Atom:** It is generally true that the orbital electrons in the outer unfilled shell are the most important in predicting the metal/non-metal character of the compound as well as the expected valence. The carbon atom has two electrons in the K shell and four in the L shell ($1s^2\, 2s^2\, 2p_x{}^1\, 2p_y{}^1$). It might be expected to lose four electrons to produce the electronic configuration of the noble element helium, or gain four electrons to produce the electronic configuration of the noble element neon. For the most part it shares electrons to complete the L shell. Thus it may be said to have a valence of 4 (see below).

4. **Bond Hybridization:** The orbital electrons of the carbon atom consist of two electrons in the $1s$ orbital, two electrons in the $2s$ orbital and one electron each in the $2p_x$ and $2p_y$ orbitals. (This may be written as $1s^2 2s^2 2p_x{}^1 2p_y{}^1$.) It exhibits a valence of 4. In simple compounds such as methane, four equivalent covalent bonds are formed. This may be considered to occur by raising one of the $2s$ orbital electrons to the $2p_z$ orbital and then forming four hybridized orbitals from the three $2p$ orbitals and the one remaining $2s$ orbital. These hybridized orbitals are sp^3 orbitals. The four covalent bonds in methane are the result of overlap of the one orbital electron of each of four hydrogen atoms with one sp^3 hybridized orbital electron of the carbon atom. These four bonds are called sigma bonds.

In a compound such as ethylene (ethene), however, there are pi as well as sigma bonds. Two of the three $2p$ orbital electrons are hybridized with the remaining $2s$ orbital electron. Thus there are three equivalent sp^2 hybridized orbital electrons for each carbon atom. These participate in the covalent sigma bond between the two carbon atoms and in the covalent sigma bonds between the carbon atom and the hydrogen atoms. The remaining $2p$ orbital electron in each carbon atom participates in the weaker second bond between the two carbon atoms (a pi bond).

Compounds such as acetylene (ethyne) have a triple bond, consisting of one sigma bond and two pi bonds. In each carbon atom participating in a triple bond, there is contribution of two hybridized *sp* orbital electrons to produce two pi bonds. The stronger sigma bond between the carbon atoms is produced by the contribution of one 2*p* electron from each carbon atom. In acetylene itself there is another sigma bond between the carbon atom and a hydrogen atom; this bond is produced by the overlap of a 2*p* orbital from the carbon atom and the sole electron from the hydrogen atom.

5.   Stereochemistry: Chemical compounds with the same molecular formula but different structural formulas are termed *isomers*. Those having atoms joined in a different order are *structural isomers* (e.g., 2-propanol and 1-propanol). Those having their atoms joined in the same order are termed *stereoisomers*. Stereoisomers that are mirror images of each other are termed *enantiomers*. Stereoisomers that are not enantiomers are called *diastereomers*.

```
    H—C=O              H—C=O              H—C=O
      |                  |                  |
    H—C=OH             H—C—OH            HO—C—H
      |                  |                  |
   HO—C—H             HO—C—H             H—C—OH
      |                  |                  |
    H—C—OH             HO—C—H             H—C—OH
      |                  |                  |
    H—C—OH              H—C—OH            HO—C—H
      |                  |                  |
    CH₂OH              CH₂OH              CH₂OH

   D-glucose          D-galactose        L-galactose
```

D-Glucose and D-galactose are diastereomers. D-galactose and L-galactose are enantiomers.

To possess optical activity a compound must have a chiral center. A *chiral center* is a carbon atom that is attached to four different substituents. A compound possessing a chiral center may still not possess optical activity if there is a plane of symmetry in the molecule.

Light ordinarily oscillates in all planes. If it is passed through a polarizer, its oscillation is reduced to only one plane. If this plane-polarized light is allowed to pass through a solution of an optically active compound, the plane of the light will be rotated. If it is rotated to the right, the rotation is termed dextrorotatory or (+). If it is rotated to the left, the rotation is termed levorotatory or (−). The specific rotation [α] is characteristic of an optically active compound:

$$[\alpha] = \frac{\alpha}{(c)(l)}$$

where α = observed degrees of rotation
c = concentration, grams per milliliter
l = length of light path, decimeters

For comparison in the literature, the D line of sodium as the incident light and a temperature of 25°C have been agreed upon as standard.

A mixture of equal amounts of two enantiomers (called a *racemic* mixture) will have a rotation of zero. The rotations are opposite in sign and equal in numerical value, canceling each other.

The Alkanes

Alkanes are saturated noncyclic compounds of carbon and hydrogen. If carbon atoms are arranged in a straight chain sequence

C–C–C–C

and hydrogen atoms are added to account for each carbon atom's valence of four, we produce a compound like this:

$$\begin{array}{cccc} & H & H & H & H \\ & | & | & | & | \\ H\dot{C} & - \dot{C} & - \dot{C} & - \dot{C}H \\ & | & | & | & | \\ & H & H & H & H \end{array}$$

This compound is *n*-butane. The *n* designates the straight chain character. Another compound with the same numbers of carbon and hydrogen atoms is isobutane (or 2-methylpropane).

$$\begin{array}{c} H_3C-CH-CH_3 \\ | \\ CH_3 \end{array}$$

It is useful to learn the names of many of the alkanes. With modification these names are an integral part of the names of the derivatives of alkanes.

Chain Length	Name	Chain Length	Name
1	Methane	11	Undecane
2	Ethane	12	Dodecane
3	Propane	13	Tridecane
4	Butane	14	Tetradecane
5	Pentane	15	Pentadecane
6	Hexane	16	Hexadecane
7	Heptane	17	Heptadecane
8	Octane	18	Octadecane
9	Nonane	19	Nonadecane
10	Decane	20	Eicosane

The IUPAC rules for nomenclature require that a compound that is not a straight chain be named on the basis of its longest chain. Thus, the following compound is 2-methyl-4-ethylheptane:

$$\begin{array}{c} H_3C-CH-CH_2-CH-CH_2-CH_2-CH_3 \\ \quad\quad | \quad\quad\quad\quad | \\ \quad\quad CH_3 \quad\quad\quad CH_2 \\ \quad\quad\quad\quad\quad\quad\quad\quad | \\ \quad\quad\quad\quad\quad\quad\quad\quad CH_3 \end{array}$$

1. Synthesis—Wurtz Reaction:

$$2RBr + 2Na \longrightarrow RR + 2NaBr$$

(R will often be used to refer to an unspecified alkyl group.) More specifically:

$$2CH_3Br + 2Na \longrightarrow CH_3 - CH_3 + 2NaBr$$

If a mixture of two alkyl bromides is used, a mixture of three possible products is expected.

2. Reactions:

The alkanes are not very reactive, but they will undergo some reactions.

a. *Halogenation*

$$Cl_2 + \begin{array}{c} H \quad H \\ | \quad | \\ H\dot{C}-\dot{C}H \\ | \quad | \\ H \quad H \end{array} \xrightarrow[\substack{u.v. \\ light}]{heat} \begin{array}{c} H \quad H \\ | \quad | \\ H\dot{C}-\dot{C}-Cl \\ | \quad | \\ H \quad H \end{array} + HCl$$

Reaction may continue and produce a more highly chlorinated product.

b. *Oxidation*

Alkanes may be oxidized to produce CO_2, water and energy.

The Cycloalkanes

The small ring cycloalkanes (cyclopropane and cyclobutane) are strained and are more reactive. Cyclopropane is planar, and the bond angles must be 60°. The normal bond angle is 109°28'. Five- and six-membered rings are not appreciably strained. Larger rings were once thought to be unstable because of the strain (Baeyer), but puckering allows relative freedom from strain.

Example:

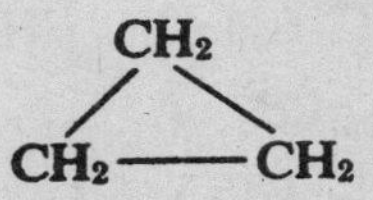

$$\overset{\displaystyle CH_2}{\underset{\displaystyle CH_2 \rule{1cm}{0.4pt} CH_2}{\diagdown \diagup}} \qquad \text{cyclopropane}$$

The Alkenes

The alkenes may be considered as alkanes from which hydrogen has been removed, producing a carbon-to-carbon double bond. The simplest example of this series is ethene (ethylene).

$$H_2C=CH_2 \qquad \qquad \text{ethene}$$

$$H_2C=CH-CH_2-CH_3 \qquad \text{1-butene}$$

$$\underset{\displaystyle H}{\overset{\displaystyle H}{H_3C-C=C-CH_3}} \qquad \textit{trans}\text{-2-butene}$$

$$\overset{\displaystyle H \quad H}{H_3C-C=C-CH_3} \qquad \textit{cis}\text{-2-butene}$$

1. Synthesis:

a. *Dehydrohalogenation*

$$H_3C-CH_2Br + \text{alcoholic KOH} \longrightarrow H_2C=CH_2 + H_2O + KBr$$

b. *Dehydration*

$$H_3C-CH_2OH \xrightarrow[H_2SO_4]{\text{heat}} H_2C=CH_2 + H_2O$$

c. *Dehalogenation*

$$Br-CH_2-CH_2-Br + Zn \longrightarrow H_2C=CH_2 + ZnBr_2$$

d. *Cracking* (relatively nonspecific decomposition reactions)

$$H_3C-(CH_2)_4-CH_3 \xrightarrow[\text{cracking}]{\text{heat}} H_2C=CH_2 + H_3C-CH_2-CH_2-CH_3$$

2. Reactions:

a. *Addition of HX to the double bond*

$$H_3C-CH=CH_2 + HBr \longrightarrow \underset{\displaystyle Br}{\overset{\displaystyle H}{H_3C-C-CH_3}}$$

The Markownikoff Rule says that in the addition of an acid across a double bond, the double-bonded carbon having the most hydrogen will receive the H of HX. The above is true for ionic addition, but in the presence of peroxides we see a free radical anti-Markownikoff addition:

$$H_3C-CH=CH_2 + HBr \xrightarrow{\text{peroxide}} H_3C-CH_2-CH_2Br$$

b. *Hydrogenation* (catalyst such as Pt, Pd, or Ni)

$$H_2C=CH_2 + H_2 \xrightarrow{\text{Pt}} H_3C-CH_3$$

$$3H_2C=CH-CH=CH_2 + 4H_2 \xrightarrow{\text{Pt}} H_3C-CH=CH-CH_3$$
$$+ H_2C=CH-CH_2-CH_3$$
$$+ H_3C-CH_2-CH_2-CH_3$$

c. $H_2C=CH_2 + Br_2 \longrightarrow BrCH_2-CH_2Br$

d. $H_2C=CH_2 \xrightarrow{\text{catalyst}}$ polymer (polyethylene in this case)

The Alkynes (derivatives of acetylene)

$HC\equiv CH$ acetylene or ethyne

1. Synthesis:

a. $CaC_2 + H_2O \longrightarrow C_2H_2 + CaO$

b. *Dehydrohalogenation*

$$H_3C-CHBr_2 + \text{alcoholic } 2KOH \longrightarrow HC\equiv CH + 2H_2O + 2KBr$$

c. *Dehalogenation*

$$HCBr_2-CBr_2H + 2Zn \longrightarrow HC\equiv CH + 2ZnBr_2$$

2. Reactions:

a. *Hydrogenation*

$$HC\equiv CH + H_2 \xrightarrow{\text{Pt}} H_2C=CH_2 + H_2 \xrightarrow{\text{Pt}} CH_3-CH_3$$

b. *Hydrohalogenation*—see reactions of alkenes

c. *Halogenation*—see reactions of alkenes

d. *Reaction of active hydrogen*

$$H_3C-C\equiv CH + Ag^+ \longrightarrow H_3C-C\equiv CAg + H^+$$

$$H_3C-C\equiv CH + NaNH_2 \longrightarrow H_3C-C\equiv CNa + NH_3$$

$$H_3C-C\equiv CNa + CH_3Br \longrightarrow H_3C-C\equiv C-CH_3 + NaBr$$

Aromatic Compounds

Aromatic compounds consist of benzene and compounds whose chemical reactions are similar to those of benzene. Almost all aromatic compounds that you would be expected to recognize as such are derivatives of benzene; there are other unrelated aromatic compounds.

1. Nature of Benzene—Resonance: Although we may draw benzene as having three discrete double bonds and three discrete single bonds in conjugation, this does not adequately describe its structure. It may be shown as two structures in resonance:

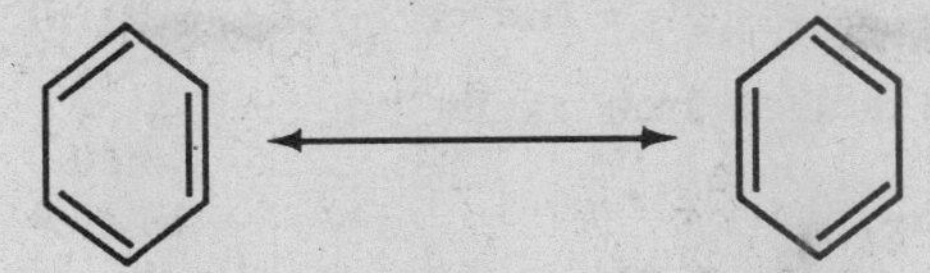

In reality, however, it appears that each carbon atom has three discrete covalent bonds, and the fourth bonding electron of each carbon atom is delocalized in electron clouds around the ring.

2. Synthesis of the Aromatic Ring: This is unusual; in general one will only be interested in reactions of compounds containing the benzene ring rather than in the synthesis of the aromatic ring.

3. Reactions: (ϕ is sometimes used as a shorthand designation for the phenyl group. Thus, benzene could be indicated as ϕ-H.)

    a. *Monosubstitution*

$$\phi\text{-H} + HNO_3 \longrightarrow \phi\text{-}NO_2 + H_2O$$
$$\phi\text{-H} + H_2SO_4 \longrightarrow \phi\text{-}SO_3H + H_2O$$
$$\phi\text{-H} + Br_2 \xrightarrow{\text{Fe}} \phi\text{-Br} + HBr$$

    b. *Friedel-Crafts reaction*

$$\phi\text{-H} + RCl \xrightarrow{AlCl_3} \phi\text{-R} + HCl$$

$$\phi\text{-H} + R\overset{\overset{\displaystyle O}{\|}}{-C}\text{-Cl} \xrightarrow{AlCl_3} \phi\overset{\overset{\displaystyle O}{\|}}{-C}\text{-R} + HCl$$

    c. *Substitution in a benzene ring that already has one substituent*

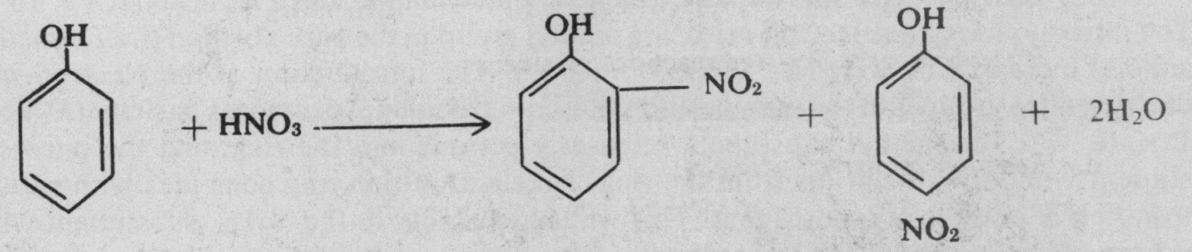

The placement of the second substituent is ordained by the first substituent. The OH substituent, as shown above, is an ortho, para-directing group. Other ortho, para-directing substituents include the CH_3 group and the halogens. The halogens deactivate the ring and also direct ortho, para. Many electrophilic substituents are said to be meta-directing: NO_2, CN, SO_3H, COOH, and so forth.

The above meta-directing substituents also deactivate the ring.

Note that the reactions above *do* balance. In many cases below, we will write organic reactions that do not balance. This is done for the sake of simplicity and to emphasize the desired products.

   d. *Diazotization of amines*

$$\phi-NH_2 + HNO_2 \longrightarrow \phi-N_2^+$$

   e. *Reactions of diazonium salts* (see above)

$$\phi-N_2^+ + CuBr \longrightarrow \phi-Br$$

$$\phi-N_2^+ + CuCN \longrightarrow \phi-CN$$

$$\phi-N_2^+ + H_2O \xrightarrow{H^+} \phi-OH$$

$$\phi-N_2^+ + \phi-OH \longrightarrow \phi-N=N-\phi-OH \text{ (Coupling)}$$

$$\phi-N_2^+ + H_2 \xrightarrow{Pt} \phi N \overset{H}{\underset{|}{-}} NH_2$$

4. Acidity and Basicity:

   a. *Acidity*. Phenol will ionize as an acid with a K_a of about 1×10^{-10}. A methyl substituent in the ortho position will lower the K_a (and the acidity) to about 6×10^{-11}. The electron-releasing methyl substituent contributes electrons to the ring and depresses release of H^+. A nitro substituent in the ortho position, conversely, increases the acidity (K_a about 7×10^{-8}) by withdrawing electrons from the ring.

   b. *Basicity*. Aniline (aminobenzene or phenylamine) has a K_b of about 4×10^{-10}. The introduction of an electron-releasing methyl group in the para position (i.e., *p*-methyl-aniline) increases basicity (K_b about 1×10^{-9}). The introduction of the electron-withdrawing nitro group into the para position (i.e., *p*-nitroaniline) decreases basicity (K_b about 1×10^{-13}). The methyl substituent releases electrons into the ring, and the nitro substituent withdraws electrons from the ring. An electron-rich ring coincides with an electron-rich N in the NH_2 substituent. This will add stability to the NH_3^+ substituent which is formed by reaction of the NH_2 substituent with a proton, and the tendency of the NH_3^+ group to ionize by releasing the proton is decreased.

The Grignard Reagent

The Grignard reagent is one of the most important and versatile in organic chemistry. We will try to outline only a few of its reactions.

1. Synthesis: The Grignard reagent is synthesized by the reaction of an alkyl halide with elemental magnesium in the presence of anhydrous ether.

Example:

$$H_3C-CH_2Br + Mg \xrightarrow[\text{ether}]{\text{anhydrous}} H_3C-CH_2MgBr$$

or

$$RBr + Mg \xrightarrow[\text{ether}]{\text{anhydrous}} RMgBr$$

2. Reactions:

a. Reaction with active hydrogen. A Grignard reagent will react with any compound having active hydrogen (e.g., H_2O, an alcohol, an acid, or a 1-alkyne) to form a hydrocarbon.

$$RMgBr + H_2O \longrightarrow RH + MgBrOH$$

b. Reaction with aldehydes and ketones

$$RMgBr + HCHO \xrightarrow[\text{ether}]{\text{anhydrous}} R-CH_2OMgBr \xrightarrow{H^+}$$
$$RCH_2OH \text{ (primary alcohol)}$$

$$RMgBr + R'CHO \xrightarrow[\text{ether}]{\text{anhydrous}} \underset{H}{\overset{R'}{R\underset{|}{\overset{|}{C}}-OMgBr}} \xrightarrow{H^+} \underset{H}{\overset{R'}{R\underset{|}{\overset{|}{C}}-OH}}$$
(secondary alcohol)

$$RMgBr + \overset{R''}{R'-\underset{|}{\overset{|}{C}}=O} \xrightarrow[\text{ether}]{\text{anhydrous}} \underset{R}{\overset{R''}{R'-\underset{|}{\overset{|}{C}}-OMgBr}} \xrightarrow{H^+}$$
$$\underset{R}{\overset{R''}{R'-\underset{|}{\overset{|}{C}}-OH}}$$
(tertiary alcohol)

c. Reaction with CO_2

$$RMgBr + CO_2 \xrightarrow[\text{ether}]{\text{anhydrous}} R-\overset{O}{\overset{||}{C}}-OMgBr \xrightarrow{H^+} RCOOH$$

d. Reaction with an ester or an acyl halide

$$RMgBr + R'COOR'' \xrightarrow[\text{ether}]{\text{anhydrous}} R'-\overset{O}{\overset{||}{C}}-R$$

$$RMgBr + R'COBr \xrightarrow[\text{ether}]{\text{anhydrous}} R'-\overset{O}{\overset{||}{C}}-R$$

Alcohols

Alcohols may be designated as ROH. The simplest alcohol is CH_3OH and is named methanol (i.e., methan-ol) as a derivative of the one-carbon hydrocarbon, methane. Other alcohols are similarly named as derivatives of hydrocarbons. The compound below is named 2-pentanol or 2-hydroxypentane.

$$H_3C—CH_2—CH_2—\underset{\underset{OH}{|}}{CH}—CH_3$$

The alcohols are very weak acids, even weaker than water. Polarity and hydrogen bonding cause short chain alcohols to be soluble in water.

1. **Synthesis:**
   a. *Hydration of alkenes*

   $$H_2C{=}CH_2 + H_2O \overset{H^+}{\rightleftharpoons} H_3C—CH_2OH$$

   b. *Using Grignard reagents—discussed elsewhere*
   c. *Hydrolysis of alkyl halides*

   $$R—I + H_2O \overset{KOH}{\rightleftharpoons} ROH + I^-$$

   d. *Reduction of aldehydes and ketones*

   $$R—CHO + NaBH_4 \overset{H_2O}{\longrightarrow} R—CH_2OH$$

2. **Reactions:**

   a. *Oxidation to form aldehydes or ketones*

   $$R—CH_2OH + K_2Cr_2O_7 \overset{H^+}{\longrightarrow} R—CHO$$

This is useful only if the aldehyde may be removed (sometimes by distillation) before further oxidation to the carboxylic acid. A ketone may not be easily oxidized further, but chain rupture is possible.

   b. *Dehydration to form alkenes—discussed elsewhere*
   c. *Formation of esters*

   $$R—COOH + R—CH_2OH \overset{H^+}{\rightleftharpoons} R—COOCH_2—R$$

   d. *Conversion to halides*

   $$ROH + HI \rightleftharpoons RI + H_2O$$

Amines

Amines have the structure $R—NH_2$. The simplest example is methylamine (or aminomethane):

$$H_3CNH_2$$

1. **Synthesis:**
   a. $RX + NH_3 \longrightarrow R—NH_2$
   b. $RCN + LiAlH_4 \longrightarrow R—CH_2—NH_2$
   c. *Hofmann degradation*

   $$R—CONH_2 \overset{Br_2, NaOH}{\longrightarrow} RNH_2$$

2. **Reactions:**

$$R—NH_2 + HONO \xrightarrow{H_2O} ROH + N_2$$

a. (This is the reaction for a primary alkyl amine)

b. $R—NH_2 + HONO \longrightarrow RN_2^+$

(This is the reaction for a primary aromatic amine. The diazonium salt is stable at the temperatures of ice water. It is capable of numerous further reactions under appropriate conditions.)

c. $R—NH_2 + R'—COOH + dicyclohexylcarbodiimide \longrightarrow R—NH—COR'$

(an amide)

Amides

Amides have the structure $R—NH—COR$.
A simple example is acetanilide, $\phi—NH—CO—CH_3$.

1. **Synthesis:**

a. $R—NH_2 + R'—COCl$ (an acyl chloride) $\longrightarrow R—NH—\overset{\displaystyle O}{\overset{\|}{C}}—R'$

b. $R—NH_2 + (R—CO)_2O$ (an anhydride) $\longrightarrow R—NH—\overset{\displaystyle O}{\overset{\|}{C}}—R'$

c. $R—NH_2 + R'—COOH + dicyclohexylcarbodiimide \longrightarrow R—NH—\overset{\displaystyle O}{\overset{\|}{C}}—R'$

(Primary amines are shown, but secondary amines may also be used.)

2. **Reaction:**

$$R—NH—COR' + H_2O \xrightarrow{H+} R—NH_3^+ + R' – COOH$$

(The reaction may also be accomplished in an aqueous base.)

Aldehydes and Ketones

1. **Synthesis:**

a. *Reaction of a Grignard reagent with a carboxylic ester or an acyl halide to form a ketone* (outlined above under "Grignard Reagent"—Section 2;d)

b. *Mild oxidation of an alcohol* (often feasible in the synthesis of ketones and sometimes in the synthesis of aldehydes)

$$RCH_2OH \xrightarrow{Cu, \triangle} R–CHO \text{ (aldehyde)}$$

$$\underset{\displaystyle \underset{H}{|}}{\overset{\displaystyle \overset{R'}{|}}{R–C}}OH \xrightarrow{Cu, \triangle} R–\overset{\displaystyle \overset{R'}{|}}{C}{=}O \text{ (ketone)}$$

c. *Friedel-Crafts acylation to produce aromatic ketones* (see "Aromatic Compounds" —Section 3;b)

d. *Decarboxylation of acids to produce ketones*

$$2RCOOH \xrightarrow{ThO_2, \triangle} R–\overset{\displaystyle O}{\overset{\|}{C}}–R + CO_2$$

e. *Oxidation of diols to form aldehydes*

$$\underset{\underset{\displaystyle \text{R-CH-CH-R}'}{|\quad\;|}}{\overset{\text{OH OH}}{}} \xrightarrow{\text{HIO}_4 \text{ or Pb(OAc)}_4} \text{R-CHO} + \text{R}'\text{-CHO}$$

$$\underset{\underset{\displaystyle \text{R-CH-CH-CH-R}'}{|\quad\;|\quad\;|}}{\overset{\text{OH OH OH}}{}} \xrightarrow{\text{HIO}_4 \text{ or Pb(OAc)}_4} \text{R-CHO} + \text{R}'\text{-CHO} \\ + \text{HCOOH}$$

$$\underset{\underset{\displaystyle \text{R-CH-CH}_2\text{-CH-R}'}{|\qquad\qquad\;|}}{\overset{\text{OH}\qquad\;\;\text{OH}}{}} \xrightarrow{\text{HIO}_4 \text{ or Pb(OAc)}_4} \text{No reaction}$$

2. Reactions:

a. *Reaction with Grignard reagents*

$$\underset{\displaystyle \text{R-C-R}'}{\overset{\text{O}}{\|}} + \text{R}''\text{MgBr} \xrightarrow[\text{ether}]{\text{anhydrous}} \underset{\underset{\displaystyle \text{R}''}{|}}{\overset{\text{OMgBr}}{\underset{\displaystyle \text{R-C-R}'}{|}}} \xrightarrow{\text{H}_2\text{O}} \underset{\underset{\displaystyle \text{R}''}{|}}{\overset{\text{OH}}{\underset{\displaystyle \text{R-C-R}'}{|}}}$$

$$\text{R-CHO} + \text{R}'\text{MgBr} \xrightarrow[\text{ether}]{\text{anhydrous}} \underset{\displaystyle \text{R-CH-R}'}{\overset{\text{OMgBr}}{|}} \xrightarrow{\text{H}_2\text{O}} \underset{\displaystyle \text{R-CH-R}'}{\overset{\text{OH}}{|}}$$

$$\text{HCHO} + \text{RMgBr} \xrightarrow[\text{ether}]{\text{anhydrous}} \text{R-CH}_2\text{-OMgBr} \xrightarrow{\text{H}_2\text{O}} \text{R-CH}_2\text{OH}$$

b. *Reaction of aldehydes or ketones with HCN*

$$\text{R-CHO} + \text{HCN} \longrightarrow \underset{\underset{\displaystyle \text{H}}{|}}{\overset{\text{OH}}{\underset{\displaystyle \text{R-C-CN}}{|}}} \xrightarrow{\text{H}_2\text{O, H}^+} \underset{\underset{\displaystyle \text{H}}{|}}{\overset{\text{OH}}{\underset{\displaystyle \text{R-C-COOH}}{|}}}$$

c. *Reaction of aldehydes or methyl ketones with NaHSO₃*

$$\text{R-CHO} + \text{NaHSO}_3 \longrightarrow \underset{\underset{\displaystyle \text{H}}{|}}{\overset{\text{OH}}{\underset{\displaystyle \text{R-C-SO}_3^-\text{Na}^+}{|}}}$$

d. *Reaction with alcohols*

$$\text{R-CHO} + \text{R}'\text{-OH} \xrightarrow{\text{H}^+} \underset{\underset{\displaystyle \text{H}}{|}}{\overset{\text{OH}}{\underset{\displaystyle \text{R-C-OR}}{|}}} \xrightarrow{\text{R}'\text{OH, H}^+} \underset{\underset{\displaystyle \text{H}}{|}}{\overset{\text{OR}'}{\underset{\displaystyle \text{R-C-OR}'}{|}}}$$

(a hemiacetal) (an acetal)

$$\underset{\displaystyle \text{R-C-R}'}{\overset{\text{O}}{\|}} + \text{R}''\text{OH} \xrightarrow{\text{H}^+} \underset{\underset{\displaystyle \text{OR}''}{|}}{\overset{\text{OH}}{\underset{\displaystyle \text{R-C-R}'}{|}}} \xrightarrow{\text{R}''\text{OH, H}^+} \underset{\underset{\displaystyle \text{OR}''}{|}}{\overset{\text{OR}''}{\underset{\displaystyle \text{R-C-R}'}{|}}}$$

(a hemiketal) (a ketal)

e. *Reaction of ketones and aldehydes with hydroxylamine*

$$R-CHO + NH_2OH \xrightarrow{H^+} R-\overset{\overset{\displaystyle H}{|}}{C}=NOH$$

(an oxime)

f. *Reaction of ketones and aldehydes with hydrazine or hydrazine derivatives*

$$R-CHO + NH_2NH_2 \xrightarrow{H^+} R-\overset{\overset{\displaystyle H}{|}}{C}=N-NH_2$$

(a hydrazone)

g. *Oxidation of aldehydes*

$$R-CHO + Ag(NH_3)_2^+ \xrightarrow{OH^-} R-\overset{\overset{\displaystyle O}{\|}}{C}-O^- + Ag$$

(Tollens' reagent)   (silver mirror)

$$R-CHO + Cu^{++} \xrightarrow{OH^-,\,citrate} R-\overset{\overset{\displaystyle O}{\|}}{C}-O^- + Cu_2O$$

(Benedict's reagent)   (red ppt.)

h. *Haloform reaction with acetaldehyde or methyl ketones*

$$R-\overset{\overset{\displaystyle O}{\|}}{C}-CH_3 \xrightarrow{IO^-} RCO^- + CHI_3$$

i. *Aldol condensation* (requires alpha-hydrogen). Further reaction can also lead to polymers.

$$2CH_3-CHO \xrightarrow{OH^-} H_3C-\overset{\overset{\displaystyle OH}{|}}{\underset{\underset{\displaystyle H}{|}}{C}}-CH_2-CHO$$

j. *Cannizzaro reaction* (for aldehydes having no alpha-hydrogen)

$$2\,\emptyset-CHO \xrightarrow{OH^-} \emptyset-CH_2OH + \emptyset-\overset{\overset{\displaystyle O}{\|}}{C}-O^-$$

Carboxylic Acids

The carboxylic acids are organic compounds that ionize to produce free protons and carboxylate anions. The simplest example is formic acid, $H-\overset{\overset{\displaystyle O}{\|}}{C}-OH$

1. **Synthesis:**

a. *Addition of carbon dioxide to a Grignard reagent*

$$R\,MgBr + CO_2 \rightarrow R-\overset{\overset{\displaystyle O}{\|}}{C}-OMgBr \xrightarrow{H^+} R-\overset{\overset{\displaystyle O}{\|}}{C}-OH$$

b. *Oxidation of alkene*

$$R-\overset{\overset{\displaystyle H}{|}}{C}=\overset{\overset{\displaystyle H}{|}}{C}-R' + KMnO_4 \rightarrow R-\underset{\underset{\displaystyle OH}{|}}{\overset{\overset{\displaystyle H}{|}}{C}}-\underset{\underset{\displaystyle OH}{|}}{\overset{\overset{\displaystyle H}{|}}{C}}-R'$$

$$R-\overset{\overset{H}{|}}{\underset{\underset{OH}{|}}{C}}-\overset{\overset{H}{|}}{\underset{\underset{OH}{|}}{C}}-R' + KMnO_4 \rightarrow RCOOH + R'COOH$$

c. *Oxidation of primary alcohol*

$$R-CH_2OH + KMnO_4 \rightarrow RCOOH$$

d. *Hydrolysis of nitrile*

$$RCN \xrightarrow{\ H_2O,\ H^+\ } RCOOH$$

e. *Hydrolysis of esters*

$$R-\overset{\overset{O}{\|}}{C}-O-R' + H_2O \overset{H^+}{\rightleftharpoons} R-COOH + R'OH$$

f. *Saponification of esters*

$$R-\overset{\overset{O}{\|}}{C}-O-R' + NaOH \rightleftharpoons R'OH + R-\overset{\overset{O}{\|}}{C}-ONa \xrightarrow{H^+} R-COOH$$

2. Reactions:

a. *Neutralization of base*

$$RCOOH + NaOH \rightarrow R\overset{\overset{O}{\|}}{C}-O-Na^+ + H_2O$$

b. *Esterification*

$$RCOOH + R'OH \overset{H^+}{\rightleftharpoons} R-\overset{\overset{O}{\|}}{C}-OR' + H_2O$$

c. *Formation of acylhalide*

$$RCOOH \xrightarrow{PBr_3} R\overset{\overset{O}{\|}}{C}-Br$$

d. *Formation of anhydride*

$$2RCOOH \longrightarrow R-\overset{\overset{O}{\|}}{C}-O-\overset{\overset{O}{\|}}{C}-R + H_2O$$

e. *High-temperature decomposition*

$$2RCOOH \xrightarrow{ThO_2,\ \Delta} R-\overset{\overset{O}{\|}}{C}-R + CO_2 + H_2O$$

Esters

Esters may be formed from the reaction between an acid and an alcohol. Upon hydrolysis the products are an acid and an alcohol. We often think first of carboxylic acid esters, but they are not the only ones known. Phosphate esters are common in biochemistry.
The simplest carboxylic acid ester is methyl formate,

$$H-\overset{\overset{O}{\|}}{C}-O-CH_3$$

1. **Synthesis:**

a. $R-COCl + R'-OH \rightarrow R-\overset{\overset{\textstyle O}{\|}}{C}-OR'$

b. $(R-\overset{\overset{\textstyle O}{\|}}{C})_2O + R'-OH \rightarrow R-\overset{\overset{\textstyle O}{\|}}{C}-OR'$

c. $R-COOH + R'-OH \underset{}{\overset{H^+}{\rightleftharpoons}} R-\overset{\overset{\textstyle O}{\|}}{C}-OR' + H_2O$

An equilibrium will be established. Removal of water by an appropriate method such as azeotropic separation will produce good yields. High yields based on one reactant can also be achieved by adding large quantities of the other reactant.

2. **Reactions:**

a. *Acid hydrolysis*

$$R-COOR' + H_2O \overset{H^+}{\longrightarrow} R-COOH + R'OH$$

b. *Saponification*

$$R-COOR' + H_2O \overset{OH^-}{\longrightarrow} R-COO^- + R'OH$$

Ethers

1. **Synthesis:**

a. *Dehydration. (Remember that the choice of conditions determines whether the ether or the unsaturated hydrocarbon, in this case ethylene, is the major product.)*

$$2CH_3-CH_2OH \xrightarrow{H_2SO_4 \ \Delta} CH_3-CH_2-O-CH_2-CH_3$$

b. *Williamson synthesis.* Much more useful than the dehydration method if an unsymmetrical ether is desired.

$$RONa + R'Br \longrightarrow ROR'$$

2. **Reactions:** Ethers are generally unreactive compounds. They are often useful as solvents in organic reactions because of their unreactive nature. They may be cleaved by heated halogen acids:

$$ROR + HI \xrightarrow{heat} RI + ROH$$

The ROH which is formed may react with HI to form an additional RI.

Final Remarks

As stated earlier, you cannot learn organic chemistry from a brief presentation such as this. We recognize that we have been able to present only some of the more important points. It is our intent that you use this material (and the questions and answers in the practice tests) to review the organic chemistry you have learned in your coursework. If you find areas of weakness in your preparation, we would recommend that you study those areas in your organic chemistry textbook.

Biochemistry

Biochemistry or biological chemistry may be seen as an attempt to better understand life by studying the chemicals that are important in living cells and organisms. One must consider the amounts and identities of a variety of chemicals, as well as the ways in which they are transformed during different life processes. Perhaps it should not be surprising that biochemistry calls upon the background of other areas of chemistry, including organic chemistry, analytical chemistry, inorganic chemistry, and physical chemistry.

In these few pages we can only touch lightly on a few concepts in biochemistry. Those of you who continue in the life sciences, such as medicine, dentistry, or pharmacy, will be taught a great deal more about this fascinating area. Here we can only begin to delineate the forest, leaving you to study the trees at a later time. For those who have had little or no exposure to biochemistry, this brief introduction will help to prepare you for the Medical College Admission Test and will also lay the groundwork for your course in professional school. For those who have already taken a course in biochemistry, this material will assist in consolidating the information you already possess.

Areas of Biochemistry

Although there are a number of ways of subdividing biochemistry, there are substantial similarities among them. The subdivision is done according to similarities in the properties of the compounds within each subdivision and/or similarities in the techniques for the study of compounds within each subdivision. A biochemist usually specializes in the study of one of these subdivisions:

I. pH and Buffers
II. Amino Acids, Peptides, and Proteins
   A. Amino Acids
   B. Peptides and Proteins
III. Enzymes
   A. Nomenclature
   B. Cofactors
   C. Energy
   D. Velocity and Inhibition
IV. Carbohydrates
   A. Chemistry
   B. Functions
   C. Metabolism
      1. Glycolysis
      2. Krebs Cycle
      3. Hexose Monophosphate Shunt
V. Lipids
   A. Chemistry
   B. Metabolism
      1. Hydrolysis to Produce Fatty Acids
      2. Oxidation of Fatty Acids in the Mitochondria
      3. Synthesis of Fatty Acids
      4. Synthesis of Glycerides
VI. Nucleotides and Nucleic Acids; Biosynthesis of Nucleic Acids and Proteins
   A. Nucleotides
   B. Nucleic Acids
   C. Biosynthesis of Nucleic Acids and Proteins

pH and Buffers

The concepts of pH and buffers presented on page 109 under acids and bases are used also in biochemistry. The biochemist applies these principles in the context of the human body.

The human body (and other animal bodies) requires that the pH be maintained over a rather small range. The pH of human blood is ordinarily maintained from 7.36 to 7.42. Buffers prevent greater fluctuation, which could occur in response to loss or gain of acid or base.

The buffer pairs used in human blood include HCO_3^-/H_2CO_3; base/acid species of oxygenated hemoglobin; and base/acid species of deoxygenated hemoglobin. The phosphate pair $HPO_4^{2-}/H_2PO_4^-$ would offer a possible buffer, but little is present in the blood.

Amino Acids, Peptides, and Proteins

Amino Acids: The naturally occurring amino acids are primarily α-amino acids of the general structure

$$
\begin{array}{c}
NH_2 \\
| \\
R-C-COOH \\
| \\
H
\end{array}
$$

If R does not represent H, then it will be noted that an asymmetric center exists, allowing for L and D isomers. The ones commonly found in nature, especially in higher animals, are usually of the L series. (The amino acid having no asymmetric center, and thus devoid of optical activity, is glycine.)

Although approximately 300 amino acids are found in nature, some are relatively rare. About 20 amino acids occur in all organisms. Amino acids can serve as biological active compounds in their own right (e.g., neurotransmitters), but we tend to think of them most often as the monomers of which the polymeric peptides and higher molecular weight proteins are composed.

Subdivisions of Amino Acids. It is possible to subdivide the amino acids based on their R groups. This is useful in predicting such things as the folding of a protein in a lipoprotein membrane; it is also helpful in remembering the different amino acids. Thus, they may be subdivided into aliphatic, hydroxy, sulfur, aromatic, dicarboxy (or dicarboxy with one carboxyl as an amide), diamino, and imino on the basis of the R groups.

They may also be subdivided into acidic, basic, and neutral. Those having a second amino function are basic (two basic functional groups and only one carboxyl). Those having a second proton-releasing functional group are acidic. (This second group could be a carboxyl. It could also be the more weakly ionized phenolic or sulfhydryl group.) The neutral amino acids contain only a single acidic and a single basic group, thus canceling each other.

Essential Amino Acids. Although many amino acids may be synthesized in the animal body, certain animals are unable to synthesize sufficient quantities of particular amino acids, called *essential amino acids.* (The term indicates no judgment of the importance of these amino acids compared to that of the other amino acids. It simply indicates that for optimal health these amino acids must be supplied in the diet.) In humans, ten amino acids are usually called essential: phenylalanine, valine, tryptophan, threonine, isoleucine, methionine, histidine, arginine, leucine, and lycine. Of these, histidine and arginine may be required in the diet only of infants or under special circumstances.

Forms of an Amino Acid. A simple amino acid such as glycine can exist in three forms. At a low pH such as 1, the amino group is protonated (and carrying a charge of +1); the carboxyl is not ionized or charged; and the net charge is +1. At an intermediate pH such as 7, the amino function and the carboxyl function carry equal and opposite charges of +1 and −1, and the net is a charge of zero. At a still higher pH such as 12, the carboxyl is ionized and the amino not ionized, resulting in a net of −1. The mean of the pK_a of these two ionizable groups is the pH at which the amino has no net charge and will not move in an electrical field. This pH is defined as the *isoionic point* and designated as p*I*.

Peptides and Proteins: Peptides are linear chains of amino acids with the carboxyl group of one amino acid attached in amide (specifically peptide) linkage to the amino group of the next amino acid.

$$H_3N^+ - \underset{\underset{H}{|}}{\overset{\overset{R_3}{|}}{C}} - \overset{\overset{O}{\|}}{C} - \underset{}{\overset{\overset{H}{|}}{N}} - \underset{\underset{H}{|}}{\overset{\overset{R_2}{|}}{C}} - \overset{\overset{O}{\|}}{C} - \overset{\overset{H}{|}}{N} - \underset{\underset{H}{|}}{\overset{\overset{R}{|}}{C}} - COO^-$$

Proteins are larger assemblies of amino acids. The linear sequence of amino acids in a chain is called the *primary structure*. The orientation of the peptide chain (e.g., the alpha helix) is called the *secondary structure*. The relationship of portions of the polypeptide chains to one another is called the *tertiary structure*. In some cases there are dimers, trimers, tetramers, etc., of the polypeptide chains. This is called the *quaternary structure*. Sometimes the units are identical, sometimes not. In the enzyme lactate dehydrogenase, two different monomers are assembled into an active tetramer. Five different active lactate dehydrogenase tetramers are possible and are separable by electrophoresis.

The primary structure of a peptide or protein may be determined by a combination of procedures. The carboxy terminal amino acid may be determined by its enzymatic release by carboxypeptidases. The rate of release allows determination of the sequence of a small number of amino acids at the carboxy terminal end. Another method, the Edman degradation, utilizes reaction of the amino terminus with phenylisothiocyanate, hydrolysis of the derivative of this amino acid from the peptide chain, and identification of the amino acid derivative. This Edman degradation allows determination of a number of amino acids in sequence at the amino terminal end.

Determination of a number of amino acids at each end of a peptide chain would not allow determination of the sequence of a long peptide chain. Fortunately there are also other enzymes (endopeptidases) that perform internal cleavage with a high degree of specificity. The smaller peptides thus formed may be separated and sequenced. By utilizing different endopeptidases, it is possible to prepare a series of overlapping peptides. When they are sequenced, it is possible to determine the sequence of the intact peptide.

By other methodology it is also possible to synthesize peptides. This procedure, referred to as the Merrifield synthesis, utilizes a solid material with a functional group to which the peptide chain is attached.

Enzymes

In 1926 Sumner isolated the enzyme urease from jack beans and claimed the enzyme to be a protein. Few believed this initially, and the claim was not accepted until about 1935.

Now, over 2600 enzymes have been isolated. Although biological in origin and protein in nature, enzymes are simply catalysts, serving to increase the rate of reactions in which they are involved.

Nomenclature: Some enzymes are given trivial names, such as the proteolytic enzymes trypsin or pepsin, names that provide no information unless one is familiar with these specific enzymes. Others have names that identify the substrate and type of reaction;

examples are histidine decarboxylase (decarboxylating histidine to produce CO_2 and histamine), urease (breaking down urea to produce CO_2 and NH_3), and alcohol dehydrogenase (removing hydrogen and electrons from an alcohol to produce a reduced coenzyme and an aldehyde).

Since about 1965 (with a revision in 1972) there has been an attempt to confer more systematic nomenclature and classification on enzymes. An enzyme commision (EC) number is given as four numbers separated by periods. The first of these numbers indicates the main class.

1. Oxidoreductases—oxidation-reduction reactions
2. Transferases—transfer intact groups of atoms from donors to acceptors
3. Hydrolases—cleave by hydrolysis
4. Lyases—cleave C-C, C-O, C-N, and other bonds without hydrolysis or oxidation. (Hydration and dehydration reactions are included in this class.)
5. Isomerases—interconvert isomers, such as *cis → trans*;
6. Ligases—form bonds as a result of condensation of two different substances with energy provided by ATP.

An example of EC nomenclature and numbering is alcohol: NAD^+ oxidoreductase (EC1.1.1.1). The first number identifies it as an oxidoreductase; the second number identifies its subclass; the third number identifies its sub-subclass; and the final number is a serial listing within the sub-subclass. EC1.1.1.1 is more commonly known as alcohol dehydrogenase.

Cofactors: In addition to the protein portion, many enzymes need cofactors or coenzymes. The protein enzyme without cofactor is known as an *apoenzyme*; the complete enzyme with cofactor or coenzyme is called a *holoenzyme*. The term coenzyme is usually given to an organic cofactor. A cofactor may serve by altering the three-dimensional structure of the enzyme and/or the bound substrate, or it may participate effectively as a second substrate. Thus, the enzyme lactate dehydrogenase catalyzes the oxidation of lactate to pyruvate as the coenzyme NAD^+ is reduced to $NADH + H^+$.

Energy: Enzymes are often looked upon as defying or contradicting the laws of chemistry. This is not true, of course. The free energy of the substrate initially must be higher than the free energy of the products or the reaction will not occur (without net input of energy). In this case we say that the reaction is thermodynamically unfavorable. Indeed, in this case, the reverse reaction would be thermodynamically favorable.

In the case of a thermodynamically favorable reaction, however, input of energy may still be necessary. This energy input, called the *energy of activation*, will be released again as the energy of the system proceeds to the lower energy level of the final products. (This is sometimes compared to a large stone being rolled from one valley into a valley of lower elevation. The energy expended in rolling the stone to the crest of the intervening hill will be released as the stone proceeds downhill. In addition to the release of energy equal to the input of energy to reach the crest, there is also release of energy related to the difference in elevation of the starting and the ending positions.) The role of the enzyme or of other catalysts is seen as lowering the activation energy of the reaction, thus increasing the rate.

Velocity and Inhibition: In the study of enzymes several relationships must be considered: (1) the rate of the reaction will increase with temperature until there is partial denaturation of the enzyme; (2) rates of reactions of enzymes are affected by pH and will ordinarily exhibit a pH range over which maximal activity is seen; (3) reaction rates ordinarily increase linearly with substrate concentration up to the point of maximum velocity, where it is considered that all enzyme molecules have substrate bound at the same time; (4) reaction rates ordinarily increase linearly with enzyme concentration.

The determination of maximum velocity is somewhat difficult since a plot of velocity versus substrate *approaches* the maximum velocity with a reasonable substrate concentration. A more accurate method for determining maximum velocity involves a double reciprocal plot:

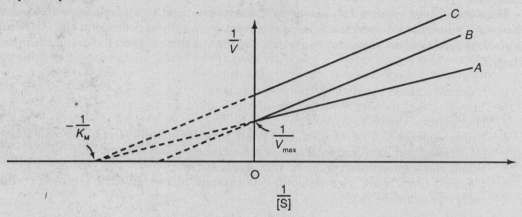

In this graph A is a plot of an uninhibited enzyme; B is a plot of the same enzyme in the presence of a competetive inhibitor; C is a plot of the enzyme in the presence of a noncompetetive inhibitor; v represents velocity and [S] represents substrate concentration. Note that the y-intercept is the reciprocal of maximal velocity, and the x-intercept is the negative of the reciprocal of the Michaelis constant, K_M, a characteristic of the individual enzyme. Note that the maximal velocity in the presence of a competetive inhibitor is the same as for the uninhibited enzyme. The maximal velocity in the presence of a noncompetetive inhibitor is lower (as noted by the fact that the reciprocal is higher).

Carbohydrates

Chemistry: Carbohydrates are a group of polyhydroxy aldehydes, polyhydroxy ketones, and closely related compounds. They may exist as monomers (monosaccharides), dimers (disaccharides), or polymers (polysaccharides).

D-glucose

α-D-glucopyranose

D-fructose

α-D-fructofuranose

D-Glucose and D-fructose are two of the most common monosaccharides found in the human body. They are shown above in straight-chain form and in ring form (as they are usually found in solution). Note that in the ring structure a hemiacetal or a hemiketal has been formed.

Disaccharides such as sucrose and lactose are formed by reaction of monosaccharides. Sucrose hydrolysis will produce equal quantities of D-glucose and D-fructose. Lactose hydrolysis will produce equal quantities of D-galactose and D-glucose.

Polysaccharides are polymers of ring-form monomers. Animal glycogen and plant starch are polymers of α-D-glucopyranose. Cellulose is a polymer of β-D-glucopyranose.

Functions: Carbohydrates play a number of roles in nature. For example, they are metabolized for energy (4 kcal/g), metabolized for production of other required compounds such as certain amino acids, serve as components of nucleic acids (ribose in RNA and deoxyribose in DNA), serve as a structural element (cellulose of plants and cell walls of bacteria), serve as components of lubricants of bone joints, serve as cellular antigens, and are components of heparin.

Metabolism: Many pathways of carbohydrate metabolism could be considered here. We will confine ourselves to comments about glycolysis, the Krebs cycle (also known as the citric acid cycle or the tricarboxylic acid cycle), and the hexose monophosphate shunt (also known as the pentose phosphate pathway).

The complete metabolism of a molecule of glucose proceeds in a series of linked reactions, as shown below. Energy associated with the bonds of glucose is eventually transferred to bonds of adenosine triphosphate (ATP) molecules, which are the molecules used most often to release this energy for work in the cell. Several of the steps shown in the diagram produce ATP directly; however, most ATPs made in the cell carry energy brought to them via "carrier" molecules, either NADH (reduced nicotinamide adenine dinucleotide) or $FADH_2$ (reduced flavin adenine dinucleotide), both of which are made in the reactions shown below. Glycolysis occurs in the cytoplasm; the Krebs cycle, in the mitochondria.

Glycolysis. Glycolysis, in a series of reactions, converts glucose to pyruvic acid (or to lactic acid under conditions of oxygen deficiency). Thus, there is a net formation of 2 moles of ATP from the anaerobic glycolysis of 1 mole of glucose.

Krebs Cycle. Pyruvic acid may be converted to acetyl coenzyme A, producing 3 moles of ATP for each mole of pyruvate. The Krebs cycle may then metabolize the acetyl CoA through a series of reactions to produce 12 moles of ATP for each mole of acetyl CoA. Since the Krebs cycle is often studied with carbohydrate metabolism, many people unconsciously associate them. It should be recognized, however, that acetyl CoA is produced in metabolism of fatty acids and amino acids as well. Acetyl CoA from these other sources is also metabolized in the Krebs cycle.

The Krebs cycle, unlike glycolysis, cannot operate under anaerobic conditions. Oxygen and a functioning electron transport system are required for regeneration of oxidized FAD and NAD^+ (from reduced $FADH_2$ and NADH), but they are also required to produce and capture most of the energy that is realized from the Krebs cycle.

Hexose Monophosphate Shunt. The hexose monophosphate shunt is a series of reactions that serve primarily to produce NADPH and the pentoses (D-ribose and D-deoxyribose). NADPH is important in numerous biosynthetic reactions, including those for biosynthesis of fatty acids and cholesterol. As noted earlier, the pentoses are required for biosynthesis of the nucleic acids (DNA and RNA).

Some Major Steps in Glycolysis and the Citric Acid Cycle*

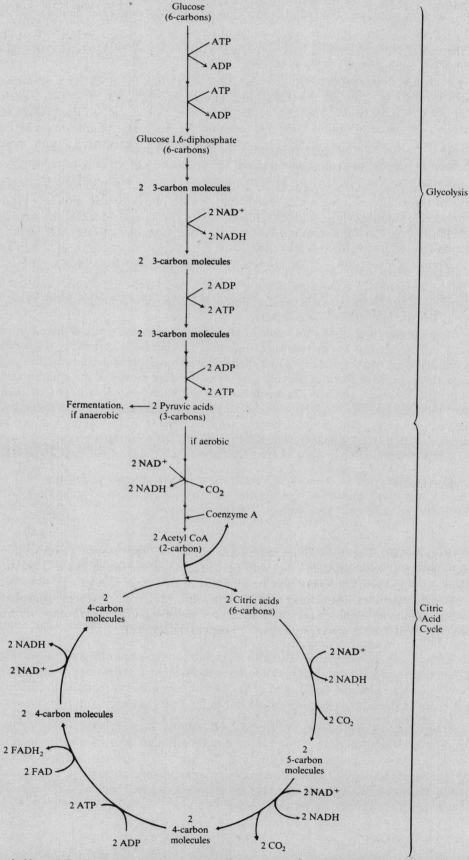

Lipids

Chemistry: Lipids are defined as compounds that may be extracted from biological materials with nonpolar solvents and that are insoluble in aqueous polar solvents. This includes the neutral glycerides (largely triglycerides), the phosphoglycerides, the sphingo-lipids, the steroids, the eicosanoids (particularly the prostaglandins), free fatty acids, and the lipid-soluble vitamins (A, D, E, and K).

Fatty acids are components of many lipids, thus suggesting the need for a discussion of their structure. Fatty acids are generally long, unbranched hydrocarbons with a carboxyl group at one terminus. In the simplest case there are no carbon-to-carbon double bonds, but unsaturation (presence of double bonds) is common. When double bonds are present, they are usually in a *cis*-configuration and in a methylene-interrupted sequence (if more than one double bond is present).

Neutral Glycerides. Neutral glycerides, or acylglycerols, are simply glycerol in ester linkage with one to three fatty acid molecules. Esterification with one fatty acid molecule produces a monoglyceride (monoacylglycerol); esterification with two fatty acid molecules produces a diglyceride (diacylglycerol); and esterification with three molecules of fatty acid produces a triglyceride (triacylglycerol). As previously stated, the triglycerides represent the principal form of storage of excess food. This appears to be a wise arrangement because triglyceride produces 9 kcal/g during metabolism, compared to 4 kcal/g for either carbohydrate or protein, and triglyceride is stored in a substantially water-free state, compared to the hydrated carbohydrates and proteins.

triglyceride

a fatty acid (linoleic acid)

Phosphoglycerides. The phosphoglycerides are similar to the neutral glycerides, but a phosphate group is substituted for the fatty acid that would be found in the 3-position in a triglyceride. Various substituents may be attached to the phosphate group, thus forming other phosphoglycerides. Attachment of choline, for example, produces phosphatidyl-choline; ethanolamine → phosphatidylethanolamine; serine → phosphatidylserine; inositol → phosphatidylinositol; and glycerol produces phosphatidylglycerol.

phosphatidic acid

Sphingolipids. The sphingolipids are based on a long-chain amino alcohol, sphingosine, rather than on glycerol.

$$H_3C-(CH_2)_{12}-\overset{\overset{\displaystyle H}{|}}{C}=\overset{\overset{\displaystyle H}{|}}{C}-\overset{\overset{\displaystyle OH}{|}}{\underset{\underset{\displaystyle H}{|}}{C}}-\overset{\overset{\displaystyle NH_2}{|}}{\underset{\underset{\displaystyle H}{|}}{C}}-CH_2OH$$

sphingosine

$$R-\overset{\overset{\displaystyle OH}{|}}{\underset{\underset{\displaystyle H}{|}}{C}}-\overset{\overset{\displaystyle H}{|}}{\underset{\underset{\displaystyle NH}{|}}{C}}-CH_2O-X$$
$$\underset{\underset{\displaystyle R'}{|}}{C}=O$$

a sphingolipid

In the preceding formula, R represents an unsaturated hydrocarbon chain, R′ represents another hydrocarbon chain (from an R′—COOH that has reacted with the NH_2 to form an amide linkage). X can represent phosphorylcholine in phosphodiester linkage, giving us sphingomyelin. It can also represent a simple glucose (giving us a glucocerebroside), or it can represent a more complex carbohydrate containing sialic acid (giving us a ganglioside).

Steroids. The term steroid is understood by the layperson to designate a natural or synthetic hormone. As used by the biochemist and other professionals in this field, however, it refers to the structure only and does not signify hormonal activity. The structure of a steroid is based on the cyclopentanoperhydrophenanthrene nucleus or steroid nucleus:

An example of a steroid is the sterol cholesterol:

cholesterol

In addition to the sterols, the steroid group includes the bile acids, vitamin D, and the steroid hormones (estrogens, androgens, adrenal corticosteroids, and progesterone).

Eicosanoids. Some fatty acids, including linoleic acid, are very important to mammalian health, but cannot be synthesized in the body. These are therefore called *essential fatty acids.* Among the products of linoleic acid are the prostaglandins, 20-carbon fatty acids that include a 5-carbon ring. Prostaglandins are active in a variety of physiologically important ways and are sometimes used pharmacologically.

prostaglandin E_1
(PGE_1)

Free Fatty Acids. Free fatty acids may sometimes be found in small amounts in various tissues. Fatty acids are also found in unesterified form in blood plasma, but in this case they are ordinarily bound noncovalently to plasma proteins, particularly albumin.

Lipid-soluble Vitamins. The lipid-soluble vitamins A, D, E, and K may also be classified as lipids, based on their solubility. They are stored in the body, and, in contrast to water-soluble vitamins, *steady* dietary intake of these vitamins is not vitally important.

Metabolism:

Hydrolysis to Produce Fatty Acids. Neutral glycerides may be hydrolyzed by lipases such as pancreatic lipase or hormone-sensitive lipase, thus releasing free fatty acids. Fatty acids may also be released from phosphoglycerides by hydrolysis that is catalyzed by phospholipase A_1 and phospholipase A_2.

Oxidation of Fatty Acids in the Mitochondria. Fatty acids may then be oxidized via B-oxidation to produce acetyl CoA + reduced flavin adenine dinucleotide ($FADH_2$) and reduced nicotinamide adenine dinucleotide ($NADH + H^+$). Thus a molecule of fatty acid $16:0$ would produce 8 molecules of acetyl CoA, 7 molecules of $FADH_2$, and 7 molecules of $NADH + H^+$. Each molecule of acetyl CoA can be metabolized in the Krebs cycle to produce 12 molecules of ATP. Each molecule of $FADH_2$ can produce 2 molecules of ATP when it is oxidized in the electron transport chain, and each molecule of $NADH + H^+$ can produce 3 molecules of ATP when oxidized in the electron transport chain.

Synthesis of Fatty Acids. Synthesis of fatty acids occurs in the nonparticulate cytoplasm. The pathway is not simply a reversal of β-oxidation; it requires biotin and carbon dioxide in addition to acetyl CoA. The carbon dioxide, however, is not incorporated into the fatty acid. Also the reducing equivalents required for the synthesis are derived from $NADPH + H^+$.

Synthesis of Glycerides. The neutral glycerides require L-3-glycerol phosphate in their biosynthesis. This glycerol phosphate may be formed by the enzymatic phosphorylation of glycerol or by the enzymatic reduction of dihydroxyacetone phosphate, which is produced in glycolysis.

Nucleotides and Nucleic Acids; Biosynthesis of Nucleic Acids and Proteins

Nucleotides: Both deoxyribonucleic acid (DNA) and ribonucleic acid (RNA) are polymers of nucleotides. A nucleotide consists of a nitrogen base (either a purine or a pyrimidine), a pentose (ribose or 2-deoxyribose), and a phosphate group. Deoxyribose is found in DNA; ribose, in RNA.

The nitrogen bases include the purines (adenine and guanine) in both DNA and RNA. The pyrimidines include cytosine and thymine in DNA; cytosine and uracil are present in RNA. Other nitrogen bases are found in small quantities. Some synthetic nitrogen bases are used in the treatment of cancer and certain viral infections.

Nucleic Acids: As mentioned above, DNA and RNA are polymers of appropriate nucleotides. The attachment between nucleotides is phosphate–pentose-phosphate-pentose–, etc. This leaves the nitrogen base as an appendage from the linear chain. In double-stranded DNA there are two strands that are paired and linked (noncovalently) through their nitrogen bases. Adenine pairs with thymine, and cytosine pairs with guanine. Methods are available to allow determination of the primary structures of both DNA and RNA.

Biosynthesis of Nucleic Acids and Proteins: It is recognized that DNA codes for its own duplication, as well as for RNA synthesis. Messenger RNA, in turn, codes for the biosynthesis of polypeptide chains. Since there is a triplet code without commas, there are $4 \times 4 \times 4 = 64$ possibilities and sequences for specification of a single amino acid. Only about 21 amino acids, however, are known to have codes. It turns out that some codes give other instructions (e.g., initiation or termination of a peptide chain biosynthesis) and some amino acids have more than one code for their placement. Arginine, for example, has six different codons that can specify its placement.

Mutations in the DNA chain can occur, of course, as a result of errors in duplication, spontaneous changes in DNA, or changes resulting from radiation or mutagenic chemicals. A point mutation results in the presence of a different nitrogen base. This may, in turn, cause problems, or it may be a silent mutation. It would be silent if the base change resulted in no difference in the amino acid or if it resulted in the substitution of a very similar amino acid.

A frame shift mutation is likely to be more serious. Consider that insertion or deletion of a nitrogen base will change the sequence of bases following it in the chain. (Remember that there are no commas.) This may be a lethal mutation.

Mutations can be repaired by a number of mechanisms. For example, sometimes an affected area is removed and replaced by a strand that is duplicated again from the complementary DNA strand. Specific cellular enzymes exist to aid in identifying and repairing mutations.

PHYSICS—FREQUENTLY ENCOUNTERED PHYSICS PROBLEMS AND THEIR ANSWERS

Accelerated Motion

Example: A boat accelerates uniformly from 15 mi/hr to 45 mi/hr in 10 sec.

1. Calculate acceleration.

$$a = \frac{v_2 - v_1}{t}$$

a = acceleration
v_1 = initial speed *or* velocity
v_2 = final speed *or* velocity
t = time

$$a = \frac{45 \text{ mi/hr} - 15 \text{ mi/hr}}{10 \text{ sec}} = \frac{30 \text{ mi/hr}}{10 \text{ sec}} = 3 \text{ mi/hr/sec, or } 3 \text{ mi/hr·sec}$$

2. Calculate average speed.

$$v = \frac{v_1 + v_2}{2}$$

v = average velocity

$$v = \frac{15 \text{ mi/hr} + 45 \text{ mi/hr}}{2} = 30 \text{ mi/hr}$$

3. Distance covered?

s = distance covered

$$s = vt$$

Recall: There are 5280 ft/mi and 3600 sec/hr. In 30 mi, 158,400 ft are covered. So,

$$\frac{158,400 \text{ ft}}{3600 \text{ sec}} = 44 \text{ ft/sec}$$

Since the boat was in motion for 10 sec,

distance covered = 44 ft/sec × 10 sec = 440 ft

Example: An object is accelerated from rest to 600 mi/hr in 30 sec; the object has been subjected to an acceleration of 29 ft/sec^2

A convenient unit for acceleration is feet per second squared (ft/sec^2). First, convert the velocity units:

$$\frac{600 \text{ mi}}{\text{hr}} \times \frac{5280 \text{ ft}}{\text{mi}} \times \frac{\text{hr}}{3600 \text{ sec}} = 880 \text{ ft/sec}$$

Then

$$a = \frac{v}{t}$$

$$a = \frac{880 \text{ ft/sec}}{30 \text{ sec}} = 29 \text{ ft/sec}^2$$

Another way of expressing this type of phenomenon is to solve a problem as follows:

Example: A car is traveling at a speed of 31 mi/hr and accelerates for 8 sec to reach a speed of 55 mi/hr. Its rate of acceleration was 3 mi/hr/sec. Mathematically expressed:

$$a = \frac{\textbf{Final Velocity} - \textbf{Initial Velocity}}{\textbf{Time}}$$

$$a = \frac{55 \text{ mi/hr} - 31 \text{ mi/hr}}{8 \text{ sec}}$$

$$a = \frac{24 \text{ mi/hr}}{8 \text{ sec}} = 3 \text{ mi/hr/sec, or 3 mi/hr·sec}$$

Falling Objects—Gravity Acceleration

Recall: $g = 32$ ft/sec^2 or 980 cm/s^2 or 9.8 m/s^2

Example: An object in free fall travels for 1 sec.

1. Calculate speed (velocity) obtained, when the body is released from rest.

$$v_2 = v_1 + at$$
$$v_2 = 0 + (32 \text{ ft/sec}^2)(1 \text{ sec})$$
$$v_2 = 32 \text{ ft/sec}$$

v_1 = initial speed = 0
v_2 = final speed
a = acceleration
t = time

2. **The above body started from rest; the distance covered in the time was?**

$$s = v_1 t + \frac{1}{2} at^2$$

$$s = 0 + \frac{1}{2}(32 \text{ ft/sec}^2)(1 \text{ sec})^2$$

$$s = 16 \text{ ft}$$

v_1 = initial speed = 0
t = time
s = distance traversed
a = acceleration

Example: A rocket traveling upward is going 400 ft/sec when its fuel is exhausted. Then:

1. The distance covered after 1 sec is?

$$s = v_1 t + \frac{1}{2} a t^2 \qquad \begin{aligned} v_1 &= 400 \text{ ft/sec} \\ a &= -32 \text{ ft/sec}^2 \\ t &= 1 \text{ sec} \end{aligned}$$

$$s = (400 \text{ ft/sec})(1 \text{ sec}) + \frac{1}{2}(-32 \text{ ft/sec}^2)(1 \text{ sec})^2$$

$$s = 384 \text{ ft}$$

2. **Calculate the speed obtained after 1 sec.**

$$v_2 = v_1 + at$$

$$v_2 = 400 \text{ ft/sec} + (-32 \text{ ft/sec}^2)(1 \text{ sec})$$

$$v_2 = 368 \text{ ft/sec}$$

v_1 = **initial velocity**

v_2 = **final velocity**

a = **acceleration**

t = **time**

Example: a. At the end of 1 sec a falling object will attain a velocity of 32 ft/sec.

$$v_f = at = 32 \text{ ft/sec} \times 1 \text{ sec} = 32 \text{ ft/sec} \qquad v_f = \text{final velocity}$$

b. During this 1 sec of falling, however, an object previously at rest will have covered a distance of 16 ft.

$$s = v_0 t + \frac{at^2}{2}$$

$$s = (0 \text{ ft})(1 \text{ sec})$$

$$+ \frac{(32 \text{ ft/sec}^2)(1 \text{ sec})^2}{2} = 16 \text{ ft}$$

s = **distance traversed**

v_0 = **velocity at rest**
    = **initial velocity = 0**

t = **time**

Uniform Velocity

Example: a car travels with a constant velocity of 30 mi/hr for 40 mi. What time is needed to travel this distance?

$$t = \frac{s}{v}$$

$$t = \frac{40 \text{ mi}}{30 \text{ mi/hr}}$$

$$t = 1.33 \text{ hr}$$

v = velocity = 30 mi/hr

s = distance traversed = 40 mi

t = time

Nonuniform Motion

Example: A rocket with an initial velocity of 25 m/s is accelerated at 75 m/s² for 10 s.

1. The rocket covers a distance of how many meters during the period of acceleration?

$$s = v_0 t + \frac{1}{2} a t^2 \qquad\qquad s = \text{distance traversed}$$

$$s = (25 \text{ m/s})(10 \text{ s}) + \frac{1}{2}(75 \text{ m/s}^2)(10 \text{ s})^2$$

$$s = 250 \text{ m} + \frac{7500 \text{ m}}{2}$$

$$s = 250 \text{ m} + 3750 \text{ m}$$

$$s = 4000 \text{ m}$$

2. **How far would the rocket travel if it started from rest?**

$$x = \frac{1}{2}(75 \text{ m/s}^2)(10 \text{ s})^2$$

$$x = 3750 \text{ m}$$

Uniform Deceleration

Example: A train travels at 60 mi/hr (88 ft/sec); the brakes are applied for 2 sec, and it decelerates at a rate of 22 ft/sec². Calculate its final velocity.

$$v = v_0 - at$$

$$v = 88 \text{ ft/sec} - (22 \text{ ft/sec}^2)(2 \text{ sec})$$

$$v = 44 \text{ ft/sec (or 30 mi/hr)}$$

Free Fall

Example: A construction worker drops a brick while working at a height of 900 ft.

$$v_0 = 0$$

$$g = 32 \text{ ft/sec}^2$$

$$t = 3 \text{ sec}$$

$$y = \text{distance traversed}$$

1. What distance does the brick cover in 3 sec?

$$s = v_0 t + \frac{1}{2} g t^2$$

$$s = \frac{1}{2} g t^2$$

$$s = \frac{1}{2}(32 \text{ ft/sec}^2)(3 \text{ sec}^2)$$

$$s = 144 \text{ ft}$$

2. **How long does it take for the brick to land on the ground?**

$$s = \frac{1}{2} gt^2$$

$$t = \left(\frac{2s}{g}\right)^{1/2}$$

$$t = \left(\frac{(2)(900 \text{ ft})}{32 \text{ ft/sec}^2}\right)^{1/2}$$

$$t = (56/\text{sec}^2)^{1/2}$$

$$t = 7.5 \text{ sec}$$

3. **What is the velocity of the brick at 2 sec of travel?**

$$v = gt$$

$$v = (32 \text{ ft/sec}^2)(2 \text{ sec})$$

$$v = 64 \text{ ft/sec}$$

Forces and Motion

Forces and Acceleration

Newton's Second Law: Force = Mass × Acceleration OR $f = ma$
Newton's Third Law: For every acting force there exists a reacting force of equal magnitude but in the opposite direction, that is, $F(\text{action}) = -F(\text{reaction})$.

$$f = \text{force}$$

$$m = \text{mass}$$

$$a = \text{acceleration}$$

Recall: A unit of force applied is the *dyne*; 1 dyne is the force that will impart to a 1-gram mass an acceleration of 1 cm/s², that is, $1 \text{ dyne} = 1 \frac{g \cdot cm}{s^2}$

Example: A force of 2000 dynes is applied to a mass of 250 g. Calculate the acceleration obtained.

$$a = \frac{f}{m}$$

$$a = \frac{2000 \text{ dynes}}{250 \text{ g}}$$

$$a = \frac{2000 \text{ g} \cdot \text{cm/s}^2}{250 \text{ g}}$$

$$a = 8 \text{ cm/s}^2$$

Example: What is the force exerted on the surface of an asteroid by a man of 70-kg mass if the acceleration due to gravity of the asteroid is 2.5 m/s²?

$$F = mg$$

$$F = 70 \text{ kg} \times 2.5 \text{ m/s}^2 = 175 \text{ N}$$

(A newton, abbreviated as N, is a unit of force expressed in kilograms × meter/second².)

Weight and Acceleration

$$F = \frac{w}{g}a \text{ OR } f = ma$$

$$w = mg$$

F or f = force

a = acceleration

w = weight

m = mass

g = acceleration due to gravity

Example: A force of 30 lb. is applied to a weight of 30 lb. Calculate the acceleration produced.

$$F = \frac{w}{g}a; \, a = \frac{Fg}{w}$$

$$a = \frac{30 \text{ lb} \times 32 \text{ ft/sec}^2}{30 \text{ lb}}$$

$$a = 32 \text{ ft/sec}^2$$

Example: A 180-lb. astronaut is accelerated upward by his rocket at 80 ft/sec². Calculate the force that the seat exerts on him.

$$F = \frac{w}{g}a$$

$$F = \frac{(180 \text{ lb})(80 \text{ ft/sec}^2)}{32 \text{ ft/sec}^2}$$

$$F = 450 \text{ lb}$$

This is the net accelerating force. The seat is also supporting his weight, so the total force is

$$F = 450 \text{ lb} + 180 \text{ lb} = 630 \text{ lb}$$

Example: A 20-kg mass located on a frictionless table is acted upon by a horizontal force of 240 N.

1. **Calculate the acceleration of the object.**

$$F = ma$$

$$a = \frac{F}{m}$$

$$a = \frac{240 \text{ N}}{20 \text{ kg}}$$

$$a = 12 \text{ m/s}^2$$

2. **Calculate the distance the mass will travel in 10 sec.**

$$s = v_0 t + \frac{1}{2}at^2$$

$$s = 0 + \frac{1}{2}(12 \text{ m/s}^2)(10 \text{ s})^2$$

$$s = \frac{1200 \text{ m}}{2}$$

$$s = 600 \text{ m}$$

Negative Acceleration

Example: A test vehicle weighing 3000 lb travels at 60 mi/hr (88 ft/sec). Its stopping distance is 300 ft.

1. Calculate the negative acceleration.

$$v^2 = v_0^2 + 2ax$$

$$a = \frac{v^2 - v_0^2}{2x}$$

$$a = 0 - \frac{(88 \text{ ft/sec})^2}{2(300 \text{ ft})}$$

$$a = -12.9 \text{ ft/sec}^2$$

2. **What is the mass?**

$$m = \frac{w}{g}$$

$$m = \frac{3000 \text{ lb}}{32 \text{ ft/sec}^2}$$

$$m = 94 \text{ lb sec}^2/\text{ft or slugs}$$

3. What force is required to stop the vehicle?

$$F = ma$$

$$F = (93.75 \text{ slugs}) \times (-12.9 \text{ ft/sec}^2)$$

$$F = -1210 \text{ lb}$$

Example: A crane is lowering a 5000 kg air conditioning unit, and the tension in the cable is 40,000 N as the unit begins to go downward.

1. Net force on the unit?

The weight of the unit is

$$w = mg = (5000 \text{ kg})\left(\frac{9.8 \text{ m}}{s^2}\right) = 49,000 \text{ N}$$

So the net downward force is

$$49,000 \text{ N} - 40,000 \text{ N} = 9000 \text{ N}$$

2. Acceleration of unit?

$$a = \frac{F}{m} = \frac{9000 \text{ N}}{5000 \text{ kg}} = 1.8 \text{ m/s}^2$$

3. How long will it take the unit to reach a speed of 4 m/s?

$$t = \frac{v}{a} = \frac{4 \text{ m/s}}{1.8 \text{ m/s}^2} = 2.2 \text{ s}$$

Resultant Forces

a. Forces Acting Upon Each Other at Right Angles.
Example: If a force of 12 lb and a force of 16 lb acted upon each other at right angles, the resultant would be 20 lb. The answer is obtained by utilizing the formula:

$$R = \sqrt{(\text{Force 1})^2 + (\text{Force 2})^2}$$

Thus,

$$R = \sqrt{(12 \text{ lb})^2 + (16 \text{ lb})^2}$$

$$R = \sqrt{144 \text{ lb} + 256 \text{ lb}}$$

$$R = \sqrt{400 \text{ lb}}$$

$$R = 20 \text{ lb}$$

b. Forces Acting in the Same Direction.
Example: The resultant of two forces of 3 dynes and 10 dynes acting in the same direction is 13 dynes. Any combination of forces acting upon the same object in the same direction will result in an addition of the forces and the result will be equal to the sum of the forces.

Equilibrium States

An object is in equilibrium when all forces on it add to zero.

Example: An instrument weighing 35 N is placed in a stream, suspended by a rope that makes an angle of 40° with the vertical. A scale inserted in the rope reads 28 N. Find the force of buoyancy and the force exerted on the instrument by the current.

1. Determine the vertical and horizontal components of the tension in the rope.

$$T_{\text{vert}} = (28 \text{ N})(\cos 40°) = 21 \text{ N}$$

$$T_{\text{hor}} = (28 \text{ N})(\sin 40°) = 18 \text{ N}$$

2. Set all upward forces equal to all downward forces.

$$\text{Weight} = \text{Buoyancy } (B) + \text{Upward Component}$$

$$B = 35 \text{ N} - 21 \text{ N} = 14 \text{ N}$$

3. Set upstream forces equal to downstream forces.

$$\text{Horizontal Component} = \text{Current Force } (C)$$

$$C = 18 \text{ N}$$

Example: A 28-kg packing case is on a ramp inclined at 25° to the horizontal, and is pulled uphill at constant speed with a force of 160 N. Determine the coefficient of friction.

1. Determine the weight of the case.

$$w = mg = (28 \text{ kg})(9.8 \text{ m/s}^2) = 247 \text{ N}$$

2. Find the components of the weight parallel and perpendicular to the ramp.

$$W_{\text{par}} = (274 \text{ N})(\sin 25°) = 116 \text{ N}$$

$$W_{\text{perp}} = (274 \text{ N})(\cos 25°) = 248 \text{ N}$$

3. Find the friction by setting uphill forces equal to downhill forces.

$$160\text{ N} = 116\text{ N} + F$$

$$F = 44\text{ N}$$

4. Find the coefficient of friction.

$$\mu = \frac{\text{friction}}{\text{normal force}} = \frac{44\text{ N}}{248\text{ N}} = 0.18$$

Projectile Motion

$$v = \text{initial velocity}$$

$$\theta = \text{angle with horizontal}$$

$$v_h = \text{horizontal component of path} = v\cos\theta$$

$$v_v = \text{vertical component of path} = v\sin\theta$$

Example: A canonball travels with a speed of 200 ft./sec. with a 30° horizontal projection.

1. Determine the height the ball reaches. Look up the sine and cosine in a standard table or use a scientific calculator.

$$\sin 30° = 0.5;\ v_v = v\sin\theta = (200\text{ ft/sec})(\sin 30°) = 100\text{ ft/sec}$$

$$\cos 30° = 0.866;\ v_h = v\cos\theta = (200\text{ ft/sec})(\cos 30°) = 173\text{ ft/sec}$$

Utilize the equation:

$$v_2{}^2 - v_1{}^2 = 2as \qquad v_1 = 100\text{ ft/sec}$$

$$v_2 = 0$$

$$a = -32\text{ ft/sec}^2$$

Thus we have:

$$0 - (100\text{ ft/sec})^2 = 2(-32\text{ ft/sec}^2)s$$

$$s = \frac{10,000\text{ ft}^2/\text{sec}^2}{64\text{ ft/sec}^2}$$

$$s = 156\text{ ft}$$

2. Calculate the time necessary to reach maximum height.

$$v_2 - v_1 = at$$

$$0 - 100\text{ ft/sec} = (-32\text{ ft/sec}^2)t$$

$$t = \frac{100\text{ ft/sec}}{32\text{ ft/sec}^2}$$

$$t = 3.1\text{ sec}$$

3. The ball will return to the earth in what time? If 3.12 sec are used for ascending, $2t$ should be required. The answer is 6.24 sec.

4. Determine the range (R) of the ball.

$$R = v_h t$$
$$R = (173 \text{ ft/sec})(6.24 \text{ sec})$$
$$R = 1080 \text{ ft}$$

Friction

$$\text{Formula } \mu = \frac{F}{N} \qquad \mu = \text{coefficient of friction}$$

$$F = \text{frictional force}$$
$$N = \text{normal or perpendicular force}$$

Example: A 2500-lb force draws a 30,000-lb railroad car at constant speed on level terrain.

1. Determine the coefficient of friction.

$$\mu = \frac{F}{N}$$

$$\mu = \frac{2500 \text{ lb}}{30,000 \text{ lb}} = 0.08$$

(The coefficient of friction is the ratio of the frictional force to the perpendicular force pressing the two surfaces together.)

2. The railroad car is pulled on a horizontal track at constant speed by a steel cable that makes a 30° angle above the horizontal. The tension in the cable is 300 lb. Determine the coefficient of friction.

$$F \text{ (parallel frictional force)} = F = 300 \text{ lb} \times \cos 30°$$
$$= 300 \text{ lb} \times 0.866$$
$$= 259.8 \text{ lb}$$

The normal force N—which is the weight of the car—is 30,000 lb. However, the vertical component of tension must be subtracted from it.

$$N = 30,000 \text{ lb} - 300 \text{ lb} \times \sin 30°$$
$$= 30,000 \text{ lb} - 150 \text{ lb}$$
$$= 29,850 \text{ lb}$$
$$\mu = \frac{F}{N}$$
$$\mu = \frac{259.8 \text{ lb}}{29,850 \text{ lb}}$$
$$\mu = 0.009$$

Work and Power

Work (*W*) equals the force (*F*) times the displacement (*d*) in the direction of the force, that is, $W = Fd$.

Example: A machine is pushed 50 ft on a level floor. The frictional force is determined as 300 lb. Calculate the work performed.

$$W = Fd$$

$$W = (300 \text{ lb})(50 \text{ ft})$$

$$W = 15,000 \text{ ft-lb}$$

Example: Instead of being pushed, the above machine is dragged via a steel cable at an angle of 30° with the floor and a force on the cable of 300 lb. The work performed is?

$$W = (F \cos 30°)d$$

$$W = 300 \text{ lb.} \times 0.866 \times 50 \text{ ft}$$

$$W = 13,000 \text{ ft-lb}$$

Work and Energy

Example: A man pushes his snowblower with a constant force of 50 lb. The shaft makes an angle of 45° with the horizontal. The work done by the man in 150 ft is?

$$W = Fd \cos 45°$$

$$W = (50 \text{ lb})(150 \text{ ft})(0.707)$$

$$W = 5300 \text{ ft-lb}$$

Power and Power Units

$$\text{Power} = \frac{\text{Work}}{\text{Time}} \text{ or } P = \frac{W}{t}$$

Units: 1 watt = 10^7 ergs/sec = 1 joule/sec
1 horsepower (hp) = 550 ft-lb/sec = 746 watts
1 kilowatt = 1000 watts = 1.34 hp

Example: By means of its steel pulleys, a crane raises a machine weighing 500 lb to a height of 100 ft in 200 sec. The average horsepower necessary is?

$$P = \frac{W}{t}$$

$$P = \frac{\text{Force} \times \text{Distance}}{\text{Time}}$$

$$P = \frac{(500 \text{ lb})(100 \text{ ft})}{200 \text{ sec}}$$

$$P = 250 \text{ ft-lb/sec}$$

$$P = \frac{250 \text{ ft-lb/sec}}{550 \dfrac{\text{ft-lb/sec}}{1 \text{ hp}}}$$

$$P = 0.45 \text{ hp}$$

Example: A man weighing 180 lb is taking a stress test. The test equals the activity of climbing stairs a vertical distance of 30 ft in 5 sec. Calculate the horsepower he develops.

$$P = \frac{W}{t}$$

$$P = \frac{180 \text{ lb} \times 30 \text{ ft}}{5 \text{ sec}}$$

$$P = \frac{5400 \text{ ft-lb}}{5 \text{ sec}}$$

$$P = 1080 \text{ ft-lb/sec}$$

$$P = \frac{1080 \text{ ft-lb/sec}}{550 \dfrac{\text{ft-lb/sec}}{1 \text{ hp}}}$$

$$P = 1.96 \text{ hp}$$

Example: To take the MCAT examination you must climb stairs to a height of 60 ft, and you weigh 180 lb. The work you do against the force of gravity is 10,800 ft-lb.

$$W = F \times D$$

$$W = 180 \text{ lb} \times 60 \text{ ft} = 10,800 \text{ ft-lb}$$

Energy

Potential Energy

Potential energy (PE)—or energy of position—is the product of the weight (w) of an object and the height (h) to which the object is elevated, or the work done in elevating it: $PE = wh$.

Example: A machine weighing 5000 lb is raised onto the roof of a building 150 ft high. Calculate the increase in potential energy or the work done in lifting the machine.

$$PE = wh$$

$$PE = (5000 \text{ lb})(150 \text{ ft})$$

$$PE = 750,000 \text{ ft-lb}$$

Kinetic Energy

Kinetic energy = energy of motion.

Formulas: 1. $KE = \dfrac{1}{2} \dfrac{w}{g} v^2$ w = weight in lb.

2. $KE = \dfrac{1}{2} m v^2$ $g = $ ft/sec^2

$v = $ ft/sec

$KE = $ ft-lb

Example: Determine the kinetic energy of a locomotive weighing 250,000 lb. and traveling at a speed of 30 mi/hr (44 ft/sec).

$$KE = \frac{1}{2} \frac{w}{g} v^2$$

$$KE = \frac{1}{2} \frac{(250,000 \text{ lb})(44 \text{ ft/sec})^2}{32 \text{ ft/sec}^2}$$

$$KE = 7,600,000 \text{ ft-lb}$$

Recall: The joule (J) is a unit of energy. It is a N·m, the work done by a force of 1 N through a distance of 1 m. It is the heat produced by an ampere flowing against an ohm for one second. One joule is equal to 10^7 ergs, and 4.185 J are equal to one calorie.

Example: A rocket with a mass of 2000 kg is fired vertically upward with an initial velocity of 100 m/s.
1. Calculate the change in kinetic energy at maximum height reached.

$$\Delta K = K - K_0$$

$$-K_0 = -\frac{1}{2} mv_0^2$$

$$-K_0 = -\frac{1}{2}(2000 \text{ kg})(100 \text{ m/s})^2$$

$$\Delta K = -K_0 = -10,000,000 \text{ J}$$

K = kinetic energy at maximum height = 0

K_0 = initial kinetic energy

V_0 = initial velocity

Answer: At maximum height reached, the rocket has lost 10,000,000 J of kinetic energy.

2. Calculate the potential energy at maximum height, and the change in kinetic energy upon return to lift-off point.

a. $\quad v^2 = v_0^2 - 2gy$

$$y = \frac{v_0^2}{2g}$$

$$y = \frac{(100 \text{ m/s})^2}{2(9.8 \text{ m/s}^2)}$$

$$y = \frac{10,000 \text{ m}^2/\text{s}^2}{19.6 \text{ m/s}^2}$$

$$y = 510 \text{ m}$$

v_0 = initial velocity

y = maximum height

g = gravitational acceleration

b. $\quad PE = mgh$

$$PE = (2000 \text{ kg})(9.8 \text{ m/s}^2)(510 \text{ m})$$

$$PE = 10,000,000 \text{ J}$$

The increase in potential energy, then, is 10,000,000 J, and one can deduce that the rocket returns to its lift-off point with the same velocity it had at the beginning. The rocket had gained 10,000,000 J of kinetic energy on the original flight, but lost this amount in potential energy and, therefore, the total change in potential energy was zero. The KE and PE balance each other and are constant; the principle of conservation of energy is demonstrated.

Momentum

Momentum is the product of the mass and velocity of an object:

$$p = mv \qquad p = \text{momentum}$$
$$m = \text{mass}$$
$$v = \text{velocity}$$

The change of momentum is equal to the force applied times time. You may use $\dfrac{w}{g}$ in place of m (mass), since $m = \dfrac{w}{g}$ (see p. 143).

Example: A 180-lb man is shot out of a cannon at the speed of 30 ft/sec. What is his momentum?

$$p = \frac{w}{g} v$$

$$p = \frac{180 \text{ lb}}{32 \text{ ft/sec}^2} (30 \text{ ft/sec})$$

$$p = 1.69 \text{ lb-sec}$$

Example: On landing, a plane is traveling at 60 mi/hr. Brakes are applied, and the plane comes to a stop in 10 sec. Assuming the average weight to be 160 lb, what is the force of the seat belts on each passenger?

Step 1   Calculate the change in momentum.

$$p = -mv_0 = -\frac{w}{g} v_0$$

$$p = -\left(\frac{160 \text{ lb}}{32 \text{ ft/sec}^2} \right) 88 \text{ ft/sec}$$

$$p = -440 \text{ lb-sec}$$

Step 2   Now calculate the force applied by the seat belt on a passenger.

$$F = \frac{p}{t}$$

$$F = \frac{-440 \text{ lb-sec}}{10 \text{ sec}}$$

$$F = -44 \text{ lb}$$

Uniform Circular Motion

Centripetal Acceleration

Example: A subway car traveling at a speed of 30 mi/hr (44 ft/sec) negotiates a curve whose radius is 600 ft. What is its acceleration?

$$a = \frac{v^2}{r}$$
a = acceleration
v = velocity
r = radius

$$a = \frac{(44 \text{ ft/sec})^2}{600 \text{ ft}}$$

$$a = \frac{1936 \text{ ft}^2/\text{sec}^2}{600 \text{ ft}}$$

$$a = 3.22 \text{ ft/sec}^2$$

Circular Motion

Recall: $\dfrac{360°}{2\pi} = 1 \text{ rad} = 57.3°$

$$360° = 2\pi \text{ rad}; \quad 180° = \pi \text{ rad}; \quad 90° = \frac{\pi}{2} \text{ rad}$$

The radian is a unit of measurement equal to the angle obtained at the center of a circle making an arc equal to the length of the radius.

Example: An airplane has its automatic pilot fly a circular route at a constant speed of 60 mi/hr. The route has a diameter of 10,000 ft.

1. Calculate the plane's angular speed.

$$\omega = \frac{v}{r}$$

$$\omega = \frac{88 \text{ ft/sec}}{5000 \text{ ft}}$$

$$\omega = 0.0176 \text{ rad/sec}$$

ω = angular speed

v = velocity = 60 mi/hr = 88 ft/sec

d = diameter = 10,000 ft

r = radius = $\dfrac{d}{2}$ = 5,000 ft

2. Calculate the angular distance and the arc length flown in 45 sec.

Angular distance $\theta = t$

$$\theta = (0.0176 \text{ rad/sec})(45 \text{ sec})$$

$$\theta = 0.792 \text{ rad}$$

$$\text{Arc length } s = r\theta$$

$$s = (5000 \text{ ft}) (0.792 \text{ rad})$$

$$s = 3960 \text{ ft}$$

OR

$$s = vt$$

$$s = (88 \text{ ft/sec}) (45 \text{ sec})$$

$$s = 3960 \text{ ft}$$

Centripetal Force

Centripetal force may be expressed as mass times velocity squared divided by the radius, that is, $F_c = \dfrac{mv^2}{r}$ or $F_c = \dfrac{w}{g} \times \dfrac{v^2}{r}$.

Example: The previously cited subway car weighs 300,000 lb, travels at 30 mi/hr, and rounds the above radius of 600 ft. Its centripetal force is?

$$F_c = \frac{w}{g} \times \frac{v^2}{r} \qquad \begin{aligned} w &= 300,000 \text{ lb} \\ g &= 32 \text{ ft/sec}^2 \\ v &= 30 \text{ mi/hr } (44 \text{ ft/sec}) \\ r &= 600 \text{ ft} \end{aligned}$$

$$F_c = \frac{300,000 \text{ lb}}{32 \text{ ft/sec}^2} \times \frac{(44 \text{ ft/sec})^2}{600 \text{ ft}}$$

$$F_c = 30,250 \text{ lb}$$

Example: A satellite is in circular orbit at an altitude of 5.0×10^2 km. One complete revolution takes 95 minutes.

1. Calculate the tangential velocity.

   Radius of earth = 6400 km

   Radius of orbit, r = 6400 km + 500 km = 6900 km, or 6.9×10^6 m

$$v = \frac{s}{t} = \frac{2\pi r}{t} = \frac{2\pi(6.9 \times 10^6 \text{ m})}{5700 \text{ s}} = 7600 \text{ m/s}$$

2. Calculate the angular speed

$$\omega = \frac{\theta}{t} = \frac{2\pi}{5700 \text{ s}} = 1.10 \times 10^{-3} \text{ rad/s}$$

   To get the tangential speed from this:

$$v = r\omega = (6.9 \times 10^6 \text{ m})(1.10 \times 10^{-3} \text{ rad/s}) = 7600 \text{ m/s}$$

3. Calculate the centripetal acceleration, due to gravity:

$$a_c = \frac{v^2}{r} = \frac{(7600 \text{ m/s})^2}{6.9 \times 10^6 \text{ m}} = 8.4 \text{ m/s}^2$$

Centrifugal Force

$$F_r = \frac{mv^2}{r} \quad \text{or} \quad F_r = \frac{w}{g} \times \frac{v^2}{r}$$

Example: An astronaut weighing 160 lb is being spun in a centrifuge with a radius of 120 ft at a speed of 60 mi/hr. What is the centrifugal force on the astronaut?

$$F_r = \frac{mv^2}{r} \qquad w = mg$$

$$m = \frac{160 \text{ lb}}{32 \text{ ft/sec}^2} = 5 \text{ slugs}$$

$$F = \frac{5 \text{ slugs } (88 \text{ ft/sec})^2}{120 \text{ ft}}$$

$$F = 320 \text{ lb}$$

Example: A 0.5-kg object is traveling in a circular orbit 20 m in diameter at a speed of 2 m/s. The cord is subjected to a force of 0.2 N. What is the centrifugal force on the cord?

$$F = \frac{mv^2}{r} = \frac{(0.5 \text{ kg})(2 \text{ m/s})^2}{10 \text{ m}} = 0.2 \text{ N}$$

Since the mass is expressed in kilograms, velocity in meters per second, and distance in meters, the unit of force will be the newton. Note that the diameter of the circle was given, but the radius is required in the equation.

Fluids at Rest

Pressure

$$P = \frac{F}{A} \qquad P = \text{Pressure}$$

$$F = \text{Force}$$

$$A = \text{Area}$$

Example: The end of a pillar of a building has an area of 400 in². The air hammer applies a force of 600 lb as the pillar is driven into the ground. What is the pressure under the pillar?

$$P = \frac{F}{A}$$

$$P = \frac{600 \text{ lb}}{400 \text{ in}^2}$$

$$P = 1.5 \text{ lb/in}^2$$

Example: A man weighs 185 lb; his shoes have a surface area of 13 in², and therefore, the pressure exerted because of his weight is 14 lb/in². The formula to be employed is:

$$P = \frac{F}{A}$$

$$P = \frac{185 \text{ lb}}{13 \text{ in}^2} = 14 \text{ lb/in}^2$$

Density

Density is the mass per unit volume of a substance.

$$P = hdg$$

$P = $ pressure

$h = $ height

$d = $ density

$g = $ acceleration due to gravity

Example: A tank $10 \times 10 \times 10$ ft is filled with gasoline (weight-density 42 lb/ft^3). Weight density $d_w = dg$.

1. Calculate the pressure at the bottom of the tank in lb/ft^2 and lb/in^2.

$$P = hd_w$$
$$P = 10 \text{ ft} \times 42 \text{ lb/ft}^3$$
$$P = 420 \text{ lb/ft}^2$$
$$P = \frac{420 \text{ lb/ft}^2}{144 \text{ in}^2/\text{ft}^2}$$
$$P = 2.92 \text{ lb/in}^2$$

2. Calculate the force at the bottom of the tank.

$$P = \frac{F}{A}$$
$$F = PA$$
$$F = (420 \text{ lb/ft}^2)(100 \text{ ft}^2)$$
$$F = 42,000 \text{ lb}$$

Example: Find the pressure due to a column of mercury 100 cm high.

$P = hdg$

$P = (100 \text{ cm})(13.6 \text{ g/cm}^3)(980 \text{ cm/s}^2)$

$P = 1,330,000 \text{ dynes/cm}^2$

$h = 100$ cm

$d = 13.6$ g/cm^3 (given)

$g = 980$ cm/s^2

Specific Gravity

$$\text{Specific Gravity} = \frac{d}{d_?}$$

$d = $ density of a substance

$d_? = $ density of a standard substance, usually water (d_w)

Example: A metal bar is suspended from a spring scale that reads 300 oz in air and 200 oz when submerged in water.

1. Calculate the specific gravity.

$$\text{Specific Gravity} = \frac{\text{Weight in Air}}{\text{Weight Lost in Water}}$$

$$\text{Specific Gravity} = \frac{300 \text{ oz}}{100 \text{ oz}}$$

$$\text{Specific Gravity} = 3$$

2. **Calculate the weight-density of the metal.**

$$d_w = 62.4 \text{ lb/ft}^3$$

$$d = \text{Specific Gravity} \times d_w$$

$$d = (3)(62.4 \text{ lb/ft}^3)$$

$$d = 187.2 \text{ lb/ft}^3$$

Buoyancy

Example: A balloon on a transatlantic flight is operating where the weight-density of air is 0.050 lb/ft³. It weighs 300 lb, has a volume of 8000 ft³, and is filled with helium, with a d of 0.011 lb/ft³. What load can it support?

Step 1. $w = Vd$ $w = $ weight
$V = $ volume
$d = $ density

Weight of Air Displaced $= 8000 \text{ ft}^3 \times 0.050 \text{ lb/ft}^3 = 400 \text{ lb}$
Weight of Helium $= 8000 \text{ ft} \times 0.011 \text{ lb/ft}^3 = 88 \text{ lb}$
Weight of Balloon $= 300 \text{ lb}$

Step 2. $L = w_a - w_h - w_b$ $L = $ load balloon can support
$L = 400 \text{ lb} - 88 \text{ lb} - 300 \text{ lb}$ $w_a = $ weight of air displaced
$L = 12 \text{ lb}$ $w_h = $ weight of helium
$w_b = $ weight of balloon

The load the balloon can support is 12 lb.

Gravity

All objects in the universe attract each other with a force equal to

$$F_{grav} = \frac{Gm_1 m_2}{r^2}$$

where m_1 and m_2 are the two masses, r is the distance between them, and G is the universal constant of gravitation, equal to $6.67 \times 10^{-11} \text{ N} \cdot \text{m}^2/\text{kg}^2$.

Example: What is the force of attraction between a 10-metric-ton wrecking ball and a 50-kg man if they are 6 m apart?

$$F = \frac{(6.67 \times 10^{-11} \text{ N} \cdot \text{m}^2/\text{kg}^2)(10 \times 10^3 \text{ kg})(50 \text{ kg})}{(6 \text{ m})^2} = 9 \times 10^{-7} \text{ N}$$

Example: What is the mass of the earth? The force on 1 kg at the surface (6400 km from the center) is 9.8 N.

$$m_2 = \frac{Fr^2}{Gm_1} = \frac{(9.8 \text{ N})(6.4 \times 10^6 \text{ m})^2}{(6.67 \times 10^{-11} \text{ N} \cdot \text{m}^2/\text{kg}^2)(1 \text{ kg})} = 6.0 \times 10^{24} \text{ kg}$$

Temperature Calculations and Measurement

Recall:

	Freezing Point	Boiling Point of Water
Celsius	0°	100°
Fahrenheit	32°	212°
Kelvin	273	373

Formulas: $C = \dfrac{5}{9} \times (F - 32°)$

$$F = \dfrac{9}{5} C + 32°$$

Example: A Celsius thermometer records a temperature of 37°C in a patient. What is the temperature on the Fahrenheit scale?

$$F = \dfrac{9}{5} \times 37° + 32°$$

$$F = 66.6° + 32°$$

$$F = 98.6°F$$

Example: An indoor arena is kept at a temperature of 72°F. What is the corresponding reading on the Celsius scale?

$$C = \dfrac{5}{9} \times (72° - 32°)$$

$$C = \dfrac{5}{9} \times 40°$$

$$C = 22°C$$

Absolute Scale: Absolute zero (0 on the Kelvin scale) is the theoretical temperature at which all molecular motion ceases. The Kelvin scale, therefore, has no negative degrees. Celsius temperatures can be expressed on the Kelvin scale ($K = 273 + C$).

Example: 40°C and −40°C can be expressed on the Kelvin scale as follows:

a. $K = 273 + 40$

$K = 313$ K

b. $K = 273 + (-40)$

$K = 233$ K

Heat

Heat is expressed in British thermal units or in calories. One British thermal unit (Btu) is the amount of heat required to raise the temperature of one pound of water one Fahrenheit degree, and one calorie (cal) is the amount of heat necessary to raise the temperature of one gram of water one Celsius degree. One British thermal unit equals about 250 calories.

Specific Heat

Example: How much heat is required to raise the temperature of 10 lb of ethylene glycol (0.528 cal/g · °C or Btu/lb · °F) from 70°F to 140°F?

$$H = (10 \text{ lb})(0.528 \text{ Btu/lb} \cdot °F)(140° - 70°F)$$

$$H = (10 \text{ lb})(0.528 \text{ Btu/lb} \cdot °F)(70°F)$$

$$H = 370 \text{ Btu}$$

Heat Lost = Heat Gained

Example: Five hundred lb of steel at 300°F are cooled in 700 lb of water at 100°F. The temperature obtained in the water is 125°F. Calculate the specific heat of the steel. Remember that the heat lost by the steel equals the heat gained by the water.

$$M_B = \text{weight of first object (steel)}$$

$$S_B = \text{specific heat of first object}$$

$$\Delta t_B = \text{initial temperature of first object}$$
$$- \text{final temperature of first object}$$

$$M_w = \text{weight of second object (water)}$$

$$S_w = \text{unit of heat (1 Btu/lb} \cdot °F)$$

$$\Delta t_w = \text{final temperature of second object}$$
$$- \text{initial temperature of second object}$$

$$M_B S_B \, \Delta t_B = M_w S_w \, \Delta t_w$$

$$(500 \text{ lb}) S_B (300°F - 125°F) = (700 \text{ lb})(1.00 \text{ Btu/lb} \cdot °F)(125°F - 100°F)$$

$$S_B = \frac{(700 \text{ lb})(1.00 \text{ Btu/lb} \cdot °F)(25°F)}{(500 \text{ lb})(175°F)}$$

$$S_B = 0.20 \text{ Btu/lb} \cdot °F$$

Heat of Vaporization

Example: How much heat is necessary to change 100 lb of ice at 10°F to steam at 212°F? Ice, 0.51 Btu/lb · °F; heat of fusion of ice, 144 Btu/lb; water, 1.00 Btu/lb · °F; heat of vaporization of water, 970 Btu/lb.

Step 1.   Heat required to raise the temperature of ice to melting point

$$= M_i S_i (32°F - 10°F)$$

$$= (100 \text{ lb})(0.51 \text{ Btu/lb} \cdot °F)(22°F)$$

$$= 1122 \text{ Btu}$$

Step 2.   Heat required to melt ice

$$= (100 \text{ lb})(144 \text{ Btu/lb})$$

$$= 14,400 \text{ Btu}$$

Step 3.   Heat required to bring water to its boiling point

$$= (100 \text{ lb})(1 \text{ Btu/lb} \cdot °F)(212° - 32°F)$$

$$= 18,000 \text{ Btu}$$

Step 4.   Heat required to vaporize water

$$= (100 \text{ lb})(970 \text{ Btu/lb})$$

$$= 97,000 \text{ Btu}$$

Step 5.   Total heat required:

$$1,122 \text{ Btu}$$
$$14,400 \text{ Btu}$$
$$18,000 \text{ Btu}$$
$$\underline{97,000 \text{ Btu}}$$
$$130,000 \text{ Btu}$$

Thermodynamics

Work and Heat

The following conversion values of mechanical energy to heat should be utilized:

$$4.18 \times 10^7 \text{ ergs equals 1 cal}$$
$$4.18 \text{ J equals 1 cal}$$
$$1 \text{ J equals 0.239 cal}$$
$$778 \text{ ft-lb equals 1 Btu}$$
$$1055 \text{ J equals 1 Btu}$$

$$W = J \text{ (constant) } H \qquad \begin{array}{l} W = \text{work} \\ J = \text{constant} \\ H = \text{heat} \end{array}$$

Example: Water drops 300 ft over the horseshoe falls at Niagara. Calculate the rise in temperature of the water if its potential energy were converted into heat.

Step 1.   Energy transformed per pound of water

$$= (1.00 \text{ lb})(300 \text{ ft})$$

$$= 300 \text{ ft-lb}$$

Step 2.   Heat produced

$$= \frac{300 \text{ ft-lb}}{778 \text{ ft-lb/Btu}}$$

$$= 0.39 \text{ Btu}$$

Step 3.   Rise in temperature:

Δt = rise (change) in temperature

H = heat change in material

M = mass (1 lb of water)

S = energy or units of work (Btu), or the specific heat of

a substance (heat/unit mass-degree change in temperature)

$$\Delta t = \frac{H}{MS}$$

$$\Delta t = \frac{0.39 \text{ Btu}}{(100 \text{ lb})(1.00 \text{ Btu/lb} \cdot {}^\circ\text{F})}$$

$$\Delta t = 0.39{}^\circ\text{F}$$

Example: A compressed gas at a constant pressure of 75 lb/in² enters a cylinder 2 in diameter and pushes a piston 5 in. The work done by the gas is?

$W = P \Delta V$ $\quad\quad\quad\quad\quad$ $P = 75$ lb/in²

$W = (75 \text{ lb/in}^2)(5\pi \text{ in}^3)$ $\quad\quad$ $\Delta V = \pi r^2 s$

$W = 1200$ in-lb $\quad\quad\quad\quad\quad$ $= \pi(1.0 \text{ in})^2 \times 5 \text{ in}$

$W = 100$ ft-lb $\quad\quad\quad\quad\quad\quad$ $= 5\pi$ in³

Efficiency of a Boiler

Recall: The maximum efficiency of a heat engine supplied with heat at temperature T_1 and delivering heat to a reservoir at temperature T_2 can be calculated as follows:

$$E = \frac{T_1 - T_2}{T_1} = 1 - \frac{T_2}{T_1}$$

Example: An engine driven by a boiler receives steam at 300°C. Its exhaust temperature is 100°C. Its efficiency is?

$$E = \frac{T_1 - T_2}{T_1}$$

$$E = \frac{(300 + 273)\text{ K} - (100 + 273)\text{ K}}{(300 + 273)\text{ K}}$$

$$E = \frac{573 \text{ K} - 373 \text{ K}}{573 \text{ K}}$$

$$E = 0.349$$

$$E = 34.9\%$$

Example: A heat engine removes 6000 J per cycle of heat energy from the heat chamber and exhausts 1000 J to a cold chamber.

1. What is the thermal efficiency of the engine?

$$E = 1 - \frac{T_{cold}}{T_{hot}} \text{ or } \frac{Q_{cold}}{Q_{hot}}$$

$$E = 1 - \frac{1000 \text{ J}}{6000 \text{ J}}$$

$$E = 1 - 0.17$$

$$E = 83\%$$

2. **What is the work done by the engine?**

$$W = Q_{hot} - Q_{cold}$$

$$W = 6000 \text{ J} - 1000 \text{ J}$$

$$W = 5000 \text{ J}$$

Electrostatics

The Electric Force

A positive and a negative charge attract each other; two similar charges repel each other. The force is given by Coulomb's Law:

$$F_{elec} = \frac{kq_1 q_2}{r^2}$$

where q_1 and q_2 are electric charges in coulombs (C), r is the distance between them, and k is the electric constant of free space, equal to $9.0 \times 10^9 \text{ N} \cdot \text{m}^2/\text{C}^2$.

Example: What is the electric force between two plastic spheres, carrying charges of 20 nC and 12 nC, respectively, if they are 15 cm apart?

$$F = \frac{(9.0 \times 10^9 \text{ N} \cdot \text{m}^2/\text{C}^2)(20 \times 10^{-9} \text{ C})(12 \times 10^{-9} \text{ C})}{(0.15 \text{ m})^2} = 9.6 \times 10^{-5} \text{ N}$$

Since the charges are alike, the force is a force of repulsion.

The Quantum of Charge

All electric charges are integral multiples of the charge on an electron, 1.60×10^{-19} C.

Example: How many electrons are there in a charge of 12 nC?

$$\frac{12 \times 10^{-9} \text{ C}}{1.60 \times 10^{-19} \text{ C}} = 7.5 \times 10^{10}$$

Electric Field

A positive charge in an electric field experiences a force in the direction of the field; a negative charge gets a force in the opposite direction. The magnitude of the force is

$$F_{elec} = \mathscr{E}q$$

where $\mathscr{E}$ is the electric field in newtons per coulomb.

Example: How strong an electric field will exert a force of 2.0×10^{-16} N on the electron?

$$\mathscr{E} = \frac{F_{elec}}{q} = \frac{2.0 \times 10^{-16} \text{ N}}{1.60 \times 10^{-19} \text{ C}} = 1250 \text{ N/C}$$

Example: How strong is the field at a distance of 30 cm from a point charge of 20 μC? The field is the force per coulomb of charge in the field. From Coulomb's law

$$\frac{F}{q^2} = \frac{kq_1}{r^2} = \frac{(9.0 \times 10^9 \text{ N} \cdot \text{m}^2/\text{C}^2)(20 \times 10^{-6} \text{ C})}{(0.30 \text{ m})^2} = 2.0 \times 10^6 \text{ N/C}$$

which is the electric field strength.

Electric Potential Difference

The electric potential difference between two points in an electric field is the energy change in moving a unit charge from one point to the other. The unit is the joule per coulomb, called a volt (V).

$$V = \frac{E_{elec}}{q}$$

Example: The potential difference between the terminals of an autombile battery is 12 V. If the battery is charged using 1800 J of energy, how much charge is transferred from one terminal to the other?

$$q = \frac{E_{elec}}{V} = \frac{1800 \text{ J}}{12 \text{ V}} = 150 \text{ C}$$

Example: In a uniform electric field of 650 N/C, what is the potential difference between two points that are 20 cm apart in the direction of the field?

1. Determine the force on a coulomb in the field.

$$F = \mathscr{E}q = (650 \text{ N/C})(1 \text{ C}) = 650 \text{ N}$$

2. Determine the work done in moving the charge.

$$W = Fs = (650 \text{ N})(0.20 \text{ m}) = 130 \text{ J}$$

This is the electric energy difference between the points.

3. Determine the potential difference.

$$V = \frac{E_{elec}}{q} = \frac{130 \text{ J}}{1\text{C}} = 130 \text{ V}$$

Electricity

Ohm's Law

In a metal conductor at constant temperature, the ratio of the voltage to the current is a constant, that is,

$$R \text{ (a constant)} = \frac{V}{I}$$

The constant is called resistance, measured in ohms = volts per ampere.

Example: The difference in potential between two terminals is 10 volts. A current of 5 A passes; calculate the resistance.

$$R = \frac{V}{I}$$

$$R = \frac{10 \text{ volts}}{5 \text{ A}}$$

$$R = 2 \text{ ohms}$$

Example: Increase the difference of the above potential to 20 volts. Calculate the current that passes. Remember that according to Ohm's law, the resistance (R) will remain the same when the voltage is increased—it is constant.

$$I = \frac{V}{R}$$

$$I = \frac{20 \text{ volts}}{2 \text{ ohms}}$$

$$I = 10 \text{ A}$$

Example: A motor needs a current of 8 A and has a resistance of 40 ohms. What voltage is necessary for the operation?

$$V = IR$$

$$V = 8 \text{ A} \times 40 \text{ ohms}$$

$$V = 320 \text{ volts}$$

Example: A 150-watt bulb operates on a potential difference of 110 volts.

1. Calculate the current drawn.

$$P = IV$$

$$I = \frac{P}{V}$$

$$I = \frac{150 \text{ watts}}{110 \text{ volts}}$$

$$I = 1.36 \text{ A}$$

2. Calculate the resistance.

$$V = IR$$

$$R = \frac{V}{I}$$

$$R = \frac{110 \text{ volts}}{1.36 \text{ A}}$$

$$R = 80. \text{ ohms}$$

Example: A current of 10 A flows through a wire for 45 min. The charge that passes through a cross section of the wire may be calculated as follows:

$$I = \frac{q}{t}$$

$$q = It$$

$$q = (10 \text{ A})(2700 \text{ sec})$$

$$q = 27,000 \text{ A} \cdot \text{sec or coulombs}$$

Electric Circuits

Electromotive Force (emf) and Internal Resistance

$$V = E - Ir$$

V = **terminal potential difference**
E = no-load potential difference or emf
r = **internal resistance**
I = **current**

Example: A battery powering a portable television has an emf of 10 volts and an internal resistance of 0.20 ohm. It supplies a current of 6 A. Calculate the terminal potential difference.

$$V = E - IR$$

$$V = 10 \text{ volts} - (6 \text{ A} \times 0.20 \text{ ohm})$$

$$V = 10 \text{ volts} - 1.2 \text{ volts}$$

$$V = 8.8 \text{ volts}$$

Resistors in Series

Example: A direct-current circuit is wired with resistances of 3 ohms, 6 ohms, and 2 ohms in series. These resistances could be replaced by one resistor of 11 ohms to produce equivalent resistance.

Example: Three lamps are connected in series and exhibit a resistance of 15, 10, and 5 ohms, respectively. How much current is produced by a potential difference of 100 volts across its terminals?

1. Determine the current in the lamp.

$$R = (15 + 10 + 5) \text{ ohms}$$

$$R = 30 \text{ ohms}$$

$$I = \frac{V}{R}$$

$$I = \frac{100 \text{ volts}}{30 \text{ ohms}}$$

$$I = 3.33 \text{ A}$$

2. Determine the voltage across each lamp; it is the product of its resistance and the current.

$$v_1 = (3.33 \text{ A})(15 \text{ ohms}) = 50 \text{ volts}$$

$$v_2 = (3.33 \text{ A})(10 \text{ ohms}) = 33 \text{ volts}$$

$$v_3 = (3.33 \text{ A})(5 \text{ ohms}) = 17 \text{ volts}$$

Resistors in Parallel

$$\frac{1}{R} = \frac{1}{R_1} + \frac{1}{R_2} + \frac{1}{R_3}$$

Recall that addition to a circuit of resistors in series increases the resistance while addition to a circuit of resistors in parallel decreases the resistance.

Example: Using the example of 3, 6, and 2 ohms, the equivalent resistance can be calculated as follows:

$$\frac{1}{R_{eq}} = \frac{1}{R_1} + \frac{1}{R_2} + \frac{1}{R_3}$$

$$\frac{1}{R_{eq}} = \frac{1}{3 \text{ ohms}} + \frac{1}{6 \text{ ohms}} + \frac{1}{2 \text{ ohms}}$$

$$= \frac{2}{6 \text{ ohms}} + \frac{1}{6 \text{ ohms}} + \frac{3}{6 \text{ ohms}} = \frac{6}{6 \text{ ohms}}$$

$$\frac{1}{R_{eq}} = 1 \text{ ohm, OR, } R_{eq} = 1 \text{ ohm}$$

Example: A circuit has resistances of 15, 10, and 5 ohms. If these are wired in parallel what is their combined resistance?

$$\frac{1}{R} = \frac{1}{R_1} + \frac{1}{R_2} + \frac{1}{R_3}$$

$$\frac{1}{R} = \frac{1}{15 \text{ ohms}} + \frac{1}{10 \text{ ohms}} + \frac{1}{5 \text{ ohms}}$$

$$\frac{1}{R} = (0.07 + 0.1 + 0.2) \text{ ohm}$$

$$\frac{1}{R} = 0.37 \text{ ohm}$$

$$R = \frac{1}{0.37} \text{ ohm}$$

$$R = 2.7 \text{ ohms}$$

Example: Find the current in a series circuit with two energy sources ($E_1 = 12$ volts, $E_2 = -4$ volt) and two resistors ($R_1 = 15$ ohms, $R_2 = 10$ ohms).

$$E_1 + E_2 = I_1(R_1 + R_2) \text{ or } V_1 + V_2 = I_1 (R_1 + R_2)$$

$$I_1 = \frac{E_1 + E_2}{R_1 + R_2} \text{ or } \frac{V_1 + V_2}{R_1 + R_2}$$

$$I_1 = \frac{(12 - 4) \text{ volts}}{(15 + 10) \text{ ohms}}$$

$$I_1 = \frac{8 \text{ volts}}{25 \text{ ohms}} = 0.32 \text{ A}$$

Example: A circuit has three resistors—of 2 ohms, 4 ohms, and 8 ohms.

1. **What is the resistance of these three resistors when connected in series?**

$$R_s = R_1 + R_2 + R_3$$

$$R_s = (2 + 4 + 8) \text{ ohms}$$

$$R_s = 14 \text{ ohms}$$

2. **What is their resistance when connected in parallel?**

$$\frac{1}{R_p} = \frac{1}{R_1} + \frac{1}{R_2} + \frac{1}{R_3}$$

$$\frac{1}{R_p} = \frac{1}{2 \text{ ohms}} + \frac{1}{4 \text{ ohms}} + \frac{1}{8 \text{ ohms}}$$

$$\frac{1}{R_p} = \frac{4}{8 \text{ ohms}} + \frac{2}{8 \text{ ohms}} + \frac{1}{8 \text{ ohms}}$$

$$\frac{1}{R_p} = \frac{7}{8 \text{ ohms}}$$

$$R_p = \frac{8}{7} \text{ ohms}$$

3. **How much current would be drawn from a 12-volt battery?**

SERIES

$$I = \frac{V}{R_s} = \frac{12 \text{ volts}}{14 \text{ ohms}} = 0.857 \text{ A}$$

Potential drop in each resistor:

$$V_1 = IR_1 = (0.857 \text{ A})(2 \text{ ohms})$$
$$= 1.7 \text{ volts}$$

$$V_2 = IR_2 = (0.857 \text{ A})(4 \text{ ohms})$$
$$= 3.4 \text{ volts}$$

$$V_3 = IR_3 = (0.857 \text{ A})(8 \text{ ohms})$$
$$= 6.9 \text{ volts}$$

PARALLEL

$$I = \frac{V}{R_p} = \frac{12 \text{ ohms}}{8/7 \text{ ohms}} = 10.5 \text{ A}$$

Current in each resistor:

$$I_1 = \frac{V}{R_1} = \frac{12 \text{ volts}}{2 \text{ ohms}} = 6 \text{ A}$$

$$I_2 = \frac{V}{R_2} = \frac{12 \text{ volts}}{4 \text{ ohms}} = 3 \text{ A}$$

$$I_3 = \frac{V}{R_3} = \frac{12 \text{ volts}}{8 \text{ ohms}} = 1.5 \text{ A}$$

$$I_i = I_1 + I_2 + I_3 = 10.5 \text{ A}$$

The drop equals the voltage rise
in the battery:

$V_i = V_1 + V_2 + V_3$

$V_i = 12$ volts

Cells in Series

Example: Three cells are connected in series; each has an emf of 10 volts and a resistance of 2 ohms. Calculate the current after the combination is connected to an external resistance of 20 ohms.

$$\text{Total emf} = 10 \text{ volts} + 10 \text{ volts} + 10 \text{ volts}$$

$$= 30 \text{ volts}$$

$$\text{Total Resistance } (R) = 2 \text{ ohms} + 2 \text{ ohms} + 2 \text{ ohms} + 20 \text{ ohms}$$

$$= 26 \text{ ohms}$$

$$\text{Total Current} = \frac{\text{Total emf}}{\text{Total Resistance}}$$

$$\text{Total Current} = \frac{30 \text{ volts}}{26 \text{ ohms}}$$

$$\text{Total Current} = 1.15 \text{ A}$$

Cells in Parallel

Example: Consider the following three arrangements:

    a. A single cell
    b. Two cells in series
    c. Two cells in parallel

Compare the currents maintained in a 5-ohm resistor under each condition. Each cell has an emf of 3 volts and negligible internal resistance. The emf of (a) is 3 volts, of (b) 6 volts, and of (c) 3 volts.

(a): $I_{\text{total}} = \dfrac{E_{\text{total}}}{R_{\text{total}}}$

$$I_a = \frac{3 \text{ volts}}{5 \text{ ohms}}$$

$$I_a = 0.6 \text{ A}$$

(b): $I_b = \dfrac{6 \text{ volts}}{5 \text{ ohms}}$

$$I_b = 1.2 \text{ A}$$

(c): $I_c = \dfrac{3 \text{ volts}}{5 \text{ ohms}}$

$$I_c = 0.6 \text{ A}$$

In each cell, however, the current is 0.3 A.

Electric Energy

Joule's Law

$$\text{Voltage} = \frac{\text{Energy}}{\text{Charge}} \qquad V = \text{volts}$$

$$V = \frac{W}{Q} \qquad W = \text{usually in joules}$$

$$\text{OR } VIt = I^2Rt \qquad Q = \text{usually in coulombs}$$

Rewriting $W = VQ$, we can make the substitutions $Q = It$ and $V = IR$. Then, the basic equation for electric energy may be $W = VQ = VIt = I^2Rt$. This equation indicates that one joule must be expanded in maintaining for one second a current of one ampere in a circuit of one-ohm resistance.

Example: A motor is used for 45 min to drive a conveyor belt. It uses 35 A at 110 volts. Calculate the electric energy used.

$$W = VIt$$

$$W = (110 \text{ volts})(35 \text{ A})(2700 \text{ sec})$$

$$W = 10,395,000 \text{ J}$$

$$W = 10.4 \times 10^6 \text{ J}$$

Example: How many calories are produced in a central electric resistance heating system in 5 min as it draws 30 A connected to a 220-volt line?

Recall: 1 cal = 4.18 J

$$H = \frac{VIt}{J} \text{ or } H = \frac{W}{J}$$

$$H = \frac{(220 \text{ volts})(30 \text{ A})(300 \text{ sec})}{4.18 \text{ J/cal}}$$

$$H = \frac{1,980,000}{4.18 \text{ J/cal}}$$

$$H = 470,000 \text{ cal}$$

Power and Resistance

Example: The above furnace operating at 220 volts requires 2 hp. What are the current and the resistance of the unit?

1. Current

$$P = 2 \text{ hp} \times 746 \frac{\text{watts}}{\text{hp}}$$

$$P = 1492 \text{ watts}$$

$$P = VI$$

$$1492 \text{ watts} = 220 \text{ volts} \times I$$

$$I = 6.78 \text{ A}$$

2. Resistance

$$R = \frac{V}{I}$$

$$R = \frac{220 \text{ volts}}{6.78 \text{ A}}$$

$$R = 32 \text{ ohms}$$

Alternating Current

Effective Values

In a sine-wave varying current, the average power is half the maximum power. The average power is $I_{rms}^2 R$, where I_{rms} is the root-mean-square, or effective, value of the current.

Example: A sine-wave alternating current with a peak current of 60 A is passing through a resistance of 2.0 Ω. Find the peak power, average power, effective current, and effective potential difference.

1. The peak power is $I_{max}^2 R$:

$$P_{max} = (60 \text{ A})^2 (2.0 \ \Omega) = 7200 \text{ W}$$

2. The average power is half the maximum, 3600 W.
3. The effective current produces the average power:

$$I_{rms}^2 R = 3600 \text{ W}$$

$$I_{rms} = \sqrt{\frac{3600 \text{ W}}{2.0 \ \Omega}} = 42 \text{ A}$$

4. Effective potential difference:

$$V_{rms} = I_{rms} R = (42 \text{ A})(2.0 \ \Omega) = 84 \text{ V}$$

Example: An effective potential difference of 120 V supplies a resistance of 40 Ω. Find the maximum potential difference and current.

1. Maximum is RMS value times the square root of 2:

$$V_{max} = (120 \text{ V})\sqrt{2} = 170 \text{ V}$$

2. Effective current is

$$I_{rms} = \frac{V_{rms}}{R} = \frac{120 \text{ V}}{40 \ \Omega} = 3.0 \text{ A}$$

3. Maximum current is

$$(3.0 \text{ A})\sqrt{2} = 4.2 \text{ A}$$

Machines and Mechanical Advantage

Actual Mechanical Advantage (AMA) $= \dfrac{F_o}{F_i}$,

where F_o = output force and F_i = input force.

Theoretical Mechanical Advantage (TMA) $= \dfrac{d_i}{d_o}$

Efficiency (E) $= \dfrac{F_o/F_i}{d_i/d_o} = \dfrac{AMA}{TMA} = \dfrac{\text{Output Work}}{\text{Input Work}}$

Example: A man pushing down with a force of 50 lb lifts a 200-lb crate by utilizing a lever system. The lever arms are 6 and 1.2 ft, respectively.

1. Calculate the AMA.

$$AMA = \dfrac{F_o}{F_i}$$

$$AMA = \dfrac{200 \text{ lb}}{50 \text{ lb}}$$

$$AMA = 4$$

2. Calculate the TMA.

$$TMA = \dfrac{d_i}{d_o}$$

$$TMA = \dfrac{6 \text{ ft}}{1.2 \text{ ft}}$$

$$TMA = 5$$

3. What is the efficiency?

$$E = \dfrac{AMA}{TMA}$$

$$E = \dfrac{4}{5}(100\%)$$

$$E = 80\%$$

Example: A car weighing 1500 lb is pushed up a 50-ft ramp exhibiting an incline of 30°. A parallel force of 1000 lb is used to accomplish this task.

1. What is the AMA?

$$AMA = \dfrac{F_0}{F_i} = \dfrac{1500 \text{ lb}}{1000 \text{ lb}} = 1.5 \text{ lb}$$

2. What is the efficiency of the system?

$$TMA = \dfrac{50 \text{ ft}}{50 \text{ ft sin } 30°}$$

$$= \dfrac{1}{0.5} = 2$$

$$E = \dfrac{1.5}{2}$$

$$E = 75\%$$

Simple Harmonic Motion

Period and Frequency

The motion of an oscillating object is described by its:

displacement—distance from central position
amplitude—maximum displacement
period (T)—time for one full cycle
frequency (v, Greek nu)—cycles per unit time. One cycle per second is called a hertz (Hz)

Frequency is the reciprocal of period.

Example: What is the frequency of a vibrating rod that completes each cycle in 1/20 s?

$$v = \frac{1}{T} = \frac{1}{1/20 \text{ s}} = 20/\text{s} = 20 \text{ Hz}$$

Phase

Phase is the time difference, in fractions of a cycle, between two objects oscillating with the same frequency. One cycle is 360°.

Example: What is the phase difference between two identical pendulums with periods of 1.5 s if one reaches its maximum displacement 0.2 s before the other?

$$\text{Phase difference} = \left(\frac{0.2 \text{ s}}{1.5 \text{ s}}\right)(360°) = 48°$$

Waves

A wave is a system of oscillating particles or fields, in which each point transmits energy to the next point in turn. The next point follows with a slight time delay, so the phase varies continuously.

crest—a point of maximum displacement that appears to travel through the medium
trough—a traveling point of negative maximum displacement
wave velocity—speed of travel of crests and troughs
wavelength (λ, Greek lambda)—distance between successive points in phase.

Frequency, Wavelength and Phase

Wavelength depends on frequency and velocity:

$$v = \lambda v.$$

Example: If a wave in a rope travels at 4.6 m/s and the rope is shaken at one end with a frequency of 2.0 Hz, what is the wavelength of the wave in the rope?

$$\lambda = \frac{v}{v} = \frac{4.6 \text{ m/s}}{2.0/\text{s}} = 2.3 \text{ m}$$

Example: If a 120-Hz wave of vibration in a steel rail travels at 840 m/s, how far apart are two points that are 90° out of phase?

1. Find the wavelength.

$$\lambda = \frac{v}{\nu} = \frac{840 \text{ m/s}}{120/\text{s}} = 7.0 \text{ m}$$

2. Each phase cycle corresponds to a wavelength, so

$$\frac{90°}{360°} \times 7.0 \text{ m} = 1.75 \text{ m}$$

Interference

When two identical waves arrive simultaneously at a point, their displacements add. If they arrive out of phase, the interference is *destructive*, and a *node*, a point of no vibration, is formed. If they arrive in phase, the interference is *constructive*, and an *antinode*, a point of maximum vibration, develops.

Standing Waves

A standing wave in a string has alternate nodes and antinodes, spaced 1/4 wavelength apart.

Example: In the fundamental mode, a string vibrates with a node at each end and an antinode in the middle. What is the frequency of vibration if the string is 25 cm long and the wave in it travels at 390 m/s?

1. Find the wavelength. Since there is a node at each end, the string is a half-wavelength long.

$$\lambda = 2 \times 25 \text{ cm} = 0.50 \text{ m}$$

2. Now find the frequency.

$$v = \frac{v}{\lambda} = \frac{390 \text{ m/s}}{0.50 \text{ m}} = 780 \text{ Hz}$$

Example: At a higher mode, there are 5 antinodes in the string of the preceding problem. What is the frequency at this mode?

1. Find the wavelength. Since there are 2 antinodes in each wavelength, there are 2½ wavelengths in the string.

$$\lambda = \frac{25 \text{ cm}}{2.5} = 10 \text{ cm}$$

2. Find the frequency.

$$v = \frac{v}{\lambda} = \frac{390 \text{ m/s}}{0.10 \text{ m}} = 3900 \text{ Hz}$$

Sound Waves

A vibrating object sets the adjacent air into vibration. This starts a longitudinal wave traveling through the air, a sound wave.

Pitch and Frequency

The *pitch* of the sound is its apparent tonal level, as defined by musical scales. An increase of 1 octave represents doubling the frequency.

Example: When the oboe sounds 440-A, what is the frequency of the tuba, sounding A two octaves lower? One octave lower is 220 Hz, the next octave below is 110 Hz.

In the equal-tempered chromatic scale, each increase of a half tone represents a frequency increase by a factor of $2^{1/12} = 1.05946$.

Example: What is the frequency of high C, which is 3 halftones above A?

$$\text{Frequency} = 440 \text{ Hz} \times 1.05946^3 = 523.2 \text{ Hz}$$

Intensity

The intensity, or loudness, of a sound in bels is the order of magnitude of its energy as compared with the softest audible sound. Thus, 3 bels (B), or 30 decibels (dB), has 10^3 times the zero level.

Example: If a rock band produces sound at 80 dB, how does the energy of this sound compare with that of the softest audible sound?
The value of 80 dB is 8 B, so the loudest sound has 10^8 times the energy of 0 B.

Speed of Sound

The speed of a sound wave depends on the nature of the medium in which it travels. It travels faster in liquids than in gases, and much faster in elastic solids. In air, the speed of sound depends on the temperature and can be calculated from the following formula:

$$v_{air} = 331 \, \frac{m}{s} + 0.6 \, T \frac{m}{s \cdot °C}$$

Example: How far away is a wall if an echo is received from it 3.9 s after the sound is produced when the temperature is 26°C?

1. Find the speed of sound.

$$v_{air} = 331 \, \frac{m}{s} + \left(0.6 \, \frac{m}{s \cdot °C} \right)(26°C) = 346.6 \text{ m/s}$$

2. Calculate the distance the sound traveled:

$$s = vt = (346.6 \text{ m/s})(3.9 \text{ s}) = 1352 \text{ m}$$

3. Since the sound had to travel both ways, the distance of the wall is half this distance, or 676 m.

Beats

Two sound waves of different frequencies arriving at a point will interfere, alternating constructive and destructive interference. The beat frequency is the difference between the frequencies of the two sounds.

Example: As an orchestra tunes up, the oboe sounds 440-A. If the clarinetist hears 3 beats per second when he plays A, what is the frequency of the clarinet's A?
It could be either 443 Hz or 437 Hz.

Doppler Effect

If a sound source is moving away from an observer, the frequency heard is lower than the frequency emitted, and conversely.

$$v = v_s \frac{v}{v + v_s}$$

where v is the observed frequency, v_s is the frequency of the source, v is the speed of sound, and v_s is the speed of the source as it moves away from the observer.

Example: With the temperature at $-10°C$, a train moving toward the observer at 32 m/s sounds its horn at 380 Hz. What frequency does the observer hear?

1. Find the speed of sound.

$$v = 331\frac{m}{s} + \left(0.6\frac{m}{s \cdot °C}\right)(-10°C) = 325 \text{ m/s}$$

2. Apply the formula; v_s is negative because the source is moving toward the observer:

$$v = (380 \text{ Hz})\frac{325 \text{ m/s}}{(325 - 32)\text{m/s}} = 421 \text{ Hz}$$

Light Rays

Light travels in straight lines (rays) unless deflected by reflection or refraction.

Reflection

In specular reflection, the angle of reflection is equal to the angle of incidence. Angles are measured with respect to the perpendicular to the surface (the normal).

Example: If a light ray strikes a mirror at an angle of incidence of 22°, what is the angle between the incident and reflected rays?

Since the angles are measured from the normal, there are 44° between the incident and reflected rays.

Refraction

When a light ray goes from one medium into another, it will bend. The speeds of light in the two media are proportional to the sines of the angles the rays make with the normal.

Example: A light ray in air enters a piece of glass, in which light travels at 2.20×10^6 m/s. If the angle of incidence is 25°, which is the angle of refraction?

$$\frac{\sin \theta_{glass}}{\sin 25°} = \frac{2.20 \times 10^8 \text{ m/s}}{3.00 \times 10^8 \text{ m/s}}$$

$$\theta_{glass} = 18°$$

Index of Refraction

The index of refraction (n) of a medium is the ratio between the speed of light in vacuum and the speed in the medium.

Example: What is the index of refraction of the glass in the preceding example?

$$n_{glass} = \frac{c}{v_{glass}} = \frac{3.00 \times 10^8 \text{ m/s}}{2.20 \times 10^8 \text{ m/s}} = 1.36$$

Refraction between Two Media

If light passes from medium A to B, or vice versa,

$$\frac{\sin \theta_A}{\sin \theta_B} = \frac{n_B}{n_A}$$

Example: A ray of light passes from crown glass ($n = 1.62$) into water ($n = 1.33$), making an angle of incidence of 40°. What is the angle of refraction?

$$\frac{\sin \theta_{glass}}{\sin \theta_{water}} = \frac{n_{water}}{n_{glass}}$$

$$\sin \theta_{water} = \sin 40° \left(\frac{1.62}{1.33}\right)$$

$$\theta_{water} = 52°$$

Total Internal Reflection

If a ray passes into a medium of higher index of refraction, the calculated angle of refraction may exceed 90°. Then the ray is totally reflected.

Example: What is the largest angle of incidence (the critical angle) at which a ray of light can pass from crown glass into water (constants given above)?

$$\frac{\sin i_c}{\sin 90°} = \frac{n_{water}}{n_{glass}} = \frac{1.33}{1.62}$$

$$i_c = 55°$$

Mirrors

Plane Mirrors

In a plane mirror, the image is virtual, erect, the same size as the object, and just as far behind the mirror as the object is in front of it.

Example: The image in a plane mirror of a book is 25 cm high when the book is 50 cm from the mirror. How high is the image if the book is moved to 150 cm?

The answer is 25 cm; the size of the image is always the same as the size of the object.

Convex mirrors

In a convex mirror, the focal length is half the radius of curvature and the image distance obeys the rule

$$\frac{1}{f} = \frac{1}{D_o} + \frac{1}{D_i}$$

where f is focal length, D_o is object distance, and D_i is image distance. The focal length is negative. The image is always erect, virtual, smaller than the object, and behind the mirror.

Example: A convex mirror has a radius of curvature of 60 cm. Where is the image of a lamp that is 180 cm from the mirror?
1. Find the focal length; it is half the radius of curvature, 30 cm.
2. Use the formula to find the image distance.

$$\frac{1}{-30 \text{ cm}} = \frac{1}{180 \text{ cm}} + \frac{1}{D_i}$$

$$\frac{1}{D_i} = \frac{-180 \text{ cm} - 30 \text{ cm}}{(180 \text{ cm})(30 \text{ cm})}$$

$$D_i = -26 \text{ cm}$$

A negative sign indicates that the image is behind the lens. The sizes of the object (S_o) and of the image (S_i) are in the same ratio as the respective distances.

Example: If the lamp in the preceding example is 40 cm tall, how tall is the image?

$$S_i = S_o \left(\frac{D_i}{D_o} \right) = 40 \text{ cm} \left(\frac{-26 \text{ cm}}{180 \text{ cm}} \right) = -5.8 \text{ cm}$$

The negative sign indicates that the image is virtual.

Concave Mirrors

Focal length is half the radius of curvature and positive. Image is either real, inverted, and in front of the lens, or virtual, erect, and behind the lens.

Example: (Object distance greater than focal length) A convex mirror has a radius of curvature of 80 cm. Find the size and location of the image of a lamp that is 60 cm high and 180 cm from the mirror.

1. Find the focal length; it is half the radius of curvature, 40 cm.
2. Apply the formula to find the image distance.

$$\frac{1}{D_i} = \frac{1}{f} - \frac{1}{D_o} = \frac{1}{40 \text{ cm}} - \frac{1}{180 \text{ cm}}$$

$$D_i = \frac{(40 \text{ cm})(180 \text{ cm})}{180 \text{ cm} - 40 \text{ cm}} = 51 \text{ cm}$$

3. Set the sizes proportional to the distances.

$$S_i = (60 \text{ cm}) \left(\frac{51 \text{ cm}}{180 \text{ cm}} \right) = 17 \text{ cm}$$

Example: (Object distance less than focal length) A can 15 cm high is placed 25 cm in front of the same mirror as above. Find the size and location of the image.

1. Find the image distance.

$$\frac{1}{D_i} = \frac{1}{f} - \frac{1}{D_o} = \frac{1}{40 \text{ cm}} - \frac{1}{25 \text{ cm}}$$

$$D_i = \frac{(25 \text{ cm})(40 \text{ cm})}{25 \text{ cm} - 40 \text{ cm}} = -67 \text{ cm}$$

The image is behind the mirror.

2. Solve for the size.

$$S_i = (15 \text{ cm})\left(\frac{-67 \text{ cm}}{25 \text{ cm}}\right) = -40 \text{ cm}$$

The image is enlarged and virtual.

Lenses

Concave Lenses

Lenses that are thinner in the middle than at the edges form the same kinds of images as convex mirrors. They obey the same equations, and the focal length is negative.

Example: Find the size and location of the image formed in a lens of focal length -40 cm of a book 25 cm high placed 30 cm from the lens.

1. Find the image distance:

$$\frac{1}{D_i} = \frac{1}{f} - \frac{1}{D_o} = \frac{1}{-40 \text{ cm}} - \frac{1}{30 \text{ cm}}$$

$$D_i = \frac{(-40 \text{ cm})(30 \text{ cm})}{(30 \text{ cm}) - (-40 \text{ cm})} = -17 \text{ cm}$$

The negative sign shows that the image is behind the mirror.

2. Find the image size.

$$S_i = S_o\left(\frac{D_i}{D_o}\right) = (25 \text{ cm})\left(\frac{-17 \text{ cm}}{30 \text{ cm}}\right) = -14 \text{ cm}$$

The image is virtual.

Convex Lenses

Lenses that are thicker in the middle than at the edges form the same kinds of images as concave mirrors. They obey the same equations, and the focal length is positive.

Example: (Object distance less than focal length) Find the size and position of the image formed in a $+12.0$-cm lens of a postage stamp 2.4 cm high placed 10.0 cm from the lens.

1. Find the image position.

$$\frac{1}{D_i} = \frac{1}{f} - \frac{1}{D_o} = \frac{1}{12.0 \text{ cm}} - \frac{1}{10.0 \text{ cm}}$$

$$D_i = \frac{(10.0 \text{ cm})(12.0 \text{ cm})}{(10.0 \text{ cm}) - (12.0 \text{ cm})} = -60 \text{ cm}$$

The negative sign shows that the image is in front of the lens.

2. Find the image size.

$$S_i = S_o\left(\frac{D_i}{D_o}\right) = 2.4 \text{ cm}\left(\frac{-60 \text{ cm}}{10.0 \text{ cm}}\right) = -14 \text{ cm}$$

The image is enlarged and virtual.

Example: (Object distance greater than focal length) What focal-length lens is needed to form a real image 35 mm high of a man 2.0 m tall when the man is 1.7 m from the lens?

1. Find the image distance in centimeters.

$$D_i = D_o\left(\frac{S_i}{S_o}\right) = 170 \text{ cm}\left(\frac{3.5 \text{ cm}}{200 \text{ cm}}\right) = 3.0 \text{ cm}$$

The image is real.

2. Find the focal length.

$$\frac{1}{f} = \frac{1}{D_o} + \frac{1}{D_i} = \frac{1}{280 \text{ cm}} + \frac{1}{3.0 \text{ cm}}$$

$$f = \frac{(170 \text{ cm})(3.0 \text{ cm})}{170 \text{ cm} + 3.0 \text{ cm}} = 2.9 \text{ cm}$$

The image is real and small.

Combinations of Lenses

The power of a lens, in diopters, is the reciprocal of its focal length in meters. When lenses are combined, their powers add.

Example: What is the focal length of a combination of a $+50$-cm convex lens and a -20-cm concave lens?

1. Find the powers of the two lenses.

$$\frac{1}{+0.50 \text{ m}} = +2.0 \text{ diopters} \qquad \frac{1}{-0.20 \text{ m}} = -5.0 \text{ diopter}$$

2. Add the powers.

$$2.0 - 5.0 = -3.0 \text{ diopter}$$

3. Find the focal length.

$$\frac{1}{-3.0 \text{ diopter}} = -0.33 \text{ m}, \quad \text{or} \quad -33 \text{ cm}$$

Any number of lenses can be combined in this way.

Composition of the Atom

Subatomic Particles

Recall that the nucleus of an atom is composed of neutrons (no charge) and protons (positive electric charge). The total number of particles equals the mass number; the number of protons equals the atomic number. In an atom, the number of protons equals the number of electrons. The number of neutrons can be found by subtracting the atomic number from the mass number.

Example: How many particles of each type are there in an atom of $^{35}_{17}Cl$?

The atomic number is 17, so the element is chlorine (Cl). There are 17 protons in the nucleus and 17 electrons outside it. The number of neutrons in the nucleus is $(35 - 17) = 18$.

Isotopes

Isotopes of the same element have the same atomic number, but different mass numbers (because of different numbers of neutrons).

Example: Of the following, which are isotopes of the same element?

$$^{65}_{29}Cu \qquad ^{65}_{30}Zn \qquad ^{60}_{29}Cu \qquad ^{60}_{28}Ni$$

There are two isotopes of copper (Cu), both with atomic number 29.

Nuclear Reactions

In any nuclear reaction, the mass numbers and the electric charges must be the same on both sides of the equation.

Example: When aluminum atoms are bombarded with helium nuclei, which isotope is produced along with a neutron?

$$^{27}_{13}Al + ^{4}_{2}He \rightarrow ^{30}_{15}P + ^{1}_{0}n$$

An isotope of phosphorus is produced along with the neutron. The mass numbers are $27 + 4 = 30 + 1$. The electric charge (on the protons) is $13 + 2 = 15 + 0$.

Radioactivity

Large nuclei are unstable and break down, releasing particles and energy. There are two kinds of radioactivity in nature: alpha and beta.

Alpha Decay

In alpha decay, the nucleus releases an alpha particle, which is a nucleus of helium, $^{4}_{2}He$.

Example: What nucleus results from the alpha decay of a nucleus of radon-210?

$$^{210}_{86}Rn \rightarrow ^{4}_{2}He + ^{206}_{84}Po + \gamma$$

The γ (gamma ray) is a high-energy photon, which always accompanies alpha decay. The mass numbers agree: $210 = 4 + 206$. The electric charges agree: $86 = 2 + 84$.

Beta Decay

In beta decay, a neutron emits an electron, turning into a proton. It also produces a chargeless, massless particle called a neutrino.

Example: What is the result of the beta decay of radium-227?

$$^{227}_{88}Ra \rightarrow ^{227}_{89}Ac + ^{0}_{-1}e + \gamma$$

Since the electron and the neutrino have negligible mass, there is no change in the mass number; $227 = 227 + 0$. The atomic number increases by 1, and the electric charge balance is $88 = 89 - 1$.

Half-life

The half-life of a nucleus is the time required for half of any given sample to undergo radioactive decay.

Example: The half-life of radon-214 is 2.5 seconds. If a sample of this gas contains 200 g, how much will be left at the end of 10 seconds?

Ten seconds is 4 half-lives, so the mass drops to half 4 times. The amount left will be

$$(200 \text{ g})(0.5)^4 = 13 \text{ g}$$

Example: What is the half-life of a radioactive nucleus if it takes 4 billion years for 40 g to decay down to 10 g?

The mass of the sample has dropped to half twice, so the half-life is 2 billion years.

Nuclear Energy

The mass of a nucleus is less than the sum of the masses of the protons and neutrons that compose it. The difference is called the mass deficit of the nucleus, which corresponds to the binding energy ($E = mc^2$).

Units of Measure

The mass of nuclei is measured in atomic mass units, or daltons.

6.02×10^{26} daltons (D1) = 1 kg
6.25×10^{18} electron-volts (eV) = 1 J
931 megaelectron volts (MeV) = 1 D1

Example: If the mass deficit of a nucleus is 0.0067 D1, how much energy will be needed to separate it into protons and neutrons?

$$0.0067 \text{ D1} \times \frac{931 \text{ MeV}}{\text{D1}} = 6.2 \text{ MeV}$$

Example: If a nuclear reaction yields 6.5×1012 J of energy, how much mass disappears?

$$m = \frac{E}{c^2} = \frac{6.5 \times 10^{12} \text{ J}}{(3.0 \times 10^8 \text{ m/s})^2} = 7.2 \times 10^{-5} \text{ kg, or 72 mg}$$

Fusion Reactions

When two small nuclei combine, their binding energy must be released.

Example: How much energy is released when lithium-6 combines with deuterium to form two helium nuclei (deuterium is hydrogen-2)?

1. Write the equation.

$$^6_3\text{Li} + ^2_1\text{H} \rightarrow 2^4_2\text{He}$$

The mass numbers are $6 + 2 = 2 \times 4$. The electric charge numbers are $3 + 1 = 2 \times 2$.

2. Add the nuclear masses on each side of the equation to find the mass deficit.

Li-6:   6.01512 D1
H-2:   2.0140 D1
        8.02912 D1
He-4: 2×4.00260 D1 = 8.00520 D1

The mass deficit is $8.02912 - 8.00520 = 0.0239$ D1.

3. Determine the energy equivalent of the mass deficit:

$$0.0239 \text{ D1}\left(\frac{930 \text{ MeV}}{\text{D1}}\right) = 22 \text{ MeV}$$

Nuclear Fission

When a very large nucleus splits into two medium-sized nuclei, the combined mass of the two fragments is less than the mass of the original nucleus. Thus, energy is released.

Example: When Uranium-235 is split by impact with a slow neutron, how many neutrons are produced?

$$^{235}_{92}\text{U} + ^{1}_{0}\text{n} \rightarrow ^{92}_{36}\text{Kr} + ^{141}_{56}\text{Ba} + ?^{1}_{0}\text{n}$$

Barium and krypton result. To balance the mass numbers, three neutrons must be produced. These neutrons can split additional uranium nuclei, producing a chain reaction.

Photons

Light has a dual nature; it can be described as a wave or a stream of particles (photons).

Wave Property of Light

As a wave, light obeys the equation

$$c = \lambda v$$

where c is the speed of the wave (3.00×10^8 m/s); λ (lambda) is the wavelength, and v (nu) is the frequency.

Example: What is the frequency of yellow light of wavelength 570 nm (nanometers)?

$$v = \frac{c}{\lambda} = \frac{3.00 \times 10^8 \text{ m/s}}{570 \times 10^{-9} \text{ m}} = 5.26 \times 10^{14}/\text{s} = 5.26 \times 10^{14} \text{ Hz}$$

Photon Energy

The energy of a photon obeys the equation

$$E = hv = \frac{hc}{\lambda}$$

where h is Planck's constant, 4.14×10^{-15} eV · s.

Example: What is the energy of a photon of red light with wavelength 730 nm?

$$E = \frac{hc}{\lambda} = \frac{(4.14 \times 10^{-15} \text{ eV} \cdot \text{s})(3.00 \times 10^8 \text{ m/s})}{730 \times 10^{-9} \text{ m}} = 1.70 \text{ eV}$$

Photoelectric Effect

A photon may release an electron from a metal surface. The energy of the electron is equal to the energy of the photon minus the work function of the metal.

Example: What is the maximum energy of an electron emitted by a metal whose work function is 2.60 eV if the incident light is ultraviolet with a wavelength of 370 nm?

1. Find the energy of the photon.

$$E = hv = h\frac{c}{\lambda} = \frac{(4.14 \times 10^{-15} \text{ eV} \cdot \text{s})(3.00 \times 10^8 \text{ m/s})}{370 \times 10^{-9} \text{ m}} = 3.36 \text{ eV}$$

2. Subtract the work function of the metal.

$$3.36 \text{ eV} - 2.60 \text{ eV} = 0.76 \text{ eV}.$$

Example: What is the longest wavelength of light that will release an electron from a metal whose work function is 3.61 eV?

The minimum energy of the photon is the work function of the metal, so

$$\lambda = \frac{hc}{E} = \frac{(4.14 \times 10^{-15} \text{ eV} \cdot \text{s})(3.00 \times 10^8 \text{ m/s})}{3.61 \text{ eV}} = 3.4 \times 10^{-7} \text{ m}$$

or 340 nm, in the ultraviolet.

Atomic Energy Levels

The electrons in the outer shells of an atom can be raised from ground state to excited states in quantized steps.

Spectra

When an electron falls to a lower energy state, it loses a definite amount of energy by emitting a photon having that energy. The spectrum of the light emitted by a substance contains only photons of certain definite energies.

Example: What is the wavelength of the light emitted when an electron drops from a 4.70-eV excited state to a 3.22-eV state?

1. The energy of the photon is 4.70 eV − 3.22 eV = 1.48 eV.

2. The wavelength of the photon is

$$\lambda = \frac{hc}{E} = \frac{(4.14 \times 10^{-15} \text{ eV} \cdot \text{s})(3.00 \times 10^8 \text{ m/s})}{1.48 \text{ eV}} = 8.39 \times 10^{-7} \text{ m}$$

which is the wavelength of an infrared photon, at 839 nm.

Spectrum of Atomic Hydrogen

The single electron of a hydrogen atom occupies quantum states which can be represented by the expression $-13.6 \text{ eV}/n^2$, where n is any whole number.

Example: What is the wavelength of a photon that is emitted when a hydrogen electron drops from the fifth to the second state?

1. Find the energy levels of the two states.

$$\frac{-13.6 \text{ eV}}{2^2} = -3.40 \text{ eV} \qquad \frac{-13.6 \text{ eV}}{5^2} = -0.54 \text{ eV}$$

2. Subtract to get the energy of the photon.

$$-0.54 \text{ eV} - (-3.40 \text{ eV}) = 2.86 \text{ eV}$$

3. Find the wavelength of the photon:

$$\lambda = \frac{hc}{E} = \frac{(4.14 \times 10^{-15} \text{ eV} \cdot \text{s})(3 \times 10^8 \text{ m/s})}{2.86 \text{ eV}} = 4.34 \times 10^{-7} \text{ m}$$

Example: What is the wavelength of a photon that will ionize a hydrogen atom in its ground state?

1. The energy needed is enough to raise the total energy level to zero:

$$0 - \frac{(-13.6 \text{ eV})}{1^2} = 13.6 \text{ eV}$$

2. Calculate the wavelength of this photon:

$$\lambda = \frac{hc}{E} = \frac{(4.14 \times 10^{-15} \text{ eV} \cdot \text{s})(3.00 \times 10^8 \text{ m/s})}{13.6 \text{ eV}} = 9.1 \times 10^{-8} \text{ m or 91 nm}$$

Mathematics Review

An understanding of basic mathematical skills is essential for the science and quantitative skills test questions. This section reviews the most important mathematical concepts that may be present in these tests. This presentation does not attempt to cover all areas in great depth. Rather, it should be used in conjunction with texts so that the student will be prepared for mathematically oriented test questions.

Arithmetic

Operations on Numbers

Whole numbers are the counting numbers, 1, 2, 3, 4, 5, . . . *Integers* are the positive and negative whole numbers and zero: . . . , $-3, -2, -1, 0, 1, 2, 3, $ . . . A *mixed number* consists of an integer combined with a fraction, for example, $3\frac{1}{8}$. Many questions call for rounding off an answer "to the nearest integer." To round off a mixed number to the nearest integer, drop the fraction part of the number; if the fraction part is $\frac{1}{2}$ or more than $\frac{1}{2}$, increase the integer by 1; if the fraction part is less than $\frac{1}{2}$, keep the original integer. For example, $4\frac{7}{8}$ rounded off to the nearest integer is 5, but $3\frac{1}{8}$ rounded off to the nearest integer is 3.

Questions often require that decimal answers be rounded off to some specified degree of precision, for example, to the nearest tenth, or to the nearest hundredth, or to the nearest thousandth. To answer such a question, drop all digits in the decimal which are to the right of the specified digit; if the first digit dropped is 5 or more, increase the last digit retained by 1; if the first digit dropped is less than 5, keep the last digit retained at its present value. As examples, 81.698 rounded to the nearest tenth is 81.7; 81.698 rounded to the nearest hundredth is 81.70 (note that the zero is retained to show a hundredths place); 45.639 rounded to the nearest tenth is 45.6.

The rules for rounding off decimals also apply to rounding off whole numbers to a specified degree of precision. For example, 102,681 rounded off to the nearest thousand is 103,000; 102,681 rounded off to the nearest hundred is 102,700; 49,294 rounded off to the nearest thousand is 49,000.

Precision and Significant Digits

All measurements are approximate. Consider a measurement said to be 43 grams to the nearest gram. The unit of measure is the smallest unit indicated by the number and is the unit which was applied in the measurement. In the illustration, the unit is the gram and the maximum possible error is one-half that unit. Thus 43 grams to the nearest gram means the true measure is between 43 ± 0.5 grams. A measure of $28\frac{1}{2}$ feet means that the unit of measure is $\frac{1}{2}$ foot and the maximum error is therefore $\frac{1}{4}$ foot. A measure of $28\frac{1}{2}$ feet could represent a true measure of anywhere between $28\frac{1}{4}$ feet and $28\frac{3}{4}$ feet. A measurement of 2.05 inches means that the unit of measure is 0.01 inch (that is, $\frac{1}{100}$ of an inch), and the 2.05 may represent a true measure anywhere between 2.045 and 2.055 inches.

If an approximate number is multiplied by some number greater than 1, the precision of the result is reduced since the maximum error is also multiplied by that number. If the approximate measure of $28\frac{1}{2}$ feet, which has a maximum error of $\frac{1}{4}$ foot, is multiplied by 5, the result is $5 \times 28\frac{1}{2}$ or $142\frac{1}{2}$ feet with a maximum error of $5 \times \frac{1}{4}$ or $1\frac{1}{4}$ feet. Thus, the $142\frac{1}{2}$ foot approximation really represents a measure anywhere between $141\frac{1}{4}$ feet and $143\frac{3}{4}$ feet.

If an approximate number is represented as a decimal, every digit starting from the leftmost non-zero digit and extending through the digit which represents the unit of measure is a *significant digit*. Thus, 2345 has 4 significant digits, 23.45 also has 4 significant digits, 0.00023 has 2 significant digits, and 2300 may have either 2, 3 or 4 significant digits depending on whether the two zeroes represent accurate measures in the tenths and units places or are merely used as "fillers" to locate the decimal point. Note that the position of the decimal point has nothing to do with the number of significant digits. The speed of light is 186,272 mi/sec; this figure has 6 significant digits; if we talk about the speed of light being 186,000 mi/sec., the figure used has only 3 significant digits.

Performing mathematical operations on approximate numbers cannot increase the number of significant digits. If two approximate numbers are multiplied together or divided, you should carry out the multiplication or division and then round off your answer to the number of significant digits in the number with the *fewest* significant digits. Note that in the case of multiplication and division, the position of the decimal point has nothing to do with the number of significant digits in the answer. The situation in addition and subtraction is very different. If 231.2 is added to 15.623, the sum becomes 246.823, but digits beyond 246.8 are not significant since 231.2 was accurate to the nearest tenth only. Thus, in adding or subtracting approximate numbers, you should first carry out the operation and then round the answer to the first place where the *last* significant digit of any of the numbers is found. Note also that if 231.2 had been added to 15.673, the sum would first be 246.873, which would be rounded off to 246.9.

Percent and Percentage

Problems involving percent, actually involve three quantities: the base, the percent (or rate), and the percentage. The *percent* (expressed as a decimal such as .20 or as a part of 100 such as 20%) is the ratio of one quantity (the percentage) to another (the base). The number of which the percent is taken is the *base*; the result after the percent of the base is taken is the *percentage*. For example, if we say that 40% of the 2000 bacteria in a certain culture are spirochetes, then there are 800 spirochetes present in the culture. 40% or .40 is the percent or rate, 2000 is the base, and 800 is the percentage. The best way to solve any problem involving percent or percentage is to write an equation based on the formula $p = br$, that is, percentage equals base times rate. Thus, if asked to find what percent of the 2000 bacteria in a culture is represented by the 800 spirochetes, the equation $800 = 2000r$ is solved. If asked to find the number of bacteria in a culture in which 800 spirochetes are known to represent 40%, the equation $800 = b(.40)$ is solved. If asked to find how many spirochetes there are in a culture containing 2000 bacteria of which 40% are spirochetes, the equation $p = 2000(.40)$ is used.

Algebra

Ratio and Proportion

Ratio: A comparison of two values that are expressed in the same units. It may be expressed as an indicated division or as two numbers separated by a colon.

Example: A comparison of the length of two insects might be expressed as $2 \, \text{cm} : 3 \, \text{cm}$, that is, as $2:3$ or as $\frac{2 \, \text{cm}}{3 \, \text{cm}}$, that is, as $\frac{2}{3}$. Note that in each case, the name of the units cancels and the ratio consists of two pure numbers, $2:3$ or $\frac{2}{3}$. The units involved must be the same, however; the ratio of 3 inches to 2 yards is not $3:2$, but 3 inches to 72 inches, that is $3:72$ or $\frac{3}{72}$ or $\frac{1}{24}$.

Proportion: A statement that two ratios are equal. For example, $1:2 = 4:8$ or $\frac{1}{2} = \frac{4}{8}$ represents a proportion.

The first and last terms of a proportion are called the *extremes* and the second and third terms of a proportion are called the *means*. In the proportion $\frac{1}{2} = \frac{4}{8}$, 1 and 8 are the extremes and 2 and 4 are the means. A most important relation used to solve problems involving proportions is this: In any proportion, the product of the means equals the product of the extremes.

Example: If two substances, A and B, are to be mixed in the ratio of 2 parts of A to 3 parts of B, how many milliliters of A must be mixed with 15 milliliters of B to make the proper mixture?

Let x = the number of milliliters of A.

Since the ratio of A to B equals the ratio 2:3, a proportion is formed:

$$\frac{x}{15} = \frac{2}{3}$$

In a proportion, the product of the means equals the product of the extremes (cross multiply):

$$3x = 2(15)$$
$$3x = 30$$
$$x = 10$$

If the means in a proportion are equal, either of the means is called the *mean proportional* between the two extremes. Thus, in the proportion $\frac{1}{3} = \frac{3}{9}$, 3 is the mean proportional between 1 and 9.

Example: Find the mean proportional between 4 and 16.

If x is the mean proportional, then:

$$\frac{4}{x} = \frac{x}{16}$$

In a proportion, the product of the means equals the product of the extremes (cross multiply):

$$x^2 = 4(16)$$
$$x^2 = 64$$

Take the square root of both sides of the equation: $x = \pm 8$.

Note that every positive number has two square roots, one positive and one negative. In a practical problem, one of the roots (usually the negative one) may have to be rejected as meaningless (for example, if x represents a length).

Equations

Equations Containing Fractions: These are solved by multiplying all terms on both sides of the equation by the Least Common Denominator of all the fractions.

Example: Find a if $\frac{a}{4} - \frac{a}{6} = \frac{1}{2}$.

The least common denominator for 4, 6, and 2 is 12. Multiply all terms on both sides of the equation by 12:

$$12\left(\frac{a}{4}\right) - 12\left(\frac{a}{6}\right) = 12\left(\frac{1}{2}\right)$$
$$3a - 2a = 6$$
$$a = 6$$

Quadratic Equations: Second-degree equations may often be solved by factoring.

Example: Solve $2x^2 + 5x = 3$.

Rewrite the equation so that all terms are on one side in descending order of exponents, equal to 0:

$$2x^2 + 5x - 3 = 0$$

The quadratic trinomial on the left factors into two binomials. The factors of the first term, $2x^2$, become the first terms of the binomials:

$$(2x \quad)(x \quad) = 0$$

The factors of the last term, -3, become the second terms of the binomials, but they must be chosen in such a way that the product of the inner terms added to the product of the outer terms equals the middle term of the original trinomial, $+5x$. Try -1 and $+3$ as the factors of -3:

$$-x = \text{inner product}$$

$$(2x - 1)(x + 3) = 0$$

$$6x = \text{outer product}$$

Since $(-x) + (6x) = +5x$, these are the correct factors:

$$(2x - 1)(x + 3) = 0$$

Set each factor equal to zero:

$$2x - 1 = 0 \quad \text{OR} \quad x + 3 = 0$$

$$2x = 1 \qquad\qquad x = -3$$

$$x = \frac{1}{2}$$

The solution is $x = \frac{1}{2}$ or -3.

If a quadratic equation cannot be solved by factoring, the *quadratic formula* may be used: In a quadratic equation of the form $ax^2 + bx + c = 0$,

$$x = \frac{-b \pm \sqrt{b^2 - 4ac}}{2a}$$

Example: Solve $x^2 - 4x - 3 = 0$

Here $a = 1$, $b = -4$ and $c = -3$:

$$x = \frac{-(-4) \pm \sqrt{(-4)^2 - 4(1)(-3)}}{2(1)}$$

$$x = \frac{4 \pm \sqrt{16 + 12}}{2}$$

$$x = \frac{4 \pm \sqrt{28}}{2}$$

$$x = \frac{4 \pm \sqrt{(4)(7)}}{2}$$

$$x = \frac{4 \pm 2\sqrt{7}}{2}$$

$$x = 2 \pm \sqrt{7}$$

Radical Equations: Equations in which the variable appears under a radical sign. They may be solved by isolating the radical on one side of the equation and then squaring both sides.

Example: Solve $\sqrt{x^2 - 8} - x = 4$

Isolate the radical on one side of the equation:

$$\sqrt{x^2 - 8} = x + 4$$

Square both sides of the equation:

$$x^2 - 8 = (x + 4)^2$$
$$x^2 - 8 = x^2 + 8x + 16$$
$$-8 - 16 = 8x$$
$$-24 = 8x$$
$$-3 = x$$

The process of squaring may introduce an *extraneous root*; therefore, radical equations solved by squaring must always have the solution(s) checked to see if any are extraneous; checking must be done by substituting in the *original* equation:

$$\sqrt{(-3)^2 - 8} - (-3) \stackrel{?}{=} 4$$
$$\sqrt{9 - 8} + 3 \stackrel{?}{=} 4$$
$$1 + 3 \stackrel{?}{=} 4$$
$$4 = 4 \checkmark$$

-3 is a true root.

Equations Containing Decimals: Such equations are best solved by removing all decimals by multiplying each term in the equation by the highest power of 10 that will remove all the decimals:

Example: Solve $153 + 0.085x = 0.85x$

Multiply each term by 1000:

$$153,000 + 85x = 850x$$
$$153,000 = 850x - 85x$$
$$153,000 = 765x$$
$$200 = x$$

Formulas

Questions may be asked requiring you to transform a given formula so that it is solved for a specified variable in terms of the others. This is accomplished in the same manner as the solution of a literal equation; the specified variable must be isolated on one side of the equation with all terms not containing this variable on the other side.

Example: The formula for obtaining the Fahrenheit temperature, F, when the Celsius temperature, C, is known is $F = \frac{9}{5}C + 32$. Find an expression for C in terms of F.

To solve for C, first multiply both sides by 5:

$$5F = 9C + 160$$

Isolate the term containing C on the right side:

$$5F - 160 = 9C$$

Divide both sides by 9:

$$\frac{5F - 160}{9} = C$$

Factor out a 5 in the numerator:

$$\frac{5(F - 32)}{9} = C$$

In another form:

$$C = \frac{5}{9}(F - 32)$$

Scientific Notation

Scientific notation is a method of writing a number as the product of a power of 10 and a decimal number whose whole number part is between 1 and 10. For example, 3.6903×10^4 is in scientific notation. Scientific notation is a convenient method for designating very large or very small numbers. It is particularly useful when only a small number of significant digits are used in the number. For example, the speed of light is said to be 186,000 mi/sec. The only significant digits are "186" since the three zeroes are merely used to indicate the placement of the decimal point. The speed of light is expressed more meaningfully in scientific notation as 1.86×10^5 mi/sec. Scientific notation makes the number easier to handle and also makes it clear that the zeros are not significant digits.

Questions may involve conversion from scientific notation to ordinary notation or vice versa. Since multiplication by 10 results in moving the decimal point one digit to the right, the number 1.25×10^4 becomes 12,500 in ordinary notation (the decimal point is moved 4 places to the right). Similarly, 10 raised to a negative exponent indicates division by 10 that many times. Division by 10 results in moving the decimal point to the left one place. Thus, 1.25×10^{-2} is equivalent to 0.0125 in ordinary notation. 81,250 in ordinary notation becomes 8.125×10^4 in scientific notation, and 0.002728 becomes 2.728×10^{-3}.

Exponents and Logarithms

Positive Exponents: A positive exponent is a number which indicates the number of times a quantity is to be used as a factor in a power. For example, 2^4 means $(2)(2)(2)(2)$ or 16.

Zero Exponents: By definition $x^0 = 1$ for all values of x except $x = 0$, which is undefined. Thus, $5^0 = 1$ and $(-3)^0 = 1$.

Negative Exponents: By definition, $x^{-n} = \dfrac{1}{x^n}$ provided $x \neq 0$. Thus, $3^{-2} = \dfrac{1}{3^2} = \dfrac{1}{9}$.

Fractional Exponents: By definition $x^{m/n} = \sqrt[n]{x^m}$ or $(\sqrt[n]{x})^m$ provided $n \neq 0$. Thus, $x^{1/2} = \sqrt{x}$, and $8^{2/3} = (\sqrt[3]{8})^2 = 2^2 = 4$.

Law of Exponents:

For multiplication: $(x^a)(x^b) = x^{a+b}$ Example: $y^3 \cdot y^4 = y^7$
For division: $x^a \div x^b = x^{a-b}$ Example: $y^6 \div y^2 = y^4$
For powers: $(x^a)^b = x^{ab}$ Example: $(y^2)^3 = y^6$
For roots: $\sqrt[b]{x^a} = x^{a \div b}$ Example: $\sqrt{y^6} = y^3$

Exponential Equations: An exponential equation is an equation in which the variable appears in an exponent. Simple exponential equations may be solved by expressing both sides of the equation as powers of the same base.

Example: Solve $3^{x-1} = 9$

Express both sides of the equation as powers of the same base, in this case, 3:

$$3^{x-1} = 3^2$$

Since the bases are the same, the exponents must be equal:

$$x - 1 = 2$$
$$x = 2 + 1$$
$$x = 3$$

If it is impossible to express both sides of the equation as powers of the same base, logarithms must be used to solve an exponential equation (see next section).

Logarithms: The logarithm of a number is the exponent to which a given base must be raised to produce the number. The given base for *common logarithms* is 10.

Thus, $\log_{10} 100 = 2$ since $10^2 = 100$
$\log_{10} 10,000 = 4$ since $10^4 = 10,000$
$\log_{10} 50 = 1.6990$ since $10^{1.6990} = 50$
$\log_{10} 10 = 1$ since $10^1 = 10$

In writing common logarithms, the base, 10, is generally omitted. Thus, we say log 100 = 2, log 10,000 = 4, log 50 = 1.6990, and log 10 = 1.

Of course, log 50 = 1.6990 cannot be found readily. Like all common logarithms, it consists of two parts. The whole number part, or *characteristic,* is positive and is 1 less than the number of digits before the decimal point if the number is 1 or greater. Thus, the characteristic for log 839 would be 2. If the number is a positive number less than 1, the characteristic is negative and its absolute value is 1 more than the number of zeroes between the decimal point and the first significant digit. Thus, the characteristic for log 0.0072 would be −3.

The *mantissa,* or decimal part of the logarithm, is found in the Table of Common Logarithms. The mantissa is always positive and is the same for the same sequence of significant digits. Thus, the mantissas for 365, 36.5, and 0.0365 are the same. The mantissa for log 50 is found by looking for the sequence of digits, 500; the table shows the mantissa for this sequence to be .6990. The characteristic for log 50 is 1, so log 50 = 1.6990. Since the mantissa is always positive and the characteristic may be negative, the log for a number such as 0.00372 must be written as 7.5705 − 10.

Interpolation: If we have a Table of Common Logarithms that provides entries for numbers with a sequence of only 3 digits, we must interpolate to find a mantissa of a number having 4 significant digits. To find the mantissa for log 183.6, we look for the mantissa for the sequence 183 (it is .2625) and for the mantissa for the sequence 184 (it is .2648). Since 1836 lies between 1830 and 1840, its mantissa will lie at a proportionate distance between their mantissas.

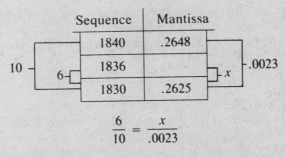

$$\frac{6}{10} = \frac{x}{.0023}$$

The product of the means equals the product of the extremes (cross multiply):

$$10x = 6(.0023)$$
$$10x = .0138$$
$$x = .00138 \text{ or } .0014$$

Mantissa for log 1836 is .2625 + .0014 = .2639
Log 183.6 is 2.2639 since the characteristic for 183.6 is 2.

Laws of Logarithms: Since logarithms are exponents, they obey the same laws of exponents:

For multiplication: $\log (ab) = \log a + \log b$
   Example: $\log 8 = \log (4 \cdot 2) = \log 4 + \log 2$

For division: $\log \left(\dfrac{a}{b}\right) = \log a - \log b$

   Example: $\log \left(\dfrac{12}{4}\right) = \log 12 - \log 4$

For powers: $\log a^n = n \log a$
   Example: $\log 2^3 = 3 \log 2$

For roots: $\log \sqrt[n]{a} = \dfrac{1}{n} \log a$

   Example: $\log \sqrt{5} = \dfrac{1}{2} \log 5$

Solving Exponential Equations by Logarithms:

Example: Solve for x: $3^x = 17$.

Since both sides cannot be written as powers of the same base, take logarithms of both sides of the equation:

$$x \log 3 = \log 17$$

$$x(0.4771) = 1.2304$$

$$x = \frac{1.2304}{0.4771}$$

The solution is completed by dividing 1.2304 by 0.4771.

Natural or Naperian Logarithms: Common logarithms use the base 10. In more advanced mathematics and in many scientific applications, it is more effective to use logarithms with a base called the natural number and represented by e; e is approximately 2.718. Logarithms using the base e are called natural or Naperian logarithms and are designated by ln. Thus, $\ln 100 = 4.605$ since $e^{4.605} = 100$

$$\ln 10{,}000 = 9.210 \quad \text{since } e^{9.210} = 10{,}000$$

$$\ln e = 1.000 \quad \text{since } e^1 = e$$

$$\ln 1 = 0 \quad \text{since } e^0 = 1$$

Using either base 10 or base e, a negative logarithm indicates a number between 0 and 1. There are no logarithms for negative numbers.

Natural logarithms obey the same laws as common logarithms since both are exponents. For example, $\ln 65 = \ln (5 \cdot 13) = \ln 5 + \ln 13$.

Variation

Direct Variation: Many physical variables are so related that an increase in one will produce an increase in the other. For example, the pressure of a confined gas will increase as the temperature of the gas is increased. If the values of two variables bear a constant ratio to each other, they are said to be in direct variation; sometimes it is said that "y varies as x" or "y varies directly with x." Direct variation can be expressed in symbols as $\dfrac{y}{x} = k$ or $y = kx$, where k is called the constant of variation.

Example: If the work done, y, by a constant force varies directly as the distance, d, through which the force acts, and if $y = 16$ when $x = 3$, find y when $x = 9$.

Use the formula $y = kx$. Substitute 16 for y and 3 for x:

$$16 = 3k$$

Solve for k, the constant of variation:

$$\frac{16}{3} = k$$

Since k is a constant, substitute the new value of x in $y = \frac{16}{3}x$:

$$y = \frac{16}{3}(9)$$

$$y = 48$$

Inverse Variation: In many sciences, two variables are related so that their product is constant; when one gets larger, the other gets smaller. In an electrical circuit of constant voltage, for example, the product of the current and the resistance is constant. Current and resistance are said to vary inversely. Inverse variation involves a relationship of the form $xy = k$ or $y = \frac{k}{x}$, where k is the constant of variation.

Example: The volume, y, of a gas at a constant temperature is inversely proportional to the pressure, x. If $y = 30$ when $x = 2$, find y when $x = 12$.
  Substitute in $xy = k$ to find the constant, k:

$$(2)(30) = k$$

$$60 = k$$

Since k is a constant and equal to 60, now substitute 12 for x in $xy = 60$:

$$12y = 60$$

$$y = 5$$

Joint Variation: Some physical phenomena involve the variation of more than two variables. If y varies directly with both x and z, then the basic relationship may be expressed as $y = kxz$. If y varies directly with x but inversely as the square of z, then the basic relationship may be expressed as $y = \frac{kx}{z^2}$.

Trigonometry and the Right Triangle

The Pythagorean Theorem

Many problems involving right triangles can be solved by use of the Pythagorean Theorem, which states that in any right triangle, the square of the length of the hypotenuse equals the sum of the squares of the lengths of the legs. In the diagram shown, where a and b are the lengths of the legs and c is the length of the hypotenuse, $a^2 + b^2 = c^2$. Thus, if the lengths of any two sides of a right triangle are known, the length of the third side can be found.

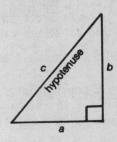

Example: If the hypotenuse of a right triangle is 7 feet, and the length of one leg is 4 feet, find the length of the other leg.

If b is the length of the other leg, apply the Pythagorean Theorem:

$$4^2 + b^2 = 7^2$$

$$16 + b^2 = 49$$

$$b^2 = 49 - 16$$

$$b^2 = 33$$

Take the square root of both sides of the equation:

$$b = \pm\sqrt{33}$$

Reject the negative value as meaningless for a length:

$$b = \sqrt{33}$$

Pythagorean Triples

Certain special cases result in right triangles in which the ratio of the lengths of the sides can be represented by integers. They are the 3-4-5, 5-12-13, and 8-15-17 right triangles. Note that in every case the largest number in the triple represents the hypotenuse; the other two represent the legs. These triples should be committed to memory as they make the solutions of many right triangles extremely easy.

Example: Find the remaining leg of a right triangle whose hypotenuse is 15 and one of whose legs is 12.

The hypotenuse, 15, is equal to 3 times 5 and the leg, 12, is equal to three times 4. Hence the triangle is a 3-4-5 right triangle with all the values multiplied by 3. The remaining leg is three times 3 or 9.

45°-45°-90° and 30°-60°-90° Triangles

The MCAT includes questions that may require knowledge of the relationships among the sides of two special right triangles, the 45°-45°-90° triangle and the 30°-60°-90° triangle. The relationships can all be determined by use of the Pythagorean Theorem and certain facts from plane geometry, but it is recommended that the student commit to memory the two diagrams below and use the values shown as formulas to apply in solving either of these special triangles.

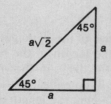
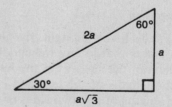

Example: Find the leg of an isosceles right triangle whose hypotenuse is $5\sqrt{2}$.

An isosceles right triangle is a 45°-45°-90° triangle. Applying the formulas from the diagram above, the hypotenuse is $a\sqrt{2}$:

$$a\sqrt{2} = 5\sqrt{2}$$

$$a = 5$$

From the diagram above, the length of a leg is a:

$$\text{leg} = 5$$

Example: If the hypotenuse of a 30°-60°-90° triangle is 6, find the length of the leg opposite the 30° angle and the length of the leg opposite the 60° angle.

The formula for the hypotenuse of a 30°-60°-90° triangle is $2a$:

$$2a = 6$$
$$a = 3$$

The formula for the leg opposite 30° is a:

$$a = 3$$

The formula for the leg opposite 60° is $a\sqrt{3}$:

$$a\sqrt{3} = 3\sqrt{3}$$

Trigonometric Functions

The three basic trigonometric functions are defined for acute angles from ratios in a right triangle:

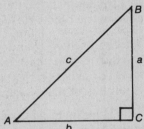

$$\sin A = \frac{\text{opposite side}}{\text{hypotenuse}} = \frac{a}{c}$$

$$\cos A = \frac{\text{adjacent side}}{\text{hypotenuse}} = \frac{b}{c}$$

$$\tan A = \frac{\text{opposite side}}{\text{adjacent side}} = \frac{a}{b}$$

A convenient way to remember these definitions is by memorizing the mnemonic *soh-cahtoa*. Split into three parts, *soh,cah,toa*, where "*s*" stands for sine, "*o*" for opposite, "*h*" for hypotenuse, etc., the mnemonic gives all three definitions. Note that sin is an abbreviation for sine, cos for cosine, and tan for tangent. When any 2 parts from among the two acute angles and the three sides of a right triangle are known, any of the other parts can be found.

Example: In the right triangle shown, find the length of side $\overline{EG}$.

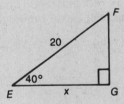

$\overline{EG}$ is the side adjacent to the 40° angle and 20 is the hypotenuse. Hence the cosine is used:

$$\cos 40° = \frac{\text{adjacent leg}}{\text{hypotenuse}}$$

From the Table of the Values of Trigonometric Functions, $\cos 40° = 0.7660$:

$$0.7660 = \frac{x}{20}$$

Multiply both sides of the equation by 20:

$$20(0.7660) = x$$
$$15.32 = x$$

A student taking the MCAT will be expected to know the sines and cosines of 0°, 90°, and 180°. These are shown in tabular form below:

	0°	90°	180°
sin	0	1	0
cos	1	0	−1
tan	0	∞	0

The sines, cosines, and tangents of 0° and 90° are deduced from consideration of what happens as angle A in the diagram of $\triangle ABC$ collapses toward 0°. BC will approach 0, and thus the sin 0° and the tan 0° will both be 0. As angle A collapses, the hypotenuse $\overline{AB}$ will approach $\overline{AC}$, and hence $\dfrac{AB}{AC}$ will equal 1 at 0°, or cos 0° = 1. The values for 90° are deduced in a similar manner; those for 180° are the result of an extension of the definitions of the trigonometric functions to values beyond the acute angles found in a right triangle.

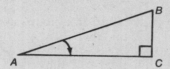

MCAT candidates are also expected to know the sines, cosines, and tangents of 30°, 45°, and 60°. If the candidate commits to memory the formulas for the sides as recommended in the section of this book on the 45°-45°-90° triangle and the 30°-60°-90° triangle, these values need not be memorized since they can be obtained by applying the definition of the sine, cosine, or tangent to the expressions in the formulas. For example, sin 45° $= \dfrac{\text{opposite side}}{\text{hypotenuse}} = \dfrac{a}{a\sqrt{2}} = \dfrac{1}{\sqrt{2}}$. The value $\dfrac{1}{\sqrt{2}}$ can be used for sin 45° or it can be changed to $\dfrac{1}{2}\sqrt{2}$, obtained by multiplying numerator and denominator by $\sqrt{2}$. As another example, cos 60° $= \dfrac{a}{2a} = \dfrac{1}{2}$. For the convenience of those candidates who would prefer to memorize the values of the sine, cosine, and tangent of 30°, 45°, and 60°, a table of these values is also given here:

	30°	45°	60°
sin	$\dfrac{1}{2}$	$\dfrac{1}{2}\sqrt{2}$	$\dfrac{1}{2}\sqrt{3}$
cos	$\dfrac{1}{2}\sqrt{3}$	$\dfrac{1}{2}\sqrt{2}$	$\dfrac{1}{2}$
tan	$\dfrac{1}{3}\sqrt{3}$	1	$\sqrt{3}$

Systems of Measurement

The MCAT candidate will be expected to understand and operate in either the metric system of measurement or in the system of common British units. It may be required to perform conversions from one system to the other, but in all such cases, the conversion factor will be supplied with the question.

The Common British System

The following equivalences and abbreviations should be known:

$$1 \text{ yard (yd)} = 3 \text{ feet (ft)} = 36 \text{ inches (in)}$$
$$1 \text{ foot} = 12 \text{ inches}$$
$$1 \text{ mile (mi)} = 5280 \text{ feet} = 1760 \text{ yards}$$
$$1 \text{ pound (lb)} = 16 \text{ ounces (oz)}$$
$$1 \text{ ton (T)} = 2000 \text{ pounds}$$
$$1 \text{ gallon (gal)} = 4 \text{ quarts (qt)} = 8 \text{ pints (pt)}$$
$$1 \text{ quart} = 2 \text{ pints}$$
$$1 \text{ pint} = 16 \text{ fluid ounces (oz)}$$

This table of equivalences permits conversions within the British system.

Example: How many ounces are there in 3 tons?

$$3 \text{ tons} \times \frac{2000 \text{ lbs}}{\text{ton}} \times \frac{16 \text{ oz}}{\text{lb}}$$

$$3 \times 2000 \times 16 \text{ oz} = 96,000 \text{ oz}$$

Note that names of units which appear once in a numerator and a denominator are cancelled. For example, tons ÷ tons = 1 and lbs ÷ lbs = 1. This leaves only the name of the units in which the answer is denoted.

Balancing Equations Containing Physical Units: The preceding comment on cancelling the names of units in an equation points up the importance of balancing the names of units on both sides of an equation that deals with physical units.

Example: Given that the distance, d, that a body falls if dropped from rest is $\frac{1}{2}$ the acceleration due to gravity, a, times the time, squared, t^2, find the distance in meters that a body will drop in 3 minutes.

The given equation is:

$$d = \frac{1}{2} at^2$$

We cannot substitute 16 ft/sec² for a, or 3 min for t and expect to get a distance in meters because the units involved will not balance:

$$d(\text{meters}) \neq \frac{1}{2} \cdot \frac{16 \text{ ft}}{\text{sec}^2} (60 \text{ min})^2$$

Since 1 min = 60 sec, we can replace $(60 \text{ min})^2$ by $(60)^2(\text{sec})^2$, and since 1 ft = 0.3 meter, we can replace 16 ft by 16(0.3 meter):

$$d(\text{meters}) = \frac{1}{2} \cdot \frac{16(0.3 \text{ meter})}{\text{sec}^2} (60)^2(\text{sec})^2$$

Cancelling names of units wherever possible shows that both sides of the equation are in meters only:

$$d(\text{meters}) = \frac{1}{2} \cdot \frac{16(0.3 \text{ meter})}{\text{sec}^2} (60)^2(\text{sec})^2$$

If the units in an equation cannot be balanced in this way, it is an indication that there is an error somewhere in the equation.

The Metric System

The basic units for the metric system are:

For length: meters (abbreviated m)
For volume: liters (abbreviated l or L)
For mass: grams (abbreviated g)

The following prefixes are attached to the names of the basic units to denote other units whose size equals the basic unit multiplied or divided by a power of 10:

$$\text{pico (p)} = 10^{-12}$$
$$\text{nano (n)} = 10^{-9}$$
$$\text{micro } (\mu) = 10^{-6}$$
$$\text{milli (m)} = 10^{-3}$$
$$\text{centi (c)} = 10^{-2}$$
$$\text{deci (d)} = 10^{-1}$$
$$\text{deka (da)} = 10$$
$$\text{hecto (h)} = 10^{2}$$
$$\text{kilo (k)} = 10^{3}$$
$$\text{mega (M)} = 10^{6}$$

Thus, a kilometer (km) is 10^3 or 1000 times as large as a meter. A centimeter (cm) is 10^{-2} times a meter or $\frac{1}{100}$ the size of a meter. A milligram (mg) is 10^{-3} times the size of a gram or $\frac{1}{1000}$ the size of a gram.

Conversions may be made within the metric system simply by moving the decimal point. Thus, 53 cm = 0.53 m.(since a meter is 10^2 centimeters). Similarly, 8.3 kg = 8300 g (since a kilogram is 10^3 grams).

Elementary Probability

The probability of an event occurring $= \dfrac{\text{the number of favorable cases}}{\text{the total possible number of cases}}$.

For example, the chance of a tossed coin landing heads up is $\frac{1}{2}$ or 0.5, since there is 1 favorable case, heads, out of a total possible number of 2 cases, either heads or tails. The probability of drawing a king on a single draw from a pack of 52 cards is $\frac{1}{13}$. The number of favorable cases is 4 (there are 4 kings) and the total possible number of cases is 52; $\frac{4}{52} = \frac{1}{13}$.

The probability of two or more independent events occurring is the product of their separate probabilities. Thus, the probability of tossing 3 coins and having them all land heads up is $\left(\frac{1}{2}\right)\left(\frac{1}{2}\right)\left(\frac{1}{2}\right) = \left(\frac{1}{2}\right)^3 = \frac{1}{8}$ or 0.125.

If a coin has been tossed 3 times and has landed heads up each time, what is the probability that a fourth toss will result in a head? The answer is still $\frac{1}{2}$ since the fourth result is not affected by the three previous cases (it is said that "coins and cards have no memory"). The probability that all of four tossed coins will land heads up is $\left(\frac{1}{2}\right)\left(\frac{1}{2}\right)\left(\frac{1}{2}\right)\left(\frac{1}{2}\right) = \left(\frac{1}{2}\right)^4 = \frac{1}{16} = 0.0625.$

In a medical situation, suppose that a patient requires ear surgery for which the success rate is 90%. Note that this is equivalent to saying that the probability of success is $\frac{9}{10}$ or 0.9. If the patient requires surgery on both ears, what is the probability of a successful outcome for both?

$$(0.9)(0.9) = 0.81 = 81\%$$

Note that in these calculations, the assumption has been made that the events are independent, that is, that one event does not influence another. Thus, it is assumed that the surgical patient is a normal patient and that success of surgery on one ear does not make success on the other ear more nor less probable.

In a compound probability situation, be sure to examine the number of favorable cases and the total possible number of cases for each of the separate situations.

Example: What is the probability of drawing 2 blue marbles from a bag containing 4 red and 6 blue marbles if the first marble is not replaced before the second one is drawn?

The probability of drawing a blue marble on the first draw is $\frac{6}{10}$. But since this first blue marble is not replaced, there are now only 5 blue marbles in the bag out of a total of only 9 marbles. Therefore, the probability of drawing a blue marble on the second draw is $\frac{5}{9}$. The probability of the two events occurring one after the other is $\frac{6}{10} \times \frac{5}{9}$ or $\frac{30}{90}$ or $\frac{1}{3}$.

Statistics

Some Measures of Central Tendency

Suppose you are asked to examine the fasting blood glucose concentrations of several patients in a hospital and obtain the results in mg/dl as 100, 80, 100, 90, 100, 120, and 125.

The *range* (the distance between the extreme values) is from 80 to 125, or 45.

The *mode* (the most common value in the series) is 100.

The *arithmetic mean* or *average* is the sum of all the values divided by the number of values:

$$\frac{100 + 80 + 100 + 90 + 100 + 120 + 125}{7} = 102.1$$

The *median* (the middle value when they are arranged in order of size) is 100 since arrangement in order of size gives 80, 90, 100, 100, 100, 120, 125, and the middle number is 100. If there were an even number of items in the series, there would be no single middle number; in such a case, the median is taken as the value half way between the two middle values.

The Standard Deviation

The standard deviation is a statistical measure that indicates the dispersion or spread of the values in a set of data. You will not be expected to calculate it on the MCAT, but you must be able to interpret it. In the previous illustration, the standard deviation is 15.8. You should know that in a normal distribution, 68% of the values will fall within the arithmetic mean ± 1 standard deviation, and 96% of the values will fall within the arithmetic mean ± 2 standard deviations. Thus, in the example shown, 68% of the values would be expected to lie between 102.1 − 15.8 or 86.3, and 102.1 + 15.8 or 117.9. The fact that only 4 out of the 7 values fall in this range $\left(\frac{4}{7} = 57.1\%\right)$ is due to the sample being so small. 96% of the values would be expected to fall between 102.1 − 31.6 or 70.5, and 102.1 + 31.6 or 133.7. Actually, all 7, that is 100% of them, do so.

Correlation

Suppose two variables change at random. The *coefficient of correlation* is a statistical measure of the degree to which the variation in one imitates the variation in the other. On the MCAT, you will not be expected to calculate a coefficient of correlation, but you will be expected to understand the nature of this measure.

The coefficient of correlation may have values between -1 and $+1$ inclusive; for example, values of $+.86$ or $-.23$ are typical. A correlation of $+1$ is a perfect positive correlation; the two variables involved move up and down together although they may be measured in different units and the moves may be of different magnitudes. A correlation of -1 is a perfect negative correlation; the variables involved move at the same times and to the same degree but in opposite directions (one decreases when the other increases). A correlation of 0 means that there is no relation between the variations in the two.

The output of a factory and its direct costs would tend to move together to some degree; hence the correlation between these two could be expected to be positive although not nearly as great as $+1$. It is usually true that the higher the price, the lower the sales; if there is a price increase, sales tend to drop; hence price and sales can be expected to be negatively correlated.

The three graphs below represent "scatter diagrams" obtained by plotting random readings of two variables, x and y. Graph A shows no association between x and y and hence the correlation would probably be close to 0. Graph B shows a generally negative correlation (y decreases when x increases), and Graph C shows a positive correlation.

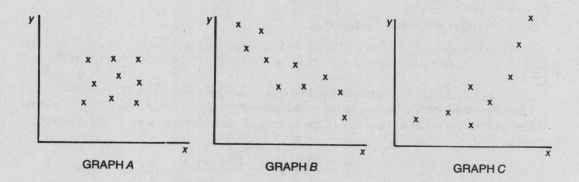

GRAPH A   GRAPH B   GRAPH C

Graphic Representation of Data and Functions

Medical and other scientific publications use graphic representation of data and of algebraic functions to make relationships clear and also to deduce other information from such a representation.

The Rectangular or Cartesian Coordinate System

This system permits the location of any point on a plane with reference to two perpendicular axes whose point of intersection is called the *origin*. The horizontal axis is the x-axis, and the vertical axis is the y-axis. The position of a point is specified by an ordered pair of numbers in parentheses, for example, $(4,3)$, which are called the *coordinates* of the point. The x-coordinate, also called the *abscissa*, is always written first, and the y-coordinate, also called the *ordinate*, is second. The abscissa is the distance measured horizontally from the y-axis and the ordinate is the distance measured vertically from the x-axis to the point. In the diagram, P is the point $(4,3)$, Q is the point $(-2,5)$, and R is the point $(-3,-6)$.

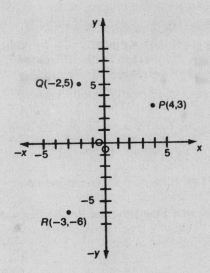

A first degree equation in two variables has an infinite number of pairs of values of x and y which satisfy it. These points may be plotted on a graph to represent the equation. A first degree equation always has a graph which is a straight line.

Example: Draw the graph of $x + 4y = 8$.
  Solve the equation for y in terms of x:

$$4y = -x + 8$$

$$y = -\frac{1}{4}x + 2$$

Choose some convenient values for x and calculate the corresponding values of y from the equation:

x	-4	0	8
y	3	2	0

Plot the points $(-4,3)$, $(0,2)$, and $(8,0)$ and draw a straight line through them. This line is the graph of $x + 4y = 8$.

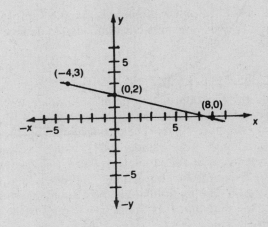

Slope of a Line: If Δy represents the change in the y-values from one point to another and Δx represents the change in the x-values of these two points, then the slope, m, of the line joining the two points is defined as $m = \dfrac{\Delta y}{\Delta x}$. If the coordinates of the two points are represented by (x_1, y_1) and (x_2, y_2), then the slope may also be defined as $m = \dfrac{y_2 - y_1}{x_2 - x_1}$. The slope is the rate of change of y with respect to x.

Example: Find the slope of the first two points plotted to draw the graph of the line $x + 4y = 8$ in the section preceding this. These are the points $(-4, 3)$ and $(0, 2)$.

Let $(-4, 3)$ be (x_1, y_1) and $(0, 2)$ be (x_2, y_2). Then $y_2 - y_1$ or Δy is $2 - 3$ or -1, and $x_2 - x_1$ or Δx is $0 - (-4)$ or 4. $m = \dfrac{-1}{4}$: The slope is $-\dfrac{1}{4}$.

The Slope-Intercept Form of a Straight Line: In the last example, notice that the slope of the line is $-\dfrac{1}{4}$ and that $-\dfrac{1}{4}$ (or m) is also the coefficient of x in the equation

$$y = -\frac{1}{4}x + 2.$$

The constant term $+2$, which we denote by b, is the y-intercept, that is, the value of y where the graph crosses the y-axis. By solving the equation of a line for y, we can put it in the form $y = mx + b$, which tells us immediately the slope and y-intercept of the line. For example, the line $y = \dfrac{2}{3}x - 4$ has a slope of $\dfrac{2}{3}$ and a y-intercept of -4. This information can be used to draw the graph of the equation instead of plotting points. Begin with the y-intercept (at the point $[0, -4]$), and move 3 units to the right and 2 units up to locate the next point on the line; continue this process for more points on the line.

Graphs of equations other than first degree do not appear as straight lines. The graphs of such equations may be drawn by preparing a table of corresponding values of x and y (obtained by substitution in the equation). These values are used to plot points whose coordinates they are; joining the points with a smooth curve produces the graph representing the equation. Figure 1 shows the graph of the equation $xy = 12$. An equation of the form $xy = k$ where k is a constant is a relationship between two variables that are *inversely proportional*; this type of relationship and its characteristic graph is common to many natural physical phenomena. Figure 2 illustrates the graph of $y = 2^x$ which is an

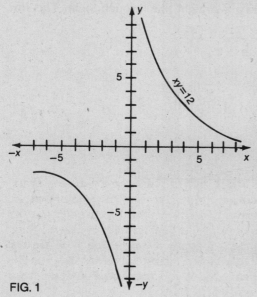

FIG. 1

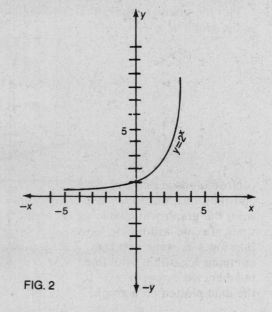

FIG. 2

exponential function; an exponential function and its characteristic graph is common in many medical and scientific areas, such as the growth of bacteria in a culture or the decay of a radioactive substance. The graphs in both Figures 1 and 2 approach certain lines but never actually reach them; such lines are called *asymptotes*. In Figure 1, both the *x*- and *y*-axes are asymptotes; in Figure 2, the *x*-axis is an asymptote.

Finding the Equation from a Graph

Suppose that readings from experiments are taken on two variables, say blood clotting time and the quantity administered of a certain anti-clotting substance. If these data are used as coordinates of points plotted on a rectangular coordinate chart, and if the points turn out to lie in a straight line, then we know that we can represent the relationship between the two variables by a first degree algebraic equation. In fact, we can write the equation; all we need do is read the value of the *y*-intercept, *b*, from the graph and figure the slope, *m*, by noting the Δy and the Δx between two of the points; substituting the values of *m* and *b* in the slope-intercept form, $y = mx + b$, gives the equation.

But suppose that points plotted from experimental data readings do not lie in a straight line. Then the equation of the graph is not a first degree equation. To find out what it is, we use other types of coordinate systems. Two of those that are especially useful with the types of equations and graphs common in medicine and other sciences are the semi-log scale and the log-log scale.

Semi-log Graphs: The rectangular coordinate system uses scales on the *x*- and *y*-axes that are arithmetic, that is, the distances on the scale from 0 to 1, from 1 to 2, from 2 to 3, etc., are always the same. The semi-log coordinate system uses an *x*-axis that has an arithmetic scale, but the distances from the origin along the *y*-axis represent the values of the logarithms of the numbers instead of the numbers themselves. Thus, the *y*-axis scale begins at 1 (since log 1 = 0). Since log 10 = 1 and log 100 = 2, the distance on the scale from 1 to 10 is the same as the distance from 10 to 100. It is also the same as the distance from 100 to 1000, etc.

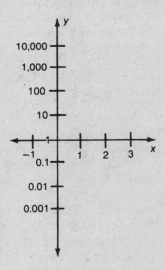

Now suppose that experimental data readings are plotted as points on a semi-log chart, and they turn out to lie in a straight line. Reading the slope, *m*, and the *y*-intercept, *b*, from the graph will enable us to write an equation, but the variable represented on the vertical scale will be log *y* instead of *y* and the intercept, *b*, will actually be log *b*. Note that log *b* is some constant. The equation will then be log $y = mx + \log b$. Since the common logarithm is defined as the exponent to which 10 must be raised to give the number, we can write $y = 10^{mx + \log b}$. Thus we have found an exponential function from the data plotted on a graph.

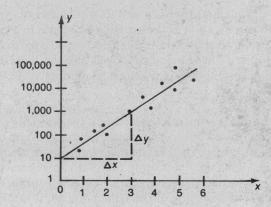

Example: The graph above, drawn on semi-log coordinate paper, shows a line obtained by plotting a scattering of points from experimental data. Find the equation of the line.

Read the y-intercept, b, from the graph: $b = \log 10 = 1$. Calculate the slope, m:

$$m = \frac{\Delta y}{\Delta x} = \frac{\log 1000 - \log 10}{3 - 0} = \frac{3 - 1}{3} = \frac{2}{3}$$

Using the slope-intercept form of the straight line, $y = mx + b$:

$$\log y = \frac{2}{3}x + 1$$

Since $\log y$ is the exponent to which 10 must be raised to equal y:

$$y = 10^{2/3x + 1}$$

Note that although for simplicity this discussion involves a y-axis scale which is for common logs (base 10), semi-log scales used in medicine could be scaled for natural logarithms (base e).

Log-log Graphs: In semi-log graphs, the x-axis has an arithmetic scale and the y-axis has a scale that is logarithmic. In log-log graphs, both the x-axis and y-axis have scales that are logarithmic.

Suppose we plot points from experimental data and find that they lie in a straight line on a log-log chart. As before, we can read the slope, m, and the y-intercept, b, and use them in the $y = mx + b$ form of the straight line to write the equation. However, the variables are now $\log y$ and $\log x$ instead of y and x, and the value we read for the y-intercept is actually $\log b$. Thus, we can write an equation, $\log y = m \log x + \log b$. Making use of the laws of logarithms, $m \log x = \log x^m$, and $\log x^m + \log b = \log (bx^m)$. Thus, our equation becomes $\log y = \log (bx^m)$. Since we have the logs of two expressions equal, the expressions themselves are equal. Thus, our equation is $y = bx^m$. Since m may be any positive or negative integer or even a fraction, we have a powerful tool for converting data readings into complicated equations of degree greater than 1.

A first degree equation in two variables can always be rewritten in the form $y = mx + b$, and its graph is *always* a straight line on rectangular coordinate graph paper. The MCAT candidate should know that one type of exponential equation is of the form $y = a^{bx + c}$, where a, b, and c are constants, and that its graph is *always* a straight line when drawn on semi-log coordinate paper. In scientific work the "a" of $y = a^{bx + c}$ is frequently equal to e, the natural number, and c is frequently equal to 0, so that the most common form of an exponential equation in medicine or other sciences is $y = e^{bx}$.

MCAT candidates should also know that an equation of the form $y = ax^n$ where a and n are constants and n may be positive, negative, or a fraction, is known as a power law; its graph is *always* a straight line when drawn on log-log coordinate paper.

Vector Addition and Subtraction

Vectors

Most quantities are *scalar* quantities, that is, they have magnitude only. The length of a line, the number of pages in this book, or your bank balance are all scalar quantities. Some quantities have both a magnitude and a direction. They are called *vector* quantities. Examples are a wind velocity of 15 mph in an easterly direction, a downward (vertical) water pressure of 20 lb/in^2, or the motion of a ship sailing northeast at 23 knots. A directed line segment called a *vector* is used to represent such quantities; its length represents the magnitude of the quantity and its orientation represents the direction.

Vector Addition

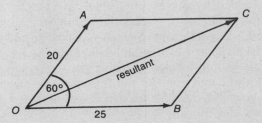

Suppose that two forces, one of 20 lb and one of 25 lb act simultaneously on a body at an angle of 60° to each other. We may represent the 20 lb force by vector $\overrightarrow{OA}$ and the 25 lb force by the vector $\overrightarrow{OB}$. Complete the parallelogram of which $\overrightarrow{OA}$ and $\overrightarrow{OB}$ are two sides. The diagonal of the parallelogram, $\overrightarrow{OC}$, is a vector which is called the sum of the vectors $\overrightarrow{OA}$ and $\overrightarrow{OB}$. $\overrightarrow{OC}$ is also called the *resultant* of the two vectors, $\overrightarrow{OA}$ and $\overrightarrow{OB}$, and $\overrightarrow{OA}$ and $\overrightarrow{OB}$ are the *components* of the force represented by $\overrightarrow{OC}$. If the object on which forces $\overrightarrow{OA}$ and $\overrightarrow{OB}$ are acting is free-moving, the object will move in the direction represented by $\overrightarrow{OC}$ and with a force whose magnitude is represented by the length of $\overrightarrow{OC}$.

If it is desired to compute the magnitude of $\overrightarrow{OC}$ in the above example, $\triangle OBC$ must be solved. Since $AOBC$ is a parallelogram, $BC = OA = 20$, and $\angle B \triangleq 120°$. By the Law of Cosines, $(OC)^2 = (OB)^2 + (BC)^2 - 2(OB)(BC)\cos \angle B$. All the quantities on the right side of the equation are known, so $(OC)^2$, and hence $\overrightarrow{OC}$, can be calculated.

Questions on the MCAT involving vector addition could involve simpler cases than the above, usually those in which the two component forces are at right angles to each other.

Example: Find the resultant force and the angle it makes with the larger component, if two component forces, one of 10 lb and one of 20 lb, act at 90° to each other.

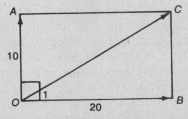

Draw vectors representing the two forces and complete the parallelogram of which they are sides. The diagonal of this parallelogram, which comes from their common origin, is the resultant or sum of the two forces. Vector $\overrightarrow{OC}$ is the resultant. In right $\triangle OBC$, $OB = 20$ and $CB = OA = 10$. By the Pythagorean Theorem, $(OC)^2 = 20^2 + 10^2$ or $(OC)^2 = 400 + 100$; since $(OC)^2 = 500$, $OC = \sqrt{500}$ or $10\sqrt{5}$. In right triangle OBC, $\tan \angle 1 = \dfrac{\text{opposite leg}}{\text{adjacent leg}} = \dfrac{10}{20} = \dfrac{1}{2} = 0.5000$. From the Tables of Trigonometric Functions, the angle whose tangent is 0.5000 is 27° to the nearest degree, so the resultant makes a 27° angle with the larger component.

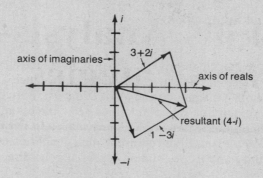

Vectors may also be added by representing them as complex numbers. The vector represented by the complex number $3 + 2i$ is the vector which extends from the origin to the point representing $3 + 2i$ graphically. Suppose we wish to add the vector represented by $3 + 2i$ to the vector represented by $1 - 3i$. As before, the resultant can be drawn as the diagonal of the parallelogram formed by using the two given vectors as sides. The complex number which is the end point of the resultant can be read from the graph; it represents the resultant vector. However, the sum can be obtained more simply by adding the two complex numbers algebraically:

$$\begin{array}{r} 3 + 2i \\ \underline{1 - 3i} \\ 4 - i \end{array}$$

The resultant is $4 - i$.

Subtraction of Vectors

To subtract one vector from another, we simply add the additive inverse of the vector to be subtracted. If the complex number representation of the vectors is used, this simply means that the signs of the vector being subtracted are changed and the resulting complex number is then added to the other vector. If the parallelogram method is used, the vector being subtracted is replaced by a vector of the same magnitude but extending in the opposite direction. This new vector is then added to the other vector by forming a parallelogram and finding the diagonal which is the resultant (see diagram).

SUBTRACTING $\vec{OB}$ FROM $\vec{OA}$

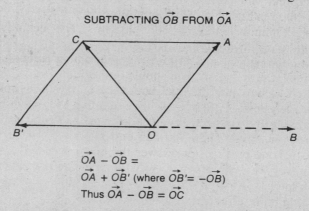

$\vec{OA} - \vec{OB} =$
$\vec{OA} + \vec{OB}'$ (where $\vec{OB}' = -\vec{OB}$)
Thus $\vec{OA} - \vec{OB} = \vec{OC}$

Reading Skills Analysis— Test-Taking Strategies

This portion of the book will focus on various techniques to help you get the most out of reading.

You can learn to read efficiently and effectively, and the more you read the better you will read. People who do not like to read generally do not read well, and most people who do not read well read too slowly. They read almost word by word and must consequently backtrack to capture the main idea. You should read as fast as you can think without the loss of comprehension, misreading or losing facts or ideas.

Learning to read rapidly takes effort, willpower and a plan. Success depends on your interest and the effectiveness of the techniques and habits you acquire. Find the time for the activities that are necessary for academic success: first things first!

A great deal of your success depends on your frame of mind. You must develop confidence in your own ability. Believe in yourself. You have been successful in the past and will be successful in the future. Confidence comes with knowledge, experience and practice.

In the MCAT Examination, reading skill is assessed by presenting to the examinee one or more paragraphs of material. The selection is followed by a variable number of questions pertaining to it. Subjects from a wide variety of areas are used to test the student's ability to analyze data accurately. The information necessary to answer the questions is in the selection, and no prior knowledge is necessary to arrive at a correct answer.

Approach to the Reading Questions

There is no one correct way to handle this section. Some people routinely read the selection first, and some read the questions first. With either approach, rapid processing of information and maximum retention are key elements. The techniques of underlining (described later in this chapter) are useful here.

If you prefer to read the selection first, use the underlining technique to highlight the details. When you finish the selection, you should immediately move on to the questions and answer them one by one while the information is still fresh in your mind.

Some people read the questions first since they feel that they have better attention to details when they know what to expect. If you choose this approach, you read the passage with specific questions in mind. Then you can either answer the questions as a group when you have finished the passage, or answer the questions as the answers appear in the selection. Whichever way you proceed, we still advocate the underlining method. If you have to go back later, the material is already grouped and easier to work with. This will make backtracking more efficient.

Do not, however, leave questions blank in the hope of returning to them later. This could be costly since rereading the entire passage may require a great deal of time. (In the knowledge sections of the examination this is not a problem because the questions are units in themselves and not based on paragraphs.) Answer all questions as best you can, marking those you are not certain of for checking if you have time at the end. Please remember that you must base your answers on the material presented in the passage, not on your own knowledge or experience.

The Quantitative questions should be approached in the same way as the Reading questions. The only difference is that in this section the information is presented in tables, graphs, charts, maps and other quantitative forms instead of straight prose. The student's ability to read and analyze the material is tested by the questions. There is no single perfect approach to this type of material. However, it is important to be sure you know what each number, axis, line or graph means before proceeding to answer the questions. Make sure that you are aware what information has been presented, what the limitations of the data are and what reasonable conclusions may be drawn from it. Do not base your answer on information that isn't there.

Ways and Means

Reading experts seem to agree that the rapid reader's comprehension is usually excellent, and the slow reader's comprehension is usually poor. This does not mean that the rapid reader never slows down for difficult material. It does mean that the rapid reader is able to find the right speed for the material, while the slow reader habitually reads more slowly than the occasion or subject matter demands.

Word-by-Word Reading: Word-by-word reading does not improve comprehension and makes concentration more difficult. Understanding and comprehension demand that you read groups of words, or ideas. As you read, you must analyze, think, group ideas and topics, spot relationships, and see similarities and differences in the passage. The word-by-word reader sees only the trees and misses the forest.

Backtracking: Most readers backtrack occasionally. This technique is not only acceptable but also part of efficient reading. All of us look back and reread a word or several words now and then. The good reader, however, does it less frequently than the poor reader. The efficient reader basically looks back only when he needs to, while the slow reader does it mechanically and out of habit. The inefficient reader usually reads most words, phrases, sentences and paragraphs more than once since he often misses the central idea or meaning the first time. The first time through, he has merely read the words and must therefore reread the selection to see how they are connected. The habit of reading single words rather than groups usually keeps you from grasping the central theme. Grouping words, sentences, and paragraphs as you go along allows you to make sense of the material and to focus on the theme and idea.

Pausing and Stopping: Inefficient readers usually allow long and frequent pauses as they proceed. This not only hinders concentration but also makes it difficult to absorb the ideas presented. If you pause after reading only a few sentences, you lose track of the author's train of thought. You may remember certain details, but the connections get lost.

Quick Skimming to Elicit the General Theme: This technique involves reading rapidly and concentrating on the key words and phrases that develop and support the theme. One might think that in this approach, the main point could be missed; however, nothing could be further from the truth. This is purposeful reading for comprehension, since its object is to grasp the central point and carefully note the key elements that support that point.

Key Words That Announce Conditions and Should Be Kept in Focus!

1. again, also, accordingly, just as
2. therefore, thus, hence, henceforth
3. for example, for instance, in other words
4. nevertheless, however, notice, but
5. always, at all times, under all circumstances, every time
6. finally, in conclusion, in brief, at last
7. never, not, no, none
8. only, specifically, significantly, importantly, decidedly
9. first, another, and, likewise, as well as, besides
10. despite, although, regardless

How is Material Usually Organized?

1.   Most selections have a *central subject* (main idea) which could be used as the *title*. In many instances, the first sentence of a paragraph will tell you this main idea.

2.   The material is usually presented in a fashion that answers a question, poses one, gives a solution, or gives a non-committal statement of fact.

3.   Key words and facts should substantiate and solidify the main idea of the reading. These are the details. Always look for key words. If you go back and read the key words, you should be able to get the essence of the passage.

4.   The details are usually of two types. The main details are directly related to the central theme, and are used to develop it. The subordinate details break down and clarify the main details, to further develop the theme. Breaking the material down this way can help you to understand it.

5.   Read in a questioning manner. This will ensure that you are actively involved. Ask *who, what, when* and *where* to elicit key elements. Ask *how* and *why* to determine reasons.

Suggested Method for Efficient Analysis of Reading Material

1.   Identify the topic or main theme and underline it with a *straight* line.

2.   Find the main details about the topic and underline the key words or phrases with a curved line.

3.   As you read the subordinate details about the details bracket them with (curved brackets).

4.   Extraneous elements or qualifiers should be bracketed with [square brackets] as they are encountered.

Don't go overboard! Focus on key elements only. This simple method will allow you to backtrack if needed, and will help you answer the questions at the end of a selection. Your information is now arranged to highlight the interrelationships of facts. While you have read, you have been forced to think and organize the material. You have formed associations that will foster recall.

A Plan for Self-Improvement

1.   Set aside a time and place specifically for reading every day even if it is only 10 minutes. You know the conditions under which you function best. No one can set them for you.

2.   Develop the habit of reading for ideas. After you have read a passage, ask yourself what the central theme was and verbalize it. The verbalization will quickly synthesize the material and draw upon relationships (similarities, differences) in the passage. The central idea will not only be highlighted but also be substantiated and amplified. Picture yourself as a critic who is writing a review that will evaluate the material for a potential reader.

3.   Read different material; become a versatile reader.

4.   Keep a record of your progress and be optimistic. A positive attitude is half the battle. Don't be discouraged by plateaus; they are common.

The Do's and Don'ts

1.   Even though *scientific* reading, unlike pleasure reading, often involves word-by-word reading, you should coordinate speed and thought processes, and you should read as fast as you think. Backtracking usually interferes with efficient assimilation and processing of information.

2.   Even though word-by-word reading is slower and more tedious, eliminate irrelevant thoughts. You don't want them to intrude just because you believe you must have something to think about. Irrelevant thoughts make concentration impossible.

3.   Usually, poor concentration will lead to poor comprehension, and unnecessarily slow reading can lead to poor concentration and poor comprehension. Read as rapidly as you can without losing comprehension. Adapt speed as necessary.

4. Don't hold back your thinking processes by unnecessarily slow reading. Do not create a gap between reading and thinking. In the same vein, do not stop and pause frequently since this also will allow gaps in your thinking to occur.

5. Remember, it's a poor reader who stops too often and pauses too long at each stop.

6. Apply the same concentration whether a selection is long or short.

7. Look for a general impression, main thoughts, and implications so that you may draw inferences. Read ideas rather than words. Identify your topics, the details about them and the details about the details. Above all, don't fail to note the important ideas.

8. Whether you are the original writer or the reader of a selection, you must approach it with the thought of a distinct design and technique to present a specific subject matter and topic. Look for special effects and results.

9. You can usually identify the main topic of a paragraph by key words or phrases that could serve as possible titles. Concentrate on why certain words are used and how they are used. By concentrating on why and how, you can establish and follow the main idea. During your reading, you should realize that the paragraph is merely a sum of its parts. In turn, look at paragraphs as key elements in the development of the ideas of the passage. Don't let minor details or sentences overshadow paragraphs or the whole selection. Where there are paragraph headings, these usually lead you to main ideas.

10. Central thoughts are usually found in the lead sentence or in the summary sentence, but they may be located in other places and may, at times, be implied rather than stated. Read to understand by focusing on central ideas and units of thought.

11. Exhibit versatility, and adjust to the material. Don't use the same technique for all material; be pliable, adapt, use common sense.

12. Most of the material you confront will be familiar and understandable to you. Don't stick too closely to the particular selection; always associate present material with previous material. Nothing is ever completely new. In this context, you must focus on detail and read for specific comprehension and specific meanings to see what is new. Whether you read for general or specific ideas, use your previous knowledge. Read for meaning. Try to determine the meaning of unfamiliar words as you reason through a selection. Don't let an unfamiliar word stump you and worry you unduly; the context will often help you determine the meaning.

13. Do not decrease speed because of fear that you might miss something, and do not fall into the trap of reading each sentence twice before you proceed. Don't reread material unless necessary, but if you need to reread, do not hesitate to spend the time to clarify meaning.

14. Do not read each sentence as a distinct unit, but use each unit to build the paragraph and the selection to create the whole.

15. As you read a selection composed of several paragraphs, reflect whether succeeding paragraphs amplify the ideas or points raised in the preceding paragraphs or whether they provide an example or illustration of them. Is a qualifier of a point introduced, or is another aspect of the same subject considered?

16. Before you answer the whole battery of questions, quickly review your underlinings to make sure you understood the point.

17. Under no circumstances should you get yourself involved more deeply than necessary with the reading selection and with the task. Don't read more into it than is there; answer the questions on the basis of only what is presented.

18. Be critical when you read; extract the important facts and see relationships and associations. Visualize descriptions accurately. Avoid misreading.

19. Avoid superficiality when you consider the selection. Don't come to a conclusion before you have read the whole passage and without sufficient thought. Don't jump to a conclusion.

Practice Reading Exercises

Exercise 1

Identify the central theme or topic, details, and details about details.

DIRECTIONS: Read the sample and underline the topic, the details of the topic, and bracket (the details about the details).

Example: Following the work of Chalmers and others, 831 geriatric and orthopedic patients in West London were reviewed for osteomalacia.

(a) The topic deals with osteomalacia.
(b) Details or key words are geriatric and orthopedic patients.
(c) Details about details are (831 patients) and (West London).

DIRECTIONS: Read the sample paragraph and underline the topic, the details about the topic, and bracket the (details about the details). Use square brackets for [extraneous material].

Example: Following the work of Chalmers and others, 831 geriatric and orthopedic patients in West London were reviewed for osteomalacia. History, relevant blood tests (calcium, phosphate, alkaline phosphatase, 24-hour urinary calcium) and radiology were assessed. Thirty-eight bone biopsies were performed. Thirty-three were positive (32 female, 1 male). Average age was 73.4 years. None had a history of gastric surgery. Twenty-eight were widows living alone. Three were sisters (spinsters) living together. Twenty-two lived on their own property. Average weekly income was $25.00. Average weekly food bill, $9.00 (mostly bread, canned meat and canned fruit). The minimum for a balanced diet was thought to be $18.00. Average milk consumption was one pint per week. None of the patients cooked regularly. Twenty-six never cooked at all. None had sought the assistance of any of the welfare organizations, through either pride, ignorance, or apathy. All showed subjective and objective improvement following calcium and Vitamin D supplementation and dietary improvement.

Method: Following the work of Chalmers and others, (831) geriatric and orthopedic patients in [West London] were reviewed for osteomalacia. History, relevant blood tests (calcium, phosphate, alkaline phosphatase, 24 hour urinary calcium) and radiology were assessed. Twenty-eight bone biopsies were performed. (Thirty-three were positive) ([32 female], 1 male). Average age was (73.4) years. [None] had a history of [gastric surgery]. (Twenty-eight) were (widows) living alone. Three were sisters (spinsters) living together. [Twenty-two] lived on their [own property]. Average weekly income was $25.00. Average weekly food bill, $9.00 (mostly bread, canned meat and canned fruit). The minimum for a balanced diet was thought to be $18.00. Average milk consumption (one pint) per week. None of the patients cooked regularly. (Twenty-six never) cooked at all. None had sought the assistance of any of the welfare organizations, through either pride, ignorance, or apathy. All showed subjective and objective improvement following calcium and Vitamin D supplementation and dietary improvement.

Method in Outline Form

(a) The topic: osteomalacia
(b) Details or key words:
    1. geriatric, orthopedic patients
    2. history, blood tests, radiology, bone biopsies
    3. age, milk consumption, week
    4. none cooked regularly, none assistance
    5. improvement, calcium, Vitamin D, dietary

    (c) Details about details:
        1. (831)
        2. (33 positive)
        3. (73.4 years)
        4. (twenty-eight widows)
        5. (one pint)
        6. (twenty-six never)
    (d) Extraneous material:
        1. [West London]
        2. [32 female]
        3. [None gastric surgery]
        4. [Twenty-two own property]

Having used the underlining technique, let us use this information to answer the type of questions used in the examination.

DIRECTIONS: Choose the best answer.

1. Osteomalacia
    (A) has a predilection for males.
    (B) occurs more frequently in females.
    (C) can only be diagnosed by bone biopsy.
    (D) has a predilection for apartment dwellers.

2. The average weekly income did not allow these people to buy more food.
    (A) True
    (B) False
    (C) They needed to save for their old age.
    (D) They spend their money on the little luxuries of life.

3. From these data we may conclude that
    (A) homeowners are more likely to develop osteomalacia than are renters.
    (B) spinsters will not develop osteomalacia if they live alone.
    (C) consumption of bread is a consistent factor in the development of osteomalacia.
    (D) there seems to be a correlation between an unbalanced diet, irregular meal consumption, and osteomalacia.

4. Given a greater income, these individuals would have
    (A) eaten more nutritious meals.
    (B) cooked at least two meals a day.
    (C) spent a greater percentage of their income on food.
    (D) The passage does not give enough information to answer this question.

5. This study
    (A) was a unique one.
    (B) utilized every technique available.
    (C) utilized a great variety of patients.
    (D) showed that at least ten percent of the elderly suffer from osteomalacia.
    (E) indicated that dietary supplementation is beneficial.

Answers

1.	**B**		4.	**D**
2.	**B**		5.	**E**
3.	**D**			

Exercise 2

Identify the central theme or topic, details, and details about details.

DIRECTIONS: Read the sample and underline the topic, the details about the topic, and bracket the (details about the details). Use square brackets for [extraneous material].

Example: The orbit is a cone-shaped bony structure with an apex directed posteriorly and a large anterior opening.

(a) The topic deals with the orbit.
(b) Details or key words are bony, apex posteriorly, anterior opening.
(c) Details about details are (cone shaped).

DIRECTIONS: Read the sample paragraph and underline the topic, the details about the topic, and bracket the (details about the details). Use square brackets for [extraneous material].

Example: The orbit is a cone-shaped bony structure with an apex directed posteriorly and a large anterior opening. It may be described as having a floor, a roof, and medial and lateral walls. The roof is formed mainly by the frontal bone anterior to a small portion of the sphenoid bone. The floor of the orbit from anterior to posterior is composed of the zygomatic, maxillary, and palatine bones. The lateral wall consists of portions of the zygomatic bone anteriorly and the sphenoid bone posteriorly. The medial wall from anterior to posterior is formed by the frontal process of the maxilla, the lacrimal bone, the ethmoid bone, and the sphenoid bone. Besides the anterior opening, the orbit communicates with other regions via nine openings. The infraorbital nerve enters the orbit through the infraorbital foramen. On its medial wall the anterior and posterior ethmoidal foramina transmit the anterior and posterior ethmoidal nerves, respectively. Posteriorly, near the apex of the orbit, the optic nerve and the ophthalmic artery enter via the optic canal. Also located near the apex, the superior orbital fissure transmits cranial nerves III, IV, and VI and the ophthalmic division of cranial nerve V.

Method: The orbit is a (cone-shaped) bony structure with an apex directed posteriorly and a large anterior opening. It may be described as having a floor, a roof, and medial and lateral walls. The roof is formed mainly by the frontal bone anterior to a small portion of the sphenoid bone. The floor of the orbit from (anterior to posterior) is composed of the zygomatic, maxillary, and palatine bones. The lateral wall consists of portions of the zygomatic bone anteriorly and the sphenoid bone posteriorly. The medial wall from anterior to posterior is formed by the frontal process of the maxilla, the lacrimal bone, the ethmoid bone, and the sphenoid bone. Besides the anterior openings, the orbit (communicates) with other regions via (nine openings). The infraorbital nerve enters the orbit through the inferior orbital fissure, then lies the infraorbital groove in the floor and exits anteriorly through the infraorbital foramen. On its medial wall the anterior and posterior ethmoidal foramina transmit the anterior and posterior ethmoidal nerves, respectively. Posteriorly, near the apex of the orbit, the optic nerve and the ophthalmic artery enter via the optic canal. Also located near the apex, the superior orbital fissure transmits the (cranial nerves) III, IV, and VI and the (ophthalmic division) of cranial nerve V.

Method in Outline Form

(a) The topic: orbit
(b) Details or key words:
  1. bony, apex posteriorly, anterior opening
  2. floor, roof, medial, lateral walls
  3. roof, frontal, sphenoid
      floor, zygomtic, maxillary, palatine
      lateral, zygomatic, sphenoid
      medial, frontal, maxilla, lacrimal, ethmoid, sphenoid
  4. infraorbital nerve, infraorbital foramen

    5. medial, anterior, posterior ethmoid foramina, nerves
    6. optic nerve, ophthalmic artery, optic canal
    7. supraorbital fissure, III, IV, VI, V
(c) Details about details:
    1. (cone shaped)
    2. (communicates)
    3. (nine openings)
    4. (cranial nerves)
    5. (ophthalmic division)

Having read the passage and used the underlining technique, let us use this information to answer the type of questions used in the examination.

DIRECTIONS: The following statements are related to the passage above. Based on the information given, select:

(A) if the statement is *supported* by the information in the passage.
(B) if the statement is *contradicted* by the information in the passage.
(C) if the statement is *neither supported nor contradicted* by the information in the passage.

1. The superior ophthalmic vein exits the orbit via the superior orbital fissure.
2. The orbit is formed by portions of seven bones.
3. The anterior margin, or entrance of the orbit, is bounded by parts of the frontal, zygomatic, and maxillary bones.
4. The lacrimal bone forms part of the lateral wall of the orbit.
5. The superior orbital fissure transmits the optic nerve.
6. The anterior ethmoidal foramen is located between the ethmoid and frontal bones.
7. The ophthalmic artery is a branch of the internal carotid artery.
8. Cranial nerves pass through the superior orbital fissure.

Answers:

1.	C		5.	B
2.	A		6.	C
3.	A		7.	C
4.	B		8.	A

Exercise 3

Identify the central theme or topic, details, and details about details.

DIRECTIONS: Read the sample and underline the topic, the details of the topic, and bracket the (details about the details).

Example: Just about anyone you talk to nowadays complains about the cost of his automobile insurance. It's about time that someone came to the defense of the insurance companies.

(a) The topic deals with automobile insurance:
(b) Details or key words are complains, cost, defense, companies.

DIRECTIONS: Read the sample selection and underline the topic, the details about the topic, and bracket the (details about the details). Use square brackets for [extraneous material] if desired.

Example: Just about anyone you talk to nowadays complains about the cost of his automobile insurance. It's about time that someone came to the defense of the insurance companies.
    We are all familiar with the effects of inflation, but most people forget that the insurance companies are affected too. An interesting point should be noted. Even though the total costs of pro-

ducing a policy have been increasing because of increased salaries, paper cost, equipment replacement, etc., the insurance companies' expense ratios have been going down.

If expenses are reduced, then why are premiums going up? Let's look at what makes up the rates that the insurance companies must charge. Automobile repair rates for labor have risen about 20 percent in the last year and a half. In addition, it has been shown that a new automobile costing $5000 would cost $20,000 if it were to be repaired with replacement parts (not including the engine). During this same period, a semiprivate hospital room has increased in cost over 22 percent and physicians' and surgeons' fees have increased 20 percent. Lawyers continue to ask for larger awards, and the courts are granting them. How can insurance companies continue to pay amounts inflated in this manner without reflecting the increase in their rates?

It is a real shame that the insurance companies don't make these facts known more widely to their customers. A widespread advertising campaign would help to explain their position and make it more tolerable when that next bill comes and has once again increased.

Method: Just about anyone you talk to nowadays complains about the cost of his automobile insurance. It's about time that someone came to the defense of the insurance companies.

We are all familiar with the effects of inflation, but most people forget that the insurance companies are affected too. An interesting point should be noted. Even though the total costs of producing a policy have been increasing because of (increased salaries, paper cost, equipment replacement, etc.) the insurance companies' expense ratios have been going down.

If expenses are reduced, then why are premiums going up? Let's look at what makes up the rates that the insurance companies must charge. Automobile repair rates for labor have risen about (20 percent) in the last year and a half. In addition, it has been shown that a new automobile costing ($5000) would cost ($20,000) if it were to be repaired with replacement parts (not including the engine). During this same period, a semiprivate hospital room has increased in cost over (22 percent) and physicians' and surgeons' fees have increased (20 percent). Lawyers continue to ask for larger awards, and the courts are granting them. How can insurance companies continue to pay amounts inflated in this manner without reflecting the increase in their rates?

It is a real shame that the insurance companies don't make these facts known more widely to their customers. A widespread advertising campaign would help to explain their position and make it more tolerable when the next bill comes and has once again increased.

Method in Outline Form

(a) The topic: automobile insurance
(b) Details or key words:
    1. complains, cost
    2. defense, companies
    3. inflation, policy, increasing
    4. expense ratios, down
    5. premiums, up
    6. repair, risen, replacement parts
    7. hospital, physicians, increased
    8. lawyers, awards, courts, granting
    9. advertising campaign, tolerable, next bill, increased
(c) Details about details:
    1. (20 percent)
    2. ($5000), ($20,000)
    3. (22 percent), (20 percent)

Having read the passage and used the underlining technique, let us use this information to answer the type of questions used in the examination.

DIRECTIONS: The following statements are related to the passage above. Based on the information given, select:

(A) If the statement is *supported* by the information in the passage.

(B)   if the statement is *contradicted* by the information in the passage.

(C)   if the statement is *neither supported nor contradicted* by information in this passage.

1.   Insurance companies' expense ratios are continuing to rise with inflation.
2.   A car repaired with replacement parts would cost four (4) times as much as a new car.
3.   The public is fully aware of why their insurance premiums are increasing.
4.   Automobile insurance premiums have risen mainly because of larger awards in lawsuits.
5.   Inflation is affecting the insurance industry and the rates that are charged.
6.   Insurance companies are involved in a widespread advertising campaign to make their customers aware of the inflationary problems that have caused rates to rise.

Answers

1.	B	4.	C
2.	A	5.	A
3.	B	6.	C

Exercise 4

Identify the central theme or topic, details, and details about details.

DIRECTIONS: Read the sample and underline the topic, the details of the topic, and bracket the (details about the details).

Example: The blood vessels of the mammalian brain normally provide a barrier that blocks the passage of certain molecules which readily penetrate other body tissues.

a)   The topic deals with blood vessels, brain, barrier.
b)   Details or key words are passage, molecules, other, tissues.

DIRECTIONS: Read the sample selection and underline the topic, the details about the topic, and bracket the (details about the details). Use square brackets for [extraneous material].

Example: The blood vessels of the mammalian brain normally provide a barrier that blocks the passage of certain molecules which readily permeate other body tissues. This unique property of the brain vasculature is referred to as the blood-brain barrier and in normal functional states this property prevents the entrance of numerous intravascular probes such as horseradish peroxidase into the substance of the brain. However, in experimental studies of brain dysfunction, such as seen in mechanical brain injury, a disruption of the blood-brain barrier occurs, and experimental probes such as horseradish peroxidase can enter the brain's substance. The mechanism of this blood-brain barrier dysfunction in brain injury is poorly understood. Some contend that the mechanical stress of the injury physically disrupts the vessels and permits peroxidase leakage through defects in the vascular walls. Others argue that brain injury activates cellular mechanisms which allow the blood vessels to rapidly take up substances such as horseradish peroxidase, and then deposit them within and ultimately flood the substance of the brain tissue.

To date few substantive experimental data have been advanced to support any of the above-stated theories of blood-brain barrier dysfunction in instances of mechanical brain injury. However, research continues, for medical scientists realize that any rational therapeutic treatment of brain-injured patients is totally dependent upon the elucidation of those mechanisms involved in blood-brain barrier dysfunction.

Method: The blood vessels of the mammalian brain normally provide a barrier that blocks the passage of certain molecules which readily permeate other body tissues. This unique property of the brain vasculature is referred to as the blood-brain barrier and in normal functional states this property prevents the entrance of numerous (intravascular probes) such as horseradish peroxidase into the substance of the brain. However, in (experimental studies) of brain dysfunction, such as seen in mechanical brain injury, a disruption of the blood-brain barrier occurs, and experimental probes such as horseradish peroxidase can enter the brain's substance. The (mechanism) of this blood-brain barrier dysfunction in brain injury is poorly understood. Some contend that the mechanical stress of the injury physically disrupts the vessels and permits peroxidase leakage through defects in the vascular walls. Others argue that brain injury activates cellular mechanisms which allow the blood vessels to rapidly take up substances such as horseradish peroxidase and then deposit them within and ultimately flood the substance of the brain tissue.

To date few substantive experimental data have been advanced to support any of the above-stated theories of blood-brain barrier dysfunction in instances of mechanical brain injury. However, research continues, for medical scientists realize that any rational therapeutic treatment of brain injured patients is totally dependent upon the elucidation of those mechanisms involved in blood-brain barrier (dysfunction).

Method in Outline Form

(a) Topic: blood vessels, brain, barrier
(b) Details or key words:
    1. certain molecules, readily permeate, other tissues
    2. unique, vasculature, prevents, entrance horseradish peroxidase
    3. injury, disruption, barrier, horseradish peroxidase
    4. barrier, poorly understood
    5. mechanical stress, disrupts, permits leakage
    6. injury, cellular mechanisms, allow, deposit, flood tissue
    7. few data, support
    8. treatment, injured, totally dependent, mechanisms
(c) Details about details:
    1. (intravascular probes)
    2. (experimental studies)
    3. (mechanisms)
    4. (dysfunction)

Having read and used the underlining technique let us use this information to answer the type of questions used in the examination.

DIRECTIONS: The following statements are related to the passage. Based on the information given, select:

(A) if the statement is *supported* by the information in the passage.
(B) if the statement is *contradicted* by the information in the passage.
(C) if the statement is *neither supported nor contradicted* by the information in the passage.

1. The blood-brain barrier is a structural rather than a physiological barrier.
2. The mechanisms responsible for blood-brain barrier dysfunction in brain injury have been identified and it is apparent that blood-brain barrier dysfunction is related to vasogenic shock.
3. This passage implies that the appropriate therapeutic management of the head-injured patient awaits the elucidation of the mechanisms responsible for blood-brain barrier dysfunction in brain trauma.
4. The blood vessels of the human brain normally provide a barrier which blocks the passage of certain substances which readily permeate the body tissues.
5. Mechanical brain injury may physically disrupt the integrity of the brain's vasculature.

Answers:

1. C
2. B
3. A

4. A
5. C

Exercise 5

Identify the central theme or topic, details, and details about details.

DIRECTIONS: Read the sample and underline the <u>topic</u>, the <u>details of the topic</u>, and bracket the (details about the details).

Example: Evolutionary evidence supports the freshwater theory of origin of the chordates. Some scientists believe that the ancestors of the chordates migrated from the sea to a freshwater or brackish water habitat during the Cambrian period.

a)   The topic deals with the <u>freshwater origin</u> of the <u>chordates</u>.
b)   Details or key words are <u>evidence</u>, <u>supports</u>, <u>migrated</u>, <u>sea</u>, <u>freshwater</u>.
c)   Details about details are (Cambrian period).

DIRECTIONS: Read the sample selection and underline the <u>topic</u>, the <u>details about the topic</u>, and bracket the (details about the details). Use square brackets for [extraneous material].

Example: Evolutionary evidence supports the freshwater theory of the origin of the chordates. Some scientists believe that ancestors of the chordates migrated from the sea to a freshwater or brackish water habitat during the Cambrian period.

Prochordate ancestors of these early vertebrates inhabited the oceans of the pre-Cambrian period. They were in a state of constant osmotic equilibrium with their environment, which had a salinity equivalent to about one-half the salinity of the present-day oceans. Since these prochordates were in equilibrium with the surrounding environment, they did not face a problem of internal water regulation, and the kidney of these forms was principally concerned with regulation of nitrogenous wastes.

Migration of the earliest chordate ancestors into fresh water was the result of an attempt on their part to escape the giant marine cephalopods which ruled the oceans of the Ordovician period. Concomitant with their migration into a freshwater habitat, these early vertebrate ancestors were faced with a two-fold problem: (1) dilution of body fluids through absorption of excess water from a hypo-osmotic environment and (2) retention of physiologically important materials that were not readily obtainable from the environment. Whereas chordate ancestors could remove nitrogenous wastes by merely secreting these substances into a tubular excretory network, migration of early chordate forms into fresh water necessitated the development of a pressure system for removal of excess water. In these forms the glomerular filtration system evolved as a means of coping with the problem of excess dilution of body fluids. However, the glomerulus did not provide a perfect osmoregulatory mechanism. In addition to its ability to filter out excess water from body fluids, it also removed a number of metabolically important substances such as glucose, phosphates, etc. Thus the problem of removal of water and retention of important elements developed secondarily as a result of glomerular evolution. The problem of conserving important substances in the glomerular filtrate was solved with the evolution of tubular reabsorptive mechanisms capable of selective reabsorption of metabolites, through the reabsorption of salt and the elaboration of urine that was hypotonic to the blood.

In early anamniotes, the primitive kidneys were relatively inefficient when some species attempted to move into a more isosmotic or hyperosmotic environment. Thus these early vertebrates were confined to an entirely freshwater habitat.

With the evolution of the Agnathostomes (lampreys, hagfish, and slime eel) during the Silurian period, the crust of the earth was undergoing a major diastrophic change which compelled the freshwater vertebrates to diverge along two courses of evolution. Some forms became trapped in a freshwater habitat and became the ancestors of the freshwater fish and higher vertebrates. Others moved back to the oceans and became ancestors of marine teleosts. Movement of the ancestors of the marine teleosts back into a hypertonic environment forced new osmotic problems on these species. Having evolved osmoregulatory mechanisms designed to cope with a hypo-osmotic environment, they were faced with a problem of dehydration from osmotic loss of water through the glomerulated excretory system and the body surface. The result of their secondary invasion of a marine habitat was the evolution of two means of coping with the extremes of the environment. A number of species of ancestral marine teleosts underwent degeneration of the glomerular portions of the excretory system and retention of an aglomerular system that evolved specialized secretory mechanisms for removal of wastes and ingested inorganic materials. Another regulatory mechanism evolved through specialization of cells in the gill surfaces to secrete salts but retain water and thereby reduce the tendency of body fluids to become hypertonic to the body tissues.

The results of the digression of teleost ancestors into freshwater and saltwater species has been the basis for the wide diversity in the morphology of the renal system of this class of vertebrates.

Method: Evolutionary evidence supports the freshwater theory of origin of the chordates. Some scientists believe that ancestors of the chordates migrated from the sea to a freshwater or brackish water habitat during the Cambrian period.

Prochordate (ancestors) of these (early) (vertebrates) inhabited the oceans of the pre-Cambrian period. They were in a state of constant osmotic equilibrium with their environment, which had a salinity equivalent to about one-half the salinity of the present-day (oceans). Since these prochordates were in equilibrium with the surrounding environment, they did not face a problem of internal water regulation, and the kidney of these forms was (principally) concerned with regulation of nitrogenous wastes.

Migration of the (earliest chordate) ancestors into fresh water was the result of an attempt on their part to escape the (giant marine) cephalopods which ruled the oceans of the [Ordovician] period. Concomitant with their migration into a freshwater habitat, these early vertebrate ancestors were faced with a two-fold problem: (1) the dilution of body fluids through absorption of excess water from a (hypo-osmotic) environment and (2) retention of physiologically important materials that were not readily obtainable from the environment. Whereas chordate ancestors could remove nitrogenous wastes by merely secreting these substances into a (tubular excretory network), migration of early chordate forms into fresh water (necessitated) the development of a pressure system for (removal of excess water). In these forms the glomerular filtration system evolved as a means of (coping) with the problem of (excess dilution) of body fluids. However, the glomerulus did not provide a perfect osmoregulatory mechanism. In addition to its ability to filter out excess water from body fluids, it also removed a number of metabolically important substances such as (glucose, phosphates), etc. Thus the problem of removal of water and retention of important elements developed (secondarily) as a result of the glomerular evolution. The problem of conserving important substances in the glomerular filtrate was solved with the evolution of tubular reabsorptive mechanisms capable of (selective) reabsorption of metabolites, through the reabsorption of salt and the elaboration of urine that was (hypotonic to the blood).

In early anamniotes, the primitive kidneys were relatively inefficient when some species attempted to move into a more (isosmotic or hyperosmotic) environment. Thus these (early) vertebrates were confined to an entirely freshwater habitat.

With the evolution of the (Agnathostomes) (lampreys, hagfish, and slime eel) during the (Silurian period), the crust of the earth was undergoing a major diastrophic change which compelled the freshwater vertebrates to diverge along two courses of evolution. Some forms became (trapped) in a (freshwater habitat) and became the ancestors of the freshwater fish and higher vertebrates. Others (moved back) to the oceans and became ancestors of marine teleosts. Movement of the ancestors of the marine teleosts back into a (hypertonic environment) forced new osmotic problems on these species. Having evolved osmoregulatory mechanisms designed to cope with (a hypo-osmotic environment), they were faced with a problem of dehydration from (osmotic loss of water) through the glomerulated excretory system and the body surface. The result of their secondary invasion of a marine habitat was the evolution of two means of coping with the extremes of the environment. A number of species of ancestral marine teleosts underwent degeneration of the glomerular portions of the excretory system and retention of an aglomerular system that evolved specialized secretory mechanisms for removal of wastes and ingested inorganic materials. Another regulatory mechanism evolved through specialization of cells in the gill surfaces to secrete salts but retain water and thereby reduce the tendency of body fluids to become hypertonic to the body tissues.

The result of the digression of teleost ancestors into freshwater and saltwater species has been the basis for the wide diversity in the morphology of the renal system of this class of vertebrates.

Method in Outline Form

(a) Topic: fresh-water, origin, chordates
(b) Details or key words:
  1. evidence, support, migrated
  2. sea to freshwater
  3. prochordate, inhabited, oceans
  4. constant osmotic equilibrium
  5. one-half, salinity, present-day
  6. did not, problem, water, regulation
  7. kidney, regulation, nitrogenous
  8. migration, fresh water, escape, cephalopods
  9. migration, dilution, body fluids, excess water
  10. chordate ancestors, remove, nitrogenous
  11. migration, chordate, fresh water, development, pressure system
  12. glomerulus, filtration, evolved
  13. glomerulus, not, osmoregulatory
  14. removed, substances
  15. removal, water, retention, elements
  16. solved, tubular, mechanism
  17. reabsorption, metabolites, salt
  18. elaboration, urine
  19. anomniotes, kidneys, inefficient
  20. vetebrates, confined, freshwater
  21. freshwater, vertebrates, two courses
  22. ancestors, freshwater fish, higher vertebrates
  23. oceans, ancestors, marine teleosts, dehydration
  24. secondary invasion, degeneration, glomerular, retention, aglomerular
  25. gill, secrete salts, reduce body fluids, hypertonic
  26. diversity, renal system, vertebrates
(c) Details about details:
  1. (ancestors), (early), (vertebrates), (principally oceans)
  2. (earliest chordate), (giant marine)
  3. (hypo-osmotic)
  4. (tubular excretory network)
  5. (necessitated), (removal of excess water)
  6. (coping), (excess dilution)
  7. (glucose), (phosphates)
  8. (selective), (hypotonic to the blood)
  9. (early vertebrates), (entirely freshwater)
  10. (Agnathostomes)
  11. (Silurian period)
  12. (trapped), (freshwater habitat)
  13. (moved back), (hypertonic), (hypo-osmotic environment), (osmotic loss of water)

Having read the passage and used the underlining technique, let us use this information to answer the type of questions used in the examination.

DIRECTIONS: The following statements are related to the passage above. Based on the information given select:

(A) if the statement is *supported* by the information in the passage.
(B) if the statement is *contradicted* by the information in the passage.
(C) if the statement is *neither supported nor contradicted* by information in the passage.

1. All scientists have embraced the theory of the origin of chordates.

2. Life originated in the sea.
3. It is proposed that prochordates were in osmotic equilibrium with their surroundings.
4. The kidneys of prochordates faced severe fluid regulation problems.
5. Small cephalopods ruled the oceans.
6. The glomerular filtration apparatus evolved as a result of chordate migration into a freshwater environment.
7. Selectivity of tubular reabsorption solved many evolutionary filtration phenomena.
8. Once the migration into freshwater had taken place only refinements in the adaptation of the glomerular filtration apparatus were necessary.
9. Gills played an important role in the evolution of vertebrates.
10. The morphology of the kidney is relatively similar in all living forms.

Answers

1.	B	6.	A
2.	C	7.	A
3.	A	8.	B
4.	B	9.	C
5.	B	10.	B

Writing the Essay

Since 1985, the Association of American Medical Colleges (AAMC) has been trial-testing an essay topic on the MCAT. This project was in response to a study about the professional preparation of the physician. The 1989 administrations of the MCAT included 60 minutes for the writing of two essays. The essay will become a permanent part of the MCAT in 1991. Until then, it will remain part of the examination for research purposes. Essays written between now and 1991 may be used retroactively for admission purposes.

Medical school faculties have long felt that writing skills are essential for a physician. Many have expressed the opinion that present-day students are somewhat weak in these skills. The goal of the essay topic is to see if the student has the ability and skill to write under standardized conditions. The students should be able to:

1. develop a central theme
2. synthesize material
3. separate major from minor issues
4. propose alternative solutions
5. present a theme in a flowing and logical manner
6. write in correct English

No specific college courses to obtain essay writing skills have been advocated by anyone. The essay portion of the examination will take 60 minutes. It will be administered following the Science Problems Subtest and prior to the lunch break.

The AAMC has proposed the following guidelines for topic developments:

1. The topic should have *no* relationship to the application process or the candidate's career choice.
2. The topic should not deal with health care or religious themes.
3. Social subjects that may prejudice an evaluator due to opinions or judgmental statements made by the examinee should be avoided.
4. Questions should come from sources which would allow any candidate to respond fully despite recognized differences in social, ethnic and geographic background.
5. Formal course content, especially in the sciences, should be avoided.

Scoring Method

During the pilot program, selected essays were scored by an experienced group of readers. Two readers rated each essay on a six-point scale. A third reader was used if the two original scores differed by more than one point. Presently, essay scores are not included in the MCAT score report.

Plan for Writing an Acceptable Essay

There are proper ways to present material in essay form. A person who has mastered the basic techniques will generally be successful while one who has not, usually does not give the reader an accurate representation of his basic fund of knowledge.

Several techniques should be considered:

1. Read every essay question asked before you develop a game plan and start to answer. Note what is included and excluded in the questions.
2. Decide exactly what is being asked. Are you asked to describe, discuss, compare, illustrate or give an opinion?

3. Formulate your plan and make an outline, preferably in writing. The outline will help you to organize your presentation. It will aid you in including relevant material and minimize the tendency to forget important points in the heat of battle. Most importantly, it will provide you with a coherent train of thought that will aid in the recall of material.

4. Write to the point, stress your key facts, and be specific.

5. Present your ideas clearly and organize them to show that you understood the question.

Pay attention to key words that guide your answer.

1. Words that require a specific answer are: state, cite, name, list, mention, identify, give, define.

2. Words that require a certain amount of description are: describe, discuss, review, illustrate, develop, outline.

3. Words that should focus your attention on associations, similarities and differences are: differentiate, compare, contrast, analyze, distinguish.

4. Words that suggest that an opinion is desired are: assess, evaluate, comment, criticize, interpret.

Practice Essay Topic

John F. Kennedy made the following comment: "The credit belongs to the man who is actually in the arena. Whose face is marred by dust, sweat and blood: who knows the enthusiasm, the great devotion, and spends himself in a worthy cause. Who at best if he wins knows the thrill of high achievement and if he fails at least fails while daring greatly so that his place shall never be with those cold and timid souls, who know neither victory nor defeat."

Explain what the author means when he comments on the man in the arena. Relate the concept of the passage to an area with which you are familiar.

Answer Sheet–Model Test A

SCIENCE KNOWLEDGE

Biology

1. Ⓐ Ⓑ Ⓒ Ⓓ Ⓔ   11. Ⓐ Ⓑ Ⓒ Ⓓ Ⓔ   21. Ⓐ Ⓑ Ⓒ Ⓓ Ⓔ   30. Ⓐ Ⓑ Ⓒ Ⓓ Ⓔ
2. Ⓐ Ⓑ Ⓒ Ⓓ Ⓔ   12. Ⓐ Ⓑ Ⓒ Ⓓ Ⓔ   22. Ⓐ Ⓑ Ⓒ Ⓓ Ⓔ   31. Ⓐ Ⓑ Ⓒ Ⓓ Ⓔ
3. Ⓐ Ⓑ Ⓒ Ⓓ Ⓔ   13. Ⓐ Ⓑ Ⓒ Ⓓ Ⓔ   23. Ⓐ Ⓑ Ⓒ Ⓓ Ⓔ   32. Ⓐ Ⓑ Ⓒ Ⓓ Ⓔ
4. Ⓐ Ⓑ Ⓒ Ⓓ Ⓔ   14. Ⓐ Ⓑ Ⓒ Ⓓ Ⓔ   24. Ⓐ Ⓑ Ⓒ Ⓓ Ⓔ   33. Ⓐ Ⓑ Ⓒ Ⓓ Ⓔ
5. Ⓐ Ⓑ Ⓒ Ⓓ Ⓔ   15. Ⓐ Ⓑ Ⓒ Ⓓ Ⓔ   25. Ⓐ Ⓑ Ⓒ Ⓓ Ⓔ   34. Ⓐ Ⓑ Ⓒ Ⓓ Ⓔ
6. Ⓐ Ⓑ Ⓒ Ⓓ Ⓔ   16. Ⓐ Ⓑ Ⓒ Ⓓ Ⓔ   26. Ⓐ Ⓑ Ⓒ Ⓓ Ⓔ   35. Ⓐ Ⓑ Ⓒ Ⓓ Ⓔ
7. Ⓐ Ⓑ Ⓒ Ⓓ Ⓔ   17. Ⓐ Ⓑ Ⓒ Ⓓ Ⓔ   27. Ⓐ Ⓑ Ⓒ Ⓓ Ⓔ   36. Ⓐ Ⓑ Ⓒ Ⓓ Ⓔ
8. Ⓐ Ⓑ Ⓒ Ⓓ Ⓔ   18. Ⓐ Ⓑ Ⓒ Ⓓ Ⓔ   28. Ⓐ Ⓑ Ⓒ Ⓓ Ⓔ   37. Ⓐ Ⓑ Ⓒ Ⓓ Ⓔ
9. Ⓐ Ⓑ Ⓒ Ⓓ Ⓔ   19. Ⓐ Ⓑ Ⓒ Ⓓ Ⓔ   29. Ⓐ Ⓑ Ⓒ Ⓓ Ⓔ   38. Ⓐ Ⓑ Ⓒ Ⓓ Ⓔ
10. Ⓐ Ⓑ Ⓒ Ⓓ Ⓔ   20. Ⓐ Ⓑ Ⓒ Ⓓ Ⓔ

To score add from Science Problems questions: 1–3; 10–12; 16–18; 28–30; 49–54; 58–60.

Chemistry

1. Ⓐ Ⓑ Ⓒ Ⓓ Ⓔ   11. Ⓐ Ⓑ Ⓒ Ⓓ Ⓔ   21. Ⓐ Ⓑ Ⓒ Ⓓ Ⓔ   30. Ⓐ Ⓑ Ⓒ Ⓓ Ⓔ
2. Ⓐ Ⓑ Ⓒ Ⓓ Ⓔ   12. Ⓐ Ⓑ Ⓒ Ⓓ Ⓔ   22. Ⓐ Ⓑ Ⓒ Ⓓ Ⓔ   31. Ⓐ Ⓑ Ⓒ Ⓓ Ⓔ
3. Ⓐ Ⓑ Ⓒ Ⓓ Ⓔ   13. Ⓐ Ⓑ Ⓒ Ⓓ Ⓔ   23. Ⓐ Ⓑ Ⓒ Ⓓ Ⓔ   32. Ⓐ Ⓑ Ⓒ Ⓓ Ⓔ
4. Ⓐ Ⓑ Ⓒ Ⓓ Ⓔ   14. Ⓐ Ⓑ Ⓒ Ⓓ Ⓔ   24. Ⓐ Ⓑ Ⓒ Ⓓ Ⓔ   33. Ⓐ Ⓑ Ⓒ Ⓓ Ⓔ
5. Ⓐ Ⓑ Ⓒ Ⓓ Ⓔ   15. Ⓐ Ⓑ Ⓒ Ⓓ Ⓔ   25. Ⓐ Ⓑ Ⓒ Ⓓ Ⓔ   34. Ⓐ Ⓑ Ⓒ Ⓓ Ⓔ
6. Ⓐ Ⓑ Ⓒ Ⓓ Ⓔ   16. Ⓐ Ⓑ Ⓒ Ⓓ Ⓔ   26. Ⓐ Ⓑ Ⓒ Ⓓ Ⓔ   35. Ⓐ Ⓑ Ⓒ Ⓓ Ⓔ
7. Ⓐ Ⓑ Ⓒ Ⓓ Ⓔ   17. Ⓐ Ⓑ Ⓒ Ⓓ Ⓔ   27. Ⓐ Ⓑ Ⓒ Ⓓ Ⓔ   36. Ⓐ Ⓑ Ⓒ Ⓓ Ⓔ
8. Ⓐ Ⓑ Ⓒ Ⓓ Ⓔ   18. Ⓐ Ⓑ Ⓒ Ⓓ Ⓔ   28. Ⓐ Ⓑ Ⓒ Ⓓ Ⓔ   37. Ⓐ Ⓑ Ⓒ Ⓓ Ⓔ
9. Ⓐ Ⓑ Ⓒ Ⓓ Ⓔ   19. Ⓐ Ⓑ Ⓒ Ⓓ Ⓔ   29. Ⓐ Ⓑ Ⓒ Ⓓ Ⓔ   38. Ⓐ Ⓑ Ⓒ Ⓓ Ⓔ
10. Ⓐ Ⓑ Ⓒ Ⓓ Ⓔ   20. Ⓐ Ⓑ Ⓒ Ⓓ Ⓔ

To score add from Science Problems questions: 4–6; 13–15; 22–27; 34–36; 40–42; 46–48.

Physics

1. Ⓐ Ⓑ Ⓒ Ⓓ Ⓔ
2. Ⓐ Ⓑ Ⓒ Ⓓ Ⓔ
3. Ⓐ Ⓑ Ⓒ Ⓓ Ⓔ
4. Ⓐ Ⓑ Ⓒ Ⓓ Ⓔ
5. Ⓐ Ⓑ Ⓒ Ⓓ Ⓔ
6. Ⓐ Ⓑ Ⓒ Ⓓ Ⓔ
7. Ⓐ Ⓑ Ⓒ Ⓓ Ⓔ
8. Ⓐ Ⓑ Ⓒ Ⓓ Ⓔ
9. Ⓐ Ⓑ Ⓒ Ⓓ Ⓔ
10. Ⓐ Ⓑ Ⓒ Ⓓ Ⓔ
11. Ⓐ Ⓑ Ⓒ Ⓓ Ⓔ
12. Ⓐ Ⓑ Ⓒ Ⓓ Ⓔ
13. Ⓐ Ⓑ Ⓒ Ⓓ Ⓔ
14. Ⓐ Ⓑ Ⓒ Ⓓ Ⓔ
15. Ⓐ Ⓑ Ⓒ Ⓓ Ⓔ
16. Ⓐ Ⓑ Ⓒ Ⓓ Ⓔ
17. Ⓐ Ⓑ Ⓒ Ⓓ Ⓔ
18. Ⓐ Ⓑ Ⓒ Ⓓ Ⓔ
19. Ⓐ Ⓑ Ⓒ Ⓓ Ⓔ
20. Ⓐ Ⓑ Ⓒ Ⓓ Ⓔ
21. Ⓐ Ⓑ Ⓒ Ⓓ Ⓔ
22. Ⓐ Ⓑ Ⓒ Ⓓ Ⓔ
23. Ⓐ Ⓑ Ⓒ Ⓓ Ⓔ
24. Ⓐ Ⓑ Ⓒ Ⓓ Ⓔ
25. Ⓐ Ⓑ Ⓒ Ⓓ Ⓔ
26. Ⓐ Ⓑ Ⓒ Ⓓ Ⓔ
27. Ⓐ Ⓑ Ⓒ Ⓓ Ⓔ
28. Ⓐ Ⓑ Ⓒ Ⓓ Ⓔ
29. Ⓐ Ⓑ Ⓒ Ⓓ Ⓔ
30. Ⓐ Ⓑ Ⓒ Ⓓ Ⓔ
31. Ⓐ Ⓑ Ⓒ Ⓓ Ⓔ
32. Ⓐ Ⓑ Ⓒ Ⓓ Ⓔ
33. Ⓐ Ⓑ Ⓒ Ⓓ Ⓔ

To score add from Science Problems questions: 7–9; 19–21; 31–33; 37–39; 43–45; 55–57.

SCIENCE PROBLEMS

1. Ⓐ Ⓑ Ⓒ Ⓓ Ⓔ
2. Ⓐ Ⓑ Ⓒ Ⓓ Ⓔ
3. Ⓐ Ⓑ Ⓒ Ⓓ Ⓔ
4. Ⓐ Ⓑ Ⓒ Ⓓ Ⓔ
5. Ⓐ Ⓑ Ⓒ Ⓓ Ⓔ
6. Ⓐ Ⓑ Ⓒ Ⓓ Ⓔ
7. Ⓐ Ⓑ Ⓒ Ⓓ Ⓔ
8. Ⓐ Ⓑ Ⓒ Ⓓ Ⓔ
9. Ⓐ Ⓑ Ⓒ Ⓓ Ⓔ
10. Ⓐ Ⓑ Ⓒ Ⓓ Ⓔ
11. Ⓐ Ⓑ Ⓒ Ⓓ Ⓔ
12. Ⓐ Ⓑ Ⓒ Ⓓ Ⓔ
13. Ⓐ Ⓑ Ⓒ Ⓓ Ⓔ
14. Ⓐ Ⓑ Ⓒ Ⓓ Ⓔ
15. Ⓐ Ⓑ Ⓒ Ⓓ Ⓔ
16. Ⓐ Ⓑ Ⓒ Ⓓ Ⓔ
17. Ⓐ Ⓑ Ⓒ Ⓓ Ⓔ
18. Ⓐ Ⓑ Ⓒ Ⓓ Ⓔ
19. Ⓐ Ⓑ Ⓒ Ⓓ Ⓔ
20. Ⓐ Ⓑ Ⓒ Ⓓ Ⓔ
21. Ⓐ Ⓑ Ⓒ Ⓓ Ⓔ
22. Ⓐ Ⓑ Ⓒ Ⓓ Ⓔ
23. Ⓐ Ⓑ Ⓒ Ⓓ Ⓔ
24. Ⓐ Ⓑ Ⓒ Ⓓ Ⓔ
25. Ⓐ Ⓑ Ⓒ Ⓓ Ⓔ
26. Ⓐ Ⓑ Ⓒ Ⓓ Ⓔ
27. Ⓐ Ⓑ Ⓒ Ⓓ Ⓔ
28. Ⓐ Ⓑ Ⓒ Ⓓ Ⓔ
29. Ⓐ Ⓑ Ⓒ Ⓓ Ⓔ
30. Ⓐ Ⓑ Ⓒ Ⓓ Ⓔ
31. Ⓐ Ⓑ Ⓒ Ⓓ Ⓔ
32. Ⓐ Ⓑ Ⓒ Ⓓ Ⓔ
33. Ⓐ Ⓑ Ⓒ Ⓓ Ⓔ
34. Ⓐ Ⓑ Ⓒ Ⓓ Ⓔ
35. Ⓐ Ⓑ Ⓒ Ⓓ Ⓔ
36. Ⓐ Ⓑ Ⓒ Ⓓ Ⓔ
37. Ⓐ Ⓑ Ⓒ Ⓓ Ⓔ
38. Ⓐ Ⓑ Ⓒ Ⓓ Ⓔ
39. Ⓐ Ⓑ Ⓒ Ⓓ Ⓔ
40. Ⓐ Ⓑ Ⓒ Ⓓ Ⓔ
41. Ⓐ Ⓑ Ⓒ Ⓓ Ⓔ
42. Ⓐ Ⓑ Ⓒ Ⓓ Ⓔ
43. Ⓐ Ⓑ Ⓒ Ⓓ Ⓔ
44. Ⓐ Ⓑ Ⓒ Ⓓ Ⓔ
45. Ⓐ Ⓑ Ⓒ Ⓓ Ⓔ
46. Ⓐ Ⓑ Ⓒ Ⓓ Ⓔ
47. Ⓐ Ⓑ Ⓒ Ⓓ Ⓔ
48. Ⓐ Ⓑ Ⓒ Ⓓ Ⓔ
49. Ⓐ Ⓑ Ⓒ Ⓓ Ⓔ
50. Ⓐ Ⓑ Ⓒ Ⓓ Ⓔ
51. Ⓐ Ⓑ Ⓒ Ⓓ Ⓔ
52. Ⓐ Ⓑ Ⓒ Ⓓ Ⓔ
53. Ⓐ Ⓑ Ⓒ Ⓓ Ⓔ
54. Ⓐ Ⓑ Ⓒ Ⓓ Ⓔ
55. Ⓐ Ⓑ Ⓒ Ⓓ Ⓔ
56. Ⓐ Ⓑ Ⓒ Ⓓ Ⓔ
57. Ⓐ Ⓑ Ⓒ Ⓓ Ⓔ
58. Ⓐ Ⓑ Ⓒ Ⓓ Ⓔ
59. Ⓐ Ⓑ Ⓒ Ⓓ Ⓔ
60. Ⓐ Ⓑ Ⓒ Ⓓ Ⓔ

SKILLS ANALYSIS: READING

1. Ⓐ Ⓑ Ⓒ Ⓓ Ⓔ
2. Ⓐ Ⓑ Ⓒ Ⓓ Ⓔ
3. Ⓐ Ⓑ Ⓒ Ⓓ Ⓔ
4. Ⓐ Ⓑ Ⓒ Ⓓ Ⓔ
5. Ⓐ Ⓑ Ⓒ Ⓓ Ⓔ
6. Ⓐ Ⓑ Ⓒ Ⓓ Ⓔ
7. Ⓐ Ⓑ Ⓒ Ⓓ Ⓔ
8. Ⓐ Ⓑ Ⓒ Ⓓ Ⓔ
9. Ⓐ Ⓑ Ⓒ Ⓓ Ⓔ
10. Ⓐ Ⓑ Ⓒ Ⓓ Ⓔ
11. Ⓐ Ⓑ Ⓒ Ⓓ Ⓔ
12. Ⓐ Ⓑ Ⓒ Ⓓ Ⓔ
13. Ⓐ Ⓑ Ⓒ Ⓓ Ⓔ
14. Ⓐ Ⓑ Ⓒ Ⓓ Ⓔ
15. Ⓐ Ⓑ Ⓒ Ⓓ Ⓔ
16. Ⓐ Ⓑ Ⓒ Ⓓ Ⓔ
17. Ⓐ Ⓑ Ⓒ Ⓓ Ⓔ

18. Ⓐ Ⓑ Ⓒ Ⓓ Ⓔ
19. Ⓐ Ⓑ Ⓒ Ⓓ Ⓔ
20. Ⓐ Ⓑ Ⓒ Ⓓ Ⓔ
21. Ⓐ Ⓑ Ⓒ Ⓓ Ⓔ
22. Ⓐ Ⓑ Ⓒ Ⓓ Ⓔ
23. Ⓐ Ⓑ Ⓒ Ⓓ Ⓔ
24. Ⓐ Ⓑ Ⓒ Ⓓ Ⓔ
25. Ⓐ Ⓑ Ⓒ Ⓓ Ⓔ
26. Ⓐ Ⓑ Ⓒ Ⓓ Ⓔ
27. Ⓐ Ⓑ Ⓒ Ⓓ Ⓔ
28. Ⓐ Ⓑ Ⓒ Ⓓ Ⓔ
29. Ⓐ Ⓑ Ⓒ Ⓓ Ⓔ
30. Ⓐ Ⓑ Ⓒ Ⓓ Ⓔ
31. Ⓐ Ⓑ Ⓒ Ⓓ Ⓔ
32. Ⓐ Ⓑ Ⓒ Ⓓ Ⓔ
33. Ⓐ Ⓑ Ⓒ Ⓓ Ⓔ
34. Ⓐ Ⓑ Ⓒ Ⓓ Ⓔ

35. Ⓐ Ⓑ Ⓒ Ⓓ Ⓔ
36. Ⓐ Ⓑ Ⓒ Ⓓ Ⓔ
37. Ⓐ Ⓑ Ⓒ Ⓓ Ⓔ
38. Ⓐ Ⓑ Ⓒ Ⓓ Ⓔ
39. Ⓐ Ⓑ Ⓒ Ⓓ Ⓔ
40. Ⓐ Ⓑ Ⓒ Ⓓ Ⓔ
41. Ⓐ Ⓑ Ⓒ Ⓓ Ⓔ
42. Ⓐ Ⓑ Ⓒ Ⓓ Ⓔ
43. Ⓐ Ⓑ Ⓒ Ⓓ Ⓔ
44. Ⓐ Ⓑ Ⓒ Ⓓ Ⓔ
45. Ⓐ Ⓑ Ⓒ Ⓓ Ⓔ
46. Ⓐ Ⓑ Ⓒ Ⓓ Ⓔ
47. Ⓐ Ⓑ Ⓒ Ⓓ Ⓔ
48. Ⓐ Ⓑ Ⓒ Ⓓ Ⓔ
49. Ⓐ Ⓑ Ⓒ Ⓓ Ⓔ
50. Ⓐ Ⓑ Ⓒ Ⓓ Ⓔ
51. Ⓐ Ⓑ Ⓒ Ⓓ Ⓔ

52. Ⓐ Ⓑ Ⓒ Ⓓ Ⓔ
53. Ⓐ Ⓑ Ⓒ Ⓓ Ⓔ
54. Ⓐ Ⓑ Ⓒ Ⓓ Ⓔ
55. Ⓐ Ⓑ Ⓒ Ⓓ Ⓔ
56. Ⓐ Ⓑ Ⓒ Ⓓ Ⓔ
57. Ⓐ Ⓑ Ⓒ Ⓓ Ⓔ
58. Ⓐ Ⓑ Ⓒ Ⓓ Ⓔ
59. Ⓐ Ⓑ Ⓒ Ⓓ Ⓔ
60. Ⓐ Ⓑ Ⓒ Ⓓ Ⓔ
61. Ⓐ Ⓑ Ⓒ Ⓓ Ⓔ
62. Ⓐ Ⓑ Ⓒ Ⓓ Ⓔ
63. Ⓐ Ⓑ Ⓒ Ⓓ Ⓔ
64. Ⓐ Ⓑ Ⓒ Ⓓ Ⓔ
65. Ⓐ Ⓑ Ⓒ Ⓓ Ⓔ
66. Ⓐ Ⓑ Ⓒ Ⓓ Ⓔ
67. Ⓐ Ⓑ Ⓒ Ⓓ Ⓔ
68. Ⓐ Ⓑ Ⓒ Ⓓ Ⓔ

SKILLS ANALYSIS: QUANTITATIVE

1. Ⓐ Ⓑ Ⓒ Ⓓ Ⓔ
2. Ⓐ Ⓑ Ⓒ Ⓓ Ⓔ
3. Ⓐ Ⓑ Ⓒ Ⓓ Ⓔ
4. Ⓐ Ⓑ Ⓒ Ⓓ Ⓔ
5. Ⓐ Ⓑ Ⓒ Ⓓ Ⓔ
6. Ⓐ Ⓑ Ⓒ Ⓓ Ⓔ
7. Ⓐ Ⓑ Ⓒ Ⓓ Ⓔ
8. Ⓐ Ⓑ Ⓒ Ⓓ Ⓔ
9. Ⓐ Ⓑ Ⓒ Ⓓ Ⓔ
10. Ⓐ Ⓑ Ⓒ Ⓓ Ⓔ
11. Ⓐ Ⓑ Ⓒ Ⓓ Ⓔ
12. Ⓐ Ⓑ Ⓒ Ⓓ Ⓔ
13. Ⓐ Ⓑ Ⓒ Ⓓ Ⓔ
14. Ⓐ Ⓑ Ⓒ Ⓓ Ⓔ
15. Ⓐ Ⓑ Ⓒ Ⓓ Ⓔ
16. Ⓐ Ⓑ Ⓒ Ⓓ Ⓔ
17. Ⓐ Ⓑ Ⓒ Ⓓ Ⓔ

18. Ⓐ Ⓑ Ⓒ Ⓓ Ⓔ
19. Ⓐ Ⓑ Ⓒ Ⓓ Ⓔ
20. Ⓐ Ⓑ Ⓒ Ⓓ Ⓔ
21. Ⓐ Ⓑ Ⓒ Ⓓ Ⓔ
22. Ⓐ Ⓑ Ⓒ Ⓓ Ⓔ
23. Ⓐ Ⓑ Ⓒ Ⓓ Ⓔ
24. Ⓐ Ⓑ Ⓒ Ⓓ Ⓔ
25. Ⓐ Ⓑ Ⓒ Ⓓ Ⓔ
26. Ⓐ Ⓑ Ⓒ Ⓓ Ⓔ
27. Ⓐ Ⓑ Ⓒ Ⓓ Ⓔ
28. Ⓐ Ⓑ Ⓒ Ⓓ Ⓔ
29. Ⓐ Ⓑ Ⓒ Ⓓ Ⓔ
30. Ⓐ Ⓑ Ⓒ Ⓓ Ⓔ
31. Ⓐ Ⓑ Ⓒ Ⓓ Ⓔ
32. Ⓐ Ⓑ Ⓒ Ⓓ Ⓔ
33. Ⓐ Ⓑ Ⓒ Ⓓ Ⓔ
34. Ⓐ Ⓑ Ⓒ Ⓓ Ⓔ

35. Ⓐ Ⓑ Ⓒ Ⓓ Ⓔ
36. Ⓐ Ⓑ Ⓒ Ⓓ Ⓔ
37. Ⓐ Ⓑ Ⓒ Ⓓ Ⓔ
38. Ⓐ Ⓑ Ⓒ Ⓓ Ⓔ
39. Ⓐ Ⓑ Ⓒ Ⓓ Ⓔ
40. Ⓐ Ⓑ Ⓒ Ⓓ Ⓔ
41. Ⓐ Ⓑ Ⓒ Ⓓ Ⓔ
42. Ⓐ Ⓑ Ⓒ Ⓓ Ⓔ
43. Ⓐ Ⓑ Ⓒ Ⓓ Ⓔ
44. Ⓐ Ⓑ Ⓒ Ⓓ Ⓔ
45. Ⓐ Ⓑ Ⓒ Ⓓ Ⓔ
46. Ⓐ Ⓑ Ⓒ Ⓓ Ⓔ
47. Ⓐ Ⓑ Ⓒ Ⓓ Ⓔ
48. Ⓐ Ⓑ Ⓒ Ⓓ Ⓔ
49. Ⓐ Ⓑ Ⓒ Ⓓ Ⓔ
50. Ⓐ Ⓑ Ⓒ Ⓓ Ⓔ
51. Ⓐ Ⓑ Ⓒ Ⓓ Ⓔ

52. Ⓐ Ⓑ Ⓒ Ⓓ Ⓔ
53. Ⓐ Ⓑ Ⓒ Ⓓ Ⓔ
54. Ⓐ Ⓑ Ⓒ Ⓓ Ⓔ
55. Ⓐ Ⓑ Ⓒ Ⓓ Ⓔ
56. Ⓐ Ⓑ Ⓒ Ⓓ Ⓔ
57. Ⓐ Ⓑ Ⓒ Ⓓ Ⓔ
58. Ⓐ Ⓑ Ⓒ Ⓓ Ⓔ
59. Ⓐ Ⓑ Ⓒ Ⓓ Ⓔ
60. Ⓐ Ⓑ Ⓒ Ⓓ Ⓔ
61. Ⓐ Ⓑ Ⓒ Ⓓ Ⓔ
62. Ⓐ Ⓑ Ⓒ Ⓓ Ⓔ
63. Ⓐ Ⓑ Ⓒ Ⓓ Ⓔ
64. Ⓐ Ⓑ Ⓒ Ⓓ Ⓔ
65. Ⓐ Ⓑ Ⓒ Ⓓ Ⓔ
66. Ⓐ Ⓑ Ⓒ Ⓓ Ⓔ
67. Ⓐ Ⓑ Ⓒ Ⓓ Ⓔ
68. Ⓐ Ⓑ Ⓒ Ⓓ Ⓔ

The MCAT
Model Examination A*

SCIENCE KNOWLEDGE

115 MINUTES
109 QUESTIONS

The following questions are based on your knowledge of science. The questions are varied; therefore, you are advised to pay careful attention to the instructions for each portion.

Biology—38 Questions   Recommended Time—25 minutes

DIRECTIONS: Each of the statements or questions is followed by suggested completions or answers. Choose the one that best completes the statement or answers the question, and mark the letter of your choice on the answer sheet.

1. Which of the following is produced by the placenta and is important in the maintenance of pregnancy?
   (A) chorionic gonadotropin
   (B) thyrotropin
   (C) androgen
   (D) estrogen
   (E) progesterone

2. Which is a biotic factor that affects the size of a population in a specific ecosystem?
   (A) the average temperature of the ecosystem
   (B) the number and kinds of soil minerals in the ecosystem
   (C) the number and kinds of predators in the ecosystem
   (D) the concentration of oxygen in the ecosystem
   (E) the average rainfall of the ecosystem

3. Which of the following plays an active role in the conversion of proteins to carbohydrates?
   (A) androgen
   (B) thyroxin
   (C) cortisol
   (D) progesterone
   (E) aldosterone

4. During replication, the strands of a double-stranded DNA molecule separate from each other when bonds are broken between their
   (A) nitrogenous bases.
   (B) 5-carbon sugars.
   (C) phosphate groups.
   (D) amino acids.
   (E) carbon atoms.

---

*Explanations for science answers can be found on p. 275.

5. Which of the following has an antidiuretic action on the kidney tubules?
   (A) renin
   (B) vasopressin
   (C) angiotensin
   (D) cortisone
   (E) thyroxine

6. A hydrolytic enzyme found in cells of the small intestine that catalyzes the formation of glucose but not other monosaccharides is
   (A) sucrase.
   (B) lactase.
   (C) pepsin.
   (D) maltase.
   (E) trypsin.

7. Epithelial cells cover and protect the body. Which of the following is a secretion of this tissue?
   (A) chitin
   (B) mucus
   (C) keratin
   (D) none of the above
   (E) all of the above

8. A fiber of striated (skeletal) muscle
   (A) possesses only one nucleus.
   (B) possesses no clear Z bands.
   (C) possesses more than one nucleus.
   (D) has the same characteristics as smooth muscle.
   (E) possesses few mitochondria.

9. The insect vector for African sleeping sickness is the
   (A) ant lion.
   (B) anopheles mosquito.
   (C) tsetse fly.
   (D) fruit fly.
   (E) fire ant.

10. Metamorphosis follows an orderly sequence. Which is the proper one?
    (A) egg → spore → adult
    (B) egg → larva → pupa → adult
    (C) egg → nymph → adult
    (D) egg → larva → pupa → nymph → adult
    (E) egg → pupa → larva → adult

11. All chordates are said to possess
    (A) a dorsal tubular nerve cord.
    (B) a vertebral column.
    (C) jaws.
    (D) appendages.
    (E) a maxilla.

12. The smallest unit possessing the capability to maintain life and to reproduce is
    (A) an organ.
    (B) a cell.
    (C) DNA.
    (D) RNA.
    (E) a nucleus.

13. Of the following, which is not considered a membranous organelle?
    (A) ribosome
    (B) endoplasmic reticulum
    (C) Golgi body
    (D) mitochondrion
    (E) lyosome

14. Cellular "digestive" or "suicide" packages is a common description or name for
    (A) mitochondria.
    (B) Golgi zones or Golgi bodies.
    (C) lysosomes.
    (D) centrosomes.
    (E) multivesicular bodies.

15. Housed in the sella tursica is the
    (A) pineal organ.
    (B) pituitary gland.
    (C) olfactory bulb.
    (D) optic chiasm.
    (E) hypothalamus.

16. Which of the following germ layers gives origin to the nervous system?
    (A) ectoderm
    (B) mesoderm
    (C) endoderm
    (D) ectoderm and endoderm
    (E) endoderm and mesoderm

17. Social stress will affect most severely the
    (A) pancreas.
    (B) pineal.
    (C) adrenal.
    (D) parathyroid.
    (E) thyroid.

18. Which of the following germ layers gives origin to the skeletal system?
    (A) ectoderm
    (B) mesoderm
    (C) endoderm
    (D) ectoderm and endoderm
    (E) ectoderm and mesoderm

19. One of the outstanding features of connective tissue is that it
    (A) has an orderly arrangement of cells into sheets.
    (B) possesses a fairly large amount of intercellular material.
    (C) comprises the majority of the ducts of secretory organs.
    (D) all of the above.
    (E) none of the above.

20. Human sperm and ova are similar in the respect that they
    (A) are haploid.
    (B) both possess flagella which give them good mobility.
    (C) are approximately the same in size.
    (D) both carry the identical genetic information.
    (E) are diploid.

21. We speak in terms of an aggregation of nerve cell bodies in the central nervous system as the site of a (an)
    (A) ganglion.
    (B) nucleus.
    (C) cranial nerve.
    (D) association area.
    (E) decussation.

22. The neurolemma of an axon is part of the
    (A) nerve cell body.
    (B) Schwann cell.
    (C) node of Ranvier.
    (D) axoplasm.
    (E) axon hillock.

23. Exchange in the lung of CO_2 and O_2 takes place in the
    (A) bronchi.
    (B) bronchioles.
    (C) alveoli.
    (D) broncho-pulmonary segment.
    (E) dust cells.

24. A common feature of sweat glands, salivary glands, and sebaceous glands is that they are
    (A) endocrine in nature.
    (B) exocrine in nature.
    (C) apocrine in nature.
    (D) merocrine in nature.
    (E) none of the above.

25. The appendix can be found by the surgeon by locating the
    (A) jejunum.
    (B) cecum.
    (C) colon (transverse).
    (D) duodenum.
    (E) right iliac fossa.

26. The process by which a cell can move a substance from a point of lower concentration to a point of higher concentration (against the diffusion gradient) is called
    (A) osmosis.
    (B) plasmolysis.
    (C) turgor pressure.
    (D) diffusion.
    (E) active transport.

27. The internal structure of a cilium or flagellum, no matter what organism, has the same arrangement. The fibrillar arrangement is
    (A) 7 outer, 2 inner.
    (B) 9 outer, 2 inner.
    (C) 11 outer, 2 inner.
    (D) 9 outer, 1 inner.
    (E) 9 outer, 3 inner.

28. The most elaborate, active, and functional system in the tapeworm is the
    (A) digestive system.
    (B) reproductive system.
    (C) sensory system.
    (D) muscular system.
    (E) cardiovascular system.

29. The incidence of tooth decay is lowered by treating drinking water with
    (A) fluorine.
    (B) chlorine.
    (C) sodium chloride.
    (D) potassium fluoride.
    (E) sodium fluoride.

30. Harmful organisms are usually killed by treating the municipal water supply with
    (A) fluorine.
    (B) sodium fluoride.
    (C) chlorine.
    (D) calcium chloride.
    (E) bromine.

31. During metaphase of mitosis
    (A) there is a dissolution of the chromosomal material.
    (B) the centrioles with asters are at the opposite poles.
    (C) the cell membrane starts to reappear.
    (D) the nuclear membrane disappears.
    (E) there is a slowdown in metabolic activity.

32. Locomotion of planaria is accomplished by
    (A) cilia.
    (B) cauda equina.
    (C) flagella.
    (D) microvilli.
    (E) pseudopodia.

33. Two types of circulatory systems are utilized by organisms: a closed and an open one. An open one as found in the crayfish denotes that
    (A) the heart has a patent foramen ovale.
    (B) the auricles receive mixed and unmixed blood.
    (C) the blood is not always encased in defined blood vessels.
    (D) blood can flow in either direction within the vessels depending on need.
    (E) none of the above.

34. The two cerebral hemispheres of the mammalian brain are connected via the
    (A) corpus callosum.
    (B) posterior commissure.
    (C) anterior commissure.
    (D) anterior peduncle.
    (E) third ventricle.

35. A human being is considered a (an)
    (A) heterotroph.
    (B) autotroph.
    (C) geotroph.
    (D) phototroph.
    (E) chemotroph.

36. Which of the following is an evolutionary mechanism that is limited to small populations?
    (A) speciation
    (B) migration
    (C) mutation
    (D) natural selection
    (E) genetic drift

37. Filtration in the kidneys results mainly from
    (A) blood flow.
    (B) reabsorption.
    (C) blood pressure.
    (D) secretion.
    (E) osmotic phenomenon.

38. If blood-sucking insects are acting as vectors for parasites, the parasites that move to a new host are most likely in the insects'
    (A) salivary glands.
    (B) blood.
    (C) tracheae.
    (D) intestines.
    (E) Malpighian tubules.

Chemistry—38 Questions   Recommended Time—46 minutes

DIRECTIONS: Each of the statements or questions is followed by suggested completions or answers. Choose the one that best completes the statement or answers the question, and mark the letter of your choice on the answer sheet.

1. Which hydrocarbon is a member of the series with the general formula $C_n H_{2n-2}$?
    (A) butane
    (B) ethene
    (C) benzene
    (D) ethyne
    (E) cyclopropane

2. One crystal of sodium chloride is added to a sodium chloride supersaturated solution. We would expect to see
    (A) the added crystal dissolve.
    (B) nothing other than the added crystal falling into the bottom of the container.
    (C) precipitation begin.
    (D) the volume decrease.
    (E) the formation of ice crystals on the surface.

3. A polymer of tetrafluoroethylene is useful because of its
    (A) flexibility.
    (B) chemical inertness.
    (C) high water solubility.
    (D) low density.
    (E) release of fluoride for water treatment.

4. Enzymes act in a reaction such as $A + B \rightarrow C + D$ to
   (A) change the equilibrium constant.
   (B) increase the rate of the forward reaction without changing the rate of the reverse reaction.
   (C) decrease the rate of the reverse reaction without changing the rate of the forward reaction.
   (D) decrease the activation energy.
   (E) increase the rate of the reverse reaction and decrease the rate of the forward reaction.

5. In comparison to β-D-glucose acid-catalyzed mutarotation, the mutarotation of the β-methyl glucoside of D-glucose will occur
   (A) more slowly.
   (B) more rapidly.
   (C) only in the presence of CaO.
   (D) only in the presence of KOH.
   (E) not at all.

6. Which class of compounds has the general formula R—O—R′?
   (A) esters
   (B) alcohols
   (C) ethers
   (D) aldehydes
   (E) ketones

7. Oxygen binds reversibly with a molecule of hemoglobin, at
   (A) a single iron atom.
   (B) nonferrous portions of heme groups.
   (C) several iron atoms.
   (D) amino acids of the alpha chains.
   (E) amino acids of the beta chains.

8. When the equation

$$\_Al + \_O_2 \rightarrow \_Al_2O_3$$

   is correctly balanced using the smallest whole numbers, the coefficient of Al is
   (A) 5
   (B) 4
   (C) 3
   (D) 2
   (E) 1

9. When energy is needed to carry out a reaction, the reaction is
   (A) endothermic.
   (B) exothermic.
   (C) incomplete.
   (D) activated.
   (E) reversible.

10. Of the functional groups listed below which is incorrectly identified?

   (A) $-NH_2$ amino group

   (D) $-\underset{\underset{O}{\|}}{C}-OH$ hydroxyl group

   (B) $-\underset{\underset{O}{\|}}{C}-CH_3$ acetyl group

   (E) $-O-\underset{\underset{O}{\|}}{\overset{\overset{OH}{|}}{P}}-OH$ phosphate group

   (C) $-\underset{\underset{O}{\|}}{C}-NH_2$ amide group

11. In electrolysis, the positively charged electrode is the
    (A) cathode.
    (B) anode.
    (C) filament.
    (D) nematode.
    (E) positron.

12. If 1-butene is reacted with HBr in the presence of peroxides, the major product is
    (A) butane.
    (B) 1-bromobutane.
    (C) 2-bromobutane.
    (D) 1,2-dibromobutane.
    (E) 2-butene.

13. A gain of electrons is known as
    (A) oxidation.
    (B) valence.
    (C) reduction.
    (D) electrolysis.
    (E) hydrolysis.

14. The eutectic temperature is the
    (A) lowest melting temperature of any alloy produced by varying the percentages of its two components.
    (B) temperature at which all motion ceases; i.e., $-273°C$.
    (C) highest temperature at which a gas may be liquefied, no matter how high the applied pressure.
    (D) most efficient temperature for electrolytic production of metals such as aluminum.
    (E) none of the above.

15. The common zinc-cased dry cell used in flashlights uses a carbon rod as the positive terminal and the zinc case as the negative terminal. One half-cell reaction during discharge is

    $$2NH_4^+ + 2e^- \rightarrow 2NH_3 + H_2$$

    and the other half-cell reaction (with electrons not indicated) is
    (A) $C + O_2 \rightarrow CO_2$
    (B) $Zn \rightarrow Zn^{2+}$
    (C) $Zn^{2+} \rightarrow Zn$
    (D) $CO_2 \rightarrow C + O_2$
    (E) $Pb^{2+} \rightarrow Pb$

16. To a solution of $AgNO_3$ is added Na_2CO_3 until no more precipitation occurs. If we know that the K_{sp} for Ag_2CO_3 is 6.2×10^{-12}, and if we find that the $[CO_3^{2-}]$ in the supernatant is 6.2×10^{-6} mole/liter, then the $[Ag^+]$ in the supernatant will be
    (A) 1×10^{-3} mole/liter.
    (B) 1×10^{-6} mole/liter.
    (C) 1×10^{-9} mole/liter.
    (D) 38×10^{-18} mole/liter.
    (E) 6.2×10^{-6} mole/liter.

17. The solubility product constant (K_{sp}) of NiS is given as 1×10^{-26}. In an experiment $Ni(No_3)_2$ solution is treated with H_2S and a precipitate forms. If the $[Ni^{2+}]$ in the supernatant is found to be 1×10^{-20} mole/liter, the $[S^{2-}]$ in the supernatant will be
    (A) $1 \times 10^{-1.4}$ mole/liter.
    (B) 1×10^{-6} mole/liter.
    (C) 1×10^{-20} mole/liter.
    (D) 1×10^{-26} mole/liter.
    (E) 1×10^{-46} mole/liter.

18. An alloy of mercury with another metal is called
    (A) a metalloid.
    (B) pollution.
    (C) an eluent.
    (D) ecology.
    (E) an amalgam.

19. Which acid could be used, in the presence of ThO_2, to produce acetone by pyrolysis?
    (A) acetic
    (B) propionic
    (C) butyric
    (D) oleic
    (E) pyruvic

20. D-glucose is an aldohexose. Not considering ring structures, how many isomeric aldohexoses are there?

(A) 6

(B) 8

(C) 10

(D) 13

(E) 17

21. Which compound listed below is used in the etching of glass?

(A) hydrofluoric acid

(B) carbolic acid

(C) boric acid

(D) ammonium nitrate

(E) nitric acid

22. Often during the oxidation of coal which contains sulfur the anhydride of sulfuric acid is produced. Which of the compounds listed is that anhydride?

(A) SO_3

(B) SO_2

(C) SO_4

(D) H_2S

(E) CS_2

23. The sum of which of the following in the shells surrounding the nucleus is equal to the atomic number for an uncharged atom?

(A) protons

(B) neutrons

(C) electrons

(D) positrons

(E) mesons

24. An atom that has lost two orbital electrons has a charge of

(A) +1.

(B) +2.

(C) −1.

(D) −2.

(E) −3.

25. A.I. Oparin suggested that in order for the complex molecules (organic molecules) to have originated and have given rise to life, the early atmosphere of the earth was probably deficient in free

(A) xenon.

(B) oxygen.

(C) hydrogen.

(D) methane.

(E) nitrogen.

26. Addition of sodium to bromobenzene in dry ether will produce

(A) naphthalene.

(B) cyclohexane.

(C) benzene.

(D) biphenyl.

(E) no reaction.

27. An individual has at his disposal benzyl chloride, benzene, aluminum chloride, and sodium, and he wishes to synthesize diphenylmethane. He should react

(A) all four compounds.

(B) benzyl chloride and sodium.

(C) benzyl chloride, benzene, and aluminum chloride.

(D) benzyl chloride, benzene, and sodium.

(E) benzyl chloride and aluminum chloride.

28. Among the properties ordinarily possessed by organic compounds can be listed those that

(A) possess mainly covalent bonds.

(B) are insoluble in water but soluble in nonpolar solvents.

(C) are generally nonconducting.

(D) all of the above.

(E) none of the above.

29. You have at your disposal benzene, bromine, nitric acid, and sulfuric acid. If you wish to produce *m*-bromonitrobenzene, you should
    (A) nitrate the benzene and then brominate.
    (B) brominate the benzene and then nitrate.
    (C) do either (A) or (B). They work equally well.
    (D) forget it. You cannot obtain the desired product with these materials.
    (E) mix all except sulfuric acid.

30. The conversion of 1,2-dichloropropane to propene may be achieved by heating with
    (A) alcoholic KOH.   (D) zinc duct in alcohol.
    (B) aqueous KOH.   (E) sodium in dry ether.
    (C) sulfuric acid.

31. In the usual commercial vulcanization process crosslinking is introduced by addition of
    (A) ethylene.   (D) sulfur.
    (B) propylene.   (E) toluene.
    (C) silicon.

32. Ethylene will react with 1,3-butadiene to produce
    (A) cyclohexene.   (D) toluene.
    (B) cyclohexane.   (E) octadiene.
    (C) benzene.

33. An uncharged atom of a particular element has an electron distribution of $1s^2, 2s^2, 2p^5$. You would expect this to be a (an)
    (A) metal.
    (B) nonmetal.
    (C) metalloid.
    (D) amalgam.
    (E) can't tell from the information given.

34. The element above would most often be expected to gain or lose electrons and thus exhibit a valence of
    (A) +1   (D) −2
    (B) +3   (E) −3
    (C) −1

35. Which of the following will react with water to form an acidic solution?
    (A) Na_2O (D) BaO
    (B) K_2O (E) P_2O_3
    (C) CaO

36. Which sugars are found in the nucleotides of nucleic acids?
    (A) D-galactose and D-ribose   (D) L-deoxyribose and D-ribose
    (B) L-ribose and D-glucose   (E) D-deoxyribose and D-ribose
    (C) L-ribose and D-ribose

37. Which of the following is NOT an anhydride?

    (A)
    $$CH_3-\overset{\overset{\displaystyle O}{\|}}{C}-Cl$$

    (B)
    $$CH_3-\overset{\overset{\displaystyle O}{\|}}{C}-O-\overset{\overset{\displaystyle O}{\|}}{C}-CH_3$$

    (C) P_2O_5

    (D)
    $$Cl-CH_2-\overset{\overset{\displaystyle O}{\|}}{C}-OH$$

    (E) SO_3

38. Ionic bonding is seen in
(A) O_2.
(B) H_2.
(C) ClF.
(D) KCl.
(E) N_2.

Physics—33 Questions   Recommended Time—44 minutes

DIRECTIONS: Each of the statements or questions is followed by suggested completions or answers. Choose the one that best completes the statement or answers the question, and mark the letter of your choice on the answer sheet.

1. In a factory, the weight of material lifted by a conveyor belt is calculated in pounds per hour. Expressed in SI base units, the weight would be given in
(A) $kg \cdot m/s^3$.
(B) kg/s.
(C) $kg \cdot m^2/s^3$.
(D) $kg \cdot s^2/m$.
(E) kg/h.

2. Which statement correctly describes a Ping-Pong ball making an elastic collision with a stone wall?
(A) Both its momentum and its kinetic energy remain unchanged.
(B) Its momentum decreases and its kinetic energy reverses direction.
(C) Its kinetic energy reverses direction and its momentum remains unchanged.
(D) Its momentum reverses direction and its kinetic energy remains unchanged.
(E) Both its momentum and its kinetic energy decrease.

3. An old satellite falls to earth, steadily increasing its speed and partially burning up as it falls through the air. What happens to the various forms of energy?
(A) Kinetic and potential decrease, thermal increases.
(B) Kinetic and thermal increase, potential decreases.
(C) All three kinds increase.
(D) All three kinds decrease.
(E) Kinetic decreases, potential and thermal increase.

4. Planet A has mass m and planet B has mass $3m$. When they are separated by a distance r, A attracts B with a force F. If the separation increases to $2r$, the force with which B attracts A is
(A) $9F/2$.
(B) $3F/4$.
(C) $F/2$.
(D) $3F/2$.
(E) $F/4$.

5. What would be the resultant, if a force of 12 pounds and a force of 16 pounds act upon each other at right angles?
(A) 14 lbs.
(B) 18 lbs.
(C) 28 lbs.
(D) 20 lbs.
(E) 192 lbs.

6. The resultant of two forces of 96 dynes and 74 dynes acting in the same direction is equal to
(A) 170 dynes.
(B) 12 dynes.
(C) 85 dynes.
(D) 7104 dynes.
(E) none of the above.

7. A man weighing 185 pounds wears a pair of thick-soled boots each with an area of 30 $inch^2$. The pressure exerted on each sole due only to his weight is
(A) 3.1 lb./in.^{2}
(B) 6.2 lb./in.^{2}
(C) 31 lb./in.^{2}
(D) 62 lb./in.^{2}
(E) 185 lb./in.^{2}

8. A ball of steel weighs 720 ounces in air; when submerged in water, its weight is recorded as 360 ounces. What is the specific gravity of this ball?

(A) 360
(B) 7
(C) 2
(D) 1
(E) 0.05

9. A test animal is partially shielded from X-rays by a 1-cm thickness of a uniform metal. If this metal shield stops 50% of the radiation, what percent of the original radiation would be stopped by a similar shield of 3-cm thickness?

(A) 50%
(B) 75%
(C) 87.5%
(D) 98%
(E) 150%

10. A flywheel of 10-cm radius is operating at a speed of 1000 rev/min. If a particle breaks away from the circumference of the wheel, what will be its linear velocity?

(A) 10,000 cm/min
(B) 60,000 cm/min
(C) 110,000 cm/min
(D) 110,000 km/s
(E) 10,000 rev/min

11. About what kind of a front or area do winds circulate in a clockwise direction in the northern hemisphere?

(A) cold front
(B) warm front
(C) stationary front
(D) high pressure area
(E) low pressure area

12. How do the size and distance of an image behind a plane mirror compare to those of the object in front of the mirror?

(A) the same size as the object and a greater distance
(B) a smaller size than the object and a lesser distance
(C) a larger size than the object and a lesser distance
(D) a larger size than the object and a greater distance
(E) none of the above

13. A 120-lb. boy scout climbed a flagpole 40 feet tall. How much work did he do against gravitational forces?

(A) 480 ft.-lb.
(B) 4800 ft.-lb.
(C) 160 ft.-lb.
(D) 4.8×10^5 ft.-lb.
(E) 220 ft.-lb.

14. A gas occupies a volume of 16 liters at STP. It is heated to 546°C and compressed to 4 atm. What volume does it now occupy?

(A) 12 liters
(B) 16 liters
(C) 8 liters
(D) 64 liters
(E) 566 liters

15. If the absolute pressure on a gas is doubled at constant temperature, the volume

(A) remains unchanged.
(B) doubles.
(C) quadruples.
(D) is halved.
(E) decreases by 25%.

16. An object is thrown upward with a vertical velocity of 128 ft./sec. It will return in

(A) 2 seconds.
(B) 4 seconds.
(C) 8 seconds.
(D) 16 seconds.
(E) 64 seconds.

17. The boiling point of any liquid at atmospheric pressure is
   (A) 3 (273) ⅓ Fahrenheit molecular weight +212.
   (B) a function of the shape and type of vessel holding the liquid.
   (C) the temperature at which sublimation takes place.
   (D) the temperature at which the vapor pressure is equal to atmospheric pressure.
   (E) all of the above.

18. In order to determine the density of an alloy, small particles (50 g) of the alloy are added to a graduated cylinder containing 100 ml of water. After adding the particles the volume reads 125 ml. The density of the alloy is
   (A) 2 g/ml.   (D) 12.5 g/ml.
   (B) 2.5 g/ml.   (E) 6.8 g/ml.
   (C) 25 g/ml.

19. To describe the properties of light, we must rely on the
   (A) assimilation model.   (D) wave model.
   (B) propagation model.   (E) wave and particle models.
   (C) dissolution model.

20. A parcel dropped from a low-flying helicopter hits the ground 8 seconds later. From what height was it dropped?
   (A) 256 ft.   (D) 64 ft.
   (B) 1024 ft.   (E) 128 ft
   (C) 512 ft.

21. An astronaut is accelerated in his spacecraft from rest to 800 mi./hr. in 60 sec. He was subjected to an acceleration of
   (A) 4800 mi./hr.^{2} (D) 48,000 mi./hr.^{2}
   (B) 1200 mi./hr.^{2} (E) 48,000 ft./sec.^{2}
   (C) 4800 ft./sec./sec.

22. In a plane two forces of 60 newtons and 40 newtons are acting on an object to produce a resultant force of 20 newtons. What is the orientation of the two forces with respect to each other?
   (A) 45°   (D) 180°
   (B) 90°   (E) 360°
   (C) 60°

23. Which of the factors listed below is NOT a type of heat transfer?
   (A) conduction   (D) radiation and absorption
   (B) convection   (E) evaporation and condensation
   (C) consumption

24. Which of the matched pairs is incorrect?
   (A) Boyle's law — $(PV = k)$ (D) 1 liter — (1.057 liquid quarts)
   (B) Torricelli's theorem — $(v = \sqrt{2\,gh})$
   (C) Avogadro's number — (6.023×10^{23}) (E) $F - \left(\dfrac{5}{9}C + 32°\right)$

25. A radioactive isotope has a half-life of 21 days; at the end of 42 days what percentage of the original radioisotope will be left?
   (A) 100%   (D) 12.5%
   (B) 50%   (E) none
   (C) 25%

26. A pin may be floated on the surface of water; the fact may be explained by which of the following?
    (A) Water is at a higher temperature than the pin.
    (B) Water is at a lower temperature than the pin.
    (C) Surface tension allows the pin to float.
    (D) Water is rich in minerals.
    (E) The temperature of the water is within 3° of 0°C.

27. About how many kilograms is the mass of a 165 lb. object?
    (A) 82
    (B) 75
    (C) 40
    (D) 100
    (E) 165

28. A locomotive accelerates at a constant rate from 10 mi./hr. to 50 mi./hr. in 20 seconds while traveling in a straight line. What is the locomotive's acceleration?
    (A) 10 mi./hr. per sec.
    (B) 2.5 mi./hr. per sec.
    (C) 5 mi./hr.^{2}
    (D) 2 mi./hr. per sec.
    (E) 5 mi./hr. per sec.

29. A 200-lb. man uses an elevator that is accelerated upward 10 ft./sec^2. The total force exerted upon him by the floor of the elevator is
    (A) 200 lb.
    (B) 20 lb.
    (C) 2000 lb.
    (D) 65.2 lb.
    (E) 263 lb.

30. Air resistance has an effect on projectiles. Which factor(s) does it influence?
    (A) speed
    (B) maximum height
    (C) range
    (D) all of the above
    (E) none of the above

31. A hot metal ball is dropped onto a large cake of ice, and 150 g of ice melts. What is the minimum information that would make it possible to determine the amount of heat lost by the metal?
    (A) heat of fusion of ice
    (B) specific heat and mass of the metal
    (C) initial temperature of the metal, its specific heat, and heat of fusion of ice
    (D) mass and specific heat of the metal and heat of fusion of ice
    (E) initial temperature and mass of the metal

32. A plastic ball with electric charge $+q$ is at the zero end of a meter bar, and another with a charge $+2q$ is at the other end. At what point would a third charged ball have to be placed in order for it to remain in equilibrium?
    (A) 80 cm
    (B) 50 cm
    (C) 33 cm
    (D) 20 cm
    (E) 15 cm

33. A radioactive element with atomic number $(A) = 89$ and atomic mass number $(Z) = 240$ emits beta particles. What are the values for the resulting breakdown product?
    (A) $A = 87, Z = 236$
    (B) $A = 90, Z = 240$
    (C) $A = 88, Z = 239$
    (D) $A = 89, Z = 239$
    (E) $A = 90, Z = 241$

SCIENCE PROBLEMS

78 MINUTES
60 QUESTIONS: Biology 21; Chemistry 21; Physics 18.

The following questions require you to use your knowledge of science to solve problems.

DIRECTIONS: The following questions or incomplete statements are in groups of three. Preceding each series of questions or statements is a paragraph or a short explanatory statement, a formula or set of formulas, or a definition. Read the written material and then answer the questions or complete the statements. Eliminate the choices that you think to be incorrect, and mark the letter of your choice on the answer sheet.

A patient is brought into the emergency room and, upon examination, a thyroid goiter is discovered. You suspect that he is suffering from a thyroid disorder, and you ask the intern for a definition of *hypothyroidism*.

1. He responds that *hypothyroidism* is the general term for syndromes that reflect
   (A) increased secretion of thyroid hormones.
   (B) decreased secretion of thyroid hormones.
   (C) no change in secretion of thyroid hormones.
   (D) increased secretion of thyroid stimulating hormone releasing factor.
   (E) increased metabolism of iodine.

2. A basal metabolism rate test is ordered that measures the rate of oxidative metabolism. In hypothyroidism, this rate is
   (A) above normal.
   (B) normal.
   (C) below normal.
   (D) not significant in your diagnosis.
   (E) a sure diagnosis.

3. Because of the hypothyroidism that you suspect, you would also consider that this patient
   1. has gained weight
   2. converts less food into energy
   3. stores more food as fat
   4. has had no shift in weight
   (A) 1, 3, 4 above
   (B) 2, 3, 4 above
   (C) 1, 2, 3 above
   (D) all of the above
   (E) none of the above

Utilize the following formulas in answering the next three questions:

$$\text{Equation 1:} \quad 6CO_2 + 6H_2O + \text{Energy} \rightarrow C_6H_{12}O_6 + 6O_2$$
$$\text{Equation 2:} \quad C_6H_{12}O_6 + 6O_2 \rightarrow 6H_2O + 6CO_2 + \text{Energy}$$
$$\text{Equation 3:} \quad C_6H_{12}O_6 \rightarrow 2C_2H_5OH + 2CO_2 + \text{Energy}$$
$$\text{Equation 4:} \quad C_6H_{12}O_6 \rightarrow 2CH_3CHOHCOOH + \text{Energy}$$

4. Which of the following combinations of the above equations listed below were exothermic reactions?
   (A) 1, 2, 3
   (B) 2, 3, 4
   (C) 1, 3, 4
   (D) 1, 2, 4
   (E) all of the above

5. Equation 1 essentially could be considered
   (A) aerobic respiration.
   (B) anaerobic respiration.
   (C) photosynthesis reaction.
   (D) butyric acid fermentation.
   (E) glycolysis.

6. **Equation 2 demonstrates**
   (A) aerobic respiration.
   (B) fermentation.
   (C) photosynthesis.
   (D) anaerobic respiration.
   (E) glycogenolysis.

Standard temperature and pressure (STP) is defined as $0°C$ (273 K) and 760 mm mercury. The specific gravity of mercury is about 14.

7. What is standard pressure, expressed in millimeters of water?
   (A) 1×10^4
   (B) 1400
   (C) 760
   (D) 54
   (E) 380

8. What would happen to a balloon containing 100 ml of air at standard pressure if it is taken to a location where the pressure is lower? (Assume no temperature change.)
   (A) It would burst.
   (B) It would become smaller.
   (C) It would exhibit no change in appearance.
   (D) It would become larger.
   (E) It would do nothing predictable.

9. A tin can is equilibrated with the atmosphere at an altitude at which the pressure is 300 mm mercury and then sealed. If the can is taken to standard pressure (assuming no change in temperature), the can may
   (A) explode.
   (B) collapse.
   (C) rust.
   (D) be noted to condense the water vapor from the contained air.
   (E) show oxidation of the tin rather than the iron.

You have been given a sample of three anhydrides:

$$H_3C-\overset{\overset{O}{\|}}{C}-O-\overset{\overset{O}{\|}}{C}-CH_3 \qquad H_3C-\overset{\overset{O}{\|}}{C}-Cl$$

1.   2.   3.

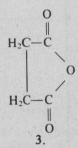

10. When all three have been hydrolyzed in water, at least one of them gives two acid products. This would be which of the above formulas?
    (A) 1
    (B) 2
    (C) 3
    (D) 1 and 2
    (E) 1 and 3

11. A mole of which of the above will give only one mole of acid product after hydrolysis?
    (A) 1
    (B) 2
    (C) 3
    (D) 1 and 2
    (E) 2 and 3

12. A mole of at least one of the above will give two moles of acid on hydrolysis, but there is chemically only one acid product. The anhydride is which of the above?
    (A) 1
    (B) 2
    (C) 3
    (D) 1 and 2
    (E) 2 and 3

For osmotic pressure, $P = cRT$ where P is osmotic pressure, c is the number of particles in solution, R is the gas constant, and T is the absolute temperature.

13. A one-molar solution of which of the following would have the greatest osmotic pressure?
    (A) NaCl
    (B) glucose
    (C) sucrose
    (D) $Ba(NO_3)_2$
    (E) HCl

14. A one-degree increase in temperature will induce the greatest percentage increase in osmotic pressure in the solution of
    (A) NaCl.
    (B) glucose.
    (C) HCl.
    (D) $Ba(NO_3)_2$.
    (E) none of the above.

15. The difference in the osmotic pressures of one molar solutions of different compounds at a given temperature results from
    (A) different values for R.
    (B) different values for Avogadro's number.
    (C) ionization to produce different numbers of particles per mole.
    (D) all of the above.
    (E) none of the above.

Black (B) is dominant over white (b); rough coat (R) is dominant over smooth (r).

16. A purebred white-rough coat male is mated to a purebred black-smooth female; their offspring are
    (A) all white with rough coat.
    (B) all white with smooth coat.
    (C) all black with smooth coat.
    (D) all agouti.
    (E) all black with rough coat.

17. When these F_1 are mated, you expect how many types of offspring?
    (A) 2
    (B) 4
    (C) 1
    (D) 16
    (E) 8

18. In what ratio will they appear?
    (A) 1:2:1
    (B) 3:1
    (C) 9:3:3:1
    (D) 2:4
    (E) 12:3:3:1

The change in length of a bar of material is given by the formula $\Delta L = \alpha L_1 \Delta t$ where ΔL is the change in length, α is coefficient of linear expansion, L_1 is the initial length, and Δt is the change in temperature.

19. If the temperature increases from 27 to 30°C, then the bar will be
    (A) three times as long as initially.
    (B) one-third as long as initially.
    (C) increased by 1/9.
    (D) increased by $3\alpha L_1$.
    (E) none of the above.

20. If length is given in centimeters and temperature in °C, the coefficient of expansion will be given in
    (A) centimeters.
    (B) cm/°C.
    (C) cm^{-1}.
    (D) $°C^{-1}$.
    (E) °C/cm

21. If thin strips of two metals are joined, an increase in temperature will cause the joined strip to
    (A) curve toward the one with the greatest α.
    (B) be longer than a similar strip of either metal alone.
    (C) curve away from the metal with the greatest α.
    (D) assume the shape of a sine wave.
    (E) none of the above.

The solubility product constant, K_{sp}, of a slightly soluble salt is given as the product of the concentrations of its ions in solution raised to the exponential powers of their coefficients in ionization.

$$BaF_2 \leftrightharpoons Ba^{2+} + 2F^- \qquad K_{sp} = [F^-]^2\,[Ba^{2+}] = 2 \times 10^{-6}$$
$$BaCO_3 \leftrightharpoons Ba^{2+} + CO_3^{2-} \qquad K_{sp} = [Ba^{2+}]\,[CO_3^{2-}] = 7 \times 10^{-9}$$

22. In the precipitation of Ba^{2+} from identical solutions in two beakers, beaker (1) contains $[F^-] = 1 \times 10^{-2}$ and beaker (2) contains $[CO_3^{2-}] = 7 \times 10^{-5}$. The higher concentration of Ba^{2+} in solution is
    (A) in beaker (1).
    (B) in beaker (2).
    (C) in neither beaker (i.e., no difference).
    (D) not possible to predict with the information given.
    (E) directly related to the difference of atmospheric pressure over the two beakers.

23. To precipitate the Ba^{2+} from a 5×10^{-4} molar solution we consider adding either F^- to produce a concentration of 0.1 molar or CO_3^{2-} to produce a concentration of 0.01 molar. The lesser concentration of Ba^{2+} left in solution will be noted after addition of
    (A) 0.1 molar F^-.
    (B) 0.01 molar CO_3^{2-}.
    (C) 0.05 molar F^-.
    (D) 0.003 molar CO_3^{2-}.
    (E) either of the above (i.e., no difference).

24. You wish to precipitate F^- from a 0.001 molar solution in a beaker or CO_3^{2-} from a 0.002 molar solution in another beaker. In which beaker will the addition of 0.1 molar Ba^{2+} result in a lower concentration of the anion mentioned?
    (A) beaker with F^-
    (B) beaker with CO_3^{2-}
    (C) neither of the above (i.e., no difference)
    (D) one of the beakers but the information is insufficient to allow prediction

The iodine number of a fatty acid is defined as the number of grams of iodine that will react with the double bonds of 100 grams of the fatty acid.

$$R-CH=CH-R' + I_2 \rightarrow R-\underset{\underset{H}{|}}{\overset{\overset{I}{|}}{C}}-\underset{\underset{I}{|}}{\overset{\overset{H}{|}}{C}}-R'$$

$$H_3C-(CH_2)_7-CH=CH-(CH_2)_5-\overset{\overset{O}{\|}}{C}-OH \qquad \text{1. molecular wt. 254}$$

$$H_3C-(CH_2)_6-CH=CH-(CH_2)_6-\overset{\overset{O}{\|}}{C}-OH \qquad \text{2. molecular wt. 254}$$

$$H_3C-(CH_2)_{14}-\overset{\overset{O}{\|}}{C}-OH \qquad \text{3. molecular wt. 256}$$

$$H_3C-(CH_2)_9-CH=CH-CH_2-CH=CH-(CH_2)_2 \qquad \text{4. molecular wt. 280}$$

$$H_3C-(CH_2)_{16}-\overset{\overset{O}{|}}{C}-OH \qquad \text{5. molecular wt. 284}$$

25. The highest iodine number in the group above would be shown by

(A) 1.
(B) 2.
(C) 3.
(D) 4.
(E) 5.

26. The lowest iodine number in the group above would be shown by

(A) 1.
(B) 2.
(C) 3.
(D) 4.
(E) more than one of the above.

27. Equal iodine numbers would be found for

(A) 1 and 3.
(B) 2 and 4.
(C) 3 and 5.
(D) 2 and 5.
(E) none of the above combinations.

The hematology laboratory reports to the surgeon that his patient's blood clumped with both anti A and anti B serum.

28. The patient's blood type is

(A) AB.
(B) A.
(C) B.
(D) O.
(E) Rh$^+$.

29. The test is based upon the presence or absence of

1. antigens (agglutinogens) in red blood cells
2. antibodies (agglutinins) in the serum
3. antigens in white blood cells
4. agglutinins in white blood cells

(A) 1 and 3 above
(B) 2 and 4 above
(C) 1 and 2 above
(D) 3 and 4 above
(E) none of the above

30. In this case, what percentage of the population would the surgeon expect to have the blood type of the patient?

(A) 47
(B) 41
(C) 9
(D) 15
(E) 3

Recall that force on any surface is the pressure on the surface times the area of the surface. The pressure exerted on a surface can be expressed as the height of an object times the specific density occupying a space. Use the diagram below in your calculations.

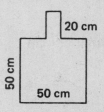

This cubical container with a narrow neck is filled with hexabromoethane, which has a specific gravity of 2.8. The cross-section of the elevated area is 15 cm^2.

31. The force exerted upon the bottom of this container is equivalent to the weight of

(A) 40 kg.
(B) 4000 kg.
(C) 4000 g.
(D) 500 g.
(E) 500 kg.

32. The area of the top of the container, below the neck, that is exposed to hexabromoethane is

(A) 2485 cm².
(B) 500 cm².
(C) 980 cm².
(D) 1200 cm².
(E) more than 3000 cm².

33. The force exerted upon the top of this container is equivalent to a weight of

(A) 1390 g.
(B) 125 g.
(C) 139 kg.
(D) 10 kg.
(E) 42 kg.

One mole of sodium, potassium, or lithium will react with an excess of ethanol to form one gram atomic weight of hydrogen. Hydrogen is also produced by the reaction of these metals with a number of alcohols, organic acids, and water.

34. At standard temperature and pressure, how many liters of hydrogen will be produced when 0.1 mole of lithium is added to excess ethanol?

(A) 0.1
(B) 0.05
(C) 0.2
(D) 1.1
(E) 11.2

35. The addition of 0.001 mole of potassium to excess ethanol produces a given quantity of hydrogen. How many milliliters of oxygen will react with that quantity of hydrogen to produce water?

(A) 5 ml
(B) 20 ml
(C) 100 ml
(D) 220 ml
(E) 11200 ml

36. If one is given a choice of adding 0.001 mole of potassium, lithium, or sodium to excess ethanol, the greatest amount of hydrogen will be produced after the addition of

(A) sodium.
(B) lithium.
(C) potassium.
(D) A or B (equal).
(E) A, B, or C (all equal).

Density is defined as the mass of a body divided by the volume of a body. The density of water is 1 g/cm³ or 62.4 lb./ft.³ Specific gravity usually is expressed as

$$\frac{\text{density or weight of a body}}{\text{density or weight of an equal volume of water}}$$

The specific gravity of water is 1. The specific gravity of a piece of steel is 8.0.

37. The density of this piece of steel in g/cm³ is

(A) 6.15
(B) less than 0.6.
(C) 0.8
(D) 8.0.
(E) more than 10.

38. The density of this piece of steel in lb./ft.³ is

(A) 499.
(B) 800.
(C) 61.5.
(D) less than 60.
(E) more than 825.

39. The weight of 35 ft.³ of this steel is

(A) 2152 lb.
(B) 17,400 lb.
(C) 2.8 × 10⁴ lb.
(D) 1.5 × 10³ lb.
(E) less than 2000 lb.

It is known that periodate will oxidize OH groups or amines on adjacent carbon atoms to form aldehydes.

$$\overset{\text{OH}}{\underset{|}{R-CH}}-\overset{\text{OH}}{\underset{|}{CH}}-R' \rightarrow R-\overset{H}{\underset{|}{C}}=O + R'-\overset{H}{\underset{|}{C}}=O$$

In the case of three adjacent alcohol or amino groups, there is oxidation to produce formic acid and two aldehydes.

$$R-\underset{\underset{OH}{|}}{C}H-\underset{\underset{OH}{|}}{C}H-\underset{\underset{OH}{|}}{C}H-R' \rightarrow R-\underset{\overset{|}{H}}{C}=O + HCOOH + R'-\underset{\overset{|}{H}}{C}=O$$

You have been given pure samples of three diol compounds, but you do not know the identity of any of them. The possible structures are

$$H_3C-\underset{\underset{OH}{|}}{C}H-\underset{\underset{OH}{|}}{C}H-CH_3 \qquad H_3C-CH_2-\underset{\underset{OH}{|}}{C}H-\underset{\underset{OH}{|}}{C}H-CH_3$$

1.   2.   3.

Each of the unknown compounds is subjected to periodate oxidation and the products are examined

40. One compound produces two different aldehydes. The structure of this compound must be

(A) 1.   (D) 1 or 2.
(B) 2.   (E) 1 or 3.
(C) 3.

41. Another compound produces one mole of aldehyde from one mole of the starting material. This compound must be

(A) 1.   (D) 1 or 2.
(B) 2.   (E) 2 or 3.
(C) 3.

42. The remaining compound yields only one aldehyde on oxidation by periodate. *Disregarding any data presented and conclusions you have reached in study of the other two compounds*, this compound must be

(A) 1.   (D) 1 or 2.
(B) 2.   (E) 1 or 3.
(C) 3.

A 10-kg piece of glass is weighed in air, and then while suspended in water. The density of the glass is 6.0 g/cm³.

43. If the piece of glass were suspended in air, it would weigh (the buoyancy of air is neglected)

(A) 10 newtons.   (D) 500 newtons.
(B) 50 newtons.   (E) 600 newtons.
(C) 100 newtons.

44. The volume of the piece of glass is

(A) 1.6 cm³.   (D) 6 cm³.
(B) 60 cm³.   (E) 1666 cm³.
(C) 166 cm³.

45. If the buoyant force of the water is equal to the weight of the water displaced, then the piece of glass suspended in water weighs

(A) 83 N.   (D) 6 N.
(B) 100 N.   (E) 50 N.
(C) 16 N.

The number of possible optical isomers of a particular organic compound is equal to 2^n (where n = the number of asymmetric carbon atoms) when no two of the asymmetric carbon atoms are attached to the same four kinds of groups.

46. Based on the above statement, how many isomers does 1,2-dibromobutane have?
    (A) 1
    (B) 2
    (C) 4
    (D) 8
    (E) none of the above

47. The number of possible isomers of 1,3-dibromobutane is
    (A) 1.
    (B) 2.
    (C) 4.
    (D) 8.
    (E) none of the above.

48. The number of possible isomers of 1,4-dibromobutane is
    (A) 1.
    (B) 2.
    (C) 4.
    (D) 8.
    (E) 12.

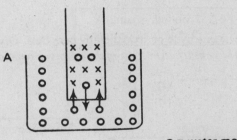 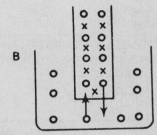

O = water molecule
x = sugar molecule

The diagrams demonstrate the principle of osmosis. As indicated, water molecules pass freely across the semipermeable membrane, while the starch molecules do not. In A, more water molecules move into the tube; the water level rises and the solution becomes more dilute. In B, osmotic equilibrium has been reached, and the same number of water molecules pass through the membrane in either direction.

49. If a cell were put into a solution of greater osmotic pressure than its protoplasm,
    (A) water would pass out through the plasma membrane faster than in.
    (B) water would pass in through the plasma membrane faster than out.
    (C) the cell would swell.
    (D) no unequal rates would be experienced.
    (E) the result could not be predicted.

50. The principle of osmosis depends upon the concentration of:
1. diffusible particles
2. nondiffusible particles
3. protons
4. starch molecules

(A) 1 and 2 above (D) 2 and 3 above
(B) 1 and 3 above (E) 3 and 4 above
(C) 1 and 4 above

51. If a red blood cell is placed in a solution and hemolysis occurs due to the osmotic relationships, we can deduce that the cell was placed in a

(A) hypertonic solution. (D) none of the above.
(B) hypotonic solution. (E) no conclusion — insufficient data.
(C) isotonic solution.

The schema of thyroxine formation is outlined below:

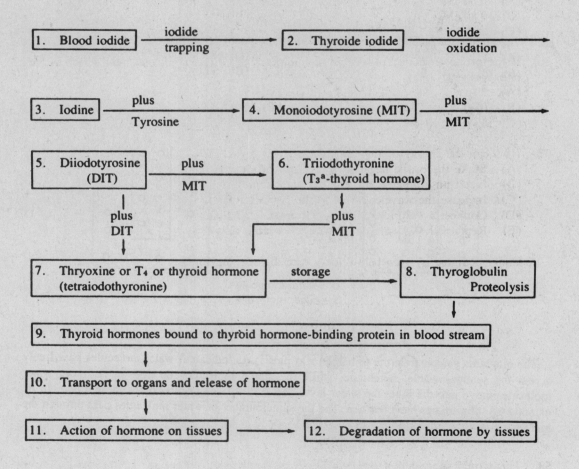

52. Chemically, thyroid hormones are
(A) iodotyrosines. (D) iodines.
(B) iodothyronines. (E) tyrosines.
(C) iodides.

53. In proceeding from compound 3 to compound 4, the amino acid tyrosine is

(A) oxidized.

(B) reduced.

(C) iodinated.

(D) synthesized.

(E) none of the above.

54. During transport thyroid hormones are inactive because they are

(A) in the form of thyroglobulin.

(B) free hormones.

(C) protein-bound.

(D) on red blood cells.

(E) deactivated.

A metal surface has a photoelectric work function of 2.2 eV and is being struck by light with a wavelength of 440 nm. The electrons are emitted at a rate of 5×10^{14} per second, and are picked up by a probe connected to the terminal of an adjustable power supply.

Constants: Speed of light $= 3.00 \times 10^8$ m/s

Electronic charge $= 1.60 \times 10^{-19}$ C

Planck's constant $= 4.14 \times 10^{-15}$ eV $\cdot$ s

55. What is the maximum energy of the emitted electrons?

(A) 0.60 eV

(B) 0.80 eV

(C) 2.2 eV

(D) 2.8 eV

(E) 4.7 eV

56. If the probe is made positive so that it picks up all the electrons, how much is the photocurrent?

(A) 2 A

(B) 0.60 A

(C) 80 μA

(D) 0.60 mA

(E) 5.0 μA

57. How can the energy of the emitted electrons be measured?

(A) Make the probe negative to cut off the current.

(B) Insert an ammeter into the current circuit.

(C) Increase the wavelength until the current stops.

(D) Connect a voltmeter to the emitter and the battery.

(E) Replace the power supply with a variable resistor.

A family pedigree is given below for a rare disorder in humans.

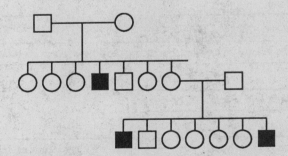

58. This would suggest that the disorder is most probably a (an)

(A) sex-linked recessive trait.

(B) sex-linked dominant trait.

(C) Y-linked trait.

(D) trisomy trait.

(E) autosomal dominant trait.

59. An example of a trait showing this inheritance is
    (A) Huntington's disease.
    (B) Tay-Sachs disease.
    (C) classical hemophilia A.
    (D) blood type A.
    (E) sickle cell disease.

60. The next most likely explanation for this disorder is
    (A) an autosomal dominant trait.
    (B) an autosomal recessive trait.
    (C) a chromosomal nondisjunction.
    (D) a trisomy trait.
    (E) a spontaneous mutation.

SKILLS ANALYSIS: READING

85 MINUTES
68 QUESTIONS

The following questions are to be answered based on your careful reading of selections from scientific writings.

DIRECTIONS: Read each passage carefully, then answer the questions following it. Consider only the material within the passage in answering the questions. Eliminate those choices that you think to be incorrect and mark the letter of your choice on the answer sheet.

Cellular regeneration has attracted great interest among both the experimenter and the clinician interested in liver disease. The liver is the largest organ of the body and is the main processing, as well as detoxification, plant of the organism. Insult and injury are common. Many of the abnormalities of liver disease are attributed to regeneration phenomena. Its absence or deficiency is responsible for many of the hepatic failures observed. Cellular hypertrophy, arrangement and distortion of the normal morphological pattern may cause portal hypertension and lead to cirrhosis. Portal hypertension may result in severe esophageal varices and necessitate the surgical creation of a porta-caval shunt. Uncontrolled regenerative hyperplasia is the hallmark of hepatic carcinoma. To study liver regeneration investigators have utilized a good animal model; after partial hepatectomy (removal of about ⅔ of liver mass) regeneration is rapid and it regains its normal size within about 20 days. The study of the specific processes has been enhanced by the development of tools such as *in vivo* techniques to measure humoral factors, transmission and scanning electron microscopy, ultra-centrifugation and analysis of subcellular fractions and radioactive tracers. The needle biopsy now allows easy access to the liver of man for study.

After partial hepatectomy or carbon tetrachloride insult, mitotic activity reaches a peak around 35 hours. The new growth encompasses not only the liver parenchymal cells but also the elements of the biliary system, reticuloendothelial system, connective tissue system and the vascular system. Utilizing ultra-centrifugation the nuclear fraction (containing DNA and RNA), the mitochondrial fraction (containing the cytochrome oxidase enzymes) and microsomal fraction (containing RNA and phospholipids) have been investigated and have yielded data that allow for a meaningful comparison of the composition and chemical processes that are prominent in normal and regenerating liver. Despite the vast amount of knowledge concerning regeneration the clinical utilization of results of animal experimentation has been very difficult because of the lack of methodology for assessing regeneration in human beings.

The following statements are related to the passage above. Based on the information given, select:
- (A) if the statement is *supported by* the information in the passage.
- (B) if the statement is *contradicted by* the information in the passage.
- (C) if the statement is *neither supported nor contradicted by* information in the passage.

1. The paragraph emphasizes liver degeneration.
2. In routine histological examinations most importance has been placed on the mitotic activity of the regenerating liver.
3. The liver is a very important functional organ.
4. Deficiency of the regenerative process may lead to liver failures.
5. A good animal model is in existence for investigators to utilize.
6. Results of animal experiments can directly be correlated with man.
7. Scanning and transmission electron microscopy are the most useful tools in the study of liver regeneration.
8. Several systems are involved in liver regeneration.
9. Mitotic activity ceases around 35 hours.

10. Partial hepatectomy and carbon tetrachloride poisoning are alike in their injury to the liver.

11. Only the nuclear fraction contains RNA.

12. Ultra-centrifugation is the most useful tool in regeneration studies.

13. Animal experimentation has yielded much information that is directly applied in clinical treatment in man.

Throughout the various phyla of the plant and animal kingdom numerous species have evolved. It is apparent that sexual reproduction plays an important role in the continuation of the species and in the expression of different phenotypes within the species. This mode of reproduction is accomplished by the fusion of two gametes which will give rise to a zygote. In order for future generations to maintain the same number of chromosomes as their parents the gametes must undergo a reduction in chromosome number. If the offspring express phenotypic traits that are different from those of their parents, there must be a rearrangement of the DNA within the chromosomes. The reduction of the number of chromosomes and mixing of the gene pool are accomplished by the process of meiosis.

The process of meiosis is characterized by a naturally occurring sequence of events which are usually artificially subdivided into ten different stages. The first five stages comprise the first or reductional division of meiosis. At the end of the reductional division the chromosomes are reduced to one-half their original number (haploid). The last five stages comprise the second or equatorial division of meiosis. Germ cells undergoing meiosis give rise to haploid gametes which contain one representative of each type of chromosome. The chromosomes of the gametes may also demonstrate variations in genetic composition due to crossing over which takes place during the first prophase.

Replication of DNA occurs during interphase before the process of meiosis begins. The condensation and coiling of chromatin to form chromosomes marks the beginning of prophase I, the first stage of meiosis. Homologous chromosomes pair with one another to form a structure called a bivalent. Next each chromosome splits lengthwise to form two chromatids. The homologous pairs of chromosomes are now composed of four chromatids which are referred to as a tetrad. The chromatids of tetrads become short and thick and breaks may occur in them. The breaks are eventually repaired but segments of different chromatids may be joined together. This process, referred to as crossing over, enables segments of two different chromatids to be joined together. This enables the gametes to receive chromosomes derived from segments of both homologous chromosomes. In the second stage of meiosis or metaphase I, the nuclear membrane disappears, a spindle apparatus forms, and the homologous pairs align along the equatorial plate of the cell. In anaphase I the homologous chromosomes migrate to opposite poles of the cell. Telophase I is characterized by the complete separation of the homologous pairs, and the spindle apparatus disappears. The nuclear membrane begins to reform and in many organisms a cytoplasmic division may occur at this stage.

After a brief interphase, prophase II begins. Prophase II is the first stage in the second or equatorial division of meiosis. It is characterized by the condensing of chromatin to form the chromosomes. During metaphase II the spindle apparatus forms and the chromosomes line up along the equatorial plate. In anaphase II the daughter chromosomes migrate to opposite poles of the cell. Anaphase II differs from the first anaphase in that the centromere divides and the two chromatids now become the daughter chromosomes. The daughter chromosomes separate completely and reach opposite poles of the cell in telophase II. Subsequent divisions of the cytoplasm result in the formation of two daughter cells which have a haploid number of chromosomes.

The two divisions of the germ cell during meiosis produce four gametes with one-half the original number of chromosomes.

14. According to this passage, at the end of the reductional division of meiosis
    (A) four haploid sets of chromosomes are produced.
    (B) the homologous pairs of chromosomes are completely separated.
    (C) the chromatin duplicates and coils.
    (D) the centromeres divide and daughter chromosomes move to opposite poles of the cell.
    (E) the chromatids of the tetrads form breaks.

15. According to this passage, crossing over occurs
    (A) during the equatorial division.
    (B) before the tetrad separates.
    (C) during anaphase I.
    (D) during prophase II.
    (E) just before the first prophase begins.

16. According to this passage, duplication of the chromatin occurs during
    (A) metaphase I.
    (B) anaphase II.
    (C) telophase I.
    (D) interphase.
    (E) the reductional division.

17. According to this passage, variation in genetic composition is made possible by
    (A) the formation of homologous pairs.
    (B) mitotic division of germ cells.
    (C) crossing over.
    (D) random mutations.
    (E) fusion of gametes to form a zygote.

18. It can be inferred from this passage that
    (A) all species in both the plant and animal kingdom are capable of sexual reproduction.
    (B) haploid cells are only found in animals.
    (C) four functional gametes are always formed by the process of meiosis.
    (D) zygote formation may produce an offspring which has the same number of chromosomes as its parents.
    (E) fusion of gametes will produce offspring that have ½ the original number of chromosomes.

Unlike skeletal muscle, smooth muscle can be stretched without developing a lasting increase in tension. When stretched slowly, smooth muscle initially contracts to resist the stretching force. However, the tension then begins to decrease and the muscle fibers adjust to new lengths without contracting against the force which continues to stretch them. This property is very useful in the case of smooth muscle in the walls of hollow visceral organs. Such organs can serve as reservoirs because, as they become filled, the smooth muscle in their walls can adapt to new lengths without raising the internal pressure of the organ. For example, the urinary bladder can contain 100 or 1000 ml of urine with approximately the same internal or intraluminal pressure. There is a limit, however, to the amount of stretch that smooth muscle can sustain before an increase in tension occurs. When this limit is reached, continued stretching stimulates the muscle to contract forcefully and consequently causes expulsion of the contents of the organ. Smooth muscle can be over-stretched, and, as is the case with skeletal muscle, once the optimal length has been exceeded the amount of tension developed will be less.

19. The main topic of this passage is
    (A) a comparison of the response of smooth and skeletal muscle to stretch.
    (B) the plasticity of smooth muscle.
    (C) the storage and release properties of hollow organs.
    (D) the contraction of smooth muscle.
    (E) the lengthening of smooth muscle.

20. By inference from this passage, skeletal muscle
    (A) can be stretched and responds by developing a lasting increase in tension.
    (B) does not develop a lasting increase in tension when stretched.
    (C) plays no role in the emptying of hollow organs.
    (D) continues to increase in tension as its optimal length is exceeded.
    (E) contracts more rapidly than smooth muscle.

21. An increase in tension does *not* occur
    (A) when skeletal muscle is stretched.
    (B) when smooth muscle is over-stretched.
    (C) as smooth muscle is initially stretched.
    (D) when the limit of stretch of smooth muscle is exceeded.
    (E) unless smooth muscle is over-stretched.

22. According to this passage, hollow visceral organs
    (A) may have skeletal muscle in their walls.
    (B) may have constant internal pressure over a wide range of internal volumes.
    (C) cannot contract if their volume is rapidly increased.
    (D) increase their internal pressure continuously as their volume increases.
    (E) do not show an initial increase in wall-tension when initially stretched.

23. It can be concluded from the passage that
    (A) skeletal muscle always responds to length increases differently than smooth muscle.
    (B) the ability of smooth muscle to adjust to increased length without increased contraction is necessary to the reservoir function of certain hollow organs.
    (C) smooth muscle does not increase the internal pressure of hollow organs.
    (D) smooth muscle has no response to stretch.
    (E) smooth muscle has a different morphology than skeletal muscle.

Migration of birds, butterflies, and fishes is still a subject of intrigue and study. Since recorded time the sounds and sights of the great migrations of birds have awed man, and we still marvel at the great distances that are covered and the accuracy of guidance that the animals possess. Migration routes of many species have been mapped as they travel south in the fall to feed and head north in the spring to breed. The fall migration seems to be triggered by the change in weather, but an endogenous factor, probably chemical in nature, is responsible for the spring migration. The question as to how the animals find their destinations with pin-point accuracy has received great attention. Experiments indicate that starlings that fly by day use the sun as a compass and actually adjust their course to the sun's changes in position. Other day fliers are capable of using landmarks such as rivers and mountains especially as they near their destination. Night fliers such as Old World warblers navigate by the stars; they seem to have an innate time clock or gyroscope which allows them to automatically know the right direction and to adjust their course during the night's flight. During adverse weather conditions when the stars are not visible, these animals become confused and their migration comes to a temporary halt. The center that controls these delicate responses and the orientation of these animals still eludes investigators.

The following statements are related to the information presented above. Based on the information given, select:
    (A) if the statement is *supported by* the information given.
    (B) if the statement is *contradicted by* the information given.
    (C) if the statement is *neither supported nor contradicted by* information given.

24. The mystery of migration has been solved.

25. Long before man learned how, birds were already flying by the sun and stars.

26. All migrating birds use the same navigational guides.

27. The fall migration is triggered by exogenous factors.

28. Migration involves every member of a species.

29. The brightest star is probably utilized by night fliers to guide them.

30. Migration routes of all species have been mapped and studied by investigators.

31. Day fliers halt their migration during bad weather.

The temporomandibular joint is characterized as a bilateral diarthroidal articulation; that is, it is capable of both rotary (hinge) and translatory (gliding) motion. This range of motion permits movement both bodily (side) and in an anterior-posterior direction of the mandibular condyle within the glenoid fossa or cavity of this joint. The functional articulation actually occurs when each condyle contacts the articular eminence of the squamous part of the temporal bone. Both the right and left joints function as one unit, but each may move somewhat independently.

Interposed between the condyle and fossa and eminence is an articular disk or meniscus which is attached to the head of the condyle posteriorly and to the joint capsule laterally. This arrangement produces upper and lower joint compartments lined by synovium. The disk consists of dense collagenous connective tissue or may be fibrocartilaginous in nature. It fuses with the joint capsule, which is composed of dense fibroelastic connective tissue. This capsule is attached to the concave surface of the fossa, the convex surface of the eminence, and inferiorly to the neck of the condyle. The thickened lateral part of the capsule forms the temporomandibular ligament.

The temporomandibular ligament functions to prevent excessive retraction of the mandible and thus limits border movements. Other ligaments attached to the joint include the sphenomandibular, the stylomandibular, and the tiny (pinto's). The sphenomandibular ligament functions to limit closure of the jaws. It becomes taut if the vertical dimension is decreased. The stylomandibular ligament functions to limit extreme mandibular protrusion and overclosure of the jaws. The tiny ligament, attached to the capsule, disk, and sphenomandibular ligament, inserts on the malleus of the ear. Tension on it may cause some change in position of the malleus.

Each synovial compartment is lined with a vascular layer of connective tissue. In areas not exposed to pressure the synovial membrane is thrown into numerous folds. There are two kinds of cells comprising the membrane. Type A cells are phagocytic in nature and are found among type B cells that are secretory in nature. The cavity is filled with synovial fluid, a transparent, yellowish, viscous material. The fluid is a dialysate of plasma and lymph consisting of a protein-mucopolysaccharide complex. Debris is removed from this lubricating and nutritional fluid by the type A cells of the membrane.

32. The main topic of this passage is
    (A) the unlimited movement capabilities of the temporomandibular joint.
    (B) the description of the functional anatomy of the joint.
    (C) the role of the ligaments in movements of the joint.
    (D) the histological characterization of various anatomic controls.
    (E) the joint is vital for the normal activity of life.

33. According to the passage, the meniscus is best described as
    (A) the layer internal to the synovial compartments.
    (B) the connective tissue separating the lower compartment from the condyle.
    (C) the fibrocartilage positioned above the upper synovial cavity.
    (D) the attachment for the head of the condyle.
    (E) none of the above.

34. Unlike the articular disk, the joint capsule
    (A) contains some connective tissue.
    (B) forms laterally into ligamentous tissue.
    (C) makes attachment with the joint.
    (D) consists of fibers and cells.
    (E) attaches to the tiny ligament.

35. It can be concluded from the passage that
    (A) border movements made by the mandible are restricted by ligamentous attachments.
    (B) overclosure of the jaws occurs frequently.
    (C) slack in one of the ligaments leads to tension in other ligaments.
    (D) protrusion involves movement of the mandible posteriorly.
    (E) retraction is common during wide opening of the mouth.

36. According to the passage, the following are correct EXCEPT which one?
    (A) Phagocytes remove foreign material from the synovial fluid.
    (B) Only Type B cells produce the synovial fluid.
    (C) Pressure flattens areas of the synovial membrane.
    (D) Blood vessels are found among the connective tissue of synovial compartments.
    (E) The composition of synovial fluid is complex.

A considerable body of knowledge concerning headaches has accumulated over the years. Progress in treatment has been largely due to the increased information from differential diagnosis of the various syndromes and types of headaches. Pain, the universal denominator, may be due to a multitude of organic and psychological disturbances and usually is the symptom that drives the sufferer to seek help. Pain may be present at the site of the lesion or it may present itself as referred pain in a distant area of the body. This phenomenon can be partly explained on the basis that the afferent components of the central nervous system at a particular spinal cord level are overloaded and at times cannot distinguish visceral pain, which travels with the autonomics, from somatic pain; therefore, pain is felt over an area that is supplied by general somatic nerves. In a differential diagnosis, the location, the nature, the frequency, the time of day or night, the severity, the duration, response of pain to drugs, and type of pain are important factors. All this information must be gathered during a thorough physical examination which includes a detailed history of the patient and his family. Once the facts have been determined, the good physician is not satisfied with the control of pain but must pry on and determine the causative factors. Most headaches are transient but the ones that drive a patient to seek help might be caused by an underlying systemic infection, head injury, tumor, eye problems, sinus infection and vascular disturbances. Often the physician is ill-equipped to handle headache problems because of lack of adequate preparation in this area of medical training. After a thorough examination several tests might be in order; these may include a radiographic examination of the skull and cervical vertebral column, an electroencephalogram, an arteriogram, a lumbar puncture, and biopsies of organs. Headaches which occur rarely may, of course, be associated with fatigue or emotional stress; headaches associated with organic disease usually are intermittent but occur daily while headaches that persist for weeks on end might be associated with psychological disturbances. Treatment should be directed toward the cure of the underlying problem. Analgesics are among the safest of drugs; tranquilizers, etc., however, must be effectively monitored.

The following statements are related to the information presented above. Based on the information given, select:
    (A) if the statement is *supported by* the information given.
    (B) if the statement is *contradicted by* the information given.
    (C) if the statement is *neither supported nor contradicted by* information given.

37. The majority of headaches are of vascular origin.

38. Before using any drug the patient should be checked for contraindications.

39. Aspirins will cure most headaches.

40. Analgesics are absolutely safe.

41. Pain usually stimulates the patient to seek help.

42. Acupuncture should be considered in the treatment of headaches.

43. A thorough history is essential to the treatment of the patient.

44. The concept of referred pain was fully explained.

45. Most common headaches are transient and probably never require a physician's treatment.

46. A radiographic examination of the skull might demonstrate a tumor.

47. All headaches that occur daily are associated with organic disease.

48. Psychological factors must be considered.

Blood transfusion has developed through the centuries from the primitive stage to the art as it is practiced today. While whole blood is still the major type of transfused product, component therapy is being increasingly practiced in order to minimize risk to the patient. Whole blood is indicated for transfusion when the patient is both anemic and hypovolemic, while packed cells are indicated only in anemic conditions. Because of supply and demand problems, most blood transfusions utilize stored blood rather than fresh blood. During storage, however, changes take place which are detrimental to the qualities of blood, such as potassium leakage into plasma, decreasing pH, increasing ammonia concentration, and increasing hemolysis of the red blood cells. The most important changes, however, are decreasing ATP and 2,3-DPG concentrations. ATP is concerned with membrane stability, and its loss is associated with increasing membrane fragility. 2,3-DPG, a glycolytic metabolite, is associated with oxygen affinity of the red cell, in that decreasing 2,3-DPG levels are associated with increasing oxygen affinity of the red blood cells. With this increased affinity, however, less tissue oxygenation occurs because the A-V (arterio-venous) O_2 concentration difference is less, and, therefore, less oxygen is liberated to the tissues. Advanced technology, however, now enables us to raise 2,3-DPG and ATP to their normal levels by biochemical alteration so that red blood cells with normal or decreased oxygen affinity can now be supplied to patients. Because of this accomplishment, tissue oxygenation immediately after transfusion is increased over that which would occur if the red cells had not been altered. This enables delivery of superior blood to the patient at a time of critical need.

49. According to the reading selection 2,3-DPG levels are
  (A) normal in stored blood.
  (B) not involved in tissue oxygenation.
  (C) able to be manipulated experimentally.
  (D) of no concern in transfusion therapy.
  (E) concerned with membrane stability.

50. It can be inferred from the reading selection that tissue oxygenation
  (A) is an object of transfusion therapy.
  (B) is not altered by 2,3-DPG levels.
  (C) does not depend on RBC oxygen affinity.
  (D) has no relation to length of storage of blood.
  (E) is of little concern.

51. It can be inferred from the reading selection that anemia is
  (A) best treated by whole blood.
  (B) influenced by quality of the RBC.
  (C) unrelated to tissue oxygenation.
  (D) best left untreated.
  (E) found more often in older persons.

52. It can be inferred from the reading selection that ATP
  (A) is directly related to 2,3-DPG levels.
  (B) doesn't decrease with time in storage.
  (C) has only a minimal effect on membrane stability.
  (D) is necessary to prevent hemolysis of the RBC.
  (E) is of no concern.

53. It can be inferred from the reading selection that patients should receive blood
  (A) with high plasma potassium levels.
  (B) consisting of only packed cells.
  (C) with high 2,3-DPG levels.
  (D) only if anemic.
  (E) only if it has not been stored.

There are probably more myths associated with the drinking of alcohol than with any other form of human behavior. The use of alcoholic beverages can be traced to prehistoric times and today 85% of the adults drink without apparent ill effects. Ethyl alcohol which is commonly consumed is nonpoisonous; it is quickly oxidized and degraded. Methyl alcohol is oxidized into a poison that damages the nervous system and often leads to blindness and death of the consumer; ethyl alcohol is oxidized in the liver to acetaldehyde which is oxidized into acetic acid and on into carbon dioxide and water.

The most pronounced physiological effect of alcohol is exerted upon the nervous system; the extent depends on the concentration in the blood and tissues. Two to three ounces (0.05% in the blood) depresses the centers of inhibition, restraint and judgement; five to six ounces (blood level of 0.1%) depresses the somewhat lower motor areas concerned with locomotion. After a consumption of ten ounces (blood level of 0.2%) the entire motor area is affected and the consumer is unable to walk; also the midbrain where emotional behavior is largely controlled is influenced and rage and tears are easily elicited. After drinking a pint (blood level of 0.3%) a person is still conscious but stupified, but when the level in the blood reaches 0.4 to 0.5% the complete perception areas of the brain are suppressed and coma results. When the concentration reaches 0.6 to 0.7%, the autonomic centers that control the heart and respiratory centers are affected and death ensues rapidly.

Ethyl alcohol may owe its toxic properties in part to its adsorption on the oxidative enzyme machinery of the brain cells which then results in the suppression of normal metabolic processes. Competition for these surfaces between ethyl alcohol and normal metabolites would be proportional to the concentration of ethyl alcohol in the system. Tissues show first an increased oxygen uptake, which normalizes relatively quickly and then starts to decrease. It is assumed that during the first phase ethyl alcohol is adsorbed on the oxidizing surfaces hitherto unoccupied, and therefore does not interfere with other metabolites, resulting in a net increase in the rate of oxygen uptake. When saturation is approached, competition with other metabolites begins and alcohol wins out because of its high concentration and easier permeability of the cell membranes, resulting in a fall in the rate of oxygen uptake.

The following statements are related to the passage above. Based on the information given, select:

(A)   if the statement is *supported by* the information in the passage.
(B)   if the statement is *contradicted by* the information in the passage.
(C)   if the statement is *neither supported nor contradicted by* information in the passage.

54.   Ethyl alcohol is a stimulant in small doses.

55.   Ethyl alcohol usually exerts a depressant effect on humans.

56.   It is suggested that the drug acts on certain specific brain cells preferentially.

57.   The rate of oxygen uptake is decreased because of the slow oxidation of ethyl alcohol.

58.   The concentration of ethyl alcohol in the blood is a determining factor of the outcome of alcohol consumption.

59.   The vascular system is directly responsible for the effects of ethyl alcohol.

60.   Lower areas of the nervous system seem to be affected earlier.

In recent years college students have come to see themselves as purchasing a service, specifically that of education. They have demanded greater accountability, asking that the remuneration of faculty members be tied to teaching effectiveness. Many faculty members agree with the concept in theory but feel that measurement of teaching effectiveness is flawed.

Teaching effectiveness is often determined through evaluations by administrators, faculty colleagues, or students, or by a combination of two or more of these evaluations. Students are usually most interested in evaluations by students, believing that they are the "consumers" who are most directly affected by the quality of the "product" called teaching.

Faculty members counter that evaluations by students are flawed, in that they are affected by the charisma (or lack of it) of the instructor, the level of difficulty of the subject matter, and the grades given in the course.

A more objective method has been suggested by various groups—the student performance at the end of the course. All students taking a particular course could be given a standard test; mean scores in sections taught by different instructors could then be compared and related to each instructor's teaching effectiveness. The results could be affected, of course, by the students' IQs, motivation, and prior instruction in the material covered by the course.

61. The main purpose of this passage is to discuss
   (A) faculty remuneration.
   (B) factors affecting the high cost of education.
   (C) the rising tide of "consumerism."
   (D) evaluation of teaching effectiveness.

62. According to the passage
   (A) all suggested methods of evaluation of teaching effectiveness are quite subjective.
   (B) the charisma of the instructor is a factor in evaluation of teaching effectiveness.
   (C) evaluations of an instructor's teaching effectiveness are unaffected by student grades.
   (D) evaluations of an instructor's teaching effectiveness are affected by the time of day when lectures are given.

63. According to the passage, greater difficulty of the course would have what effect on student ratings of teacher effectiveness?
   (A) lower ratings
   (B) higher ratings
   (C) no effect
   (D) The passage does not say.

64. The author indicates that students are most interested in ratings of teaching effectiveness when determined by
   (A) evaluation by faculty colleagues.
   (B) evaluation by administrators.
   (C) evaluation by students.
   (D) objectively determined progress of the performance of the class.

It has long been believed that one's order of birth in the family has an effect on achievement in school. A study recently reported a comparison of mathematics grades between women who were separated into three groups: (1) first born, (2) at least second born but not last born, and (3) last born, in a family. Women without siblings were excluded from the study.

The results indicate a statistical difference in mathematics grades between groups (1) and (3) but no other significant differences. Group (1) achieved higher mathematics grades than group (3).

Theories of motivation and anxiety have been advanced to explain the difference in achievement. The motivation theory states that the oldest child receives more encouragement from the parents than is given to other children. For a time the first child is the only child, an experience not shared by the other children. Particularly during this early period the parents may try very hard to help the child, thus striving to experience vicariously their own unfulfilled expectations.

The anxiety theory adds another factor to try to explain the lower achievement of the youngest child. Not only is the youngest child not pushed, as was the case with her older siblings, but this lack of parental pushing may be interpreted as lack of parental interest.

The youngest child may develop feelings of anxiety, and these may interfere with performance. Thus the youngest child may suffer as a result of less parental pressure and expectations as well as suffering from self-imposed anxiety—both contributing to lower performance.

65. This passage deals primarily with
   (A) differences in mathematics achievement between males and females.
   (B) differences in achievement of students between mathematics and other courses.
   (C) differences in achievement of females according to birth order.
   (D) the effect of parents' love on mathematics achievement.

66. Comparison of mathematics achievement between middle children and last-born children
   (A) showed higher achievement in the former.
   (B) showed higher achievement in the latter.
   (C) showed no statistically significant difference between the two groups.

67. The author suggests that anxiety
   (A) has no effect on mathematics achievement.
   (B) decreases mathematics achievement.
   (C) increases mathematics achievement.
   (D) can only be imposed by others.

68. The author introduces how many separate theories to explain a difference in mathematics achievement between first-born and last-born children?
   (A) 2   (C) 4
   (B) 3   (D) 5

SKILLS ANALYSIS: QUANTITATIVE

85 MINUTES
68 QUESTIONS

The following questions are to be answered based on your knowledge of basic mathematical principles and relationships.

DIRECTIONS: Read each passage carefully, study each table or chart, then answer the questions following it. Consider only the material presented in answering the questions. Eliminate those choices that you think to be incorrect and mark the letter of your choice on the answer sheet.

Blood samples from two groups of rats were assayed for luteinizing hormone (LH) in two separate radioimmunoassays. Half the rats were intact and half were orchidectomized. Some samples in each group were collected in the morning and some were collected in the afternoon. The data are summarized in the following table:

	Assay 1				Assay 2		
#	Intact or Orchid X.	Sampled AM or PM	LH ng/ml	#	Intact or Orchid X.	Sampled AM or PM	LH ng/ml
1	I	AM	5.0	11	I	PM	7.5
2	O	AM	50	12	O	PM	75
3	I	PM	4.8	13	I	AM	7.7
4	O	PM	480	14	O	AM	770
5	I	AM	5.2	15	I	PM	7.3
6	O	AM	52	16	O	PM	250
7	I	PM	5.1	17	I	AM	7.4
8	O	PM	350	18	O	AM	100
9	I	AM	4.9	19	I	PM	7.6
10	O	AM	100	20	O	PM	640

The following statements are related to the information presented above. Based on the information given, select:

(A) if the statement is *supported by* the information given.
(B) if the statement is *contradicted by* the information given.
(C) if the statement is *neither supported nor contradicted by* information given.

1. Orchidectomy is followed by increased levels of LH in the blood.

2. Blood LH levels are higher in the afternoon than in the morning.

3. Assays 1 and 2 are measuring different molecules.

4. The differences between LH values in these 2 assays are probably explained by interassay variations since the ratios between intact and orchidectomized levels are similar.

5. LH release in the orchidectomized rats may be occurring episodically.

6. The results of the 2 assays could be compared more precisely if some of the samples had been included in both assays.

7. Larger volumes of blood were assayed in Assay 1 than in Assay 2.

8. A significant change in LH release would be seen in intact rats had samples been taken at noon.

Ovulation in the rat can be blocked by systemic administration of drugs which depress neural function. However, ovulation depends on the response of the ovaries to LH released from the pituitary gland. In the following experiment drug X was injected subcutaneously at 13:45 hours into several groups of rats and the presence or absence of ova in the oviduct determined on the following morning. In order to pinpoint the site of action of the drug attempts were made to restore ovulation by stimulation of the brain; injection of LRF, the hormone which causes pituitary LH release; and injection of LH, which induces ovulation. The results are summarized below.

Treatment	Number of Rats Treated	Number of Rats Ovulating
Drug X	10	1
Drug X + LRF	10	5
Drug X + LH	10	5
Drug X + Brain Stimulation	10	1

The following statements are related to the information presented. Based on the information given, select:

(A)   if the statement is *supported by* the information given.
(B)   if the statement is *contradicted by* the information given.
(C)   if the statement is *neither supported nor contradicted by* information given.

9.   The testes are responsible for the production of LH.

10.   The ovaries are responsible for the production of LH.

11.   Drug X may be blocking the release of LRF from the brain and thereby preventing the activation of pituitary LH release.

12.   Drug X may be preventing pituitary LH release in response to LRF.

13.   Drug X appears to interfere with the ovarian response to LH.

14.   Drug X does not affect the brain since stimulation of the brain does not restore ovulation.

15.   Injection of drug X at 21:00 hours would be equally effective since its effect is at the ovary.

16.   The effect of drug X on the brain is greater than its effect on the ovary.

17.   Drug X would be a useful oral contraceptive in the human.

18.   Drug X functions as a competitive inhibitor of LH action on the ovary.

Use the following table as a reference to answer questions 19-21:

Country	Crude Birth Rate	Crude Death Rate
Lebanon	54	26
Egypt	50	26
India	50	25
Pakistan	49	26
USSR	43	18
East Germany	18	10
West Germany	16	16
France	35	11
Spain	19	7
Holland	45	8
Luxemburg	17	11.8
Japan	15	13

19.   Which of the countries in the table shows the most rapid population growth?
(A) Spain
(B) Holland
(C) USSR
(D) Lebanon
(E) Japan

20.   Which country can claim the lowest rate of population growth?
(A) East Germany
(B) Luxemburg
(C) Japan
(D) West Germany
(E) India

21. Which country has the longest doubling time?
    (A) India
    (B) East Germany
    (C) Japan
    (D) France
    (E) Lebanon

Female albino rats weighing between 170 and 230 g were housed in pairs in wire bottom cages and received a standard diet of rat pellets and chlorinated water *ad libitum*. Unanesthetized rats were restrained and shielded with lead so that only the head and neck regions were exposed. The animals received 6400 R of X-radiation in a single dose. Following irradiation careful check was maintained on the water and food consumption. Also, at varying intervals after exposure the animals were killed and the wet weights of their parotid salivary glands were determined. The results of these follow-ups are depicted below:

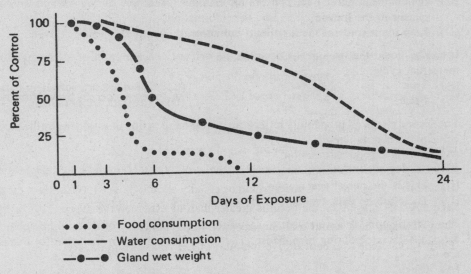

●●●●● Food consumption
---- Water consumption
—●—● Gland wet weight

22. These experiments were designed to determine if
    (A) variation in sex causes differences in rodent salivary glands.
    (B) exposure to X-radiation causes premature death in female rats.
    (C) chlorinated water *ad libitum* determines the wet weight of parotid glands.
    (D) X-radiation causes alteration in water consumption and volume of salivary glands in rats.

23. The first parameter measured in this experiment which was affected by 6400 R of X-radiation was
    (A) percent of chlorinated water given to the animals.
    (B) water consumption.
    (C) wet weight of the glands.
    (D) food intake.

24. Which of the following statements is true concerning the data obtained from this experiment?
    (A) The animals continued to consume large quantities of water up to the time of death.
    (B) An alteration in food consumption was already evident at 3 days after radiation.
    (C) Even though drinking and eating declined, the weights of the salivary glands remained unaffected until time of death.
    (D) Water consumption and wet weight of the glands first began to vary from control values at 8 days.

Levels of estrogens in the urine of the human female during the menstrual cycle, pregnancy, and the post-menopausal period were obtained from women during some routine work-ups during their visits to the ob-gyn clinic. The following data were obtained.

Time	Estriol μg/24 h	Estrone μg/24 h	Estradiol μg/24 h
Onset of menstruation	9	7	3
Ovulation peak	30	24	10
Luteal peak	20	18	9
Pregnancy, 150 days	10	1	.5
Pregnancy, term	35	4	2
Postmenopause	2	2	1

25. The object of the experiment was to
  (A) develop a technique for estrogen assay.
  (B) see if females possessed estrogens in urine.
  (C) obtain meaningful data concerning estrogen excretion during various reproductive phases of the female.
  (D) keep the records of these patients complete.

26. It can be noted that two peaks occur in the urinary concentration of estrogens during the menstrual cycle.
  (A) True.
  (B) False.
  (C) There are not sufficient data.
  (D) The data are not clear.

27. The second rise in all probability reflects an increased secretion of estrogens by the theca luteal cells of the corpus luteum.
  (A) This is a good assumption.
  (B) This is a bad assumption.
  (C) This is the purest speculation.
  (D) There are no data available at all to make such an assumption.

28. The investigators also were able to speculate as to the source of the minimal quantities of estrogens excreted during menopause. The organs most likely responsible for this estrogen are the
  (A) testes.
  (B) uterus.
  (C) adrenals (cortex).
  (D) vagina.

Twenty male New Zealand albino rabbits were divided into four groups of 5 animals each and treated as follows:

Group 1: Received a subcutaneous injection of 10×10^{-6} sheep red blood cells at two week intervals for a total of three injections.

Group 2: Received an intradermal injection of 10×10^{-6} sheep red blood cells at two week intervals for a total of three injections.

Group 3: Received a subscapular injection of 10×10^{-6} sheep red blood cells at two week intervals for a total of three injections.

Group 4: Received an intravenous injection of 10×10^{-6} sheep red blood cells at two week intervals for a total of three injections.

During the six week immunization period antibody titers against sheep red blood cells were measured and the following results obtained:

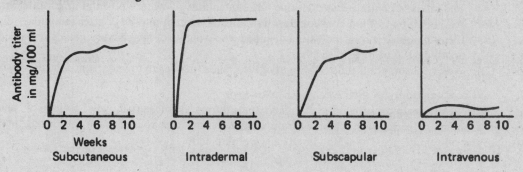

29. The purpose of this study was to
   (A) assay the rate of antigen clearance from immunized animals.
   (B) determine the effect of different routes of administration on antibody titer.
   (C) determine the effect of sheep red blood cells on total I_gG content of serum.
   (D) determine the effect of different antigen dosage on antibody titer.

30. These data show that
   (A) there is little difference in the results produced by the various routes of administration.
   (B) there is little difference between subscapular and subcutaneous injection routes.
   (C) the animals receiving intravenous red blood cells were immunologically incompetent.
   (D) antigen clearance was most rapid in the animals receiving intradermal injections.

31. It may also be seen that
   (A) intravenous administration of antigen leads to anaphylactic shock.
   (B) subscapular administration produces delayed hypersensitivity.
   (C) subcutaneous administration produces a generalized Arthus reaction.
   (D) intradermal administration produces the highest antibody titer.

An experimental drug, S24953, may maintain hepatic fatty acid oxidation at a normal rate in ethanol-treated rats. The following groups were studied at 8, 16, and 32 hours after administration of ethyl alcohol and glucose. Biochemically speaking a fatty liver is the end result of ethanol consumption.

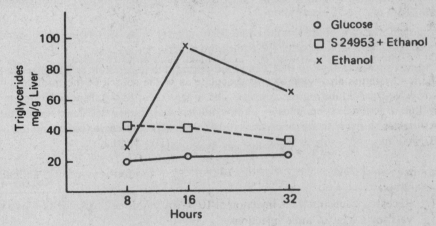

The following statements are related to the information presented above. Based on the information given, select:
   (A) if the statement is *supported by* the information given.
   (B) if the statement is *contradicted by* the information given.
   (C) if the statement is *neither supported nor contradicted by* the information given.

32. The experimental data point to a complete prevention of ethanol-induced fatty liver by S24953.

33. The peak of the ethanol-induced fatty liver was observed around 16 hours after consumption.

34. There was a 300% increase in the concentration of liver triglycerides.

35. At 32 hours the fatty liver was still present but it was reduced about 30%.

36. Liver triglyceride levels after ethanol while down at 32 hours still were about 100% above control levels.

37. Food consumption was increased at 12 to 16 hours.

38. Although S24953 prevents an ethanol-induced fatty liver, when S24953 is given alone it produces an absolute decrease in liver triglycerides.

39. Glucose and S24953 given together exhibit a synergistic effect on liver triglycerides.

A blood sample was taken from a test subject. Then a masked man came in with a gun and appeared to murder 2 persons. The test subject was visibly upset. After 30 seconds, the "victims" stood up. The subject was told of the hoax, and blood samples were taken over a period of time for counting red blood cells (RBC).

Time	RBC/mm³ of Blood
Control (before "murder")	5.5 million
30 seconds after "murder"	5.9 million
6.5 minutes after "murder"	7.0 million
14.5 minutes after "murder"	5.6 million
18.5 minutes after "murder"	5.5 million

The following statements are related to the information presented above. Based on the information given, select:

(A) if the statement is *supported by* the information given.
(B) if the statement is *contradicted by* the information given.
(C) if the statement is *neither supported nor contradicted by* information given.

40. There was an increase in the RBC/mm³ of blood of the test subject a few minutes after he thought he witnessed murder.

41. A larger change in the RBC/mm³ of blood would have been noted if the test subject had been placed in greater fear for his own life.

42. Having changed from the control value, there was no return to the control value for over 20 minutes.

43. Although a return of RBC/mm³ of blood to control value was noted, a rebound would be expected within an hour after the end of the experiment.

44. The *percentage change* in RBCs in blood during this experiment is less than the *percentage change* in white blood cells in the blood.

Production of organic compounds by photosynthesis was studied in Puerto Rico. The results are given in the table below with the theoretical yield based on percentage of light captured by the plant.

Plants	Carbohydrate Production (tons/acre)		Percentage of Sunlight Captured by Plant
	Present	Theoretical	
Kelp	2.0	14	15
Cane	0.7	0.9	1.0
Plant Z	4.1	18	20

45. The protein yield per acre would be greatest from
(A) kelp.
(B) cane.
(C) plant Z.
(D) no basis for comparison.

46. If one doubled the incident light on an acre of cultivated kelp, how would the yield of kelp compare with the yield of an acre of plant Z on which the incident light was unchanged?
(A) It would surpass the carbohydrate yield per acre.
(B) It would approach the carbohydrate yield per acre.
(C) It would surpass the protein yield per acre.
(D) It would surpass the percentage of incident light captured.

47. It is decided that sugar syrup for sweetening purposes will be made from each of the plants. When the carbohydrate content is equal, the sugar syrup from plant Z is not accepted by the tasters. This might be because of
(A) impurities with bad tastes.
(B) a large percentage of the carbohydrate of this plant is not sweet.
(C) A and/or B.
(D) none of the above.

48. Without changing the incident sunlight, the largest percentage increase that is theoretically possible is predicted for
    (A) plant Z.
    (B) kelp.
    (C) cane.

Use the following table as a reference to answer questions 49-54:

MIDDLE INCOME PEOPLE

| | Food Consumed Predominantly | | | Type of Tooth Decay (percent) | | | Type of Toothpaste Used (grams/brushing) | |
Samples	Starchy Foods	Meaty Foods	Liquids	I	II	III	I	II
1	79	6.6	8	69	61	7	23	27
2	38	27	12	35	31	7	6	7
3	9	26	40	9	5	1	2	3

The following statements are related to the information presented above. Based on the information given, select:
    (A) if the statement is *supported by* the information given.
    (B) if the statement is *contradicted by* the information given.
    (C) if the statement is *neither supported nor contradicted by* information given.

49. Considering the group classified as starch eaters, there does not seem a noticeable difference between the types of tooth decay and the sample of population.

50. The average diet consumed results in less tooth decay.

51. As shown in sample 3, the less tooth paste that was used the fewer the cavities.

52. Sample 3 exhibited less tooth decay.

53. The type of tooth decay can be correlated and based on a particular diet.

54. Amount of tooth paste used significantly influences dental problems.

Use the following graphs to answer questions 55-57:

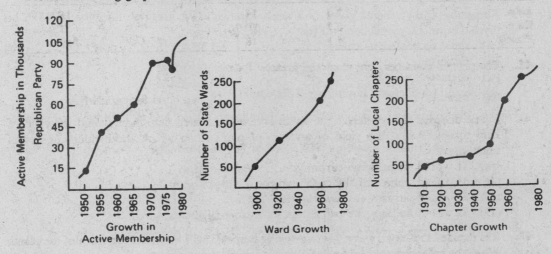

55. Based solely on the size of the membership trend and size of membership the Republican party seems to be strong.
    (A) True
    (B) False
    (C) Not enough information

56. The total number of wards and chapters, like total membership, is at an all-time high.
(A) True
(B) False
(C) Not enough information

57. There is every reason to believe that given a change in leadership this growth can be maintained and steadily increased.
(A) True
(B) False
(C) Not enough information

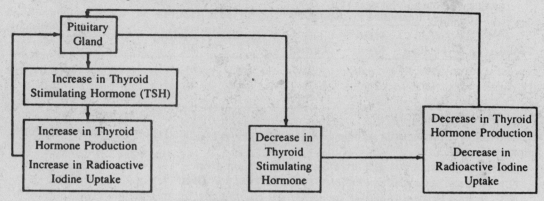

The pituitary gland is responsible for the secretion of thyroid stimulating hormone (TSH), which elicits an increased production of thyroid hormone from the gland; this thyroid hormone then may inhibit the pituitary via a negative feedback. Under hyperthyroid conditions, the following tests would give elevated values:

1. Basal metabolic rate (BMR)
2. Protein bound iodine (PBI)
3. Radioactive iodine uptake (RAI)

58. When TSH secretion falls, the secretion by the thyroid of thyroid hormone
(A) stays the same.   (C) decreases.
(B) increases.   (D) will feed back upon the pituitary.

59. According to the schema given, if a normal individual is given an injection of TSH, his thyroid hormone production will first
(A) show no noticeable change.
(B) increase.
(C) decrease.
(D) lead to a decrease in pituitary TSH output.

Use the information in the flow chart and paragraph above, and in the following graphs, to answer questions 60–62:

RAI Uptake After Administration of Thyroid Hormone

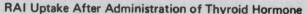
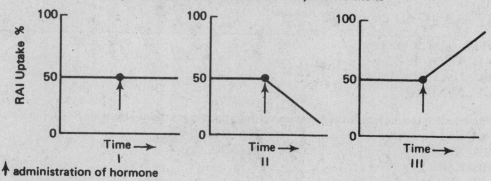

60. In which of the graphs is there evidence of thyroid malfunction?
(A) I
(B) I and II
(C) I and III
(D) III

61. Which graph(s) probably represent(s) the case of a typical hyperthyroid person?
(A) II
(B) I
(C) I and III
(D) II and III

62. Which of the graphs lead(s) you to believe that there is a breakdown in the normal thyroid-pituitary functional relationship?
(A) I and III
(B) III
(C) II
(D) II and III

The solubility of a solute varies with the temperature. All points on a solubility curve represent saturated solutions. Points below a curve represent unsaturated solutions. Solubility curves for various salts and gases are shown in the following graph.

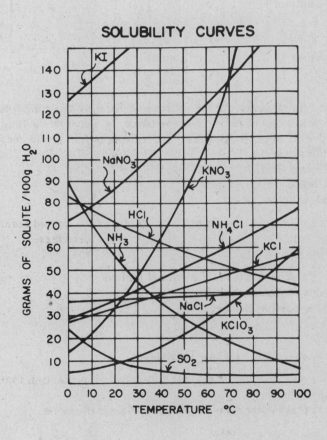

63. Which salt has the greatest solubility at 20°C?
(A) KNO_3
(B) NaCl
(C) $NaNO_3$
(D) KI
(E) $KClO_3$

64. Which salt has a solubility that is minimally affected by temperature?
(A) KCl
(B) NaCl
(C) KI
(D) $NaNO_3$
(E) $KClO_3$

65. If 80 grams of salt is dissolved in 100 grams of water at 60°C, which of the following will form an unsaturated solution?
   (A) NH_4Cl
   (B) $KClO_3$
   (C) KNO_3
   (D) NaCl
   (E) KCl

66. If 50 grams of NH_4Cl is dissolved in 100 grams of water at 70°C, approximately how many grams of salt must be added to produce a saturated solution?
   (A) 10
   (B) 20
   (C) 30
   (D) 40
   (E) 50

67. How many grams of KNO_3 must be added to 200 grams of water at 50°C to produce a saturated solution?
   (A) 32
   (B) 85
   (C) 120
   (D) 150
   (E) 170

68. If the curves for NH_3, SO_2, and HCl are typical of gases in general, which statement is correct?
   (A) Solubility of gases is unaffected by temperature.
   (B) Solubility of gases varies inversely with temperature.
   (C) Solubility of gases varies directly with temperature.

Model Test A Answers*

SCIENCE KNOWLEDGE

Biology

1. A	9. C	17. C	25. B	32. A
2. C	10. B	18. B	26. E	33. C
3. C	11. A	19. B	27. B	34. A
4. A	12. B	20. A	28. B	35. A
5. B	13. A	21. B	29. E	36. E
6. D	14. C	22. B	30. C	37. C
7. E	15. B	23. C	31. B	38. A
8. C	16. A	24. B		

Chemistry

1. D	9. A	17. B	25. B	32. A
2. C	10. D	18. E	26. D	33. B
3. B	11. B	19. A	27. C	34. C
4. D	12. B	20. E	28. D	35. E
5. E	13. C	21. A	29. A	36. E
6. C	14. A	22. A	30. D	37. D
7. B	15. B	23. C	31. D	38. D
8. B	16. A	24. B		

Physics

1. A	8. C	15. D	22. D	28. D
2. D	9. C	16. C	23. C	29. E
3. B	10. B	17. D	24. E	30. D
4. E	11. D	18. A	25. C	31. A
5. D	12. E	19. E	26. C	32. D
6. A	13. B	20. B	27. B	33. B
7. A	14. A	21. D		

SCIENCE PROBLEMS

1.	B	13.	D	25.	D	37.	D	49.	A
2.	C	14.	E	26.	C	38.	A	50.	A
3.	C	15.	C	27.	E	39.	B	51.	B
4.	B	16.	D	28.	A	40.	B	52.	B
5.	C	17.	B	29.	C	41.	C	53.	C
6.	A	18.	C	30.	E	42.	E	54.	C
7.	A	19.	D	31.	E	43.	C	55.	A
8.	D	20.	D	32.	A	44.	E	56.	C
9.	B	21.	C	33.	C	45.	A	57.	A
10.	B	22.	A	34.	D	46.	B	58.	A
11.	C	23.	B	35.	A	47.	B	59.	C
12.	A	24.	B	36.	E	48.	A	60.	B

SKILLS ANALYSIS: READING

1.	B	15.	B	29.	C	43.	A	56.	B
2.	C	16.	D	30.	B	44.	B	57.	B
3.	A	17.	C	31.	C	45.	A	58.	A
4.	A	18.	D	32.	B	46.	C	59.	B
5.	A	19.	B	33.	A	47.	B	60.	A
6.	C	20.	A	34.	B	48.	A	61.	B
7.	C	21.	B	35.	A	49.	C	62.	B
8.	A	22.	B	36.	B	50.	A	63.	D
9.	B	23.	B	37.	C	51.	B	64.	C
10.	C	24.	B	38.	C	52.	D	65.	C
11.	B	25.	C	39.	C	53.	C	66.	C
12.	C	26.	B	40.	B	54.	C	67.	B
13.	B	27.	A	41.	A	55.	A	68.	A
14.	B	28.	C	42.	C				

SKILLS ANALYSIS: QUANTITATIVE

1.	A	15.	C	29.	B	43.	C	56.	A
2.	B	16.	C	30.	B	44.	C	57.	C
3.	C	17.	C	31.	D	45.	D	58.	C
4.	A	18.	C	32.	A	46.	B	59.	B
5.	A	19.	B	33.	A	47.	C	60.	C
6.	A	20.	D	34.	A	48.	B	61.	B
7.	C	21.	C	35.	A	49.	C	62.	A
8.	C	22.	D	36.	B	50.	B	63.	D
9.	B	23.	D	37.	C	51.	C	64.	B
10.	B	24.	B	38.	C	52.	A	65.	C
11.	A	25.	C	39.	C	53.	C	66.	A
12.	B	26.	A	40.	A	54.	C	67.	E
13.	A	27.	A	41.	C	55.	A	68.	B
14.	A	28.	C	42.	B				

Explanation of Answers for Science Questions–Model Test A

SCIENCE KNOWLEDGE

Biology

1. **(A)** Chorionic gonadotropin is produced by the placenta and acts with other reproductive hormones to maintain pregnancy.

2. **(C)** A biotic factor is a living portion of the ecosystem. Predators are organisms which attack and kill other living animals. The other choices are abiotic factors.

3. **(C)** Cortisol is produced by the adrenal and is active in the conversion of proteins to carbohydrates.

4. **(A)** Replicating strands of DNA separate from each other when bonds are broken between their nitrogenous bases. The two strands of DNA are held together by weak hydrogen bonds between the bases of each strand.

5. **(B)** Vasopressin (ADH) elaborated by the hypothalamus has an antidiuretic action on the kidney tubules.

6. **(D)** Maltase, also a component of saliva, participates in starch digestion.

7. **(E)** Chitin, mucus, and keratin are products elaborated by epithelial cells.

8. **(C)** The striated muscle fiber is multinucleated.

9. **(C)** The tsetse fly transmits African sleeping sickness to humans.

10. **(B)** Complete metamorphosis comprises the following sequence:

    egg → larva → pupa → adult

11. **(A)** One of the distinguishing features of chordates is a dorsal tubular nerve cord.

12. **(B)** The cell is the basic unit of structure and function and the basis of all life; all cells come from preexisting cells.

13. **(A)** Ribosomes can be free floating or they may be attached to the endoplasmic reticulum which is then called rough endoplasmic reticulum (RER).

14. **(C)** Lysosomes contain hydrolytic enzymes and are also known as digestive bags, etc.

15. **(B)** The pituitary gland is located within the sella tursica.

16. **(A)** Ectoderm is the germ layer of origin of the nervous system.

17. **(C)** Stress and strain will have a pronounced influence on the output of epinephrine and norepinephrine by the adrenal medulla. Activation of the sympathetic portion of the autonomic nervous system will result in increased activity by the adrenal medulla which can be considered the site of the postganglionic cell bodies of that segment of the sympathetics.

18. **(B)** Mesoderm is the germ layer of origin of the skeletal system.

19. **(B)** Connective tissue, cartilage, and bone are basically supporting tissues. An abundance of nonliving-formed substance is the feature that is common to the group as a whole. Cells are interspersed in the intercellular substance and fibers are a constituent of the formed substance. Fibers and ground substance are called matrix.

20. **(A)** Human sperm and ova are similar in the respect that they both carry a haploid chromosomal complement. After fertilization the diploid composition is again found.

21. **(B)** A group of nerve cell bodies is commonly considered to be the site of a nucleus.

22. **(B)** The neurolemma of an axon is a part of the Schwann cell (outer membrane).

23. **(C)** CO_2 and O_2 exchange takes place in the alveoli of the lung.

24. **(B)** Sweat glands, salivary glands, and sebaceous glands are all exocrine glands.

25. **(B)** The appendix is a blind sac originating from the cecum of the ascending colon (large intestines).

26. **(E)** Active transport requires energy and allows a cell to move material from a point of lower concentration to a point of higher concentration.

27. **(B)** The internal structure of a cilium or flagellum is composed of 9 outer and 2 inner pairs of tubules.

28. **(B)** It is the reproductive system that is highly specialized in the tapeworm.

29. **(E)** Sodium fluoride (or other fluoride salts) is added to drinking water in very small amounts in order to reduce the incidence of tooth decay.

30. **(C)** Treatment of municipal water supplies with chlorine (i.e., chlorination) is commonly practiced to kill harmful organisms.

31. **(B)** During metaphase of mitosis the centrioles with asters are at the opposite poles; the chromosomes move to the equator of the cell and duplicate.

32. **(A)** Cilia are utilized by planaria for movement.

33. **(C)** In an open circulatory system blood is not always enclosed within well defined blood vessels.

34. **(A)** The corpus callosum connects the two cerebral hemispheres in the mammal; association fibers cross in this bundle.

35. **(A)** A heterotroph is an organism that cannot make all the complex organic molecules necessary for the metabolic machinery of the system from simple molecules such as CO_2, H_2O, etc. Humans get these complex molecules from other living organisms. Photosynthetic organisms are autotrophs.

36. **(E)** Genetic drift is change in the gene pool through random processes, whose effectiveness as an evolutionary agent is seen only in small populations.

37. **(C)** The peculiar features of renal circulation, such as the renal arteries originating directly from the aorta, the glomerulo-capillary arrangement, and differences in the calibers of the afferent and efferent vessels, indicate that blood pressure is of great functional significance for the production of urine. The vascular component probably plays an important role in the filtration process.

38. **(A)** Salivary secretions come readily into contact with the host when the latter is bitten by an insect, and parasites can be transmitted via this mode.

Chemistry

1. **(D)** The general formula C_nH_{2n-2} applies to all members of the alkyne series. The suffix for names in this series is "yne." Ethyne is the only choice that has the correct ending.

2. **(C)** Addition of a crystal is commonly employed to induce crystal formation and precipitation in a supersaturated solution.

3. **(B)** Polytetrafluoroethylene is highly prized for its chemical inertness. It is also used as a dry lubricant. One of its tradenames is Teflon.

4. **(D)** Enzymes decrease the activation energy and thereby decrease the time to reach equilibrium. The equilibrium constant is not affected.

5. **(E)** Change of specific rotation of plane-polarized light as a result of conversion of one anomer to another is called mutarotation. It can occur only if the compound is able to go from the ring form to the straight-chain form and back to the ring form. In a glycoside the anomeric OH is tied up, and the compound cannot return to the straight-chain form.

6. **(C)** Ethers have the general formula R—O—R'. The other compounds have the following general formulas:

esters $\quad R-C{\overset{\displaystyle O}{\underset{\displaystyle O-R'}{\big<}}}$

aldehydes $\quad R-C{\overset{\displaystyle O}{\underset{\displaystyle H}{\big<}}}$

alcohols $\quad$ R—OH

ketones $\quad R-\underset{\displaystyle O}{\overset{\displaystyle \|}{C}}-R'$

7. **(B)** Molecular oxygen can associate with the iron atom on each heme group. There are four hemes per molecules of hemoglobin.

8. **(B)** The given equation can be balanced by inspection as follows:

$$4Al + 3O_2 \rightarrow 2Al_2O_3$$

The coefficient of Al is 4.

9. **(A)** A reaction that requires energy is an endothermic reaction while one that liberates energy is an exothermic reaction.

10. **(D)** This configuration: $-\underset{\displaystyle O}{\overset{\displaystyle \|}{C}}-OH$ is characteristic of carboxyl groups. A hydroxyl group is identified by — OH.

11. **(B)** The anode is a positive electrode attracting negatively charged particles while the cathode is the negative electrode attracting positively charged particles.

12. **(B)** In the absence of peroxides Markovnikov's rule would predict 2-bromobutane as the major product. HBr adds with the opposite orientation in the presence of peroxides, apparently by a free-radical mechanism rather than ionic mechanism.

13. **(C)** The gain of electrons is known as reduction, while the loss of electrons is classified as oxidation.

14. **(A)** This is basically a definition of eutectic temperature.

15. **(B)** The other half-cell reaction must release the electrons required by the first half-cell reaction, $Zn \rightarrow Zn^{2+} + 2e^-$.

16. **(A)** $K_{sp} = 6.2 \times 10^{-12} = [Ag^+]^2[CO_3^{2-}]$

$$[Ag^+]^2 = \frac{6.2 \times 10^{-12}}{[CO_3^{2-}]} = \frac{6.2 \times 10^{-12}}{6.2 \times 10^{-6}} = 1 \times 10^{-6}$$

$$[Ag^+] = \sqrt{1 \times 10^{-6}} = 1 \times 10^{-3} \text{ mole/liter}$$

17. **(B)** The K_{sp} of NiS is 1×10^{-26}

$$K_{sp} = [Ni^{2+}][S^{2-}]$$

$$[S^{2-}] = \frac{1 \times 10^{-26}}{1 \times 10^{-20}} = 1 \times 10^{-6} \text{ mole/liter}$$

18. **(E)** This is the definition of an amalgam

19. **(A)** Pyrolysis of dry acetic acid in the presence of ThO_2 produces acetone and CO_2. Longer chain acids produce higher ketones.

20. **(E)** There are 4 asymmetric centers, $2^4 = 16$. The best answer given is 17.

21. **(A)** Hydrofluoric acid reacts with glass, resulting in etching. Carbolic acid is a common name for phenol.

22. **(A)** Sulfur trioxide, SO_3, is often produced by the oxidation of any fuel that contains sulfur.
$SO_3 + H_2O \rightarrow H_2SO_4$ (sulfuric acid)
$SO_2 + H_2O \rightarrow H_2SO_3$ (sulfurous acid)

23. **(C)** The atomic number represents the number of protons in the nucleus and (in the uncharged atom) the number of electrons in the shells surrounding the nucleus. Neutrons are found in the nucleus but have no charge.

24. **(B)** An atom which has lost 2 electrons has a charge of $+2$; an atom which is electrically neutral has equal numbers of protons and electrons.

25. **(B)** Oparin believed that the early atmosphere lacked free oxygen. The atmosphere consisted mainly of water vapor, carbon dioxide, nitrogen and compounds such as ammonia and methane. Hydrogen, oxygen, carbon and nitrogen make up over 99% of the tissues of living things.

26. **(D)** This is an example of the Wurtz-Fittig (or Fittig-Wurtz) Reaction. The two rings will be joined, and halogen will be lost.

27. **(C)** $\emptyset CH_2Cl + \emptyset \xrightarrow{AlCl_3} \emptyset - CH_2 - \emptyset$
Friedel-Crafts Reaction
$\emptyset CH_2Cl + Na \longrightarrow \emptyset - CH_2CH_2 - \emptyset$
Wurtz Reaction

28. **(D)** The question has listed the general properties of organic compounds.

29. **(A)** Remember that nitro groups are deactivating, meta-directing substituents and that halogens are deactivating, ortho, para-directing substituents. If bromination precedes nitration, then very little m-bromonitrobenzene will result.

30. **(D)** Halogen on adjacent carbon atoms may be removed by heating with zinc duct in alcohol, yielding an alkene. Treatment of the 1,2-dihalide with alcoholic KOH would have produced the alkyne.

31. **(D)** Charles Goodyear discovered the process of vulcanization (the chemical reaction of rubber with sulfur) in 1839. Vulcanization produces a material with greater toughness and elasticity than natural rubber. This is so because sulfur adds to the double bonds in such a manner that the chains of rubber molecules are bound together, resulting in large, cross-linked molecules.

32. **(A)** This is the classic Diels-Alder condensation between a diene and a dienophile:

1,3-butadiene   ethylene   cyclohexene
(diene)   (dienophile)

33. **(B)** The K shell $(1s)$ is filled with 2 electrons. The L shell (subshells $2s$ and $2p$) is filled with 8 electrons. This element, fluorine, is a nonmetal that is most likely to gain one electron and fill the L shell.
This will give the atom a charge (and valence) of -1.

34. **(C)** See explanation for question 33.

35. **(E)** A nonmetal oxide reacts with water to form an acid.

$$P_2O_3 + 3H_2O \rightarrow 2H_3PO_3 \quad \text{(Phosphorus Acid)}$$

36. **(E)** The two sugars found in the nucleotides of nucleic acids are D-deoxyribose and D-ribose.

37. **(D)** $Cl-CH_2-\overset{\overset{\displaystyle O}{\|}}{C}-OH$ is simply chloroacetic acid.

$CH_3-\overset{\overset{\displaystyle O}{\|}}{C}-Cl$ is a mixed anhydride.

The other formulas are for acetic anhydride, the anhydride of phosphoric acid, and the anhydride of sulfuric acid.

38. **(D)** KCl is a salt. Salts contain ionic bonding between a metal and a nonmetal. The other compounds contain only covalent bonds between nonmetals.

Physics

1. **(A)** The pound is a unit of weight, or force. The SI unit of force is the newton, which is equivalent to $kg \cdot m/s^2$. The SI unit of time is the second. A pound per hour corresponds to a newton per second.

2. **(D)** Momentum is a vector and can change direction; energy is scalar and has no directional property.

3. **(B)** Kinetic energy keeps increasing as speed increases; thermal energy keeps increasing as more heat is produced; gravitational potential energy decreases with altitude.

4. **(E)** The force (F) varies as the inverse square of the distance, so doubling the force reduces the force to $F/4$. The force of A on B is always the same as the force of B on A.

5. **(D)** If two forces act upon each other at right angles, the following formula should be used:

$$R = \sqrt{(\text{Force 1})^2 + (\text{Force 2})^2}$$
$$R = \sqrt{(12)^2 + (16)^2}$$
$$R = 20 \text{ lb.}$$

6. **(A)** Any combination of forces acting upon the same object in the same direction will result in an addition of the forces and the result will be equal to the sum of the forces.

7. **(A)** The formula for determining pressure is $Pressure = \dfrac{Force}{Area}$. In the example the man's weight of 185 pounds is the force and the area of the shoe soles is 60 inch^2. Applying the formula

$$P = \frac{185 \text{ lb.}}{60 \text{ in.}^2} = 6.1 \text{ lb./in.}^2$$

8. **(C)** Specific gravity is usually expressed as the weight of an object in air divided by the loss of weight when weighed in water. In our example:

$$\text{Sp. G} = \frac{\text{Weight in Air}}{\text{Loss of Weight}} = \frac{720 \text{ oz}}{360 \text{ oz}} = 2$$

9. **(C)** If 0.5 remains after 1 cm, then $(0.5)^3$ will remain after 3 cm.
$(0.5)^3 = 0.125$ or 12.5%
$100\% - 12.5\% = 87.5\%$ stopped

10. **(B)** $v = r\omega$ where v = linear velocity, r = radius, and ω = angular velocity in radians/time (there are 2π radians/rev).
$v = 10 (2\pi \times 1000)$
$v = 20,000 \, \pi$ cm/min
$v = 62,800$ cm/min

11. **(D)** In the northern hemisphere winds circulate about a high pressure area in a clockwise direction. In the southern hemisphere winds circulate about a high pressure area in a counterclockwise direction.

12. **(E)** The image in a plane mirror is the same size as the object and as far behind the mirror as the object is in front.

13. **(B)** Work is equal to force times distance. A mass of 120 lb. exerts a force of 120 lb. with our gravitational acceleration.
120 lb. $\times$ 40 ft. = 4800 ft.-lb.

14. **(A)** $\dfrac{P_1 V_1}{T_1} = \dfrac{P_2 V_2}{T_2}$ where P is pressure, V is volume, T is temperature in kelvins. STP (standard temperature and pressure) is 273 K and 1 atm pressure.

$$\frac{1 \times 16}{273} = \frac{4V_2}{819 \text{ K}}$$
$$V_2 = 12$$

15. **(D)** Boyle's law states that the product of volume and pressure of a gas is a constant at constant temperature.
$P_1V_1 = P_2V_2$

$$V_2 = \frac{P_1}{P_2} V_1$$

If the pressure is doubled $\dfrac{P_1}{P_2} = \frac{1}{2}$. Thus $V_2 = \frac{1}{2} V_1$

16. **(C)** Acceleration is the rate of change of velocity, and the object returns with the same speed with which it was thrown upward, but in the opposite direction:

$$32 \text{ ft/sec}^2 = \frac{v_2 - v_1}{t}$$

$$= \frac{128 \text{ ft/sec} - (-128 \text{ ft/sec})}{t}$$

which gives $t = 8$ sec

17. **(D)** The boiling point of a liquid is the temperature at which the vapor pressure of a liquid equals the external pressure to which the system is subjected.

18. **(A)** The volume of the particles is equal to the increase in liquid level (i.e., $125 - 100 = 25$)

$$\frac{50 \text{ g}}{25 \text{ ml}} = 2 \text{ g/ml}$$

19. **(E)** Neither the wave nor the particle model alone explains the properties of light, which are best explained by a combination of the two models.

20. **(B)** $s = v_0 t + \frac{1}{2} g t^2$
$s = (0)t + \frac{1}{2} (32)(8)^2$
$s = 0 + 16 (64) = 1024 \text{ ft}$

21. **(D)** $v = at; t = 60 \text{ sec} = \frac{60}{3600} \text{ hr}$

22. **(D)** The resultant force is the difference between the two forces and, therefore, the two forces must be directly opposing each other (i.e., at 180°).

23. **(C)** Conduction is the transfer of molecular energy (heat) through matter. Convection is transfer of heat by vertical movement of a fluid. Hot objects radiate and cold objects absorb energy, converting it to heat. Evaporation removes heat and subsequent condensation deposits it somewhere else. Consumption has no meaning in this context.

24. **(E)** Celsius and Fahrenheit conversions utilize the following formulas:

$$F = \frac{9}{5} C + 32°$$

$$C = \frac{5}{9} (F - 32°)$$

25. **(C)** If the half-life is 21 days, then 42 days would represent two half-lives. In the first half-life 50% will be lost, and in the second half-life 50% of the remainder will be lost.

Remainder $= 0.5^n$ and $n =$ number of half-lives.
Remainder $= (0.5)^2 = 0.25$ or 25%

26. **(C)** Surface tension explains this phenomenon. Because of surface tension the pin may be floated on water even though the metal is denser.

27. **(B)** 1 kilogram $= 2.205$ pounds, avoirdupois
Therefore, $\frac{165 \text{ lb.}}{2.205 \text{ lb./kg}} = 74.8 \text{ kg}$

28. **(D)** The acceleration is the change in speed divided by the time factor necessary to achieve the change.

$$a = \frac{50 \text{ mi./hr.} - 10 \text{ mi./hr.}}{20 \text{ sec.}} = \frac{40 \text{ mi./hr.}}{20 \text{ sec.}}$$
$a = 2 \text{ mi./hr. per sec.}$

29. **(E)** If the elevator did not move, the man would be at equilibrium and the floor would exert a force of 200 lb. upon him. To move upward *additional force* is required.

$$F = \frac{W}{g} a = \frac{(200 \text{ lb.})(10 \text{ ft./sec.}^2)}{32 \text{ ft./sec.}^2} = 62.5 \text{ lb.}$$

The total force exerted upon the man is $F = 200 + 62.5 \text{ lb.} = 262.5 \text{ lb.}$

30. **(D)** Air resistance decreases the speed, the maximum height attained and the range of a projectile.

31. **(A)** The heat lost by the metal ball is equal to the heat gained by the ice, so all you would have to know is how such heat was needed to melt 50 g of ice.

32. **(D)** Since the force varies inversely as the square of the distance, the two forces will be equal when the distance from charge $+2q$ is 4 times as great as the distance from charge $+q$.

33. **(B)** A beta particle is an electron. When it is emitted, a neutron turns into a proton. This increases the atomic number by 1, but has no effect on the mass number.

SCIENCE PROBLEMS

1-3. **(1-B)** **(2-C)** **(3-C)** The answers to questions *1-3* are self-explanatory.

4-6. **(4-B)** **(5-C)** **(6-A)** The answers to questions *4-6* are self-explanatory.

7. **(A)** The atmospheric pressure that will support a column of mercury 760 mm high will support the same weight of water.
$760 \times 14 = 10640$ or 1.0×10^4

8. **(D)** Since $P_1 V_1 = P_2 V_2$, a decreased pressure leads to an increased volume. The balloon will become larger; only if the volume change is large enough will the balloon explode.

9. **(B)** This is essentially the converse of the above question. Since the pressure has increased, the volume must decrease. This can occur in this case only by the crumpling of the can.

10. **(B)**

$$H_3C-\overset{\overset{\displaystyle O}{\|}}{C}-Cl + H_2O \rightarrow H_3C-\overset{\overset{\displaystyle O}{\|}}{C}-OH + HCl$$

Both of the products are acids.

$$H_3C-\overset{\overset{\displaystyle O}{\|}}{C}-O-\overset{\overset{\displaystyle O}{\|}}{C}-CH_3 + H_2O \rightarrow 2H_3C-\overset{\overset{\displaystyle O}{\|}}{C}-OH$$

Two moles of product are formed from one mole of starting material, but there is only one product

$$\begin{array}{c}H_2C-\overset{\overset{\displaystyle O}{\|}}{C}\\ | \qquad\qquad\diagdown\\ \qquad\qquad\quad O\\ | \qquad\qquad\diagup\\ H_2C-\overset{\underset{\displaystyle O}{\|}}{C}\end{array} + H_2O \rightarrow \begin{array}{c}H_2C-\overset{\overset{\displaystyle O}{\|}}{C}-OH\\ |\\ H_2C-\overset{\underset{\displaystyle O}{\|}}{C}-OH\end{array}$$

11. **(C)** See the preceding explanation.

12. **(A)** See the explanation above.

13. **(D)** Since the solutions are of equal molarity, there will be equal numbers of molecules. But, NaCl produces one particle (ion) per molecule; glucose does not ionize and thus gives only one particle per molecule; $Ba(NO_3)_2$ produces three particles per molecule; and HCl produces two ions per molecule. With a greater number of particles the $Ba(NO_3)_2$ solution will have the greater osmotic pressure.

14. **(E)** Since $P = cRT$, a one degree rise in T will produce the same percentage increase in all these solutions.

15. **(C)** See the answer to question 13. The value of R does not change unless we wish to change the units in which R and the remaining parts of the equation are expressed.

16. **(D)** Purebred white (bb) Rough coat (RR) mated to purebred black (BB) smooth coat (rr).

male bbRR × BBrr female

Sperms bR × Br eggs

F₁ BbRr all black with rough coats

BbRr × BbRr

sperm Br, Br, bR, br × eggs BR, Br, bR, br

17. **(B)** Four types of offspring.

18. **(C)** Black-rough 9; black-smooth 3; white rough 3; white-smooth 1.

19. **(D)** From 27 to 30°C the Δt is 3°C.
$\Delta L = \alpha L_1$, $\Delta t = \alpha L_1$ (3) or 3 αL_1.

20. **(D)** $\Delta L = \alpha L_1 \Delta t$
cm = α (cm) (°C)

$$\alpha = \frac{cm}{(cm)(°C)} = \frac{1}{°C} = °C^{-1}$$

21. **(C)** The greatest increase in length will occur with the greatest coefficient of linear expansion. This will cause the joined strip to curve away from the metal with greatest α.

22. **(A)** In beaker (1)
$$[Ba^{2+}] = \frac{2 \times 10^{-6}}{[F^-]^2} = \frac{2 \times 10^{-6}}{(1 \times 10^{-2})^2} = \frac{2 \times 10^{-6}}{1 \times 10^{-4}}$$
$$= 2 \times 10^{-2}$$

In beaker (2)
$$[Ba^{2+}] = \frac{7 \times 10^{-9}}{[CO_3^{2-}]} = \frac{7 \times 10^{-9}}{7 \times 10^{-5}} = 1 \times 10^{-4}$$

23. **(B)** With F⁻
$$[Ba^{2+}] = \frac{2 \times 10^{-6}}{(0.1)^2} = \frac{2 \times 10^{-6}}{1 \times 10^{-2}} = 2 \times 10^{-4}$$

With CO_3^{2-}
$$[Ba^{2+}] = \frac{7 \times 10^{-9}}{0.01} = \frac{7 \times 10^{-9}}{1 \times 10^{-2}} = 7 \times 10^{-7}$$

24. **(B)** In the beaker with F⁻
$$[F^-]^2 = \frac{2 \times 10^{-6}}{[Ba^{2+}]} = \frac{2 \times 10^{-6}}{1 \times 10^{-1}} = 2 \times 10^{-3}$$

and $[F^-] = 4.5 \times 10^{-3}$
In the beaker with CO_3^{2-}

$$[CO_3^{2-}] = \frac{7 \times 10^{-9}}{[Ba^{2+}]} = \frac{7 \times 10^{-9}}{1 \times 10^{-1}} = 7 \times 10^{-8}$$

Thus, the beaker with CO_3^{2-} would have the lower concentration of the α anion in question. (In the other beaker the calculations indicate there will be no precipitation of F⁻ under these conditions.)

25. **(D)** One mole of iodine (254 g) will react with one mole of fatty acid having one double bond; two moles of iodine (508 g) will react with one mole of fatty acid having two double bonds.
For compounds (1) and (2):
$$\frac{254}{254} = \frac{x}{100} \qquad x = 100 \text{ for iodine number}$$
Compound (3) does not react with iodine and thus has an iodine number of zero. For compound (4) with two double bonds

$$\frac{504}{280} = \frac{x}{100} \qquad x = 180 \text{ for iodine number}$$

26. **(C)** See answer above.

27. **(E)** See answer above. Compounds (1) and (2) have equal iodine numbers, but this combination is not one of the answers given.

28-30. **(28-A) (29-C) (30-E)** Four primary blood groups are found in humans: O (47%), A (41%), B (9%), and AB (3%). These blood groups are based on the presence or absence of antigens (agglutinogens) on red blood cells and antibodies (agglutinins) in the serum.

31. **(E)** The force exerted upon the bottom is calculated in the following fashion:
$(20 + 50)$ cm $\times$ 2.8 g/cm^3 $\times$ $(50$ cm$)^2 = 490,000$ g
$= 490$ kg

32. **(A)** The area of the top exposed to hexabromoethane is derived as follows:
$(50$ cm$)^2 - 15$ cm$^2 = 2485$ cm^2

33. **(C)** The force exerted upon the top is derived as follows:
20 cm $\times$ 2.8 g/cm^2 $\times$ 2485 cm$^2 = 139,160$ g
$= 139.2$ kg

34. **(D)** Since hydrogen gas is a diatomic molecule, one gram atomic weight will occupy a volume of
$\frac{22.4}{2} = 11.2$ liters. 0.1 mole of lithium will produce $11.2 \times 0.1 = 1.12l$ of hydrogen.

35. **(A)** See above. 0.001 mole potassium produces 0.001 gram atomic weight of hydrogen or 0.0005 mole.
$2H_2 + O_2 \rightarrow 2H_2O$
$0.0005/2 = 0.00025$ mole oxygen
$22.4 l \times 2.5 \times 10^{-4} = 5.6 \times 10^{-3} l = 5.6$ ml

36. **(E)** One mole of any of these will produce 0.5 mole of hydrogen, and 0.001 mole of either of the three will produce 0.0005 mole of hydrogen.

37. **(D)** The density of this piece of steel is arrived at in the following manner:
$8.0 \times$ density of water $= 8.0 \times 1$ g/cm$^3 = 8.0$ g/cm^3

38. **(A)** Now we use the same reasoning and substitute for 1 g/cm^3 the value 62.4 lb./ft.^{3}:
8.0×62.4 lb./ft.$^3 = 499$ lb./ft.^{3}

39. **(B)** The weight of 35 ft.^{3} of this steel is arrived at as follows:
35 ft.$^3 \times 499$ lb./ft.$^3 = 17465$ lb.

40. **(B)** On oxidation of one mole the compound represented by structure (1) will produce 2 moles of acetaldehyde; *that represented by structure (2) will produce one mole each of acetaldehyde and propionaldehyde;* and that represented by structure (3) will produce one mole of hexanedial. In the latter case the ring prevents the formation of two moles after oxidation, but there is an aldehyde functional group on each end of the chain.

41. **(C)** See explanation above. Remember that although compound (1) produces only one product, there are two moles produced.

42. **(E)** See explanations above. Both compound (1) and compound (3) produce only one product. Disregarding the earlier data on the number of moles of product from one mole of reactant, this could be either compound (1) or (3).

43. **(C)** $w = mg = (10$ kg$)(9.8$ m/s$^2) = 98$ N.

44. **(E)** The volume of the glass may be calculated as follows:
$$10,000 \text{ g} \times \frac{1 \text{ cm}^3}{6 \text{ g}} = 1666 \text{ cm}^3$$

45. **(A)** 1666 cm$^3 \times \dfrac{1 \text{ g}}{\text{cm}^3} = 1666$ g of H_2O

1.67 kg $H_2O \times 9.8$ m/s$^2 = 16.4$ N

Therefore   100 N
minus   16 N
              84 N

46. **(B)** Only the #2 carbon of this compound is asymmetric. $2^1 = 2$

47. **(B)** Only the #3 carbon of this compound is asymmetric. $2^1 = 2$

48. **(A)** There are no asymmetric carbon atoms in this compound. $2^0 = 1$

49-51. **(49-A) (50-A) (51-B)** If a cell is placed in a hypertonic solution, water from within it will cross the semipermeable membrane, leave the cell and it will shrink. If a cell is placed in a hypotonic solution, water from without will enter the cell and it will swell. In an isotonic solution, as many molecules of water will enter as will leave the cell and the cell remain the same.

52-54. **(52-B) (53-C) (54-C)** the answers to 52-54 can be found in the flow diagram of the question.

55. **(A)** The energy of the photon is

$$E = \frac{hc}{\lambda} = \frac{(4.14 \times 10^{-15}\,\text{eV} \cdot \text{s})(3.00 \times 10^{8}\,\text{m/s})}{440 \times 10^{-9}\,\text{m}}$$
$$= 2.8\,\text{eV}$$

Since at least 2.2 eV are needed to release an electron, the most energy the electron can have is $2.8 - 2.2 = 0.6\,\text{eV}$.

56. **(C)** To find the amount of current in amperes (coulombs per second), multiply the number of electrons per second by the charge on each electron.

57. **(A)** The probe that picks up electrons is negative, so the electrons must lose energy as they go through the power supply. Electron energy is measured by the negative potential on the probe that is just sufficient to cut off the current.

58. **(A)** The fact that all those affected are males and that none has an affected father suggests a sex-linked recessive trait. The heterozygous mothers are giving the affected X chromosome to half their sons (causing them to express the trait) and to half their daughters (causing them to be carriers).

59. **(C)** Classical hemophilia as seen in various families, including the royal families of Europe (e.g., Queen Victoria's descendants and the royal family in Russia), is an example of a trait showing this inheritance.

60. **(B)** The disorder could be an autosomal recessive trait, occurring by chance only in males in our small sample. It is not autosomal dominant since neither parent of an affected individual has the trait. Other explanations are unlikely.

Answer Sheet–Model Test B

SCIENCE KNOWLEDGE

Biology

1. Ⓐ Ⓑ Ⓒ Ⓓ Ⓔ
2. Ⓐ Ⓑ Ⓒ Ⓓ Ⓔ
3. Ⓐ Ⓑ Ⓒ Ⓓ Ⓔ
4. Ⓐ Ⓑ Ⓒ Ⓓ Ⓔ
5. Ⓐ Ⓑ Ⓒ Ⓓ Ⓔ
6. Ⓐ Ⓑ Ⓒ Ⓓ Ⓔ
7. Ⓐ Ⓑ Ⓒ Ⓓ Ⓔ
8. Ⓐ Ⓑ Ⓒ Ⓓ Ⓔ
9. Ⓐ Ⓑ Ⓒ Ⓓ Ⓔ
10. Ⓐ Ⓑ Ⓒ Ⓓ Ⓔ

11. Ⓐ Ⓑ Ⓒ Ⓓ Ⓔ
12. Ⓐ Ⓑ Ⓒ Ⓓ Ⓔ
13. Ⓐ Ⓑ Ⓒ Ⓓ Ⓔ
14. Ⓐ Ⓑ Ⓒ Ⓓ Ⓔ
15. Ⓐ Ⓑ Ⓒ Ⓓ Ⓔ
16. Ⓐ Ⓑ Ⓒ Ⓓ Ⓔ
17. Ⓐ Ⓑ Ⓒ Ⓓ Ⓔ
18. Ⓐ Ⓑ Ⓒ Ⓓ Ⓔ
19. Ⓐ Ⓑ Ⓒ Ⓓ Ⓔ
20. Ⓐ Ⓑ Ⓒ Ⓓ Ⓔ

21. Ⓐ Ⓑ Ⓒ Ⓓ Ⓔ
22. Ⓐ Ⓑ Ⓒ Ⓓ Ⓔ
23. Ⓐ Ⓑ Ⓒ Ⓓ Ⓔ
24. Ⓐ Ⓑ Ⓒ Ⓓ Ⓔ
25. Ⓐ Ⓑ Ⓒ Ⓓ Ⓔ
26. Ⓐ Ⓑ Ⓒ Ⓓ Ⓔ
27. Ⓐ Ⓑ Ⓒ Ⓓ Ⓔ
28. Ⓐ Ⓑ Ⓒ Ⓓ Ⓔ
29. Ⓐ Ⓑ Ⓒ Ⓓ Ⓔ

30. Ⓐ Ⓑ Ⓒ Ⓓ Ⓔ
31. Ⓐ Ⓑ Ⓒ Ⓓ Ⓔ
32. Ⓐ Ⓑ Ⓒ Ⓓ Ⓔ
33. Ⓐ Ⓑ Ⓒ Ⓓ Ⓔ
34. Ⓐ Ⓑ Ⓒ Ⓓ Ⓔ
35. Ⓐ Ⓑ Ⓒ Ⓓ Ⓔ
36. Ⓐ Ⓑ Ⓒ Ⓓ Ⓔ
37. Ⓐ Ⓑ Ⓒ Ⓓ Ⓔ
38. Ⓐ Ⓑ Ⓒ Ⓓ Ⓔ

To score add from Science Problems questions: 1–3; 22–24; 28–33; 37–39; 52–57.

Chemistry

1. Ⓐ Ⓑ Ⓒ Ⓓ Ⓔ
2. Ⓐ Ⓑ Ⓒ Ⓓ Ⓔ
3. Ⓐ Ⓑ Ⓒ Ⓓ Ⓔ
4. Ⓐ Ⓑ Ⓒ Ⓓ Ⓔ
5. Ⓐ Ⓑ Ⓒ Ⓓ Ⓔ
6. Ⓐ Ⓑ Ⓒ Ⓓ Ⓔ
7. Ⓐ Ⓑ Ⓒ Ⓓ Ⓔ
8. Ⓐ Ⓑ Ⓒ Ⓓ Ⓔ
9. Ⓐ Ⓑ Ⓒ Ⓓ Ⓔ
10. Ⓐ Ⓑ Ⓒ Ⓓ Ⓔ

11. Ⓐ Ⓑ Ⓒ Ⓓ Ⓔ
12. Ⓐ Ⓑ Ⓒ Ⓓ Ⓔ
13. Ⓐ Ⓑ Ⓒ Ⓓ Ⓔ
14. Ⓐ Ⓑ Ⓒ Ⓓ Ⓔ
15. Ⓐ Ⓑ Ⓒ Ⓓ Ⓔ
16. Ⓐ Ⓑ Ⓒ Ⓓ Ⓔ
17. Ⓐ Ⓑ Ⓒ Ⓓ Ⓔ
18. Ⓐ Ⓑ Ⓒ Ⓓ Ⓔ
19. Ⓐ Ⓑ Ⓒ Ⓓ Ⓔ
20. Ⓐ Ⓑ Ⓒ Ⓓ Ⓔ

21. Ⓐ Ⓑ Ⓒ Ⓓ Ⓔ
22. Ⓐ Ⓑ Ⓒ Ⓓ Ⓔ
23. Ⓐ Ⓑ Ⓒ Ⓓ Ⓔ
24. Ⓐ Ⓑ Ⓒ Ⓓ Ⓔ
25. Ⓐ Ⓑ Ⓒ Ⓓ Ⓔ
26. Ⓐ Ⓑ Ⓒ Ⓓ Ⓔ
27. Ⓐ Ⓑ Ⓒ Ⓓ Ⓔ
28. Ⓐ Ⓑ Ⓒ Ⓓ Ⓔ
29. Ⓐ Ⓑ Ⓒ Ⓓ Ⓔ

30. Ⓐ Ⓑ Ⓒ Ⓓ Ⓔ
31. Ⓐ Ⓑ Ⓒ Ⓓ Ⓔ
32. Ⓐ Ⓑ Ⓒ Ⓓ Ⓔ
33. Ⓐ Ⓑ Ⓒ Ⓓ Ⓔ
34. Ⓐ Ⓑ Ⓒ Ⓓ Ⓔ
35. Ⓐ Ⓑ Ⓒ Ⓓ Ⓔ
36. Ⓐ Ⓑ Ⓒ Ⓓ Ⓔ
37. Ⓐ Ⓑ Ⓒ Ⓓ Ⓔ
38. Ⓐ Ⓑ Ⓒ Ⓓ Ⓔ

To score add from Science Problems questions: 4–6; 10–18; 40–48.

Physics

1. Ⓐ Ⓑ Ⓒ Ⓓ Ⓔ	12. Ⓐ Ⓑ Ⓒ Ⓓ Ⓔ	23. Ⓐ Ⓑ Ⓒ Ⓓ Ⓔ
2. Ⓐ Ⓑ Ⓒ Ⓓ Ⓔ	13. Ⓐ Ⓑ Ⓒ Ⓓ Ⓔ	24. Ⓐ Ⓑ Ⓒ Ⓓ Ⓔ
3. Ⓐ Ⓑ Ⓒ Ⓓ Ⓔ	14. Ⓐ Ⓑ Ⓒ Ⓓ Ⓔ	25. Ⓐ Ⓑ Ⓒ Ⓓ Ⓔ
4. Ⓐ Ⓑ Ⓒ Ⓓ Ⓔ	15. Ⓐ Ⓑ Ⓒ Ⓓ Ⓔ	26. Ⓐ Ⓑ Ⓒ Ⓓ Ⓔ
5. Ⓐ Ⓑ Ⓒ Ⓓ Ⓔ	16. Ⓐ Ⓑ Ⓒ Ⓓ Ⓔ	27. Ⓐ Ⓑ Ⓒ Ⓓ Ⓔ
6. Ⓐ Ⓑ Ⓒ Ⓓ Ⓔ	17. Ⓐ Ⓑ Ⓒ Ⓓ Ⓔ	28. Ⓐ Ⓑ Ⓒ Ⓓ Ⓔ
7. Ⓐ Ⓑ Ⓒ Ⓓ Ⓔ	18. Ⓐ Ⓑ Ⓒ Ⓓ Ⓔ	29. Ⓐ Ⓑ Ⓒ Ⓓ Ⓔ
8. Ⓐ Ⓑ Ⓒ Ⓓ Ⓔ	19. Ⓐ Ⓑ Ⓒ Ⓓ Ⓔ	30. Ⓐ Ⓑ Ⓒ Ⓓ Ⓔ
9. Ⓐ Ⓑ Ⓒ Ⓓ Ⓔ	20. Ⓐ Ⓑ Ⓒ Ⓓ Ⓔ	31. Ⓐ Ⓑ Ⓒ Ⓓ Ⓔ
10. Ⓐ Ⓑ Ⓒ Ⓓ Ⓔ	21. Ⓐ Ⓑ Ⓒ Ⓓ Ⓔ	32. Ⓐ Ⓑ Ⓒ Ⓓ Ⓔ
11. Ⓐ Ⓑ Ⓒ Ⓓ Ⓔ	22. Ⓐ Ⓑ Ⓒ Ⓓ Ⓔ	33. Ⓐ Ⓑ Ⓒ Ⓓ Ⓔ

To score add from Science Problems questions: 7–9; 19–21; 25–27; 34–36; 49–51; 58–60.

SCIENCE PROBLEMS

1. Ⓐ Ⓑ Ⓒ Ⓓ Ⓔ	21. Ⓐ Ⓑ Ⓒ Ⓓ Ⓔ	41. Ⓐ Ⓑ Ⓒ Ⓓ Ⓔ
2. Ⓐ Ⓑ Ⓒ Ⓓ Ⓔ	22. Ⓐ Ⓑ Ⓒ Ⓓ Ⓔ	42. Ⓐ Ⓑ Ⓒ Ⓓ Ⓔ
3. Ⓐ Ⓑ Ⓒ Ⓓ Ⓔ	23. Ⓐ Ⓑ Ⓒ Ⓓ Ⓔ	43. Ⓐ Ⓑ Ⓒ Ⓓ Ⓔ
4. Ⓐ Ⓑ Ⓒ Ⓓ Ⓔ	24. Ⓐ Ⓑ Ⓒ Ⓓ Ⓔ	44. Ⓐ Ⓑ Ⓒ Ⓓ Ⓔ
5. Ⓐ Ⓑ Ⓒ Ⓓ Ⓔ	25. Ⓐ Ⓑ Ⓒ Ⓓ Ⓔ	45. Ⓐ Ⓑ Ⓒ Ⓓ Ⓔ
6. Ⓐ Ⓑ Ⓒ Ⓓ Ⓔ	26. Ⓐ Ⓑ Ⓒ Ⓓ Ⓔ	46. Ⓐ Ⓑ Ⓒ Ⓓ Ⓔ
7. Ⓐ Ⓑ Ⓒ Ⓓ Ⓔ	27. Ⓐ Ⓑ Ⓒ Ⓓ Ⓔ	47. Ⓐ Ⓑ Ⓒ Ⓓ Ⓔ
8. Ⓐ Ⓑ Ⓒ Ⓓ Ⓔ	28. Ⓐ Ⓑ Ⓒ Ⓓ Ⓔ	48. Ⓐ Ⓑ Ⓒ Ⓓ Ⓔ
9. Ⓐ Ⓑ Ⓒ Ⓓ Ⓔ	29. Ⓐ Ⓑ Ⓒ Ⓓ Ⓔ	49. Ⓐ Ⓑ Ⓒ Ⓓ Ⓔ
10. Ⓐ Ⓑ Ⓒ Ⓓ Ⓔ	30. Ⓐ Ⓑ Ⓒ Ⓓ Ⓔ	50. Ⓐ Ⓑ Ⓒ Ⓓ Ⓔ
11. Ⓐ Ⓑ Ⓒ Ⓓ Ⓔ	31. Ⓐ Ⓑ Ⓒ Ⓓ Ⓔ	51. Ⓐ Ⓑ Ⓒ Ⓓ Ⓔ
12. Ⓐ Ⓑ Ⓒ Ⓓ Ⓔ	32. Ⓐ Ⓑ Ⓒ Ⓓ Ⓔ	52. Ⓐ Ⓑ Ⓒ Ⓓ Ⓔ
13. Ⓐ Ⓑ Ⓒ Ⓓ Ⓔ	33. Ⓐ Ⓑ Ⓒ Ⓓ Ⓔ	53. Ⓐ Ⓑ Ⓒ Ⓓ Ⓔ
14. Ⓐ Ⓑ Ⓒ Ⓓ Ⓔ	34. Ⓐ Ⓑ Ⓒ Ⓓ Ⓔ	54. Ⓐ Ⓑ Ⓒ Ⓓ Ⓔ
15. Ⓐ Ⓑ Ⓒ Ⓓ Ⓔ	35. Ⓐ Ⓑ Ⓒ Ⓓ Ⓔ	55. Ⓐ Ⓑ Ⓒ Ⓓ Ⓔ
16. Ⓐ Ⓑ Ⓒ Ⓓ Ⓔ	36. Ⓐ Ⓑ Ⓒ Ⓓ Ⓔ	56. Ⓐ Ⓑ Ⓒ Ⓓ Ⓔ
17. Ⓐ Ⓑ Ⓒ Ⓓ Ⓔ	37. Ⓐ Ⓑ Ⓒ Ⓓ Ⓔ	57. Ⓐ Ⓑ Ⓒ Ⓓ Ⓔ
18. Ⓐ Ⓑ Ⓒ Ⓓ Ⓔ	38. Ⓐ Ⓑ Ⓒ Ⓓ Ⓔ	58. Ⓐ Ⓑ Ⓒ Ⓓ Ⓔ
19. Ⓐ Ⓑ Ⓒ Ⓓ Ⓔ	39. Ⓐ Ⓑ Ⓒ Ⓓ Ⓔ	59. Ⓐ Ⓑ Ⓒ Ⓓ Ⓔ
20. Ⓐ Ⓑ Ⓒ Ⓓ Ⓔ	40. Ⓐ Ⓑ Ⓒ Ⓓ Ⓔ	60. Ⓐ Ⓑ Ⓒ Ⓓ Ⓔ

SKILLS ANALYSIS: READING

1. Ⓐ Ⓑ Ⓒ Ⓓ Ⓔ
2. Ⓐ Ⓑ Ⓒ Ⓓ Ⓔ
3. Ⓐ Ⓑ Ⓒ Ⓓ Ⓔ
4. Ⓐ Ⓑ Ⓒ Ⓓ Ⓔ
5. Ⓐ Ⓑ Ⓒ Ⓓ Ⓔ
6. Ⓐ Ⓑ Ⓒ Ⓓ Ⓔ
7. Ⓐ Ⓑ Ⓒ Ⓓ Ⓔ
8. Ⓐ Ⓑ Ⓒ Ⓓ Ⓔ
9. Ⓐ Ⓑ Ⓒ Ⓓ Ⓔ
10. Ⓐ Ⓑ Ⓒ Ⓓ Ⓔ
11. Ⓐ Ⓑ Ⓒ Ⓓ Ⓔ
12. Ⓐ Ⓑ Ⓒ Ⓓ Ⓔ
13. Ⓐ Ⓑ Ⓒ Ⓓ Ⓔ
14. Ⓐ Ⓑ Ⓒ Ⓓ Ⓔ
15. Ⓐ Ⓑ Ⓒ Ⓓ Ⓔ
16. Ⓐ Ⓑ Ⓒ Ⓓ Ⓔ
17. Ⓐ Ⓑ Ⓒ Ⓓ Ⓔ
18. Ⓐ Ⓑ Ⓒ Ⓓ Ⓔ
19. Ⓐ Ⓑ Ⓒ Ⓓ Ⓔ
20. Ⓐ Ⓑ Ⓒ Ⓓ Ⓔ
21. Ⓐ Ⓑ Ⓒ Ⓓ Ⓔ
22. Ⓐ Ⓑ Ⓒ Ⓓ Ⓔ
23. Ⓐ Ⓑ Ⓒ Ⓓ Ⓔ
24. Ⓐ Ⓑ Ⓒ Ⓓ Ⓔ
25. Ⓐ Ⓑ Ⓒ Ⓓ Ⓔ
26. Ⓐ Ⓑ Ⓒ Ⓓ Ⓔ
27. Ⓐ Ⓑ Ⓒ Ⓓ Ⓔ
28. Ⓐ Ⓑ Ⓒ Ⓓ Ⓔ
29. Ⓐ Ⓑ Ⓒ Ⓓ Ⓔ
30. Ⓐ Ⓑ Ⓒ Ⓓ Ⓔ
31. Ⓐ Ⓑ Ⓒ Ⓓ Ⓔ
32. Ⓐ Ⓑ Ⓒ Ⓓ Ⓔ
33. Ⓐ Ⓑ Ⓒ Ⓓ Ⓔ
34. Ⓐ Ⓑ Ⓒ Ⓓ Ⓔ
35. Ⓐ Ⓑ Ⓒ Ⓓ Ⓔ
36. Ⓐ Ⓑ Ⓒ Ⓓ Ⓔ
37. Ⓐ Ⓑ Ⓒ Ⓓ Ⓔ
38. Ⓐ Ⓑ Ⓒ Ⓓ Ⓔ
39. Ⓐ Ⓑ Ⓒ Ⓓ Ⓔ
40. Ⓐ Ⓑ Ⓒ Ⓓ Ⓔ
41. Ⓐ Ⓑ Ⓒ Ⓓ Ⓔ
42. Ⓐ Ⓑ Ⓒ Ⓓ Ⓔ
43. Ⓐ Ⓑ Ⓒ Ⓓ Ⓔ
44. Ⓐ Ⓑ Ⓒ Ⓓ Ⓔ
45. Ⓐ Ⓑ Ⓒ Ⓓ Ⓔ
46. Ⓐ Ⓑ Ⓒ Ⓓ Ⓔ
47. Ⓐ Ⓑ Ⓒ Ⓓ Ⓔ
48. Ⓐ Ⓑ Ⓒ Ⓓ Ⓔ
49. Ⓐ Ⓑ Ⓒ Ⓓ Ⓔ
50. Ⓐ Ⓑ Ⓒ Ⓓ Ⓔ
51. Ⓐ Ⓑ Ⓒ Ⓓ Ⓔ
52. Ⓐ Ⓑ Ⓒ Ⓓ Ⓔ
53. Ⓐ Ⓑ Ⓒ Ⓓ Ⓔ
54. Ⓐ Ⓑ Ⓒ Ⓓ Ⓔ
55. Ⓐ Ⓑ Ⓒ Ⓓ Ⓔ
56. Ⓐ Ⓑ Ⓒ Ⓓ Ⓔ
57. Ⓐ Ⓑ Ⓒ Ⓓ Ⓔ
58. Ⓐ Ⓑ Ⓒ Ⓓ Ⓔ
59. Ⓐ Ⓑ Ⓒ Ⓓ Ⓔ
60. Ⓐ Ⓑ Ⓒ Ⓓ Ⓔ
61. Ⓐ Ⓑ Ⓒ Ⓓ Ⓔ
62. Ⓐ Ⓑ Ⓒ Ⓓ Ⓔ
63. Ⓐ Ⓑ Ⓒ Ⓓ Ⓔ
64. Ⓐ Ⓑ Ⓒ Ⓓ Ⓔ
65. Ⓐ Ⓑ Ⓒ Ⓓ Ⓔ
66. Ⓐ Ⓑ Ⓒ Ⓓ Ⓔ
67. Ⓐ Ⓑ Ⓒ Ⓓ Ⓔ
68. Ⓐ Ⓑ Ⓒ Ⓓ Ⓔ

SKILLS ANALYSIS: QUANTITATIVE

1. Ⓐ Ⓑ Ⓒ Ⓓ Ⓔ
2. Ⓐ Ⓑ Ⓒ Ⓓ Ⓔ
3. Ⓐ Ⓑ Ⓒ Ⓓ Ⓔ
4. Ⓐ Ⓑ Ⓒ Ⓓ Ⓔ
5. Ⓐ Ⓑ Ⓒ Ⓓ Ⓔ
6. Ⓐ Ⓑ Ⓒ Ⓓ Ⓔ
7. Ⓐ Ⓑ Ⓒ Ⓓ Ⓔ
8. Ⓐ Ⓑ Ⓒ Ⓓ Ⓔ
9. Ⓐ Ⓑ Ⓒ Ⓓ Ⓔ
10. Ⓐ Ⓑ Ⓒ Ⓓ Ⓔ
11. Ⓐ Ⓑ Ⓒ Ⓓ Ⓔ
12. Ⓐ Ⓑ Ⓒ Ⓓ Ⓔ
13. Ⓐ Ⓑ Ⓒ Ⓓ Ⓔ
14. Ⓐ Ⓑ Ⓒ Ⓓ Ⓔ
15. Ⓐ Ⓑ Ⓒ Ⓓ Ⓔ
16. Ⓐ Ⓑ Ⓒ Ⓓ Ⓔ
17. Ⓐ Ⓑ Ⓒ Ⓓ Ⓔ
18. Ⓐ Ⓑ Ⓒ Ⓓ Ⓔ
19. Ⓐ Ⓑ Ⓒ Ⓓ Ⓔ
20. Ⓐ Ⓑ Ⓒ Ⓓ Ⓔ
21. Ⓐ Ⓑ Ⓒ Ⓓ Ⓔ
22. Ⓐ Ⓑ Ⓒ Ⓓ Ⓔ
23. Ⓐ Ⓑ Ⓒ Ⓓ Ⓔ
24. Ⓐ Ⓑ Ⓒ Ⓓ Ⓔ
25. Ⓐ Ⓑ Ⓒ Ⓓ Ⓔ
26. Ⓐ Ⓑ Ⓒ Ⓓ Ⓔ
27. Ⓐ Ⓑ Ⓒ Ⓓ Ⓔ
28. Ⓐ Ⓑ Ⓒ Ⓓ Ⓔ
29. Ⓐ Ⓑ Ⓒ Ⓓ Ⓔ
30. Ⓐ Ⓑ Ⓒ Ⓓ Ⓔ
31. Ⓐ Ⓑ Ⓒ Ⓓ Ⓔ
32. Ⓐ Ⓑ Ⓒ Ⓓ Ⓔ
33. Ⓐ Ⓑ Ⓒ Ⓓ Ⓔ
34. Ⓐ Ⓑ Ⓒ Ⓓ Ⓔ
35. Ⓐ Ⓑ Ⓒ Ⓓ Ⓔ
36. Ⓐ Ⓑ Ⓒ Ⓓ Ⓔ
37. Ⓐ Ⓑ Ⓒ Ⓓ Ⓔ
38. Ⓐ Ⓑ Ⓒ Ⓓ Ⓔ
39. Ⓐ Ⓑ Ⓒ Ⓓ Ⓔ
40. Ⓐ Ⓑ Ⓒ Ⓓ Ⓔ
41. Ⓐ Ⓑ Ⓒ Ⓓ Ⓔ
42. Ⓐ Ⓑ Ⓒ Ⓓ Ⓔ
43. Ⓐ Ⓑ Ⓒ Ⓓ Ⓔ
44. Ⓐ Ⓑ Ⓒ Ⓓ Ⓔ
45. Ⓐ Ⓑ Ⓒ Ⓓ Ⓔ
46. Ⓐ Ⓑ Ⓒ Ⓓ Ⓔ
47. Ⓐ Ⓑ Ⓒ Ⓓ Ⓔ
48. Ⓐ Ⓑ Ⓒ Ⓓ Ⓔ
49. Ⓐ Ⓑ Ⓒ Ⓓ Ⓔ
50. Ⓐ Ⓑ Ⓒ Ⓓ Ⓔ
51. Ⓐ Ⓑ Ⓒ Ⓓ Ⓔ
52. Ⓐ Ⓑ Ⓒ Ⓓ Ⓔ
53. Ⓐ Ⓑ Ⓒ Ⓓ Ⓔ
54. Ⓐ Ⓑ Ⓒ Ⓓ Ⓔ
55. Ⓐ Ⓑ Ⓒ Ⓓ Ⓔ
56. Ⓐ Ⓑ Ⓒ Ⓓ Ⓔ
57. Ⓐ Ⓑ Ⓒ Ⓓ Ⓔ
58. Ⓐ Ⓑ Ⓒ Ⓓ Ⓔ
59. Ⓐ Ⓑ Ⓒ Ⓓ Ⓔ
60. Ⓐ Ⓑ Ⓒ Ⓓ Ⓔ
61. Ⓐ Ⓑ Ⓒ Ⓓ Ⓔ
62. Ⓐ Ⓑ Ⓒ Ⓓ Ⓔ
63. Ⓐ Ⓑ Ⓒ Ⓓ Ⓔ
64. Ⓐ Ⓑ Ⓒ Ⓓ Ⓔ
65. Ⓐ Ⓑ Ⓒ Ⓓ Ⓔ
66. Ⓐ Ⓑ Ⓒ Ⓓ Ⓔ
67. Ⓐ Ⓑ Ⓒ Ⓓ Ⓔ
68. Ⓐ Ⓑ Ⓒ Ⓓ Ⓔ

The MCAT
Model Examination B*

SCIENCE KNOWLEDGE

115 MINUTES
109 QUESTIONS

The following questions are based on your knowledge of science. The questions are varied; therefore, you are advised to pay careful attention to the instructions for each portion.

Biology—38 Questions   Recommended Time—25 minutes

DIRECTIONS: Each of the statements or questions is followed by suggested completions or answers. Choose the one that best completes the statement or answers the question, and mark the letter of your choice on the answer sheet.

1. The gastric juice in the stomach
   (A) has a neutral pH.
   (B) is alkaline.
   (C) is acidic.
   (D) contains trypsin.
   (E) contains insulin.

2. Rh-related hemolytic anemia of the newborn (erythroblastosis foetalis) may result when the
   (A) father, mother, and fetus are all Rh negative.
   (B) father and mother are Rh positive, but the fetus is Rh negative.
   (C) mother is Rh negative and the fetus is Rh positive.
   (D) mother is Rh positive and the fetus is Rh negative.
   (E) father, mother, and fetus are all Rh positive.

3. The region of the retina where vision is most acute is known as the
   (A) ciliary body.
   (B) vitreous humor.
   (C) conjunctiva.
   (D) fovea centralis.
   (E) aqueous humor.

4. If a cell is viewed under low power and then under high power, and no fine adjustment is necessary to see it clearly, the microscope is considered
   (A) achromatic.
   (B) bifocal.
   (C) parfocal.
   (D) unifocal.
   (E) apochromatic.

5. During the follicular phase of a normal menstrual cycle ovarian changes occur which are due to pituitary secretions of
   (A) FSH only.
   (B) LH only.
   (C) oxytocin.
   (D) vasopressin.
   (E) FSH and LH.

---

*Explanations for science answers can be found on p. 331.

6. Which of the following patterns would you expect to find in the blood one hour after a rich meal?

	Blood Sugar	Insulin
(A)	high	low
(B)	low	low
(C)	high	high
(D)	low	high
(E)	no change	no change

7. Which of the following type(s) of lens(es) is used to correct the vision of a near-sighted individual?
   (A) convex
   (B) biconvex
   (C) biconcave
   (D) none of the above
   (E) all of the above

8. The stage during development when the embryo is a hollow sphere of cells one cell in thickness is called the
   (A) blastula.
   (B) gastrula.
   (C) polar body.
   (D) morula.
   (E) cleavage.

9. The experiments of Miller and Urey enhanced the validity of Oparin's theory on the origin of life. They essentially
   (A) found fossil remnants in meteorites.
   (B) were able to produce a simple form of living organism after placing DNA in a mixture of hydrogen and oxygen and irradiating it.
   (C) were able to produce simple viruses.
   (D) discharged electricity into a medium consisting of water vapor, methane, ammonia, and hydrogen.
   (E) were able to produce bacteria.

10. Characteristics which are common to the Arthropod, Mollusk, Echinoderm, and Chordate lines are a(an)
    (A) coelom and a parietal eye.
    (B) endoskeleton and a coelom.
    (C) segmentation and a coelom.
    (D) compound eye and segmentation.
    (E) endoskeleton and a parietal eye.

11. Humans can become infected with trichinosis by
    (A) drinking unpasteurized milk.
    (B) cutting themselves while dressing wild game.
    (C) wading in polluted water or eating raw fish.
    (D) eating poorly cooked pork.
    (E) eating poorly cooked beef.

12. Characteristics of epithelial tissues may include
    (A) protection.
    (B) secretion.
    (C) absorption.
    (D) all of the above.
    (E) none of the above.

13. The relationship of two organisms living together for their mutual benefit is classified as
    (A) symbiosis.
    (B) commensalism.
    (C) saprophytism.
    (D) parasitism.
    (E) civilization.

14. The contractile vacuole of protozoa functions to
    (A) remove undigested food materials.
    (B) digest food materials.
    (C) regulate the pH of the internal milieu.
    (D) secrete proteins.
    (E) remove surplus water.

15. A hog breeder would use a backcross to
    (A) produce a bigger and healthier strain.
    (B) produce a larger number of offspring.
    (C) maintain a pure line of desirable traits.
    (D) determine if a particular hog is genotypically pure.
    (E) eliminate chances of congenital malformations.

16. The state of a continuously mild or partial contraction of a muscle is denoted as
    (A) tetanus.   (D) a twitch.
    (B) tonus.   (E) a reflex contraction.
    (C) an "all or none" contraction.

17. The cell bodies of the motor neurons are located in the spinal cord in
    (A) intermediolateral cell column.
    (B) dorsal root ganglia.
    (C) dorsal horn (gray matter).
    (D) ventral horn (gray matter).
    (E) ventral root ganglia.

18. Body temperature is regulated by the
    (A) thalamus.   (D) cerebellum.
    (B) medulla.   (E) hypothalamus.
    (C) pons.

19. When a physician informs a patient that his blood pressure reading is 160/90, she refers respectively to
    (A) systolic blood pressure of the left ventricle.
    (B) blood pressure in the veins of the arm.
    (C) systolic and diastolic pressures of the brachial artery.
    (D) systolic pressure of the aorta and diastolic pressure in the superior vena cava.
    (E) systolic pressure of the right ventricle.

20. Mesoderm, one of the germ layers, gives rise to a group of structures in animals. Which group includes structures of exclusively mesodermal origin?
    (A) bone, lens of the eye, pars distalis, gall bladder
    (B) muscle, outer layer of digestive tract, cartilage, bone
    (C) skin, brain, bladder, vagina
    (D) trachea, lungs, stomach, skin
    (E) none of the above

21. Vigorous exercise will cause muscle fatigue which is primarily due to
    (A) the utilization and exhaustion of ATP.
    (B) the accumulation of ADP.
    (C) the accumulation of lactic acid.
    (D) the accumulation of carbon dioxide.
    (E) a sodium and potassium imbalance.

22. A patient awaiting selective surgery presents the following symptoms. Which of them indicate(s) a heightened activity of the sympathetic portion of his autonomic nervous system?
    (A) a yearning for water due to a dry mouth
    (B) sweaty palms
    (C) pale skin
    (D) all of the above
    (E) none of the above

23. The stimulus that induces migration in animals is
    (A) hydrotrophic.
    (B) photoperiodic.
    (C) geotrophic.
    (D) hydroperiodic.
    (E) chemotrophic.

24. Follicle-stimulating hormone is to estrogen as luteinizing hormone is to
    (A) progesterone.
    (B) testosterone.
    (C) vasopressin.
    (D) luteotrophic hormone.
    (E) androgen.

25. Which of the following structures are NOT considered modifications of the cell membrane?
    (A) basement membrane
    (B) terminal bars
    (C) desmosomes
    (D) intercalated discs
    (E) microvilli

26. Administration of which of the following compound(s) increases clotting time?
    (A) heparin
    (B) aspirin
    (C) dicumarol
    (D) all of the above
    (E) none of the above

27. The functional role an organism plays in a community is referred to as its
    (A) habitat.
    (B) home range.
    (C) niche.
    (D) environment.
    (E) ecosystem.

28. All of the following may be considered as secondary sex characteristics of the male EXCEPT
    (A) increase in sex drive.
    (B) external genitalia.
    (C) pattern of hair and beard growth.
    (D) development of a deeper voice.
    (E) skin pigmentation patterns.

29. In an auto accident the driver suffers complete sectioning of several anterior (ventral) roots of spinal nerves. What would be the result of such a lesion to the regions supplied by those spinal nerves?
    (A) no neural deficit
    (B) loss of motor activity
    (C) loss of sensation
    (D) loss of sensation and motor activity
    (E) loss of temperature and pain sensation

30. The reflex arc is of utmost importance to human beings. Which of the following is NOT a component of the reflex arc?
    (A) medulla
    (B) dendrite (receptor)
    (C) synapse
    (D) ventral horn cell (effector)
    (E) axon

31. An aggregation of nerve cell bodies inside the CNS (central nervous system) is typically called a
    (A) clone.
    (B) colony.
    (C) Nissl zone.
    (D) tract.
    (E) nucleus.

32. The vital centers for control of heart rate, respiratory rate, and blood pressure are located in the
    (A) pons.
    (B) medulla.
    (C) cerebellum.
    (D) hypothalamus.
    (E) midbrain.

33. The most numerous leukocytes are the
    (A) lymphocytes.
    (B) monocytes.
    (C) eosinophils.
    (D) neutrophils.
    (E) basophils.

34. Bile, which is important in the digestion of fats, is produced by the
    (A) stomach.
    (B) liver.
    (C) duodenum.
    (D) gall bladder.
    (E) lacteals.

35. The primitive condition of the cyclostomata is indicated by their
    (A) possession of scales.
    (B) jawless mouth.
    (C) asexual reproduction.
    (D) surface slime.
    (E) toothless jaws.

36. The plasma membrane of animal cells
    (A) is usually rigid.
    (B) has selective channels made of proteins.
    (C) is too thin to be seen by the use of any microscope.
    (D) is composed only of proteins and carbohydrates.
    (E) lies just interior to the cell wall.

37. Prolonged strong contraction by a muscle is called
    (A) tonus.
    (B) refractory period.
    (C) tetanus.
    (D) twitch.
    (E) fatigue.

38. A mink breeder finds that 50% of the offspring are aa. What genotype were their parents?
    (A) aa × aa
    (B) Aa × Aa
    (C) AA × aa
    (D) Aa × aa
    (E) Aa × AA

Chemistry—38 Questions   Recommended Time—46 minutes

DIRECTIONS: Each of the statements or questions is followed by suggested completions or answers. Choose the one that best completes the statement or answers the question, and mark the letter of your choice on the answer sheet.

1. Fatty acid is to fat as glucose is to
    (A) starch.
    (B) glycogen.
    (C) cellulose.
    (D) all of the above.
    (E) none of the above.

2. The reaction of sodium alkoxide with an alkyl halide is often used to produce
    (A) an ether.
    (B) an acetal.
    (C) an ester.
    (D) a sodium halide.
    (E) none of the above.

3. The most acidic compound listed below is

   (A) CH_3OH

   (B) —OH

   (C) —OH

   (D) O_2N——OH with NO_2 groups

   (E) $HOCH_2$—CH_2OH

4. Of the compounds listed below, the one that reacts best with ethers is

   (A) HCl.
   (B) HBr.
   (C) HI.

   (D) HF.
   (E) $NaNO_3$.

5. The Hell-Volhard-Zelinsky reaction utilizes Br_2 and PBr_3 to convert a carboxylic acid to

   (A)
$$R-CH_2-\overset{\overset{\displaystyle O}{\|}}{C}-Br$$

   (B)
$$R-\underset{\underset{\displaystyle Br}{|}}{CH}-COBr$$

   (C)
$$R-\underset{\underset{\displaystyle PBr_2}{|}}{CH}-COBr$$

   (D)
$$R-CH_2-\overset{\overset{\displaystyle O}{\|}}{C}-PBr_2$$

   (E) a glycol

6. Glucose is NOT a (an)

   (A) aldose.
   (B) reducing sugar.
   (C) disaccharide.

   (D) sugar possessing optical activity.
   (E) monosaccharide.

7. The Tollens silver mirror test (ammoniacal silver nitrate) does not give a positive test with

   (A)
$$H_3C-\overset{\overset{\displaystyle O}{\|}}{C}-H$$

   (B)
$$H_3C-CH_2-\overset{\overset{\displaystyle O}{\|}}{C}-H$$

   (C)
$$H_3C-CH_2-\overset{\overset{\displaystyle O}{\|}}{C}-CH_3$$

   (D)

   (E) any of the above

8. HIO_4 will oxidize all of the following except

   (A) 1,3-propanediol.
   (B) ethylene glycol.
   (C) glycerol.

   (D) 1,2-cyclopentanediol.
   (E) B and C

9. Alcohols have higher boiling points than do alkyl halides of the same chain lengths because

   (A) alcohols are more polar.
   (B) alcohols have higher molecular weights.
   (C) alcohols form ethers.
   (D) alcohols form intermolecular hydrogen bonds.
   (E) of all of the above.

10. Catalysts

   (A) are changed and consumed during a reaction.
   (B) have virtually no effect on the overall rate of the reaction.
   (C) must be present in high concentrations.
   (D) are changed but not consumed during a reaction.
   (E) speed up the rate of the reaction.

11. Which of the following are nitrogenous metabolic waste products?
    (A) sodium chloride, potassium phosphate, and water
    (B) urea, ammonia, and creatinine
    (C) amino acids, ammonia, and DNA
    (D) glucosamine, creatine, and RNA
    (E) sugar, ammonia, and creatine

12. Margarine and shortening are made from vegetable oils and animal fats by treatment to decrease rancidity. The process is known as
    (A) oxidation.   (D) hydrolysis.
    (B) hydrogenation.   (E) reduction.
    (C) esterification.

13. The process referred to in question 12
    (A) removes high molecular weight glycerides.
    (B) increases the number of free carboxylic acids.
    (C) removes high molecular weight alcohols.
    (D) raises the melting point of the mixture.
    (E) decreases the melting point of the mixture.

14. One mole of methyl magnesium bromide will react with one mole of substrate to give the indicated product upon hydrolysis. Which substrate and product are correct?
    (A) acetaldehyde → primary alcohol   (D) ketone → secondary alcohol
    (B) carboxylic acid → tertiary alcohol (E) acetaldehyde → secondary alcohol
    (C) ester → ketone

15. If solution A is less concentrated in dissolved particle content than solution B, then solution A is said to be
    (A) hypertonic.   (D) isotonic.
    (B) hypotonic.   (E) supersaturated.
    (C) isoosmotic.

16. Compared to one mole of oxygen, how many more molecules do two moles of carbon dioxide contain?
    (A) 25×10^6 (D) 12.04×10^{23}
    (B) 12.04×10^{46} (E) 6.02×10^6
    (C) 6.02×10^{23}

17. An example of a fatty acid is

    (A) $CH_3(CH_2)_{16}CH_2OH$ (C) $CH_3(CH_2)_{12}COOH$
    (B) $CH_2 - COOH$ (D) $CH_3(CH_2)_{14}COOH_3$
        $\overset{|}{CH} - COOH$ (E) $\phi - OH$
        $\overset{|}{CH_2} - COOH$

18. Which one of the following acids does not commonly form acid salts?
    (A) $HC_2H_3O_2$ (D) H_3PO_4
    (B) H_2SO_4 (E) $HOOC - COOH$
    (C) H_2CO_3

19. One mole of acetal may be synthesized from the quantitative reaction of
    (A) one mole of alcohol and two moles of aldehyde.
    (B) two moles of alcohol and one mole of aldehyde.
    (C) one mole each of alcohol and aldehyde.
    (D) one mole each of aldehyde and ketone.
    (E) one mole each of aldehyde, ketone, and alcohol.

20. An atom undergoing neutron capture and negatron decay will produce an atom of
  (A) smaller atomic number.
  (B) greater atomic number.
  (C) greater atomic weight.
  (D) greater atomic weight and smaller atomic number.
  (E) greater atomic weight and greater atomic number.

21. Which of the statements listed below is false?
  (A) An aqueous solution in which $[H^+] > 1 \times 10^{+7}$ is said to be acidic.
  (B) Ions are atoms or groups of atoms that have lost or gained one or more electrons.
  (C) HCl is a Bronsted acid because it furnishes H^+ ion in solution.
  (D) NaOH is called a base because it furnishes Na^+ ions in solution.

22. Cholesterol is an intermediate in the biosynthesis of
  (A) essential fatty acids.
  (B) steroid hormones.
  (C) essential amino acids.
  (D) prostaglandins.
  (E) thyroglobulin.

23. The essential fatty acids are required in the human body in the biosynthesis of
  (A) ascorbic acid
  (B) bile acids.
  (C) estrogens.
  (D) prostaglandins.
  (E) androgens.

24. 2-Butyne + H_2 $\xrightarrow{\text{Pd}}$
  (A) *trans*-2-butene
  (B) *cis*-2-butene
  (C) 1,3-butadiene
  (D) 1-butyne
  (E) no reaction

25. A compound which is insoluble in concentrated sulfuric acid is
  (A) 1-pentyne.
  (B) 1,3-pentadiene.
  (C) 2-pentyne.
  (D) *n*-pentane.
  (E) none of the above.

26. Which reaction would yield 1-butene as the major product?
  (A) CH_3—CH_2—CH_2—CH_2—Br + alcoholic KOH $\xrightarrow{\text{heat}}$
  (B) CH_3—CH_2—$\overset{\overset{\displaystyle Br}{|}}{CH}$—$CH_3$ + alcoholic KOH $\xrightarrow{\text{heat}}$
  (C) $CH_3CH_2CH_2CH_2$—OH + H_2SO_4 $\xrightarrow{\text{heat}}$
  (D) $CH_3C \equiv C$—CH_3 + H_2 $\xrightarrow{\text{Pt}}$
  (E) CH_3—CH_2—CH_3—CH_3 + Na

27. In the chlorination of nitrobenzene the product recovered in greatest yield is
  (A) *o*-chloronitrobenzene.
  (B) *m*-chloronitrobenzene.
  (C) *p*-chloronitrobenzene.
  (D) *p*-dichlorobenzene.
  (E) *o*-dichloronitrobenzene.

28. The nitro group present on the benzene ring in the above question is
  (A) activating, meta-directing.
  (B) activating, para-directing.
  (C) deactivating, meta-directing.
  (D) none of the above.

29. An atom undergoing beta decay will initially produce an atom of
  (A) greater atomic number.
  (B) smaller atomic number.
  (C) greater atomic weight.
  (D) greater atomic weight and greater atomic number.
  (E) equal atomic number.

30. In the decomposition of $KClO_3$ to generate oxygen gas, MnO_2 is added in order to
    (A) increase the volume of oxygen obtained from the $KClO_3$.
    (B) produce oxygen of higher purity.
    (C) reduce the temperature at which decomposition of $KClO_3$ takes place.
    (D) decrease the volume of Cl_2 produced.
    (E) increase the temperature at which decomposition of $KClO_3$ takes place.

31. The name applied to a substance such as MnO_2 used in the reaction above is a (an)
    (A) enzyme.
    (B) catalyst.
    (C) isotope.
    (D) free radical scavenger.
    (E) cofactor.

32. Large ring compounds are difficult to prepare because
    (A) these rings are stable but the two ends of the chain must be brought close together to effect ring closure.
    (B) these rings are flat and their bond angles exceed 109.5°.
    (C) both large and small rings are highly strained.
    (D) these rings are puckered and their bond angles are compressed to less than 109.5°.
    (E) these rings are extremely unstable.

33. The species which acts as the electrophile in the bromination of benzene is
    (A) benzene.
    (B) Br^-.
    (C) $Br\cdot$.
    (D) Br^+.
    (E) $-Br^+$

34. The ionization constant for an acid, HA, may be designated as K_a. It is equal to
    (A) $\dfrac{[H^+][A^-]}{[HA]}$
    (B) $\dfrac{[H^+]}{[HA][A^-]}$
    (C) $\dfrac{[HA]}{[H^+][A^-]}$
    (D) $\dfrac{[H^+]^2}{[HA]}$

35. In the reaction

$$HSO_4^- + H_2O \rightarrow H_3O^+ + SO_4^{2-}$$

an acid-base conjugate pair is
    (A) HSO_4^- and H_2O
    (B) SO_4^{2-} and H_3O^+
    (C) SO_4^{2-} and H_2O
    (D) HSO_4^- and H_3O^+
    (E) HSO_4^- and SO_4^{2-}

36. What is the hydroxide ion concentration (in moles per liter) of a solution that has a hydronium ion concentration of 1×10^{-9} mole per liter at 298 K?
    (A) 1×10^{-1}
    (B) 1×10^{-3}
    (C) 1×10^{-5}
    (D) 1×10^{-7}
    (E) 1×10^{-9}

37. A racemic mixture contains dextrorotatory and levorotatory isomers in the proportion of
    (A) 5 : 1
    (B) 4 : 1
    (C) 3 : 1
    (D) 2 : 1
    (E) 1 : 1

38. Which is the oxidizing agent in the reaction

$$2Fe^{2+} + Cl_2 \rightarrow 2Fe^{3+} + 2Cl^-\ ?$$

    (A) Fe^{2+}
    (B) Fe^{3+}
    (C) Cl^-
    (D) Cl_2

Physics—33 Questions   Recommended Time—44 minutes

DIRECTIONS: Each of the statements or questions is followed by suggested completions or answers. Choose the one that best completes the statement or answers the question, and mark the letter of your choice on the answer sheet.

1. A 200-lb. highdiver climbed a tower 60 ft. tall. How much work did he do against gravitational forces?
   - (A)   1200 ft.-lb.
   - (B)   260 ft.-lb.
   - (C)   12,000 ft.-lb.
   - (D) 1.2×10^6 ft.-lb.
   - (E)   3.3 ft.-lb.

2. A gas occupies a volume of 4 liters at STP. It is heated to 546°C and compressed to 2 atm. It now occupies a volume of
   - (A)   4 liters.
   - (B)   2 liters.
   - (C)   6 liters.
   - (D)   12 liters.
   - (E)   8 liters.

3. Two point masses that are equal are separated by a distance of 1 meter. If one mass is doubled, the gravitational force between the two masses would be
   - (A)   one-half as great
   - (B)   two times greater
   - (C)   one-fourth as great
   - (D)   four times greater

4. An object is thrown upward with a vertical velocity of 65 ft./sec. It will return in
   - (A)   2 sec.
   - (B)   4 sec.
   - (C)   16 sec.
   - (D)   120 sec.
   - (E)   1 sec.

5. Electric current in a solid metal conductor is caused by the movement of
   - (A)   electrons, only
   - (B)   protons, only
   - (C)   both electrons and protons
   - (D)   neutrons

6. According to the kinetic molecular theory, the average kinetic energy of gaseous molecules depends on the
   - (A)   temperature and the identity of the gas molecules.
   - (B)   identity of the gas molecules and is independent of temperature.
   - (C)   third root of the absolute pressure under which the gas molecules are contained.
   - (D)   pressure and the identity of the gas molecules.
   - (E)   temperature without regard to the identity of the gas molecules.

7. Small particles (90 g) of a new alloy are added to a graduated cylinder containing 30 ml of water. After the addition the volume reads 45 ml. The density of the alloy is
   - (A)   6 g/ml.
   - (B)   7.5 g/ml.
   - (C)   9 g/ml.
   - (D)   3 g/ml.
   - (E)   15 g/ml.

8. In the absence of friction, raising a 60 kg mass to a height of 6 m directly requires
   - (A)   less work than in moving the same mass to the same vertical height on a 45° plane.
   - (B)   more work than in moving the same mass to the same vertical height on a 45° plane.
   - (C)   the same quantity of work as in moving the same mass to the same vertical height on a 30° plane.
   - (D)   more work than in moving a 70 kg mass to the same vertical height on a plane 15° to the vertical.
   - (E)   more work than the potential energy derived from the system.

9. In which type of wave is the disturbance parallel to the direction of wave travel?
    (A) torsional
    (B) longitudinal
    (C) transverse
    (D) circular

10. An object dropped from the top of a tower hits the ground 4 sec. later. How high is the tower?
    (A) 4 ft.
    (B) 16 ft.
    (C) 64 ft.
    (D) 256 ft.
    (E) 128 ft.

11. During a game of chance a gambler tossing a coin has a string of nine "heads" appearing in succession. His chances of getting another "head" on his next toss are
    (A) 1/1
    (B) 9/10
    (C) 1/2
    (D) 3/4
    (E) 9/1

12. A test pilot who is accelerated from rest to 600 mi./hr. in 30 sec. would be subjected to an acceleration of
    (A) 1200 mi./hr.^{2}.
    (B) 20 mi./hr.^{2}.
    (C) 72,000 mi./hr.^{2}.
    (D) 1200 ft./sec.^{2}.
    (E) 18,000 mi./hr.^{2}.

13. In a plane two forces of 4 newtons and 6 newtons are acting on an object to produce a resultant force of 2 newtons. What is the orientation of the two forces with respect to each other?
    (A) 45°
    (B) 90°
    (C) 180°
    (D) 360°
    (E) 270°

14. A twenty-pound cannonball is shot from a cannon horizontally at a height of three feet from the ground at the same time that an identical cannonball is dropped from a height of three feet. The cannonball which is dropped will
    (A) strike the ground with a greater vertical velocity than the other cannonball.
    (B) reach the ground at the same time as the other cannonball.
    (C) reach the ground after the other cannonball.
    (D) reach the ground before the other cannonball.
    (E) strike the ground with a lesser vertical velocity than the other cannonball.

Questions 15, 16, 17, 18:

Object X (mass 50 g) is moving at a speed of 0.2 m/s along a frictionless horizontal surface. When it strikes object Z (mass 10 g), the two objects stick together. Object Z was at rest before the collision.

15. The momentum of the system before the collision is
    (A) 10 g · m/s.
    (B) 12 g · m/s.
    (C) 6 g · m/s.
    (D) 250 g · m/s.
    (E) 100 g · m/s.

16. The momentum of the system after the collision is
    (A) 10 g · m/s.
    (B) 12 g · m/s.
    (C) 6 g · m/s.
    (D) 25 g · m/s.
    (E) 60 g · m/s.

17. The velocity of the objects after they are stuck together is
    (A) 0.2 m/s.
    (B) 0.32 m/s.
    (C) 0.17 m/s.
    (D) 0.38 m/s.
    (E) 0.01 m/s.

18. The kinetic energy of the new XZ object after they are stuck together is
    (A) $1.2 \text{ g} \cdot \text{m}^2/\text{s}/\text{s}^2$.
    (B) $0.87 \text{ g} \cdot \text{m}^2/\text{s}^2$.
    (C) $0.38 \text{ g} \cdot \text{m}^2/\text{s}^2$.
    (D) in excess of $4 \text{ g} \cdot \text{m}^2/\text{s}^2$.
    (E) none of the above.

19. If a radioactive isotope of silver has a half-life of about 7.5 days, at the end of 15 days what percentage of the original radioactive isotope will remain?
    (A) 25%
    (B) 15%
    (C) 7.5%
    (D) none
    (E) 50%

20. How does the velocity of sound in a vacuum compare to its velocity in air?
    (A) greater than
    (B) less than
    (C) the same
    (D) none of the above

21. A steel needle may be carefully floated on the surface of water
    (A) because steel is less dense than water.
    (B) because of surface tension.
    (C) only if the water is at a temperature of about 4°C.
    (D) only if the water contains detergent.
    (E) because steel is more dense than water.

22. An approaching locomotive sounds its horn. The frequency of the tone (as compared with the tone of the horn when it is stationary) will appear
    (A) to be higher.
    (B) to be lower.
    (C) to be unchanged.
    (D) to be outside the frequency range of the human ear.

23. A 0.5 kg object attached to a nylon cord outside a space vehicle is travelling in a circular orbit of 20 m diameter at a speed of 2 m/s. The cord is subjected to a force of
    (A) 0.2 newton.
    (B) 4.0 newtons.
    (C) 5.0 newtons.
    (D) 0.1 newton.
    (E) 20.0 newtons.

24. A nuclear reactor that is used for the production of electricity by a power company serves to
    (A) generate electricity directly by the photoelectric effect.
    (B) produce wind currents that turn generators.
    (C) produce heat for the generation of steam.
    (D) vaporize carbon to turn air turbines.
    (E) transform uranium into electrons.

25. A microscope with an eyepiece magnification of 10X and an objective of 97X would magnify an object on the stage
    (A) 19.7X.
    (B) 107X.
    (C) 197X.
    (D) 97X.
    (E) 970X.

26. The critical temperature of a compound is
    (A) the temperature at which a sustained chain reaction begins.
    (B) the highest temperature at which the gas may be liquefied.
    (C) the temperature at which the shell of a nuclear reactor is strongest.
    (D) none of the above.
    (E) all of the above.

27. A direct current circuit is wired with resistances of 3 ohms, 6 ohms, and 2 ohms in series. What would be the strength of one resistor with an equivalent resistance to replace the three resistances in series?
    (A) 11 ohms
    (B) 6 ohms
    (C) 1 ohm
    (D) none of the above
    (E) 36 ohms

28. If the above question had used the individual resistances (i.e., 3 ohms, 6 ohms, and 2 ohms) in parallel instead of in series, the equivalent resistance would be
    (A) 11 ohms.
    (B) 6 ohms.
    (C) 1 ohm.
    (D) 17 ohms.
    (E) 36 ohms.

29. If white light is dispersed by a prism, one sees a series of colors. Which listing of colors below is out of order?
    (A) red, yellow, green, blue
    (B) red, orange, green, blue
    (C) red, yellow, violet, blue
    (D) orange, yellow, green, violet
    (E) none of the above

30. A battery of 20 volts is attached to a series circuit containing resistances of 2 ohms, 3 ohms, and 5 ohms. The current in the circuit is
    (A) 2 A.
    (B) 3 A.
    (C) 5 A.
    (D) 10 A.
    (E) 30 A.

31. An airplane is flying through the air. According to the law of action and reaction, which of the following pairs of forces must have the same magnitude?
    (A) atmospheric drag of the air and lift on the wings
    (B) thrust of the engines pushing the plane forward and the atmospheric drag holding it back
    (C) weight of the plane and the lift produced by the air on the wings
    (D) weight of the plane and the engine thrust moving it forward
    (E) earth pulling the plane down and the plane pulling the earth up

32. Two points in an electric field have potentials 20 V and 80 V. If a charge of 5 nanocoulombs is moved from one point to the other, how much does its electric potential energy change?
    (A) 1×10^{-7} J
    (B) 3×10^{-7} J
    (C) 5×10^{-7} J
    (D) 3×10^{-4} J
    (E) 5×10^{-4} J

33. A ball is thrown horizontally from the roof of a building 60 m high with a speed of 20 m/s. If air resistance is neglected, how long will it take for the ball to reach the ground?
    (A) 1.8 s
    (B) 2.0 s
    (C) 3.0 s
    (D) 3.5 s
    (E) 6.1 s

SCIENCE PROBLEMS

78 MINUTES
60 QUESTIONS: Biology 21; Chemistry 21; Physics 18.

The following questions require you to use your knowledge of science to solve problems.

DIRECTIONS: The following questions and incomplete statements are in groups. Preceding each series of questions or incomplete statements is a paragraph or a short explanatory statement, a formula or set of formulas, or a definition. Read the written material and then answer the questions or complete the statements. Eliminate the choices that you think to be incorrect and mark the letter of your choice on the answer sheet.

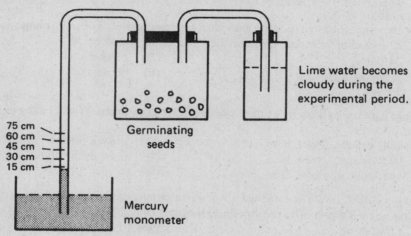

1. The process demonstrated by this experiment is
   (A) osmosis.
   (B) respiration.
   (C) metabolism.
   (D) photosynthesis.
   (E) titration.

2. The gas produced as indicated by the clouding of the lime water is
   (A) CO_2.
   (B) O_2.
   (C) N_2.
   (D) CO.
   (E) H_2.

3. If the germinating seeds used up all the air (gases) available, the mercury manometer would rise to a level of
   (A) 15 cm.
   (B) 30 cm.
   (C) 45 cm.
   (D) 4 cm.
   (E) 76 cm.

Ethanol has a boiling point of 78.3°C. When a mixture of ethanol and water is distilled, a product with a boiling point of 78.15°C is collected. This product is 95.6% ethanol by weight. If benzene is added to the initial mixture, distillation produces a ternary mixture (7.4% water, 18.5% ethanol, and 74.1% benzene) with a boiling point of 64.85°C.

4. How much pure ethanol would be produced by distillation of 1 kilogram of a 50% mixture (by weight) of ethanol and water?
   (A) 500 g
   (B) 478 g
   (C) 22 g
   (D) 92.5 g
   (E) none

5. How much pure water would be produced by distillation of 1 kilogram of a 50% (by weight) mixture of ethanol and water?
   (A) 23 g
   (B) 477 g
   (C) 500 g
   (D) 92.5 g
   (E) none

6. Increasing the amount of pure ethanol produced in the distillation of ethanol and water may be accomplished by
   (A) more efficient fractionating column.
   (B) redistillation of the product.
   (C) addition of benzene to the product.
   (D) removal of water by phase separation.
   (E) addition of benzene to the distillation mixture.

In uniformly accelerated motion the following equations hold:
$$v = v_0 + at$$
$$x = v_0 t + \tfrac{1}{2} at^2$$
where v = velocity at time t, v_0 = initial velocity, x = displacement, t = time, and a = acceleration. A smooth steel ball having a mass of 1 kg is released from rest and starts falling toward the ground.

7. Neglecting friction, what is its velocity at the end of 1 second?
   (A) 4.9 m/s
   (B) 9.8 m/s
   (C) 14.7 m/s
   (D) 19.6 m/s
   (E) none of the above

8. How far has the ball dropped in the first second?
   (A) 4.9 m
   (B) 9.8 m
   (C) 14.7 m
   (D) 19.6 m
   (E) none of the above

9. If the ball is originally 19.6 m above the ground, how long will it take to hit the ground?
   (A) 10 s
   (B) 8 s
   (C) 6 s
   (D) 4 s
   (E) 2 s

Buffer solutions are prepared from a salt of a weak acid and a weak acid. These solutions are resistant to changes in pH when acid or base is added. Buffers are generally effective within ±1 pH unit of the pK_a ($-\log K_a$) of the weak acid. According to the Henderson-Hasselbach equation

$$pH = pK_a + \log \frac{\text{salt}}{\text{weak acid}}$$

the pH of a buffer solution is defined by the pK_a and the ratio of the concentration of salt of a weak acid to the concentration of a weak acid.

10. When the salt is ten times that of the weak acid then the pH is
    (A) equal to the pK_a.
    (B) ten times the pK_a.
    (C) 1/10 the pK_a.
    (D) the pK_a plus 1.
    (E) the pK_a minus 1.

11. From the Henderson-Hasselbach equation, when pH = pK, then the salt is
    (A) zero.
    (B) equal to the weak acid.
    (C) greater than the acid concentration.
    (D) less than the acid concentration.
    (E) equal to one.

12. The pH of a 0.1 M solution of a strong acid is 1. What is the pH of a 0.1 M solution of a weak acid (pK_a 5) and 0.1 M salt?

(A) 1

(B) 5

(C) 7

(D) 9

(E) none of the above

Amino acids may be represented by the formula $R—\overset{\overset{\textstyle H}{|}}{\underset{\underset{\textstyle NH_2}{|}}{C}}—COOH$. A polypeptide is a polymer of amino acids in which the amino group of one amino acid is attached to the carboxyl of the neighboring amino acid in an amide (peptide) linkage. Ninhydrin will react with "free" amino groups (i.e., those not in amide or other linkage) to produce a purple product. In solution the intensity is proportional to the concentration of "free" amino groups.

13. Boiling a polypeptide solution in 1 N HCl prior to reacting with ninhydrin will

(A) increase the intensity of purple color compared to an equal amount of polypeptide not boiled in the presence of HCl.

(B) decrease the intensity of purple color compared to an equal amount of polypeptide not boiled in the presence of HCl.

(C) have no effect on the intensity of purple color compared to an equal amount of polypeptide not boiled in the presence of HCl.

(D) result in production of no purple color.

(E) cause reaction of ninhydrin with carboxyl groups to produce a green color.

14. Reacting a polypeptide solution with peptidase enzyme prior to reacting with ninhydrin will

(A) increase the intensity of purple color compared to an equal amount of polypeptide not reacted with peptidase.

(B) decrease the intensity of purple color compared to an equal amount of polypeptide not reacted with peptidase.

(C) have no effect on the intensity of purple color compared to an equal amount of polypeptide not reacted with peptidase.

(D) result in production of no purple color.

(E) cause reaction of ninhydrin with carboxyl groups to produce a green color.

15. What effect will addition of an inhibitor of the peptidase enzyme to the peptide solution before adding the peptidase enzyme have, as compared to a sample containing no inhibitor?

(A) increase the amount of purple color that will be produced on reacting with ninhydrin

(B) decrease the amount of purple color that will be produced on reacting with ninhydrin

(C) have no effect on the amount of purple color that will be produced on reacting with ninhydrin

(D) result in production of no purple color

(E) cause reaction of ninhydrin with carboxyl groups to produce a green color

Fatty acids may be defined as straight hydrocarbon chains terminating in a carboxyl group. The chains may be saturated or unsaturated. The unsaturation may consist of *cis* or *trans* double bonds, but the double bonds in the fatty acids of the fats of animals and higher plants are almost exclusively *cis*. *Trans* double bonds absorb light at 10.3 microns; saturated fatty acids and fatty acids containing *cis* double bonds do not absorb at this wavelength.

16. In a solution of fatty acid in solvent, absorption of light at 10.3 microns may be used to determine the concentrations of

(A) fatty acids.

(B) *cis* fatty acids.

(C) *trans* fatty acids.

(D) unsaturated fatty acids.

(E) saturated fatty acids.

17. Catalytic hydrogenation of a sample containing saturated fatty acids, *cis*-unsaturated fatty acids, and *trans*-unsaturated fatty acids will
    (A) decrease the absorption of light at 10.3 microns.
    (B) increase the absorption of light at 10.3 microns.
    (C) increase the amount of *cis*-unsaturated fatty acids.
    (D) have no effect on the absorption of light at 10.3 microns.
    (E) decrease the amount of saturated fatty acids.

18. Of the organisms listed below, the highest concentrations of *trans* fatty acids would be expected in the fats of
    (A) coconuts.
    (B) olives.
    (C) kangaroos.
    (D) bacteria.
    (E) crows.

The density of water is 1 g/cm³ and that of mercury is 13.6 g/cm³.

19. What is the mass in kg of a 30 cm³ volume of mercury?
    (A) 0.001 kg
    (B) 0.030 kg
    (C) 0.408 kg
    (D) 13.600 kg
    (E) 30.000 kg

20. What is the mass of the same volume of water?
    (A) 0.030 kg
    (B) 1.000 kg
    (C) 13.600 kg
    (D) 30.000 kg
    (E) none of the above

21. What is the specific gravity of the mercury?
    (A) 1
    (B) 13.6
    (C) 30.0
    (D) 48.0
    (E) none of the above

Ten milliliters of blood were removed from a patient, and centrifugation was utilized to separate 5 ml of plasma from the blood cells. A 3-ml sample of the plasma was extracted with 100 ml of an appropriate lipid solvent. The lipid solvent was then evaporated to 10 ml, and a 0.1 ml sample was analyzed for cholesterol. The color produced in the colorimetric analysis at 560 millimicrons was exactly equal to a standard in which 0.5 mg of cholesterol was known to be present.

22. The cholesterol concentration of the patient's plasma was
    (A) 200 mg cholesterol/100 ml plasma.
    (B) 295 mg cholesterol/100 ml plasma.
    (C) 867 mg cholesterol/100 ml plasma.
    (D) 1238 mg cholesterol/100 ml plasma.
    (E) 1665 mg cholesterol/100 ml plasma.

23. In order to make the above calculations it was NOT necessary to know
    (A) the volume of plasma separated from the blood.
    (B) the volume of plasma subjected to extraction.
    (C) the solvent volume after evaporation.
    (D) the volume of sample that was subjected to colorimetric analysis.
    (E) any of the above.

24. If the addition of twice the volume of standard produces more than twice the absorbance at 560 millimicrons, this is probably best explained by
    (A) exceeding the linear range of the method.
    (B) error in pipetting.
    (C) error in weighing to prepare the standard solution.
    (D) any or all of the above.
    (E) none of the above.

A generated water wave travels from its source with a period of 10 seconds and a wavelength of 50 meters.

25. What is the frequency of the wave?
    (A) 1/10
    (B) 1/50
    (C) 1
    (D) 5
    (E) 1/5

26. What is the velocity of the wave?
    (A) 5 m/s
    (B) 10 m/s
    (C) 1 m/s
    (D) 1/2 m/s
    (E) none of the above

27. The wave is generated at an angle to the shore such that portions of the wave nearest the shore have a decrease in velocity while the remaining portions maintain their velocity. This phenomenon is known as wave refraction and it tends to
    (A) make wave fronts normal to the shore.
    (B) make wave fronts parallel to the shore.
    (C) not change the wave approach.
    (D) decrease the wave height.
    (E) none of the above.

The following graph illustrates several phenomena that develop while a muscle is being repetitively stimulated:

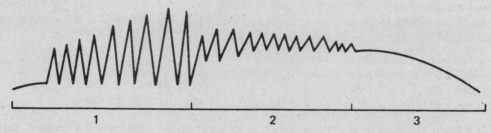

28. In the diagram above, region 1 represents
    (A) summation.
    (B) complete or fused tetanus.
    (C) repeated identical twitches.
    (D) hyperpolarization.
    (E) gradual fatiguing of the muscle.

29. What is the most likely cause of the event in region 3?
    (A) consumption of ATP stored in the muscle
    (B) loss of myosin from the muscle
    (C) gradual failure to transmit the stimulus to the contraction apparatus
    (D) loss of elasticity within the muscle
    (E) physical damage within the muscle

30. What is the major difference between regions 1 and 2?
    (A) Elastic elements have become fully stretched in region 1, but not in region 2.
    (B) Elastic elements have become fully stretched in region 2, but not in region 1.
    (C) The stimulus strength is greater in region 2.
    (D) The stimulus strength is greater in region 1.
    (E) Region 2 is isometric contraction; region 1 is isotonic contraction.

An enzyme, lactic dehydrogenase, catalyzes the oxidation of lactic acid to produce pyruvic acid. As lactic acid is oxidized, a coenzyme, NAD^+, is reduced to $NADH + H^+$. The normal serum enzyme activity is about 40-100 enzyme units/ml, but the enzyme activity is often increased after occlusion of a blood vessel which nourishes the heart.

31. If the rate of reduction of NAD⁺ (in the presence of lactic acid) in the serum of a patient suspected of having a heart attack is decreased compared to pooled normal serum, this is
   (A) evidence of a heart attack.
   (B) definite proof of a heart attack.
   (C) not evidence of a heart attack.
   (D) proof that no heart attack occurred.
   (E) proof of laboratory error.

32. The rate of production of $NADH + H^+$ by the lactic dehydrogenase in 0.1 ml of serum from patient B is 4 times the rate that is noted in 0.2 ml of serum from patient E. If the lactic dehydrogenase activity in patient E is 40 units/ml, then the activity in patient B's serum is
   (A) 40 units/ml.   (D) 320 units/ml.
   (B) 160 units/ml.   (E) 5 units/ml.
   (C) 10 units/ml.

33. What is the rate of appearance of $NADH + H^+$ in comparison to the rate of disappearance of NAD^+ in the enzymatic reaction catalyzed by lactic dehydrogenase?
   (A) unrelated to   (D) one-fourth
   (B) twice   (E) equal to
   (C) one-half

Given that the index of refraction is defined as the ratio of the speed of light in a vacuum to that of the speed of light in the medium ($n = C/S_m$), $C = 3.0 \times 10^8$ m/s, and that the speed of light in water is about 2.25×10^8 m/s.

34. What is the index of refraction of water?
   (A) 0.75   (D) 6.25
   (B) 1.00   (E) 6.75
   (C) 1.33

35. If a beam of light strikes a water surface at an angle of 45° after leaving a vacuum, then
   (A) $n_r/n_1 = 1$.   (D) $n_r/n_1 = 0$.
   (B) $n_r/n_1 > 1$.   (E) none of the above.
   (C) $n_r/n_1 < 1$.

36. If the direction of the beam is reversed and goes from the water to the vacuum, the ratio of n_r/n_1 would be less than 1 indicating that the n_1 beam would bend
   (A) toward the normal.   (D) along the boundary.
   (B) away from the normal.   (E) none of the above.
   (C) into the normal.

The following diagram represents a graduated centrifuge tube containing 10 ml of blood following 15 to 20 min. of centrifugation at a speed of 2,500 rpm. The tube had been heparinized to prevent coagulation.

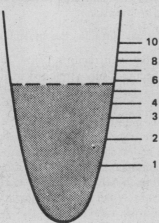

37. The lower 5.5 ml consists of predominantly
    (A) fibrin clot material.
    (B) platelets.
    (C) white blood cells.
    (D) red blood cells.

38. The hematocrit of the donor is
    (A) 45%
    (B) 55%
    (C) 4.5 ml.
    (D) 5.5 ml.
    (E) 10 ml.

39. This situation deviates from the normal in such a way that it could be due to
    (A) living at high altitude.
    (B) sickle-cell anemia.
    (C) pernicious anemia.
    (D) excessive X-ray treatment.
    (E) all of the above.

Hydrofluoric acid, HF, ionizes in water to produce H^+ and F^-. The ionization constant is 2×10^{-4}.

40. The pH of a 0.5 M aqueous solution of HF may be calculated to be
    (A) 2.
    (B) 4.
    (C) 5.
    (D) 8.
    (E) 10.

41. What is the error in pH units when one fails to consider the ionization of water in the above calculation of pH?
    (A) >0.5
    (B) 0.4
    (C) 0.2
    (D) 0.09
    (E) <0.01

42. The pH of a 0.5 N aqueous solution of HF may be calculated to be
    (A) 2.
    (B) 4.
    (C) 5.
    (D) 8.
    (E) 10.

An unidentified compound is composed solely of carbon and hydrogen. Complete combustion of 0.100 g of the compound produced 0.677 g of CO_2 and 0.138 g of water.

43. The empirical formula of this compound is
    (A) CH.
    (B) CH_2.
    (C) CH_3.
    (D) C_2H_4.
    (E) CH_4.

44. The molecular formula could be
    (A) CH_4.
    (B) C_2H_4.
    (C) C_2H_2.
    (D) C_2H_6.
    (E) C_3H_6.

45. Having determined the empirical formula, the molecular formula can be determined by information derived from
    (A) the amount of oxygen consumed during combustion.
    (B) freezing point depression when the compound is dissolved in water.
    (C) the amount of nitrogen oxides formed during combustion.
    (D) the temperature at which combustion begins.
    (E) all of the above.

To 100 ml of 0.1 M $AgNO_3$ is added sufficient solid Na_2SO_4 to begin precipitation.

46. Knowing that the solubility product constant for Ag_2SO_4 is 6.4×10^{-5}, it is possible to predict that precipitation will begin when the concentration of Na_2SO_4 reaches
    (A) $6.4 \times 10^{-7} M$.
    (B) $6.4 \times 10^{-6} M$.
    (C) $6.4 \times 10^{-3} M$.
    (D) 0.8 M.
    (E) 0.08 M.

47. If Na_2SO_4 were a weakly ionized salt, the addition of $NaNO_3$ in the above problem would be expected to
(A) cause the precipitation of $AgNO_3$.
(B) decrease the concentration of Na_2SO_4 required for precipitation to begin.
(C) increase the concentration of Na_2SO_4 required for precipitation to begin.
(D) have no effect on precipitation.
(E) change the solubility product constant for Ag_2SO_4.

48. If NaCl were substituted for $NaNO_3$ in the above question, we would expect to
(A) prevent any precipitation.
(B) increase the precipitation of $NaNO_3$.
(C) decrease but not abolish the precipitation of $NaNO_3$.
(D) precipitate $AgNO_3$.
(E) precipitate AgCl.

Given the circuit diagram below where $R_1 = 20$ ohms; $R_2 = 5$ ohms; $R_3 = 10$ ohms; and $R_4 = 15$ ohms.

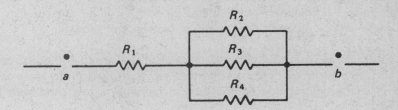

49. What is the resistance in the parallel resistors?
(A) 2.75 ohms
(B) 5.00 ohms
(C) 10.00 ohms
(D) 15.00 ohms
(E) 30.00 ohms

50. What is the total resistance in this circuit?
(A) 20.0 ohms
(B) 22.7 ohms
(C) 33.1 ohms
(D) 45.0 ohms
(E) 50.7 ohms

51. If the current through the circuit is 5 amperes, what is the potential difference from a to b?
(A) 100 volts
(B) 114 volts
(C) 220 volts
(D) 230 volts
(E) none of the above

Use the following diagram to answer questions 52–54.

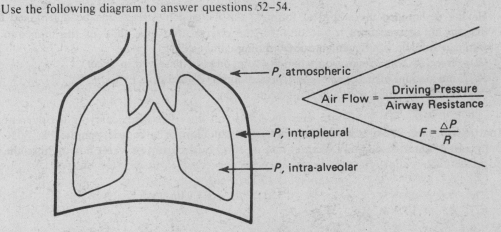

P, atmospheric

$$\text{Air Flow} = \frac{\text{Driving Pressure}}{\text{Airway Resistance}}$$

$$F = \frac{\Delta P}{R}$$

P, intrapleural

P, intra-alveolar

52. The driving pressure (ΔP) in breathing which causes air to flow into the lungs is
   (A)   atmospheric pressure (*Patm*).
   (B)   the intra-alveolar (intrapulmonary) pressure (*Palv*).
   (C)   atmospheric pressure minus the intra-alveolar pressure.
   (D)   the intrapleural pressure (*Ppl*).
   (E)   the intrapleural pressure minus the intra-alveolar pressure.

53. During inspiration, intra-alveolar pressure (*Palv*)
   (A)   transiently goes below atmospheric pressure (*Patm*).
   (B)   transiently goes above atmospheric pressure.
   (C)   equals atmospheric pressure.
   (D)   equals intrapleural pressure.
   (E)   transiently goes below intrapleural pressure.

54. The alveolar ventilation per minute refers to the amount of fresh air which reaches the alveoli of the lungs per minute. Alveolar ventilation per minute equals the
   (A)   functional residual capacity × frequency of breathing.
   (B)   physiologic dead space × frequency of breathing.
   (C)   anatomic dead space × frequency of breathing.
   (D)   tidal volume × frequency of breathing.
   (E)   (tidal volume − anatomic dead space) × frequency of breathing.

The ABO blood group is transmitted in humans as alleles A and B that are codominate, occurring at the same autosomal chromosome as a recessive allele O. In some cases it may be utilized to assist in determining paternity or in reuniting a lost child with his or her biological parents.

55. A woman of blood type O claims a child of blood type AB, and alleges that the father is a man of blood type B. The most likely explanation is that

   (A)   these are the biological parents.
   (B)   she is the mother but the man is not the father.
   (C)   neither is a possible parent of the child.
   (D)   she is not the mother but the man's blood type does not rule him out as the father.
   (E)   there is insufficient information to allow one to reach any conclusion as to the child's parentage.

56. If the man in question 55 is found to have previously fathered a child of blood type O, the chance that a child of the man and the woman in this question would be blood type O is
   (A)   zero.   (D)   50%.
   (B)   25%.   (E)   100%.
   (C)   33%.

57. With the information from question 56, the chance that any child of the man and woman would be a girl with blood type B is
   (A)   zero.   (D)   50%.
   (B)   25%.   (E)   100%.
   (C)   33%.

A large electric motor uses 60 amperes on a 550-volt line. The leads carrying the current into the motor have a combined resistance of 0.020 ohm. The motor operates at 80% efficiency and is water cooled to a temperature of 30°C by a stream of water flowing into the system at 18°C.

Constants: 4.19 J = 1 cal
   550 ft · lb/sec = 1 hp

58. At what rate is heat generated in the lead-in wires?
(A) 9 W
(B) 11 W
(C) 14 W
(D) 48 W
(E) 72 W

59. At what rate does the motor produce mechanical energy?
(A) 60 kJ/s
(B) 33 kW
(C) 33 hp
(D) 7 kW
(E) 26 kJ/s

60. What mass of water must flow through the system every second?
(A) 130 g
(B) 520 g
(C) 660 g
(D) 2.3 kg
(E) 19 kg

SKILLS ANALYSIS: READING

85 MINUTES
68 QUESTIONS

The following questions are to be answered based on your careful reading of selections from scientific writings.

DIRECTIONS: Read each passage carefully, then answer the questions following it. Consider only the material within the passage in answering the questions. Eliminate those choices that you think to be incorrect and mark the letter of your choice on the answer sheet.

As soon as any business becomes large enough for an owner to employ an assistant, a manager-subordinate relationship has been created. As the business grows even larger, we may find this subordinate having employees working for him or her so that the necessary duties are able to be performed.

The reason for having a subordinate is that the person supervising does not have the time, or in some cases, the ability to accomplish the tasks. The supervisor or manager must delegate part of his or her duties to another.

Delegation is made up of two parts—authority and responsibility. The manager or supervisor gives the subordinate the authority to do part of his or her duties so that he or she may be free to pursue other duties. The subordinate with this authority may then act independently without consulting the supervisor in the accomplishment of these tasks. Responsibility on the other hand, cannot be fully delegated. If the subordinate fails to carry out the tasks in a proper manner, it is the manager or supervisor who is held ultimately responsible for the failure.

Each level of supervision may create its own responsibility for getting the job accomplished. It can never fully be delegated, however, as there is still the upward reporting relationship back to the owner.

The important thing is to give a manager or supervisor the full authority within which to work if duties are to be delegated. Too many managers overlook this simple point and then wonder why the task is not accomplished. They also wonder why their supervisor is dissatisfied with the results over which they feel they have no control.

The following statements are related to the passage above. Based on the information given, select:
(A) if the statement is *supported by* the information in the passage.
(B) if the statement is *contradicted by* the information in the passage.
(C) if the statement is *neither supported nor contradicted by* information in the passage.

1. Managers often incompletely delegate to their subordinates freedom to carry out a total commitment.

2. Both authority and responsibility can and should be delegated to subordinates by their manager or supervisor.

3. Managers are held responsible for the acts of their employees.

4. Supervisors or managers may create their own responsibility as they delegate to their subordinates.

5. The only way to get a job accomplished is to do it yourself.

6. Responsibility and authority are the two components of delegation.

Wars have been won and lost. Men sent to the moon and back. Marriages made and divorces granted. All because of one little but very important, and often overlooked item—communication!

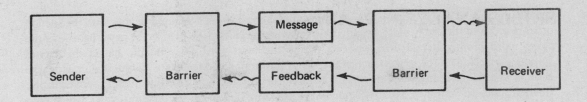

Senders will express a thought which will be influenced by their experiences, backgrounds, and personal needs. These barriers will change the way the message is expressed. The receiver is also influenced by experience, background, and personal interests; this will distort what is heard. Many times the thought expressed is completely different from what the receiver hears. By the same token, the reply that the receiver gives is influenced by these same barriers so that what is heard may be completely different from what was said. The end result could be conflict or at the very least, a misunderstanding.

When the receiver replies to the sender's statements, it becomes easier for the sender to determine if his or her message was understood. Many times this reply does not come forth. How can the sender make sure that he or she is understood? One can ask a clarifying question, but one must be careful not to phrase it "do you understand" as it is mostly likely the receiver will merely answer "yes." The sender will be more confident if he or she can phrase a question in a manner to elicit a response of "what do you understand?" that is understood. This clarification to the sender by the receiver is called "feedback." Unless the sender receives this positive feedback in one form or another, he or she can never be fully confident that the message was received as it was intended.

A simple example of how communications can break down without feedback is the parlor game where one person tells the person next to him a story. The second person repeats what was heard to the third and so on around the group until it gets back to the originator. Chances are, the story the originator receives back will be completely different from the one which was initiated.

In addition to verbal communications, there are several other types. One is physical communication. The pat on the back and handshake are examples of touch. A second type of physical communication is a visible movement of some part of the body. A nod of the head, the pointing of a finger, or a frown expresses this type of communication. Yet a third type would be symbols which we recognize. A flashing red light, newspapers or books, and traffic lights are common examples.

To summarize, we can say that communication is the transfer of some type of meaning from one person to another. Since we all wish to express ourselves, and be understood, communication becomes very important and our techniques must be continually practiced and improved.

The following statements are related to the passage above. Based on the information given, select:
(A) if the statement is *supported by* the information in the passage.
(B) if the statement is *contradicted by* the information in the passage.
(C) if the statement is *neither supported nor contradicted by* information in the passage.

7. Clear expression of a thought assures that it will be properly understood.

8. The best way to assure understanding by the receiver is to elicit feedback.

9. Communication is the interaction between individuals.

10. Our prejudices influence what we say and what we hear.

11. If the receiver returns the same message to the sender, one can always be sure that one has been understood.

12. "Feedback" is the clarification to the sender by the receiver of what the latter understood.

The sensations of pain and temperature are made possible in human beings by a neural pathway called the spinothalamic system. This system is composed of three neuron chains that extend from the spinal cord to the thalamus of the brain.

Various kinds of external receptors for pain and temperature relay impulses via myelinated and unmyelinated fibers to the first neuron in the chain that is located in the dorsal root ganglion of the dorsal (sensory) root of the spinal cord. No synapse occurs here, but these unipolar ganglion cells do send fibers to regions of the dorsal horn of the spinal cord where a synapse occurs with the second order neurons of the chain. Postsynaptic fibers from these cells cross over to the opposite side of the spinal cord (contralaterally) and ascend to the thalamus in a fiber bundle called the lateral spinothalamic tract. This tract reaches the ventroposterior lateral nucleus of the thalamus where another synapse is seen, this time with third-order neurons of this pathway. Finally, postsynaptic fibers from these neurons go to the region of the postcentral gyrus of the cerebral cortex where pain and temperature information is processed by the brain.

As one might expect, injury to the lateral spinothalamic tract results in contralateral loss of pain and temperature sensation below the level of the lesion. This fact is applied clinically since surgical sectioning of this tract is sometimes done to relieve persistent, intractable pain.

13. Pain and temperature information reaches the postcentral gyrus of the cerebral cortex by which of the following route sequences?
    (A) external receptors—dorsal root ganglion—lateral spinothalamic tract—ventroposterior nucleus of the thalamus—postcentral gyrus of cortex
    (B) dorsal root ganglion—dorsal horn of spinal cord—lateral spinothalamic tract—medial ventroposterior nucleus of the thalamus—postcentral gyrus of cortex
    (C) external receptors—dorsal root ganglion—contralateral lateral spinothalamic tract—ventroposterior lateral nucleus of the thalamus—postcentral gyrus of cortex
    (D) external receptors—dorsal root ganglion—dorsal horn of spinal cord—contralateral lateral spinothalamic tract—ventroposterior lateral nucleus of the thalamus—postcentral gyrus of the cerebral cortex

14. The cell body of origin for fibers comprising the lateral spinothalamic tract is located in the
    (A) dorsal root ganglion.
    (B) dorsal horn of the spinal cord.
    (C) external pain and temperature receptor organ.
    (D) ventroposterior lateral nucleus of the thalamus.

15. The nucleus of termination for the lateral spinothalamic tract is found in
    (A) the dorsal horn of the spinal cord.
    (B) the postcentral gyrus of the cerebral cortex.
    (C) the ventroposterior lateral thalamus.
    (D) none of the above.

16. A lesion or injury to the left lateral spinothalamic tract would probably result in
    (A) contralateral loss of pain and temperature sensation at the level of the lesion.
    (B) loss of pain and temperature sensation from regions of the left side of the body supplied by spinal cord areas below the level of the lesion.
    (C) contralateral loss of pain and temperature sensation from regions of the right side of the body supplied by spinal cord areas below the level of the lesion.
    (D) none of the above.

In order for a thoracic surgeon to visualize the heart he or she must open up the pericardium which is a sac that covers the heart. A human heart is four-chambered and is composed of right and left atria which are separated by an interatrial septum that is frequently marred by defects. In the fetus the foramen ovale is an opening in this septum and blood passes from the right atrium to the left atrium so that the pulmonary circulation may be bypassed. A patent foramen ovale may contribute to the condition known as "blue baby." Two ventricles are also present; specifically we can speak of a right ventricle which pumps deoxygenated blood to the lungs and a left ventricle which pumps oxygenated blood to the tissues of the body. Between the ventricles is located the interventricular septum. As the surgeon approaches the heart from the anterior aspect he or she finds the atrioventricular sulcus which separates the atria from the ventricles and on the anterior side lodges the right coronary artery; while on the posterior side the coronary sinus, which is the confluence of most of the venous drainage of the heart, occupies this sulcus. The parts of the heart seen in an anterior view are mainly the right atrium and ventricle; only a portion of the left ventricle is seen in an anterior view. Between the right and left ventricle the surgeon finds the anterior interventricular sulcus which is continuous posteriorly as the posterior interventricular sulcus. In the anterior interventricular sulcus is lodged the anterior interventricular branch of the left coronary artery; while in the posterior the corresponding posterior interventricular branch of the right coronary artery can be found.

The superior and inferior vena cava and the coronary sinus empty into the right atrium. From here blood passes into the right ventricle to be pumped into the lungs via the pulmonary arteries. Blood from the lungs is returned to the left atrium by the pulmonary veins; it then passes into the left ventricle to leave upon its contraction via the aorta to supply the arterial system of the body. The heart alternately contracts and relaxes, and this cardiac cycle is repeated about 75 times per minute; the duration of one cycle is about 0.8 seconds. Atrial systole (contraction) which takes about 0.1 seconds is followed by ventricular systole lasting about 0.3 seconds and absolute diastole (relaxation) follows lasting about 0.4 seconds.

The heart has an automatic rhythmic beat, but it is also under the influence of nerves which, however, serve only to change the force or frequency of the contractions of the muscle in accordance with the physiologic needs of the organism. The modification of the intrinsic rhythmicity is by way of the two parts of the autonomic nervous system; stimulation occurs through the sympathetic portion while homeostatic maintenance is mainly a function of the parasympathetic portion. Stimulation through the sympathetic nerves increases the rate and force of the heart beat; while slowing and reduction in force are the result of parasympathetic stimulation. Vasodilation of the coronary arteries is brought about by sympathetic stimulation while vasoconstriction is elicited by parasympathetic stimulation.

The following statements are related to the passage. Based on the information given, select:

(A)   if the statement is *supported by* the information in the passage.
(B)   if the statement is *contradicted by* the information in the passage.
(C)   if the statement is *neither supported nor contradicted by* information in the passage.

17.   The paragraph deals mainly with the surgical anatomy of the heart.

18.   At rest, the coronary circulation is dilated.

19.   Most of the left side of the heart probably projects posteriorly.

20.   The left ventricle is the main pumping chamber.

21.   Most of the venous drainage of the heart enters the right atrium.

22.   Venous blood brings deoxygenated blood back to the heart.

23.   All chambers of the heart contract.

24.   The actual period of rest for each chamber is 0.7 seconds for the atria and 0.5 seconds for the ventricles.

25.   The heart is at rest longer than at work.

26.   The parasympathetic portion of the autonomic nervous system slows down the activity of most organs of the body.

27.   The automatic rhythmicity of the heart cannot be altered.

28.   Heart rate may be controlled by neuronal stimulation.

29.   A defect in the valvular system may be noticed as a murmur.

Graded or nongraded elementary schools? Educational authorities today are often in obvious disagreement as to which type of system produces the better student.

Many advocates of the nongraded approach are quick to argue that the time-honored practice of pupil classification by numerical grade levels is surely a pitfall for the school-age child. Under the graded system, a specified amount of progress is standard for the year's work. The content of the work to be covered and mastered, is laid out within the grade and the students are then manipulated to fit the mold. For example, children who are above average in ability are given the same materials as the average group, for whom the system was developed, in hopes that they will adapt themselves to the slower pace without turning the boredom they experience into a problem situation. The below-average child on the other hand, is pushed along and expected to master a slightly watered down version of the material. Failure to do so usually results in the child being forced to repeat the entire year using the same materials with the philosophy that a second-go-round will solve the problem.

Not so! cry educators who strongly defend the graded system and who predict that the pendulum is, in fact, swinging back to a more traditional approach for education.

Handled properly, the graded format provides for an organized, predictable program, in which teachers can be held accountable for imparting a specific amount of material within a given time frame. They are, however, by no means limited to the prescribed amount of material and are, therefore, able to accommodate all types of students through the use of supplementary as well as remedial programs.

What of the nongraded system? Traditionalists claim that while it is unique in theory, it more often than not causes serious problems when put into practice.

Organizationally, the nongraded approach is designed to provide continuous learning experiences for each pupil, which will allow the student to achieve success at every level of instruction. Movement from level to level occurs as fast as the individual student masters the content and skills at each level of achievement. The student will not experience failure; and boredom is eliminated even for the most gifted, as students are stimulated and challenged to move to new levels whenever they are ready to do so. Therein lies the main fallacy of the system, according to opponents, for who, they ask, will decide when the child is ready?

The argument of graded versus nongraded schools is likely to continue for some time to come. Who will be the judge of the better system? Most probably it will be the institutions of higher learning which receive the final products.

The following statements are related to the passage. Based on the information given, select:

(A)   if the statement is *supported by* the information in the passage.
(B)   if the statement is *contradicted by* the information in the passage.
(C)   if the statement is *neither supported nor contradicted by* information in the passage.

30.   Authorities always agree that the nongraded approach to education is superior, because it provides for every child's specific needs.

31.   Once graduated from college or other institutions of higher learning, products of the nongraded system are able to acquire better jobs and hold them longer.

32.   Advocates of the traditional method of education claim an organized, predictable frame work as one of the main strengths of a graded system.

33.   The nongraded school system allows students to study whatever they want.

34.   Most school systems are swinging back to a more traditional educational philosophy, because they now realize that it suits the needs of the majority.

The pituitary (hypophysis) is a small gland at the base of the brain to which it is connected by the pituitary stalk. The pituitary, often referred to as the master gland, is composed of two lobes—the anterior lobe or adenohypophysis and the posterior lobe or neurohypophysis. The anterior pituitary secretes six major hormones while the neurohypophysis secretes two. Hormonal secretion by the pituitary is almost completely controlled by the hypothalamus which receives information from most of the nervous system. This incoming information then influences the regulatory control of the hypothalamus upon the pituitary. The hypothalamus synthesizes and secretes releasing factors which cause release of anterior pituitary hormones and, for three of these hormones, inhibiting factors as well. The hormones secreted by the anterior pituitary regulate metabolic functions of the body through their effect upon target glands. The target glands stimulated by the pituitary hormones subsequently release their products into the bloodstream, and the level of the products then, via a negative feedback loop, controls the output and activity of the pituitary. The anterior pituitary hormones are:

Growth hormone which stimulates body growth.

Thyrotropin which controls secretion of thyroxine by the thyroid gland. Thyroxine regulates the rates of most chemical reactions in the body.

Corticotropin regulates adrenal cortical hormone secretions which influence metabolism of proteins, carbohydrates and fats.

Follicle stimulating hormone, luteinizing hormone and *luteotrophic hormone*—all of which promote the growth and/or function of the gonads.

Two important hormones secreted by the posterior pituitary gland are synthesized directly in the hypothalamus. They are antidiuretic hormone, which regulates water excretion by the kidneys, and oxytocin, which promotes milk release during suckling. A few abnormalities of the pituitary may be agenesis (failure to develop), hyperplasia (growth to an abnormally large size), and tumors.

These anatomical deviations may result in hyperfunction or hypofunction of the pituitary gland and one or more of the target glands controlled by the specific hormone released in unusual quantities.

35. The main topic of this passage is the
  - (A) location and importance of the pituitary gland.
  - (B) role of the pituitary gland in endocrine function.
  - (C) major pituitary hormones and their target organs.

36. According to the passage,
  - (A) the glands in the body can function properly only if the pituitary secretion is normal.
  - (B) the anterior lobe of the pituitary is more important than the posterior pituitary because it secretes more hormones.
  - (C) any disease state affecting the pituitary could lead to dysfunction of endocrine glands controlled by the pituitary.

37. It cannot be inferred from the passage that
  - (A) the pituitary as the master gland is responsible for all glandular secretions.
  - (B) derangements in pituitary function may lead to extreme variations in size, e.g., giantism or dwarfism.
  - (C) hypersecretion of thyroxine by the thyroid may be caused by increased pituitary secretion of thyrotropin.

38. Corticotropin influences electrolyte balance within the system.
  - (A) The statement is supported by the passage.
  - (B) The statement is contradicted by the passage.
  - (C) The statement is neither supported nor contradicted by the passage.

There is a great deal of independence exhibited in the manner in which many systems of the body perform their functions; in contrast the cellular organization and units of the nervous system are mutually dependent upon each other to carry out their complicated integrative activities. The functioning of the nervous system depends on its receptors, pathways, neurotransmitters, synaptic terminals, polarities, and effectors. An impulse perceived must be conducted and transmitted along a series of nerve cells; it must be interpreted and processed; and finally an effector organ response must be elicited. It is this complex arrangement among receiving, transmitting, integrating, and effector stimulation and response that results in the meaningful activities visualized and characterized as behavior. To clarify the highly complex operations of the system, research by neuroanatomists, neurophysiologists, and neuroendocrinologists is necessary. The neuroanatomist might be likened to the electrical engineer who traces the telephone wires of a city while the other two groups are perhaps more interested in the switching and relay stations. The course of the peripheral and central pathways and the functional significance of the many centers of the spinal cord and brain have been determined mainly by the study of animals and humans. Certain parts of their systems had been destroyed by disease, injury, the use of chemical or physical agents, or, in animals, by experimental lesions. In recent years scientific interest has turned to the hypothalamus since many of the body's physiological and endocrine functions seem to be influenced by its activities. It is an integrative center that controls behavior patterns and many of the organism's basic life functions. The center is controlled and modulated by higher centers of the nervous system and via a direct and indirect feedback loop of the endocrine system which it influences. No direct neuronal connections exist between the hypothalamus and the pituitary gland and, therefore, hypothalamic humoral factors reach the anterior lobe of the pituitary via its blood supply. Most experts regard the hypophysial portal system as the critical link between the brain and the pituitary as far as the transport of neurosecretions are concerned. The hypothalamus secretes releasing factors or hormones which in turn elicit in the pituitary the production of pituitary tropic hormones which then influence target organs in the organism. We may illustrate this point by carrying out a subtotal thyroidectomy in an animal. We may reason that thyroid secretions should fall, thyroid hormone levels in the blood should drop, hypothalamic areas would be alerted, and the releasing factor output initiated. This then results in an increase of pituitary thyroid tropic hormone output which will lead to increased thyroid productivity and compensatory action. If, however, a subtotal thyroidectomy and electrolytic lesion in the proper hypothalamic area are carried out at the same time, the compensatory activity does not occur.

The following statements are related to the passage. Based on the information given, select:
- (A) if the statement is *supported by* the information in the passage.
- (B) if the statement is *contradicted by* the information in the passage.
- (C) if the statement is *neither supported nor contradicted by* information in the passage.

39. Successful operation of the nervous system results from the combined activity of its cells.

40. All systems of the body can function independently of one another.

41. The pituitary gland is influenced by indirect neuronal connections of the hypothalamus.

42. The hypothalamus is under the influence of a feedback mechanism.

43. Neurosecretions reach the pituitary by means of the portal system.

44. The parts of the nervous system are mutually dependent upon each other.

45. Neurotransmitters are key elements in the transmission and integration of impulses.

46. Behavior might be considered the sum total of all nervous system activity.

47. The neuroanatomist is not interested in the transmission process of an impulse.

48. Disease processes lead only to destruction.

49. The hypophysial portal system begins as capillaries which form veins; these then break up into capillaries again.

50. Thyroidectomy without electrolytic lesion leads to compensatory activity of the thyroid gland.

51. Electrolytic lesions may be used to study the functions of the nervous system.

The trigeminal nerve via its mandibular and maxillary divisions supplies innervation for general sensation to the anterior 2/3 of the tongue and the mandibular and maxillary teeth. Sensation from all the mandibular teeth is mediated by the inferior alveolar nerve, which is a branch of the mandibular division. The maxillary division gives rise to the posterior superior alveolar nerve which innervates the three maxillary molar teeth except the mesio-buccal root of the first molar. The infraorbital nerve, also a branch of the maxillary division, divides into middle and anterior superior alveolar nerves. The former innervates the first and second bicuspid teeth and the mesio-buccal root of the first molar. The remainder of the anterior teeth, the canines and incisors, are supplied by the anterior superior alveolar nerve. To provide local anesthesia to specific teeth, the nerve or nerves innervating them must be anesthetized by injecting an anesthetic drug.

The following statements are related to the passage above. Based on the information given, select:
- (A) if the statement is *supported by* the information in the passage.
- (B) if the statement is *contradicted by* the information in the passage.
- (C) if the statement is *neither supported nor contradicted by* information in the passage.

52. The maxillary nerve must be anesthetized to block the sensory innervation of the hard palate.

53. The maxillary teeth can be blocked by anesthetizing the maxillary division of the trigeminal nerve.

54. Sensation from the mandibular incisor teeth is mediated via the inferior alveolar nerve.

55. The special sense of taste from the anterior 2/3 of the tongue is perceived by the facial nerve.

56. The trigeminal nerve divides into three divisions.

57. Sensation from the second maxillary molar tooth may be blocked by anesthetizing the posterior superior alveolar nerve.

58. Inadequate anesthesia of the maxillary incisors of one side may be due to overlapping innervation from the anterior superior alveolar nerve of the opposite side.

59. Innervation of the maxillary bicuspids can be blocked by anesthetizing the anterior superior alveolar nerve.

60. A mandibular block can be accomplished by using the lingula of the mandible as a landmark.

61. The mental nerve is a branch of the inferior alveolar nerve.

The orbit is a cone-shaped bony structure with an apex directed posteriorly and a large anterior opening. It may be described as having a floor, a roof, and medial and lateral walls. The roof is formed mainly by the frontal bone anterior to a small portion of the sphenoid bone. The floor of the orbit from anterior to posterior is composed of the zygomatic, maxillary, and palatine bones. The lateral wall consists of portions of the zygomatic bone anteriorly and the sphenoid bone posteriorly. The medial wall from anterior to posterior is formed by the frontal process of the maxilla, the lacrimal bone, the ethmoid bone, and the sphenoid bone. Besides the anterior opening, the orbit communicates with other regions via nine openings. The infraorbital nerve enters the orbit through the inferior orbital fissure, then lies in the infraorbital groove in the floor and exits anteriorly through the infraorbital foramen. On its medial wall the anterior and posterior ethmoidal foramina transmit the anterior and posterior ethmoidal nerves, respectively. Posteriorly, near the apex of the orbit, the optic nerve and the ophthalmic artery enter via the optic canal. Also located near the apex, the superior orbital fissure transmits the cranial nerves III, IV, and VI and the ophthalmic division of cranial nerve V.

The following statements are related to the passage above. Based on the information given, select:
(A)   if the statement is *supported by* the information in the passage.
(B)   if the statement is *contradicted by* the information in the passage.
(C)   if the statement is *neither supported nor contradicted by* information in the passage.

62. The superior ophthalmic vein exits the orbit via the superior orbital fissure.

63. The orbit is formed by portions of seven bones.

64. The anterior margin, or entrance of the orbit, is bounded by parts of the frontal, zygomatic, and maxillary bones.

65. The lacrimal bone forms part of the lateral wall of the orbit.

66. The superior orbital fissure transmits the optic nerve.

67. The anterior ethmoidal foramen is located between the ethmoid and frontal bones.

68. The ophthalmic artery is a branch of the internal carotid artery.

SKILLS ANALYSIS: QUANTITATIVE

85 MINUTES
68 QUESTIONS

The following questions are to be answered based on your knowledge of basic mathematical principles and relationships.

DIRECTIONS: Read each passage carefully, study each table or chart, then answer the questions following it. Consider only the material presented in answering the questions. Eliminate those choices that you think to be incorrect and mark the letter of your choice on the answer sheet.

Ten adult male guinea pigs were housed in individual cages in a room at 37°C. Five of the guinea pigs were fed an ascorbic acid deficient diet while the other five were fed standard guinea pig diet. Both groups were allowed access to water *ad libitum*. At weekly intervals the serum concentration of gamma globulin and lymphocyte reactivity were measured in both the experimental and control groups. The following graphs illustrate data collected from this experiment.

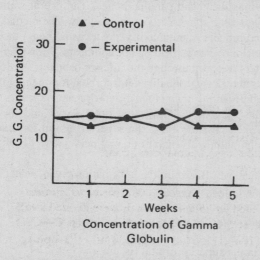

Concentration of Gamma
Globulin

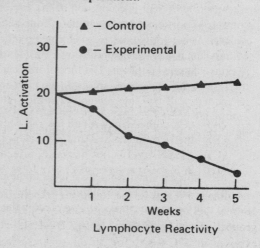

Lymphocyte Reactivity

1. The object of this experiment was to determine the effect of
    (A)   gamma globulin concentration on lymphocyte reactivity.
    (B)   ascorbic acid deficiency on the immunologic system.
    (C)   temperature on scorbutic guinea pigs.
    (D)   gamma globulin in the treatment of scurvy.

2. Another conclusion that can be reached from these data is
    (A)   there are no sex differences in the response of guinea pigs to an ascorbic acid deficient diet.
    (B)   temperature has a marked effect on gamma globulin concentration.
    (C)   lymphocyte reactivity in the scorbutic guinea pig is independent of gamma globulin concentration.
    (D)   gamma globulin concentration varies inversely with lymphocyte reactivity.

3. The experimenter may also conclude that
    (A)   the scorbutic guinea pig probably has a partial immunologic deficiency.
    (B)   lymphocyte reactivity varies widely in the normal guinea pig.
    (C)   gamma globulin concentration is affected by biological rhythms.
    (D)   there are no species differences in gamma globulin concentration.

A scientist sets up the following experiment. Ten male rats are placed in each of two cages. One cage is placed in a room regulated at a constant temperature of 37°C (group A) while the other cage is placed in a similar room kept at 45°C (group B). Food and water were provided *ad libitum* to both experimental sets. Food consumption, water consumption, ACTH blood level, and heart rate were determined for a period of ten days. The following bar graphs illustrated the results.

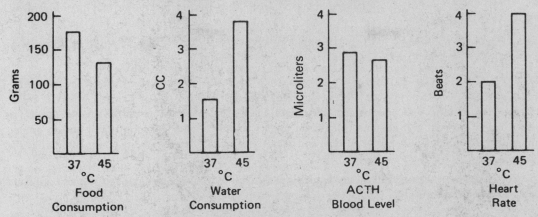

4. The objective of this experiment was to determine
   (A) food consumption in rats.
   (B) water consumption in rats.
   (C) heart rate in rats.
   (D) effect of temperature on rats.

5. The investigator after examining the four graphs can report that
   (A) at a higher temperature the rats were more active.
   (B) the rats maintained at 37°C developed a desire for water.
   (C) ACTH level is not markedly affected by the experimental conditions.
   (D) at higher temperatures more food is required.

Animals utilized in the following experiment were golden hamsters (*Mesocricetus auratus*). Normal diet consisted of Purina laboratory chow provided *ad libitum*. Animals were divided into 3 groups: group A—Control; group B—Cold exposed at 5°C ± 1°C for 5 days; group C—Cold exposed at 5°C ± 1°C for 30 days. Body weight (BW), Thyroid weight (TW), ^{131}I uptake (^{131}I), and Serum Protein Bound Iodine^{-127} (PB ^{127}I) were measured.

Groups	BW grams	TW mg/100 g BW	^{131}I Uptake 24 hours	Serum PBI μg/100 ml
A	97	5:89	5.88	4.09
B	79	5.55	15.37*	5.27*
C	110	6.25	11.06*	5.02*

*Fisher's "T" significant to .001

6. The scientist was interested to determine
   (A) whether hamsters can survive in the cold.
   (B) the basic metabolic rate of these animals.
   (C) the effect cold has on body weight.
   (D) the influence cold exposure has on several parameters used to assess thyroid function.

7. The data suggest that
   (A) the morphology of the thyroid gland was not altered since no significant weight change was recorded.
   (B) the thyroid gland is in a physiological state of hyperactivity in cold-exposed animals.
   (C) hamsters in the cold are in great distress.
   (D) the thyroid gland is in a physiological state of hypoactivity in cold-exposed animals.

8. The scientist showed that
   (A) cold exposure leads to an increased ^{131}I uptake and more thyroxine is produced.
   (B) the amount of hormone released from the thyroid is greater but probably less active.
   (C) serum ^{127}PBI differences are obvious and no statistical methods need to be employed.
   (D) cold has a significant effect on ^{131}I uptake and serum PBI.

An investigation was conducted to compare early host response to transplantable tumor, as manifested by mast cell adenine release, in golden hamsters with growing tumor and in golden hamsters immunized with tumor antigen and bacteria adjuvant. The following tables summarize the results.

Comparison of adenine release in hamsters sensitized with tumor antigen and bacteria adjuvant and adjuvant controls.

TABLE 1

Groups	No. of Animals	% Release
Tumor antigen and bacteria adjuvant	40	66.51
Bacteria adjuvant	40	11.13

Comparison of adenine release in the golden hamster with growing tumor and untreated controls.

TABLE 2

Groups	No. of Animals	% Release
Tumor transplant	40	33.50
Normal controls	40	7.50

The following statements are related to the passage above. Based on the information given, select:
(A) if the statement is *supported by* the information in the passage.
(B) if the statement is *contradicted by* the information in the passage.
(C) if the statement is *neither supported nor contradicted by* information in the passage.

9. While adjuvant controls had more histamine release than untreated controls, their group average was significantly below that of the animals actively sensitized to tumor.

10. Animals that received transplants released half as much adenine as those given tumor antigen and bacteria adjuvant.

11. There is a significant difference between the tumor-bearing animals and their controls indicating some degree of enhanced cellular sensitization.

12. The experiments indicate that the immunological system of the golden hamster can respond with adenine release upon challenge with antigen prepared from that tumor.

13. Adenine release was a good parameter in the above study.

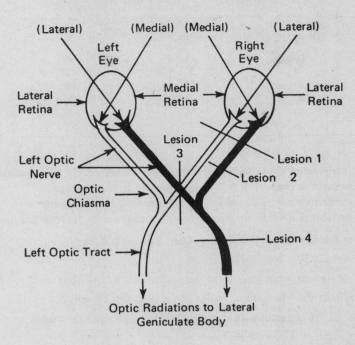

Area of Visual Field   Area of Visual Field

This diagram represents fiber pathways by which impulses from the retina are carried to the brain. Note components of each optic nerve and which retinal region, and corresponding visual field region, are carried by each optic nerve component.

Assume lesions 1-4 are functionally complete; that is, they result in complete sensory loss for a particular visual field region.

Based on location of the lesions in the preceding diagram, predict what the *visual field deficit* (black region) would be for each lesion.

14	15	16	17
Lesion 1	Lesion 2	Lesion 3	Lesion 4

(A)
(B)
(C)
(D)

The life span of poikilotherms is related to the ambient temperature. In order to investigate the process of aging in these animals one must keep meticulous records of the temperature. Various parameters, other than temperature, have been introduced into aging studies which alter the life span, and one of these, ^{60}Co gamma rays, has been widely utilized with the following results.

No. of Animals	Temp. °C	Sex	Dose rads	Life Span days ± S.D.
100	18	M	0	55 ± 1
100	18	F	0	65 ± 2
100	18	M	10,000	40 ± 1
100	18	F	10,000	65 ± 2
100	20	M	10,000	55 ± 1
100	20	F	10,000	75 ± 2
100	20	M	0	65 ± 2
100	20	F	0	75 ± 2

The following statements are related to the passage . Based on the information, select:

(A)   if the statement is *supported by* the information in the passage.

(B)   if the statement is *contradicted by* the information in the passage.

(C)   if the statement is *neither supported nor contradicted by* information in the passage.

18.   Life span of the animals is indirectly related to temperature.

19.   Females generally live longer than males.

20.   Males whose parents were long-lived generally tend to live longer.

21.   Radiation affects the life span of males more than that of females.

22.   10,000 rads of ^{60}Co gamma rays decreases the life span of males to a greater extent than a 2°C drop in temperature.

23.   Males are less radiosensitive than females.

24.   10,000 rads of ^{60}Co gamma rays do not cause any chromosome damage.

25.   Female life spans are not affected by 10,000 rads of ^{60}Co gamma rays.

The data below show the result of an experiment concerning cell cooperation in the immune response. The experiment attempts to determine if thymus and bone marrow cells are required for antibody to be produced against egg albumin. Various donor cells (thymus or bone marrow) are injected into recipient mice whose immune system has been rendered nonresponsive by X-irradiation. Antibody levels were then determined in the serum of the recipient animals.

Donor Cells Injected	Antibody Production
1) Thymocytes + egg albumin	0
2) Thymocytes	0
3) Bone marrow + egg albumin	0
4) Bone marrow	0
5) Thymocytes + bone marrow + egg albumin	+ + +
6) Spleen cells + egg albumin	+ + +
7) Lymph node cells + egg albumin	+ + +

The following statements are related to the passage above. Based on the information given, select:

(A)   if the statement is *supported by* the information in the passage.

(B)   if the statement is *contradicted by* the information in the passage.

(C)   if the statement is *neither supported nor contradicted by* information in the passage.

26.   In this system, bone marrow and thymus cells are required for a mouse to make antibody to egg albumin.

27.   Thymus cells or cells derived from the thymus are probably found in the spleen.

28.   Thymus cells or bone marrow cells or both are capable of synthesizing antibody.

29.   In the intact animal, the thymus would probably be important as a source of antibody.

A motor unit consists of the axon of a single motor neuron and all the skeletal muscle fibers it supplies. By the procedure of electromyography, membrane depolarization with resulting contraction of the muscle fibers can be detected. Briefly, electromyography involves positioning an electrode between muscle fibers and recording current flow on a suitable detection device such as an oscilloscope (CRO). Use this information and figures A and B to answer the next five questions.

Figure A

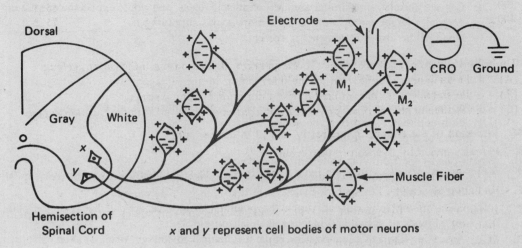

Hemisection of Spinal Cord

x and *y* represent cell bodies of motor neurons

Figure B

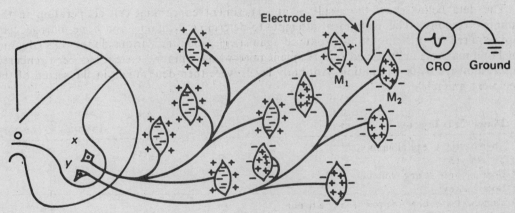

30. Which one of the following statements is correct?
   (A) Cell bodies of motor neurons are anatomically located only in the dorsal gray matter of the spinal cord.
   (B) Eleven (11) motor units are represented in figure A.
   (C) All motor units represented in figure A are inactive (resting).
   (D) A single axon supplies only a single muscle fiber.
   (E) Motor units are unilaterally associated with the spinal cord.

31. Which of the following statements is correct?
   (A) Current will flow between muscle fibers M_1 and M_2 in figure A.
   (B) Current will flow from muscle fiber M_1 toward fiber M_2 in figure B.
   (C) All motor units shown in figure B are active.
   (D) The axon of cell body *x* in figure B has fired.
   (E) The cell membrane of muscle fiber M_1 in figure B has become permeable to sodium ions (Na^+).

32. Which one of the following statements is correct?
    (A) By inference from the given information, one would expect to find smaller motor units in an extraocular muscle (eye movements) than in the biceps muscle.
    (B) By inference from the given information, one would expect to find smaller motor units in the biceps muscle than in an extraocular muscle (eye movements).
    (C) The precision of movement permitted by a muscle is probably independent of the size of its motor units.
    (D) For two muscles with similar numbers of muscle fibers, one would expect the one having generally larger motor units to have more axons supplying it.
    (E) None of the above statements is correct.

33. Skeletal muscle response can be varied (graded) by
    (A) varying the frequency at which the axons fire.
    (B) varying the number of motor units which are active.
    (C) no means, because activity of the fibers of a given muscle is all or nothing.
    (D) both methods A and B given above.
    (E) none of the above responses.

34. Which one of the following statements is correct?
    (A) The electrode shown in figure A will record electrical activity directly from axons of cell bodies x and y.
    (B) Electromyography depends upon the potential difference created between the outer membranes of active and inactive skeletal muscle fibers.
    (C) Assuming fibers of equal size and equal mechanical advantage, firing of axon y in either figure A or figure B will produce the greatest contraction.
    (D) A lesion which destroys the cell body of axon x will cause the loss of six motor units.
    (E) None of the above statements is correct.

Days on Drug	Strength of Drug	Factor 1	Factor 2	Factor 3	Factor 4	Factor 5	Factor 6
0	0	12.5	33.0	26.5	9.3	6.2	71
6	0.05	10.7	17.0	47.0	9.6	5.0	73
6	0.10	3.0	9.8	64.0	7.0	4.8	80
6	0.20	4.8	8.9	49.2	2.4	4.6	62
6	0.50	12.0	7.9	55.8	10.7	6.6	73
12	0.05	12.5	9.8	23.1	12.9	11.0	45
12	0.10	4.4	7.9	40.7	8.3	9.1	49
12	0.20	6.8	7.2	43.0	5.9	16.7	54
12	0.50	3.9	5.7	34.2	5.3	23.0	43

The following statements are related to the table presented above. Based on the information given, select:
    (A) if the statement is *supported by* the information in the table.
    (B) if the statement is *contradicted by* the information in the table.
    (C) if the statement is *neither supported nor contradicted by* information in the table.

35. There is a significant difference in the analyzed factors between the 6-day and the 12-day treatment period.

36. The percentage of Factor 3 increased and that of Factor 2 decreased.

37. If there was an increase in Factor 3 and a decrease in Factor 2, there was a resultant rise in the Factor 3/Factor 2 ratio.

38. The proportion of isolated Factor 4 did not show any consistent trend.

39. The amount of Factor 6 did not demonstrate any obvious decline from the normal in the 6-day group; in the 12-day group, a decline is noted which could be due to decreased amounts of Factors 2 and 3.

40. The level of Factor 5 varied around control values in the 6-day treatment period but showed a definite rise in the 12-day group.

41. Results of the analysis of factors are dose dependent.

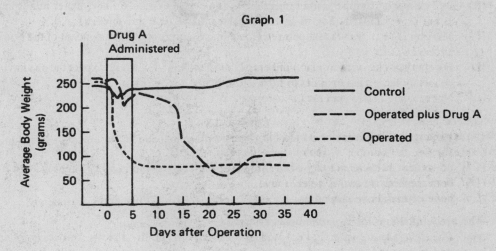

Graph 1

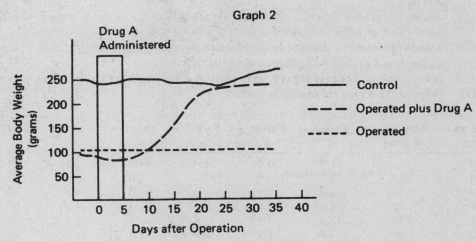

Graph 2

The following statements are related to the graphs presented above. Based on the information given, select:

(A) if the statement is *supported by* the information in the graph.
(B) if the statement is *contradicted by* the information in the graph.
(C) if the statement is *neither supported nor contradicted by* information in the graph.

42. In graph 1, the operated animals lacked a desire to eat for about 1 week, but then ate again to maintain their body weights at a reduced level.

43. In graph 1 the operated group that received drug A maintained their body weight while on the drug.

44. In graph 1, when the drug was discontinued, lack of desire to eat set in and remained until the animals' weights declined to the level of the animals that were operated on but did not receive the drug.

45. When we compare the results obtained in graph 1 to those obtained in graph 2, we note that reducing the body weight before the operation eliminated the lack of desire to eat.

46. Body weight was a significant factor in drug A action.

47. The experiments depicted were properly controlled.

The thickness of the human oral epithelium was measured in seven different areas of the oral cavity in thirty cadavers. The results are tabulated below.

Area	Average	Range
A	500μ	125-950μ
B	362μ	178-780μ
C	254μ	130-489μ
D	238μ	156-320μ
E	204μ	135-270μ
F	68μ	30-146μ
G	123μ	35-260μ

The following statements are related to the information presented above. Based on the information given, select:

(A) if the statement is *supported by* the information given.
(B) if the statement is *contradicted by* the information given.
(C) if the statement is *neither supported nor contradicted by* information given.

48. The oral epithelium has a wide range of thickness in the oral cavity.

49. The greatest range was observed in Area B.

50. The thinnest measurement was observed in Area G.

51. The results above are not valid since they were not attained from living subjects.

52. The range of thickness of the oral epithelium as observed was 30-950μ.

53. The median of the average thickness is 238μ.

Drug X is administered to a patient and a certain value is monitored. After 30 days of treatment the physician studies the following values:

% of Drug X Administered	Days	Mean Value of Y
0.000	0	6.51
0.025	3	6.61
0.05	3	7.39
0.10	3	7.90
0.20	3	8.00
0.025	15	9.02
0.05	15	9.07
0.10	15	9.27
0.20	15	9.53
0.025	30	10.80
0.05	30	11.80
0.10	30	12.00
0.20	30	12.51

The following statements are related to the information presented above. Based on the information given, select:

(A) if the statement is *supported by* the information given.
(B) if the statement is *contradicted by* the information given.
(C) if the statement is *neither supported nor contradicted by* information given.

54. The drug has an effect.

55. There is a dose relationship to the response.

56. The dose administered is of critical importance as can be deduced from the values.

57. The physician can expect the values of "Y" to continue to reflect dosage and period of treatment.

58. There were no side effects of this treatment.

59. The same values probably will be found if another patient were to be treated.

Distribution of relative amounts of radioiodinated amino acids in thyroid homogenates after administration of graded doses of PTU for three days.

Distribution of relative amounts of radioiodinated amino acids in thyroid homogenates after administration of graded doses of PTU for six days.

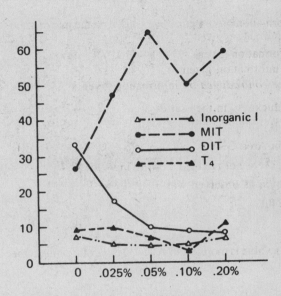
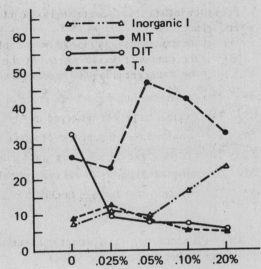

The following statements are related to the information presented above. Based on the information given, select:

(A) if the statement is *supported by* the information given.
(B) if the statement is *contradicted by* the information given.
(C) if the statement is *neither supported nor contradicted by* information given.

60. The percentage of labeled MIT increased and that of labeled DIT decreased; in the 6-day treated group there is a rise and then a decline in the MIT detected.

61. The amount of MIT rose from 26% in the controls to 64% in the 3-day experimentally treated animals.

62. A rise in the MIT/DIT ratio is observed.

63. The level of inorganic I varied around control values in the 3-day group but showed a definite rise in the 6-day group.

64. The enzymatic digest yields information on the distribution of radioactive I among the various iodinated amino acids studied.

Maloney sarcoma tumors were implanted in Brown Norway (BN), Lewis (Le), and Lewis-Brown Norway (LBN) rats. Studies were then done to determine the types and amounts of host serum antibodies produced against the protein components of the virus contained in the tumor cells. The following data are from one such experiment.

**ANTIPROTEIN 30 ACTIVITY IN SERA
OF TUMOR BEARING BN, Le, AND LBN RATS**

Host	AgB Phenotype	Mg Equivalent Day 25 Post Implant	Anti-p30 Antibody Day 31 Post Implant
BN	3/3	3.5 ± 0.8	5.3 ± 1.7
LBN	1/3	2.4 ± 0.4	4.5 ± 1.4
Le	1/1	0.4 ± 0.1	0.4 ± 0.2

The following statements are related to the information presented. Based on the information given, select:

    (A)   if the statement is *supported by* the information given.

    (B)   if the statement is *contradicted by* the information given.

    (C)   if the statement is *neither contradicted nor supported by* information given.

65. Brown Norway rats produced more anti-p30 antibody at both 25 and 31 days than the other two hosts.

66. On the basis of this information, Brown Norway rats are more resistant to cancer than either LBN or Le rats.

67. All three hosts produced more anti-p30 antibody at 31 days than they did at 25 days.

68. An AgB phenotype containing threes seems to be related to lower anti-p30 production.

Model Test B Answers*

SCIENCE KNOWLEDGE

Biology

1.	C	9.	D	17.	D	25.	A	32.	B
2.	C	10.	C	18.	E	26.	D	33.	D
3.	D	11.	D	19.	C	27.	C	34.	B
4.	C	12.	D	20.	B	28.	B	35.	B
5.	E	13.	A	21.	C	29.	B	36.	B
6.	C	14.	E	22.	D	30.	A	37.	C
7.	C	15.	D	23.	B	31.	E	38.	D
8.	A	16.	B	24.	A				

Chemistry

1.	D	9.	D	17.	C	25.	D	32.	A
2.	A	10.	E	18.	A	26.	A	33.	D
3.	D	11.	B	19.	B	27.	B	34.	A
4.	C	12.	B	20.	E	28.	C	35.	E
5.	B	13.	D	21.	D	29.	A	36.	C
6.	C	14.	C	22.	B	30.	C	37.	E
7.	C	15.	B	23.	D	31.	B	38.	D
8.	A	16.	C	24.	B				

Physics

1.	C	8.	C	15.	A	22.	A	28.	C
2.	C	9.	B	16.	A	23.	A	29.	C
3.	B	10.	D	17.	C	24.	C	30.	A
4.	B	11.	C	18.	B	25.	E	31.	E
5.	A	12.	C	19.	A	26.	B	32.	B
6.	E	13.	C	20.	D	27.	A	33.	D
7.	A	14.	B	21.	B				

SCIENCE PROBLEMS

1.	B	13.	A	25.	A	37.	D	49.	A
2.	A	14.	A	26.	A	38.	B	50.	B
3.	E	15.	B	27.	B	39.	A	51.	B
4.	E	16.	C	28.	A	40.	A	52.	C
5.	B	17.	A	29.	C	41.	E	53.	B
6.	E	18.	D	30.	B	42.	A	54.	E
7.	B	19.	C	31.	C	43.	A	55.	D
8.	A	20.	A	32.	D	44.	C	56.	D
9.	E	21.	B	33.	E	45.	B	57.	B
10.	D	22.	E	34.	C	46.	C	58.	E
11.	B	23.	A	35.	B	47.	C	59.	E
12.	B	24.	B	36.	B	48.	E	60.	A

SKILLS ANALYSIS: READING

1.	A	15.	C	29.	C	43.	A	56.	C
2.	B	16.	C	30.	B	44.	A	57.	A
3.	A	17.	B	31.	C	45.	C	58.	C
4.	A	18.	A	32.	A	46.	A	59.	B
5.	C	19.	A	33.	B	47.	B	60.	C
6.	A	20.	C	34.	C	48.	B	61.	C
7.	B	21.	A	35.	B	49.	C	62.	C
8.	A	22.	C	36.	C	50.	A	63.	A
9.	B	23.	A	37.	A	51.	A	64.	A
10.	A	24.	A	38.	C	52.	C	65.	B
11.	B	25.	B	39.	A	53.	A	66.	B
12.	A	26.	C	40.	B	54.	A	67.	C
13.	D	27.	B	41.	C	55.	C	68.	C
14.	B	28.	A	42.	A				

SKILLS ANALYSIS: QUANTITATIVE

1.	B	15.	B	29.	B	43.	A	56.	B
2.	C	16.	C	30.	C	44.	A	57.	C
3.	A	17.	B	31.	B	45.	A	58.	C
4.	D	18.	A	32.	A	46.	A	59.	C
5.	C	19.	A	33.	D	47.	B	60.	A
6.	D	20.	C	34.	B	48.	A	61.	A
7.	B	21.	A	34.	B	49.	B	62.	A
8.	D	22.	A	36.	A	50.	B	63.	A
9.	A	23.	B	37.	A	51.	C	64.	A
10.	A	24.	C	38.	A	52.	A	65.	A
11.	C	25.	A	39.	A	53.	A	66.	C
12.	A	26.	A	40.	A	54.	A	67.	B
13.	A	27.	A	41.	B	55.	A	68.	B
14.	D	28.	C	42.	A				

Explanation of Answers for Science Questions–Model Test B

SCIENCE KNOWLEDGE

Biology

1. **(C)** The gastric mucosa secretes hydrochloric acid; mucin, and the enzymes rennin, pepsin, and lipase. An average of 2 to 3 liters is secreted within a 24 hour time period. The pH of gastric juice usually varies from 0.9 to 1.5. This acidity allows pepsin to act while it inhibits ptyalin (salivary amylase). Food usually remains in the stomach for 3 to 4 hours.

2. **(C)** Multiple alleles determine the human blood types. The common blood types are: A, B, AB, and O. Red blood cells of a person classified as "Type A" contain "Agglutinogen A" and their serum contains "Agglutinin b." Type AB contains agglutinogens A and B but no agglutinins. Type O possesses no agglutinogens but the serum carries a + b agglutinins. Rhesus (Rh) agglutinogen is present in humans and is represented by a dominant gene R. The agglutinogen of an Rh positive fetus passes across the placenta, enters the maternal blood stream and elicits the production of an agglutinin (antibody) by the mother. The agglutinin passes into the circulation of the fetus and if present in sufficient concentration can produce agglutination, at times fatal to the developing fetus.

3. **(D)** Light must penetrate the retina to reach the rods and cones. The fovea centralis is the central portion of the macula lutea, it is the region of sharpest vision. It is thinner than the rest of the retina and only cones are present. Rods are absent from this area. Cones are regarded as color receptors, while rods are achromatic receptors of low intensity light.

4. **(C)** In a parfocal optical microscope the objective lenses are so constructed or mounted that one may change from one to another and the image remains focused; the lenses have focal points in the same plane.

5. **(E)** The reproductive cycle is under hormonal regulation; gonadotropic hormones of the pituitary (anterior lobe) stimulate the ovaries to produce a mature egg. The pituitary and ovaries have a reciprocal effect upon each other. FSH (follicle stimulating hormone) from the pituitary elicits estrogen production from the developing follicle. When estrogen concentration reaches a certain blood level, it inhibits FSH production. At that time the egg is discharged and the cells lining the follicle come under the influence of another gonadotropin LH (luteinizing hormone) which influences the development of the corpus luteum. The corpus luteum produces the hormone progesterone which influences the wall of the uterus in preparation for implantation. As the concentration of progesterone rises, LH production is checked. If fertilization has occurred, the production of FSH is curtailed throughout the period of gestation through the production of estrogen by the placenta and ovary. If fertilization does not occur, the cycle begins anew.

6. **(C)** Langerhans described the beta cells (within the islets of Langerhans) of the pancreas which produce insulin that affects the metabolism of glucose directly. Fat and protein are indirectly affected. After a meal the level of blood sugar rises eliciting the production of insulin which stimulates the absorption of glucose by the cells and helps in its conversion to glycogen. Insulin deficiency leads to high blood sugar levels and the disease called diabetes mellitus.

7. **(C)** Anterior-posterior diameters of eyeballs vary. A long eye is considered near-sighted or myopic; light rays come to focus before they reach the retina; therefore, a concave lens if needed for correction. A short eye results in far-sightness or hypermetropia; light rays would come to focus in back of the retina and, therefore, a convex lens is needed for correction.

8. **(A)** Development in animals results from the cleavage divisions of the zygote. The zygote divides first into two cells, then these divide into four, and so on, until it becomes a cell mass called the morula. Through more divisions the morula becomes a hollow ball of cells which is called the blastula.

9. **(D)** The mystery of the origin of life still eludes

us. Two basic concepts are proposed: 1. Vitalistic—a vital force created life; 2. Mechanistic—forces of nature were instrumental. Oparin suggested that the primitive atmosphere was made up of gases like methane, ammonia, hydrogen, and water vapor. Miller discharged electricity through the above environment and found after a week, a variety of organic compounds, including amino acids were produced. Combinations of these then could theoretically have led to the build-up of complex molecules and eventually protoplasm.

10. **(C)**   This is the general body plan, a slight modification as found in the annelids.

11. **(D)**   This is a disease which results from eating poorly cooked pork which contains *Trichinella spiralis*. Eosinophilia, nausea, fever, diarrhea, stiffness, and painful swelling of muscles are characteristic.

12. **(D)**   Epithelium is a group of cells forming a tissue. Epithelium lines the gut, the respiratory system, the genito-urinary system and forms the epidermis. It, therefore, can protect, secrete, and absorb.

13. **(A)**   Symbiosis is defined as association of organisms from which each member derives some advantage. Commensalism is defined as association of organisms which share the same food, etc. (one utilizing the leftovers from the other). Saprophytism is defined as organisms living on dead organisms or products of living ones; they bring about putrefaction or decay. Parasitism is defined as organisms that live in or on their hosts and feed on their tissues or their products.

14. **(E)**   A contractile vacuole is found in fresh-water protozoa; it periodically expels water to the outside. In this manner excess water leaves the cell. Due to its osmotic relationship with its environment, water is entering and the cell must maintain the water level of its protoplasm.

15. **(D)**   A backcross consists of crossing a dominant phenotype with a pure homozygous recessive. In this manner the breeder determines if the phenotype is heterozygous or homozygous.

16. **(B)**   Tonus refers to muscular activity in which a shortened condition is maintained for a prolonged period. Visceral muscle is the outstanding example. The word tonus can be applied to any sustained process which is the result of probable regularly repeated excitation.

17. **(D)**   The gray matter of the spinal cord is divided into two (2) components: motor and receptor. The motor part is comprised of the ventral and intermediolateral columns and gives rise to the ventral roots. Ventral horn cells supply voluntary muscles; intermediolateral cells give rise to preganglionic sympathetic fibers of the thoraco-lumbar system. The receptor portion is located in the dorsal horn. The white matter of the spinal cord is composed of nerve fibers in a network of connective tissue.

18. **(E)**   Many activities are attributed to the hypothalamus. Lesions of this area may produce diabetes insipidus, obesity, sexual dystrophy, and loss of temperature control.

19. **(C)**   Blood pressure is usually measured by placing the sphygmomanometer cuff around the arm compressing the brachial artery and vein. Maximum blood pressure is obtained during ventricular contraction (systole); in our case 160. Minimum blood pressure indicates ventricular rest (diastole); in our case 90.

20. **(B)**   Mesoderm is the middle layer of the three primary germ layers. The following are considered to be of mesodermal origin:
1. connective tissue, cartilage, and bone
2. striated and smooth muscle
3. blood and lymph cells
4. walls of the circulatory system
5. genito-urinary system
6. spleen

21. **(C)**   The cause of muscle fatigue is said to be the accumulated anaerobically produced lactic acid. Lactic acid may later be broken down into carbon dioxide and water for elimination, or it may be converted into glycogen and stored for future use.

22. **(D)**   The autonomic nervous system innervates all smooth muscle, and glands. The autonomic nervous system is divided into a sympathetic (flight and fight) component and parasympathetic (maintains homeostasis) component. It exerts important influences on the intrinsic eye musculature; skin glands; and the cardiovascular, respiratory, endocrine, and reproductive systems. Fear, rage, pain, etc., evoke sympathetic activity which mobilizes the resources of the body. Gastrointestinal activity is curtailed; heart rate and blood pressure increase; and coronary arteries and bronchioles dilate.

23. **(B)**   Alternating periods of light and darkness and the proportion thereof are extremely important to the functioning (cycles) of plant and animal life observed.

24. **(A)**   See also question 5. FSH stimulates the production of estrogen by the developing follicle. LH

stimulates the production of progesterone by the corpus luteum.

25. **(A)** Directly underlying epithelium is found a homogeneous, noncellular material, composed of reticular fibers and protein polysaccharides which serves to bind down the tissue; this structure is the basement membrane.

26. **(D)** An anticoagulant is a substance that prevents or retards coagulation of blood. Heparin is an acid mucopolysaccharide; it occurs most abundantly in the liver. Aspirin (acetylsalicylic acid) is an analgesic, antipyretic, antirheumatic compound that possesses anticoagulant properties. Dicumarol is a trademark for bishydroxycoumarin, an excellent anticoagulant.

27. **(C)** A niche is defined as the position or status that an organism occupies with respect to the other organisms with which it associates.

28. **(B)** At the time of puberty usually an increase in sex drive, beard growth, and development of a deeper voice are experienced. The external genitalia are part of the organism and will develop and grow as the organism does. They are genetically determined and are a primary characteristic of the male.

29. **(B)** The cell bodies of the motor (efferent) system are located in the ventral horns (gray matter) of the spinal cord and their fibers leave the cord via ventral (anterior) roots which join with the dorsal (sensory) roots to form a spinal nerve. If a spinal nerve were sectioned, loss of both sensation and motor activity would be experienced. In this case only motor functions were interrupted.

30. **(A)** Reception via afferent (sensory) receptors, conduction via sensory fibers to the central nervous system (spinal cord), and propagation of the impulses to the efferent (motor) system will then result in appropriate action. Usually most reflex arcs include one association neuron in the spinal cord between their afferent and efferent fibers. The medulla is not a part of the spinal cord; it is a part of the brain, and usually reflex arcs do not utilize higher centers.

31. **(E)** This is a definition and should be memorized.

32. **(B)** The medulla is a part of the brain stem and connects to the spinal cord at the foramen magnum. The following cranial nerves are associated with the medulla: a, XII—hypoglossal nerve; b, XI—spinal accessory nerve; c, X—vagus nerve; d, IX—glossopharyngeal nerve; e, VIII—stato-acoustic nerve; and f, portions of the facial nerve (VII). The vagus

nerve (X) is the most important parasympathetic nerve. Stimulation of vagal fibers slows the heart rate; constricts the smooth muscles of the bronchial tree; stimulates secretion by the bronchial mucosa; and promotes peristalsis, gastric, and pancreatic secretions. Blood pressure control also involves aortic body, carotid sinus, and carotid body receptor modulation by the glossopharyngeal (IX) and vagus (X) nerves.

33. **(D)** The percentage of white blood cells varies as listed:
Agranular cells:
1. lymphocytes   20-25%
2. monocytes   3-8%
Granular cells:
1. neutrophils   65-75%
2. eosinophils   2-5%
3. basophils   0.5% or less

34. **(B)** Bile is secreted by the liver, stored and concentrated in the gall bladder and poured into the duodenum. It contains bile salts, cholesterol, lecithin, fat, pigments, and mucin. It aids in the emulsification, digestion, and absorption of fat. It contributes to the alkalinization of the intestines.

35. **(B)** The class Cyclostomata of the phylum Chordata and sub-phylum Craniata are jawless, finless, without scales or bony plates, have a sucking mouth and possess 6-14 gill slits in the adult. The cyclostomes are the lampreys and hag-fishes.

36. **(B)** Some of the proteins embedded in the lipid layers of membranes are shaped to form channels with "gates," which open only to certain materials or under certain conditions.

37. **(C)** If more than two stimuli reach a muscle in rapid succession, a partial fusion of all contractions results. The contractions occur before relaxation can take place or is completed. If a contraction is steadily maintained and no relaxation occurs between separate stimuli, the contraction is known as tetanus.

38. **(D)** Use your genetic knowledge to show that the five suggested parental genotypes would produce the following offspring.
A: 100% aa
B: 25% AA, 50% Aa, 25% aa
C: 100% Aa
D: 50% Aa, 50% aa
E: 50% AA, 50% Aa

Chemistry

1. **(D)** Fatty acids are esterified with glycerol to form triglycerides (commonly known as fat). Fatty acid is thus a component of the larger triglyceride molecule (fat) as glucose is a component of the polysaccharides listed here (starch, glycogen and cellulose).

2. **(A)** The reaction of sodium alkoxide with alkyl halide is often used in the synthesis of ethers. This is known as the Williamson synthesis.

3. **(D)** Alcohols are not appreciably acidic. Methanol (answer A), cyclohexanol (B), and ethylene glycol (answer E) are alcohols. Phenols (C,D) are acidic as a result of resonance of the ring. Nitro substituents increase the acidity of phenols through inductive and resonance effects.

4. **(C)** Ethers are generally unreactive and for this reason often serve as the solvent in various reactions. They may, however, be cleaved with strong halogen acids (hydrogen iodide being most reactive).

5. **(B)** This reaction utilizes the activating effect of the carbonyl replacement of an alpha-hydrogen by halogen. This is a useful reaction which allows the introduction of a functional group on the alpha-carbon.

6. **(C)** Glucose is an aldohexose, a reducing sugar, and a monosaccharide. It has a number of asymmetric centers and possesses optical activity. It is *not* a disaccharide.

7. **(C)** Ammoniacal silver nitrate is reduced and produces a silver mirror in the presence of aldehydes but not ketones.

8. **(A)** HIO_4 will oxidize only vicinal hydroxyls (i.e., on adjacent carbon atoms).

9. **(D)** Hydrogen bonding occurs between alcohol molecules as between water molecules to produce the comparatively high boiling points of alcohols.

10. **(E)** A catalyst is defined as a substance which increases the velocity of a chemical reaction.

11. **(B)** Note that the question asks for *nitrogenous* metabolic waste products. The compounds in answer A are *not* nitrogenous. Amino acids, glucosamine, and nucleic acids (DNA or RNA) are not ordinarily metabolic waste products.

12. **(B)** The double bonds in the unsaturated fatty acids of margarine and shortening are susceptible to oxidative rancidity. Hydrogenation decreases the rancidity by decreasing the number of double bonds.

13. **(D)** Since more saturated fatty acids (and fats) have a higher melting point, hydrogenation raises the melting point.

14. **(C)** Under the stated conditions aldehyde (except formaldehyde) $\rightarrow$ secondary alcohol; carboxylic acid $\rightarrow$ methane + carboxylic acid; ester $\rightarrow$ ketone; ketone $\rightarrow$ tertiary alcohol.

15. **(B)** *Hypertonic:* the solution has a higher osmotic pressure than the solution with which it is compared. There is a higher concentration of solute and a lower concentration of solvent. *Hypotonic:* a lower concentration of solute and a higher concentration of solvent are present. *Isotonic:* both solutions have the same osmotic pressure.

16. **(C)** One mole of any compound contains 6.02×10^{23} molecules. Two moles of carbon dioxide would contain one mole of molecules more than that contained by one mole of oxygen.

17. **(C)** Fatty acids are the long chain monocarboxylic acids found in fats. Ordinarily they contain an even number of carbon atoms such as $CH_3(CH_2)_{12}COOH$

18. **(A)** Acid salts are formed by di- and tribasic acids. For example, H_2CO_3 can form the acid salt ($NaHCO_3$) known as sodium hydrogen carbonate or sodium bicarbonate.

19. **(B)** Acetals are formed from the reaction of two moles of alcohol with one mole of aldehyde. The reaction of equimolar quantities of alcohol and aldehyde produces a hemiacetal.

20. **(E)** The capture of a neutron by the nucleus increases the atomic weight by one and has no effect on the atomic number. Negatron decay (loss of a negative electron from the nucleus) increases the atomic number by one without appreciable effect on the atomic weight. The net effect of the two events is to increase both the atomic weight and the atomic number by one.

21. **(D)** NaOH may be called a base because it produces OH^- ions, but it is more properly called a base because it consumes H^+ ions.

22. **(B)** Cholesterol is an intermediate in the biosynthesis of steroid hormones, bile acids, and vitamin D_3. Essential fatty acids and essential amino acids must be consumed by the organism in the diet.

23. **(D)** Prostaglandins are potent compounds; they are structurally unique in the respect that they contain 20 carbon atoms and are formed from essential fatty acids. They affect the nervous system, circulation, reproductive organs, and metabolism.

24. **(B)** 2-Butyne (or dimethylacetylene) contains a triple bond between C_2 and C_3. Catalytic hydrogenation may be utilized to add hydrogen across the triple bond, creating a cis-double bond.

25. **(D)** Concentrated sulfuric acid protonates double or triple bonds to produce the polar carbonium ion. This will aid in solubilizing these unsaturated compounds (further reactions, however, may preclude simple recovery of the alkenes and alkynes). Saturated hydrocarbons do not react and are essentially insoluble.

26. **(A)** Dehydrohalogenation of an alkyl halide is a good reaction for the production of an alkene. In choosing between a primary halide and a secondary halide, remember that the adjacent carbon having the smaller number of hydrogen atoms will lose hydrogen. (That is, answer B would produce 2-butene.) Sulfuric acid dehydration of the primary alcohol produces the ether as a major product depending on conditions. Hydrogenation of the alkyne with Pt catalyst would probably not stop at the alkene, but the unsaturation is not in the right position anyway.

27. **(B)** Remember that the nitro group withdraws electrons from the ring and thus deactivates the ring to electrophilic substitution reactions. Although the ring has been deactivated, the highest electron density is in the meta-position.

28. **(C)** See explanation for question 27.

29. **(A)** Beta decay (negatron loss) converts a neutron to a proton plus a negatron. Retention of the proton by the nucleus results in an increase in atomic number (i.e., number of protons) and only a negligible decrease in atomic weight.

30. **(C)** The thermal decomposition of $KClO_3$ to produce oxygen will occur if the temperature is sufficiently high. The addition of a catalyst MnO_2 will decrease the activation energy and increase the rate at a lower temperature.

31. **(B)** See explanation for question 30.

32. **(A)** Long hydrocarbon chains have substantial flexibility. The major problem in preparing large ring compounds is that of bringing the reactive groups close enough to each other to effect ring closure. Once formed, these compounds possess a high degree of stability.

33. **(D)** In the bromination of benzene, Br^+ is the electrophile and benzene is the nucleophile.

34. **(A)** As with any reaction, the equilibrium constant is equal to the arithmetic product of the concentration of the species produced divided by the concentration of the unreacted species.

35. **(E)** According to the Bronsted-Lowry theory, a conjugate acid-base pair consists of two substances whose formulas differ by one H^+. In this reaction, HSO_4^- is the conjugate acid of the base SO_4^{2-}. Another conjugate acid-base pair in this reaction is H_3O^+ and H_2O, but this is not one of the answer choices.

36. **(C)** In all water solutions, the concentrations of hydronium ions and hydroxide ions are related as follows:

$$[H_3O^+][OH^-] = K_w = 1 \times 10^{-14}$$

where [ ] represents concentration in moles per liter. If the hydronium ion concentration is 1×10^{-9}, the hydroxide ion concentration must be 1×10^{-5}.

37. **(E)** A racemic mixture contains equal proportions of levorotatory and dextrorotatory isomers.

38. **(D)** The half-reactions for the given reaction are as follows:

oxidation: $2Fe^{2+} \rightarrow 2Fe^{3+} + 2e^-$

reduction: $Cl_2 + 2e^- \rightarrow 2Cl^-$

An oxidizing agent is defined as the substance being reduced. In this redox equation, Cl_2 is being reduced and is the oxidizing agent.

Physics

1. **(C)** Work is equal to force times distance. A weight of 200 lb exerts a force of 200 lb. 200 lb × 60 ft = 12,000 ft-lb.

2. **(C)** $\dfrac{P_1 V_1}{T_1} = \dfrac{P_2 V_2}{T_2}$ where P is pressure, V is volume, and T is temperature in kelvins. STP (standard temperature and pressure) is 273 K and 1 atm pressure.

$$\frac{1 \times 4}{273} = \frac{2V_2}{819 \text{ K}}$$

$$V_2 = 6$$

3. **(B)** According to Newton's law of universal gravitation, the gravitational force between two point masses is proportional to the product of the two masses. If one mass is doubled, the product is doubled.

4. **(B)** The acceleration due to gravity is the change in velocity divided by the time. The object returns to ground at the same speed with which it left, but in the opposite direction.

$$32 \text{ ft/sec}^2 = \frac{v_2 - v_1}{t}$$

$$= \frac{65 \text{ ft/sec} - (-65 \text{ ft/sec})}{t}$$

which gives $t = 4$ sec

5. **(A)** In a solid metal conductor the atoms are fixed in position, but some of their outer electrons are moved readily by an electric field. These moving electrons constitute the electric current in the metal.

6. **(E)** The kinetic molecular theory (or the kinetic theory of gases) tells us that the temperature (K) is a measure of the average kinetic energy of the molecules of a gas without respect to the identity of the gas.

7. **(A)** The volume of the particles is equal to the increase in liquid level (i.e., $45 - 30 = 15$)

$$\frac{90 \text{ g}}{15 \text{ ml}} = 6 \text{ g/ml}.$$

8. **(C)** In the absence of friction the horizontal component requires no work. Thus the same work is required to raise the mass the same height whether directly or on an inclined plane.

9. **(B)** A longitudinal wave is a wave in which the particles of the medium vibrate back and forth along the direction in which the energy of the wave travels. This is true of a sound wave.

10. **(D)** $s = v_0 t + \frac{1}{2} g t^2$
    $s = (0)t + \frac{1}{2}(32)(4)^2$
    $s = 0 + 16(16) = 256$ ft

11. **(C)** Only 2 factors play a role; the coin has 2 sides, 1 head and 1 tail, and the gambler's chance is 50%. No previous experience or odds apply.

12. **(C)** $v = at;$ $t = 30$ sec. $= \frac{30}{3600}$ hr.

$$600 = a \frac{30}{3600} = \frac{a}{120}$$

$a = 72,000$ mi./hr.^{2}.

In a problem like this, be sure that you convert all your units to agree (as we converted sec. to hrs. in this problem in order that all time would be in hrs.).

13. **(C)** Since the resultant force is the difference between the two forces, the two forces must be directly opposing each other (i.e., at 180°).

14. **(B)** The gravitational acceleration on a body is unaffected by the horizontal velocity. Thus the two cannonballs will strike the ground simultaneously.

15. **(A)** Momentum $= mv = m_1 v_1 + m_2 v_2 = (50)(0.2) + (10)(0) = 10$ g-m/s.

16. **(A)** Momentum is conserved.

17. **(C)** Momentum is conserved. 10 g-m/s $= (50 + 10)v.$ $v = \frac{10}{60} = 0.17$ m/s.

18. **(B)** Kinetic energy $= \frac{1}{2} mv^2 = \frac{60}{2}(0.17)^2$
    $= 30(0.0289)$
    $= 0.867$ g-m^2/s^2.

19. **(A)** If the half-life is 7.5 days, then 15 days would represent two half-lives. In the first half-life 50% will be lost, and in the second half-life 50% of the remainder will be lost.
    Remainder $= 0.5_n$ and $n =$ number of half-lives.
    Remainder $= (0.5)^2 = 0.25$ or 25%

20. **(D)** There is no sound in a vacuum.

21. **(B)** Surface tension is the explanation for the fact that a steel needle may be floated on water in spite of the fact that steel is denser. The addition of detergent decreases surface tension, and the needle will sink.

22. **(A)** This question is related to the Doppler effect. Since the point of generation of the sound is approaching, the frequency of the tone as perceived by the stationary listener will be higher. After the locomotive has passed and is moving away, the frequency perceived is lower.

23. **(A)** $F = \frac{mv^2}{r} = \frac{(0.5)(2)^2}{10} = 0.2$ Since mass is in kg, velocity in m/s^2, and distance in meters, the unit of force will be the newton. Note that the diameter of the circle was given, but the radius is required in the equation.

24. **(C)** The heat produced by a nuclear reactor is utilized in the production of steam. The steam is used to run steam turbines for the production of electricity.

25. **(E)** The magnification of a compound microscope may be calculated by multiplying the magnifications of the component lenses. In this case $10 \times 97 = 970$.

26. **(B)** The critical temperature of a compound is the highest at which its gas may be liquefied no matter what pressure is applied.

27. **(A)** In series, the equivalent resistance is equal to the sum of the individual resistances. $3 + 6 + 2 = 11$ ohms.

28. **(C)** In parallel, the equivalent resistance may be calculated as follows:

$$\frac{1}{R_{eq}} = \frac{1}{R_1} + \frac{1}{R_2} + \frac{1}{R_2}$$

$$\frac{1}{R_{eq}} = \frac{1}{3} + \frac{1}{6} + \frac{1}{2} = \frac{2}{6} + \frac{1}{6} + \frac{3}{6} = \frac{6}{6} = 1$$

$$R_{eq} = 1$$

29. **(C)** The colors in the visible spectrum are usually listed in order as red, orange, yellow, green, blue, indigo, and violet.

30. **(A)** The equivalent resistance of series resistances is the sum of their single resistances. (In this case $2 + 3 + 5 = 10$ ohms.)

$$I = \frac{E}{R} = \frac{20 \text{ volts}}{10 \text{ ohms}} = 2 \text{ A}$$

31. **(E)** The term "action and reaction" describes the interaction between two objects; any pair of forces acting on the same object cannot consist of action and reaction.

32. **(B)** The energy change is the product of charge and potential difference, which in this case is $80 - 20 = 60$ V:

$$(60 \text{ V})(5 \times 10^{-9} \text{ C}) = 3 \times 10^{-7} \text{ J}$$

33. **(D)** The horizontal velocity is irrelevant, and the initial vertical velocity is 0. Using the equation $s = \frac{1}{2}at^2$, we have

$$t = \sqrt{\frac{2s}{a}} = \sqrt{\frac{2(60 \text{ m})}{9.8 \text{ m/s}^2}} = 3.5 \text{ s}$$

SCIENCE PROBLEMS

1-3. **(1-B) (2-A) (3-E)** The experimental design illustrates the process of respiration during which oxygen is used up and carbon dioxide is produced. Lime water is commonly used to test for carbon dioxide. Only the O_2 is used up and, therefore, the mercury manometer reading will be about 15 cm since O_2 comprises about 20% of air with nitrogen contributing about 80% to the system. If all the air could be used in the above experiment the manometer reading would be 76 cm, also known as standard atmospheric pressure.

4. **(E)** The distillate would be only 95.6% ethanol. When all the ethanol had been distilled (as the major component of the 95.6% purity product), the remaining material in the distillation flask would be pure water. This could be distilled at 100°C.

5. **(B)** Since the binary azeotrope of 95.6% ethanol has the lowest boiling point, this product must be removed first. The remainder is pure water that may be recovered from the distillation flask or collected as the second fraction in distillation (100°C).

$$(0.956) X = 500 \text{ g}$$

$$X = \frac{500}{0.956}$$

$$X = 523 \text{ g of the 95.6\% mixture}$$

$$1000 \text{ g} - 523 \text{ g} = 477 \text{ g of water}$$

6. **(E)** The binary azeotrope (95.6% ethanol, 4.4% water) boils below the boiling point of pure ethanol. The binary azeotrope will be the only product until all the ethanol has been removed from the distillation flask if the beginning mixture contains at least 4.4% water. Redistillation of the 95.6% ethanol would not improve the purity but the addition of the proper amount of benzene will allow the water to be removed as the lower boiling binary azeotrope (benzene/ethanol/water), and the remaining pure ethanol may then be collected.

7. **(B)** Given $v = v_0 + at$; $x = v_0 t + \frac{1}{2}at^2$, $v_0 = 0$ and $a = 9.8 \text{ m/s}^2$, calculate v at the end of 1 second:

$$v = 0 + (9.8)(1)$$

$$v_{1s} = 9.8 \text{ m/s}$$

8. **(A)** How far has the ball dropped?

$$x = vt + \frac{1}{2}at^2$$

$$x = 0 + (\frac{1}{2})(9.8)(1)$$

$$x_{1s} = 4.9 \text{ m}$$

9. **(E)** When will the ball strike the ground if $x = 19.6$ m?

$$x = vt + \frac{1}{2}at^2$$

$$19.6 = 0 + (\frac{1}{2})(9.8)(t^2)$$

$$19.6 = 4.9t^2$$

$$t = 2 \text{ s}$$

10. **(D)** Since $pH = pK_a + \log \frac{salt}{weak\ acid}$, then $pH = pK_a + \log \frac{10}{1}$ and the log 10 is 1, so $pH = pK_a + 1$.

11. **(B)** With the Henderson-Hasselbalch equation $pH = pK + \log \frac{salt}{weak\ acid}$. The $\log \frac{salt}{weak\ acid}$ is zero which happens when the ratio of salt to weak acid is one.

12. **(B)** $pH = 5 + \log \frac{0.1}{0.1}$. Since $\frac{0.1}{0.1}$ is 1 and the log 1 is 0, the pH is 5.

13. **(A)** Ninhydrin will react with free amino groups. In a polypeptide the free amino groups are the alpha group at the amino terminal end of the chain as well as epsilon amino groups (e.g., lysine) within the polypeptide. The number of free amino groups will be increased by any reaction that hydrolyzes peptide bonds. Hydrolysis of peptide bonds may be accomplished by acid hydrolysis or by a peptidase enzyme.

14. **(A)** See answer to question 13.

15. **(B)** See previous answer. The inhibitor will decrease the activity of the peptidase enzyme. Thus the sample with enzyme and inhibitor will have fewer free amino groups than the sample with enzyme and no inhibitor.

16. **(C)** Absorption at 10.3 microns is characteristic of *trans* double bonds.

17. **(A)** Catalytic hydrogenation will convert both *cis* and *trans* unsaturated fatty acids to saturated ones.

18. **(D)** Animals and higher plants have almost exclusively *cis* double bonds in their unsaturated fatty acids. *Trans* fatty acids are more common in certain bacteria.

19. **(C)** In calculating the mass, recall the density $(\rho) = m/v$. $m = ?$. $v = 30\ cm^3$. $\rho_{Hg} = 13.6\ g/cm^3$.
$m = \rho v = (13.6)(30)$
$m = 408\ g$ (convert to kg)
$m = 408 \times 10^{-3}\ kg = 0.408\ kg$

20. **(A)** What is the mass of the same volume of water? Repeat the above calculation for water which tells us that: $m = 30\ g$ or $0.030\ kg$. Or recall that mercury is 13.6 times denser than the water and therefore the mass of an equal volume $= \frac{0.408}{13.6} = 0.030\ kg$.

21. **(B)** Specific gravity $= 13.6$ by definition.

22. **(E)** $\frac{0.5\ mg}{0.1\ ml} = \frac{X}{10\ ml}$
$X = \frac{(0.5)(10)}{0.1} = 50\ mg$

This 50 mg represents the total amount in the entire 3 ml of plasma that was extracted.
$\frac{50\ mg}{3\ ml} = \frac{X}{100\ ml}$
$X = \frac{(50)(100)}{3} = 1667\ mg/100\ ml$

23. **(A)** See the above answer. The calculation is based on 100 ml plasma rather than on whole blood.

24. **(B)** Exceeding the linear range would ordinarily lead to a lower absorbance than expected. An error in weighing to prepare the standard solution would introduce a constant error. The remaining possibility, a pipetting error, is most likely. Pipetting errors may be positive or negative.

25. **(A)** The velocity of a wave (C) is directly related to its wavelength and inversely related to its period. The frequency of a wave is inversely proportional to its period, so that in this case the period is 10 seconds and consequently the frequency is $\frac{1}{10}$ H$_2$.

26. **(A)** The velocity is simply $C = L/T$ where $L = 50$ meters and $T = 10$ seconds. $C = 5$ m/sec.

27. **(B)** Wave refraction tends to make wave trains parallel to shore fronts.

28. **(A)** The effect of repeated close-spaced stimuli is that a summation occurs: each contraction is somewhat larger than the preceding one.

29. **(C)** ATP continues to be supplied in adequate amount, even during the period of loss of contraction ability (fatigue). Some link between the stimulating event and the responding event (sliding of actins over myosins), however, gradually becomes less efficient.

30. **(B)** During the summation period each new stimulus arrives before the preceding twitch can reach the relaxation period, and elastic elements in the muscle become stretched without rebounding to their original shape. The muscle eventually reaches a steady state of nearly full contraction (region 2), when all elastic elements are fully stretched.

31. **(C)** The activity of lactic dehydrogenase may be expressed as the rate of reduction of NAD$^+$. The significance of a reduced activity of lactic dehydrogenase is not discussed here.

32. **(D)** The way the question is stated it appears that total activity is being compared between patients B and E. If 0.1 ml of serum from B has 4 times the enzymatic activity of 0.2 ml of serum from E, then the unit activity of B is 8 times that of E. $8 \times 40 = 320$ units/ml.

33. **(E)** The rate of appearance of NADH + H$^+$ must be equal to the rate of disappearance of NAD$^+$ in enzymatic reactions such as this. The only time this will not be true is when another reaction is destroying one of the forms of the coenzyme.

34. **(C)** $n = C/S_m$. $C = 3 \times 10^8$. $S_m = 2.25 \times 10^8$. n_m = index of refraction of water = 1.333

35. **(B)** The index of refraction for a vacuum = 1 because $S_m = C = 3 \times 10^8$ m/s. Therefore, $n = 1$. Snell's Law states that $\sin \theta_i/\sin \theta_r = n_r/n_i$ and so $n_r/n_i > 1$ because $n_r = 1.33$

36. **(B)** In this case n_r = vacuum = 1.0; n_i = water = 1.33. Therefore, $n_r/n_i = 1.00/1.33 = 0.75 < 1$ and the beam would bend *away* from the normal.

37-39. **(37-D) (38-B) (39-A)** The answers to questions 37-39 are self-explanatory.

40. **(A)** $K_1 = \dfrac{[H^+] [F^-]}{[HF]}$

$[H^+] [F^-] = K_1 [HF]$

Since $[H^+]$ and $[F^-]$ should be equal,

$[H^+] = \sqrt{K_1 [HF]} = \sqrt{(2 \times 10^{-4})(0.5)}$

$[H^+] = \sqrt{1 \times 10^{-4}} = 1 \times 10^{-2}$

$pH = -\log [H^+] = 2$

41. **(E)** $[H^+][OH^-] = 1 \times 10^{-14}$

$[H^+] = 1 \times 10^{-7}$

$(1 \times 10^{-2}) + (1 \times 10^{-7}) = 1.00001 \times 10^{-2}$

The logarithm of the above number is not significantly different from that in the previous question. Thus failure to include the ionization of water leads to an "error" which is substantially less than 0.001 pH units. This "error" is less than that introduced by other assumptions and simplifications.

42. **(A)** For a monoprotic acid normality and molarity are equal. See the two answers above.

43. **(A)** $4H + O_2 \rightarrow 2H_2O$

$\dfrac{X}{4} = \dfrac{0.138}{36}$

$X = 0.0153$ g of hydrogen in 0.100 g of compound $\dfrac{0.0153}{1} = 0.0153$ g atoms hydrogen in 0.100 g of compound

$C + O_2 \rightarrow CO_2$

$\dfrac{X}{12} = \dfrac{0.677}{44}$

$X = 0.185$ g of carbon in 0.100 g of compound

$\dfrac{0.185}{12} = 0.0154$ g atoms carbon in 0.100 g of compound. Obviously carbon and hydrogen appear in equal atomic amounts, and the empirical formula is CH.

44. **(C)** The molecular formula will be a multiple of the empirical formula. Since the empirical formula is CH, the molecular formula must be a multiple such as C_2H_2, C_3H_3, C_4H_4, etc.

45. **(B)** Colligative properties are those that depend on the number of particles in solution. Freezing point depression is a colligative property and could be used to determine the number of particles in a given weight (and thus determine the molecular weight). With this information the multiple to be used in converting empirical formula to molecular formula is known. In this particular problem dissolving the necessary amount of the compound (i.e., C_2H_2) in water may be difficult, but the principle is sound for use with a variety of compounds.

46. **(C)** $[Ag^+]^2[SO_4^{2-}] = 6.4 \times 10^{-5}$

$[SO_4^{2-}] = \dfrac{6.4 \times 10^{-5}}{[Ag^{+2}]} = \dfrac{6.4 \times 10^{-5}}{(0.1)^2} = 6.4 \times 10^{-3}$

47. **(C)** Na_2SO_4 is a strongly ionized salt. If it were weakly ionized (as the question supposes), the additional Na^+ ions introduced by $NaNO_3$ would depress the ionization of Na_2SO_4 and decrease the SO_4^{2-} concentration. If Na_2SO_4 were weakly ionized, however, the SO_4^{2-} concentration would already be less than what is assumed in the previous question for a strongly ionized salt.

48. **(E)** AgCl is even less soluble than Ag_2SO_4. (K_{sp} of AgCl is 2.4×10^{-10} as compared to 6.4×10^{-5} for Ag_2SO_4.)

49. **(A)** The total resistance is composed of R_1 and the resistance from the parallel resistors in the branch composed of R_2, R_3, and R_4. For resistors connected in parallel, the following statement holds: $\dfrac{1}{R} = \dfrac{1}{Ra} + \dfrac{1}{Rb} + \dfrac{1}{Rc} \cdots$ In our case:

$\dfrac{1}{R} = \dfrac{1}{5} + \dfrac{1}{10} + \dfrac{1}{15}$

$\dfrac{1}{R} = \dfrac{12 + 6 + 4}{60} = \dfrac{22}{60}$

$22R = 60$

$R_p = 2.7$ ohms

50. **(B)** $R_{tot} = R_1 + R_p = 20 + 22.7$ ohms

51. **(B)** $I = V/R$ where I = current (amperes), V = potential difference (volts), and R = resistance (ohms).

$V = RI$

$V = (5)(22.7)$

$V = 114$ volts

52-54. **(52-C) (53-B) (54-E)** The answers to questions 52-54 are self-explanatory.

55. **(D)** This woman is not the mother. She can contribute only the O gene, and this child must receive an A gene from one parent and a B gene from the other parent. The man cannot be ruled out as the father with the limited information given, since he can contribute a B gene to a child.

56. **(D)** If the man previously fathered a child with blood type O, then the man must have a genotype of BO. The woman can contribute only the O gene. Since the man has an equal chance of contributing the B or the O gene, there is a 50% chance of the child being type O (genotype OO) or type B (genotype BO).

57. **(B)** The chance of any child of this couple being type B is 50% (see explanation for question 56). The chance that any child will be a girl is 50%. Since the blood type and the sex are independent of each other, multiply their individual chances (50% × 50% = 25%).

58. **(E)** The rate of heat generation is the power consumption:

$$I^2 R = (60 \text{ A})^2 (0.020 \text{ }\Omega) = 72 \text{ W}$$

59. **(E)** The rate of mechanical energy produced must be 80% of the electric power consumed:

$$P = (0.80)IV = (0.80)(60 \text{ A})(550 \text{ V}) = 26,400 \text{ J/s}$$
$$= 26 \text{ kJ/s}$$

60. **(A)** With the efficiency at 80%, 20% of the electric energy is converted to heat. In every second, this comes to

$$(0.20)(60 \text{ A})(550 \text{ V}) = 6600 \text{ J}$$

which is $6600/4.19 = 1575$ cal. Since $H = mc\,\Delta T$ and $c = 1$,

$$m = \frac{H}{\Delta T} = \frac{1575 \text{ cal}}{12 \text{ K}} = 131 \text{ g}$$

Answer Sheet–Model Test C

SCIENCE KNOWLEDGE

Biology

1. Ⓐ Ⓑ Ⓒ Ⓓ Ⓔ   11. Ⓐ Ⓑ Ⓒ Ⓓ Ⓔ   21. Ⓐ Ⓑ Ⓒ Ⓓ Ⓔ   31. Ⓐ Ⓑ Ⓒ Ⓓ Ⓔ
2. Ⓐ Ⓑ Ⓒ Ⓓ Ⓔ   12. Ⓐ Ⓑ Ⓒ Ⓓ Ⓔ   22. Ⓐ Ⓑ Ⓒ Ⓓ Ⓔ   32. Ⓐ Ⓑ Ⓒ Ⓓ Ⓔ
3. Ⓐ Ⓑ Ⓒ Ⓓ Ⓔ   13. Ⓐ Ⓑ Ⓒ Ⓓ Ⓔ   23. Ⓐ Ⓑ Ⓒ Ⓓ Ⓔ   33. Ⓐ Ⓑ Ⓒ Ⓓ Ⓔ
4. Ⓐ Ⓑ Ⓒ Ⓓ Ⓔ   14. Ⓐ Ⓑ Ⓒ Ⓓ Ⓔ   24. Ⓐ Ⓑ Ⓒ Ⓓ Ⓔ   34. Ⓐ Ⓑ Ⓒ Ⓓ Ⓔ
5. Ⓐ Ⓑ Ⓒ Ⓓ Ⓔ   15. Ⓐ Ⓑ Ⓒ Ⓓ Ⓔ   25. Ⓐ Ⓑ Ⓒ Ⓓ Ⓔ   35. Ⓐ Ⓑ Ⓒ Ⓓ Ⓔ
6. Ⓐ Ⓑ Ⓒ Ⓓ Ⓔ   16. Ⓐ Ⓑ Ⓒ Ⓓ Ⓔ   26. Ⓐ Ⓑ Ⓒ Ⓓ Ⓔ   36. Ⓐ Ⓑ Ⓒ Ⓓ Ⓔ
7. Ⓐ Ⓑ Ⓒ Ⓓ Ⓔ   17. Ⓐ Ⓑ Ⓒ Ⓓ Ⓔ   27. Ⓐ Ⓑ Ⓒ Ⓓ Ⓔ   37. Ⓐ Ⓑ Ⓒ Ⓓ Ⓔ
8. Ⓐ Ⓑ Ⓒ Ⓓ Ⓔ   18. Ⓐ Ⓑ Ⓒ Ⓓ Ⓔ   28. Ⓐ Ⓑ Ⓒ Ⓓ Ⓔ   38. Ⓐ Ⓑ Ⓒ Ⓓ Ⓔ
9. Ⓐ Ⓑ Ⓒ Ⓓ Ⓔ   19. Ⓐ Ⓑ Ⓒ Ⓓ Ⓔ   29. Ⓐ Ⓑ Ⓒ Ⓓ Ⓔ
10. Ⓐ Ⓑ Ⓒ Ⓓ Ⓔ   20. Ⓐ Ⓑ Ⓒ Ⓓ Ⓔ   30. Ⓐ Ⓑ Ⓒ Ⓓ Ⓔ

To score add from Science Problems questions: 10–15; 25–27; 37–42; 52–57.

Chemistry

1. Ⓐ Ⓑ Ⓒ Ⓓ Ⓔ   11. Ⓐ Ⓑ Ⓒ Ⓓ Ⓔ   21. Ⓐ Ⓑ Ⓒ Ⓓ Ⓔ   31. Ⓐ Ⓑ Ⓒ Ⓓ Ⓔ
2. Ⓐ Ⓑ Ⓒ Ⓓ Ⓔ   12. Ⓐ Ⓑ Ⓒ Ⓓ Ⓔ   22. Ⓐ Ⓑ Ⓒ Ⓓ Ⓔ   32. Ⓐ Ⓑ Ⓒ Ⓓ Ⓔ
3. Ⓐ Ⓑ Ⓒ Ⓓ Ⓔ   13. Ⓐ Ⓑ Ⓒ Ⓓ Ⓔ   23. Ⓐ Ⓑ Ⓒ Ⓓ Ⓔ   33. Ⓐ Ⓑ Ⓒ Ⓓ Ⓔ
4. Ⓐ Ⓑ Ⓒ Ⓓ Ⓔ   14. Ⓐ Ⓑ Ⓒ Ⓓ Ⓔ   24. Ⓐ Ⓑ Ⓒ Ⓓ Ⓔ   34. Ⓐ Ⓑ Ⓒ Ⓓ Ⓔ
5. Ⓐ Ⓑ Ⓒ Ⓓ Ⓔ   15. Ⓐ Ⓑ Ⓒ Ⓓ Ⓔ   25. Ⓐ Ⓑ Ⓒ Ⓓ Ⓔ   35. Ⓐ Ⓑ Ⓒ Ⓓ Ⓔ
6. Ⓐ Ⓑ Ⓒ Ⓓ Ⓔ   16. Ⓐ Ⓑ Ⓒ Ⓓ Ⓔ   26. Ⓐ Ⓑ Ⓒ Ⓓ Ⓔ   36. Ⓐ Ⓑ Ⓒ Ⓓ Ⓔ
7. Ⓐ Ⓑ Ⓒ Ⓓ Ⓔ   17. Ⓐ Ⓑ Ⓒ Ⓓ Ⓔ   27. Ⓐ Ⓑ Ⓒ Ⓓ Ⓔ   37. Ⓐ Ⓑ Ⓒ Ⓓ Ⓔ
8. Ⓐ Ⓑ Ⓒ Ⓓ Ⓔ   18. Ⓐ Ⓑ Ⓒ Ⓓ Ⓔ   28. Ⓐ Ⓑ Ⓒ Ⓓ Ⓔ   38. Ⓐ Ⓑ Ⓒ Ⓓ Ⓔ
9. Ⓐ Ⓑ Ⓒ Ⓓ Ⓔ   19. Ⓐ Ⓑ Ⓒ Ⓓ Ⓔ   29. Ⓐ Ⓑ Ⓒ Ⓓ Ⓔ
10. Ⓐ Ⓑ Ⓒ Ⓓ Ⓔ   20. Ⓐ Ⓑ Ⓒ Ⓓ Ⓔ   30. Ⓐ Ⓑ Ⓒ Ⓓ Ⓔ

To score add from Science Problems questions: 4–9; 16–21; 28–33; 43–45.

Physics

1. Ⓐ Ⓑ Ⓒ Ⓓ Ⓔ
2. Ⓐ Ⓑ Ⓒ Ⓓ Ⓔ
3. Ⓐ Ⓑ Ⓒ Ⓓ Ⓔ
4. Ⓐ Ⓑ Ⓒ Ⓓ Ⓔ
5. Ⓐ Ⓑ Ⓒ Ⓓ Ⓔ
6. Ⓐ Ⓑ Ⓒ Ⓓ Ⓔ
7. Ⓐ Ⓑ Ⓒ Ⓓ Ⓔ
8. Ⓐ Ⓑ Ⓒ Ⓓ Ⓔ
9. Ⓐ Ⓑ Ⓒ Ⓓ Ⓔ
10. Ⓐ Ⓑ Ⓒ Ⓓ Ⓔ
11. Ⓐ Ⓑ Ⓒ Ⓓ Ⓔ
12. Ⓐ Ⓑ Ⓒ Ⓓ Ⓔ
13. Ⓐ Ⓑ Ⓒ Ⓓ Ⓔ
14. Ⓐ Ⓑ Ⓒ Ⓓ Ⓔ
15. Ⓐ Ⓑ Ⓒ Ⓓ Ⓔ
16. Ⓐ Ⓑ Ⓒ Ⓓ Ⓔ
17. Ⓐ Ⓑ Ⓒ Ⓓ Ⓔ
18. Ⓐ Ⓑ Ⓒ Ⓓ Ⓔ
19. Ⓐ Ⓑ Ⓒ Ⓓ Ⓔ
20. Ⓐ Ⓑ Ⓒ Ⓓ Ⓔ
21. Ⓐ Ⓑ Ⓒ Ⓓ Ⓔ
22. Ⓐ Ⓑ Ⓒ Ⓓ Ⓔ
23. Ⓐ Ⓑ Ⓒ Ⓓ Ⓔ
24. Ⓐ Ⓑ Ⓒ Ⓓ Ⓔ
25. Ⓐ Ⓑ Ⓒ Ⓓ Ⓔ
26. Ⓐ Ⓑ Ⓒ Ⓓ Ⓔ
27. Ⓐ Ⓑ Ⓒ Ⓓ Ⓔ
28. Ⓐ Ⓑ Ⓒ Ⓓ Ⓔ
29. Ⓐ Ⓑ Ⓒ Ⓓ Ⓔ
30. Ⓐ Ⓑ Ⓒ Ⓓ Ⓔ
31. Ⓐ Ⓑ Ⓒ Ⓓ Ⓔ
32. Ⓐ Ⓑ Ⓒ Ⓓ Ⓔ
33. Ⓐ Ⓑ Ⓒ Ⓓ Ⓔ

To score add from Science Problems questions: 1–3; 22–24; 34–36; 46–51; 58–60.

SCIENCE PROBLEMS

1. Ⓐ Ⓑ Ⓒ Ⓓ Ⓔ
2. Ⓐ Ⓑ Ⓒ Ⓓ Ⓔ
3. Ⓐ Ⓑ Ⓒ Ⓓ Ⓔ
4. Ⓐ Ⓑ Ⓒ Ⓓ Ⓔ
5. Ⓐ Ⓑ Ⓒ Ⓓ Ⓔ
6. Ⓐ Ⓑ Ⓒ Ⓓ Ⓔ
7. Ⓐ Ⓑ Ⓒ Ⓓ Ⓔ
8. Ⓐ Ⓑ Ⓒ Ⓓ Ⓔ
9. Ⓐ Ⓑ Ⓒ Ⓓ Ⓔ
10. Ⓐ Ⓑ Ⓒ Ⓓ Ⓔ
11. Ⓐ Ⓑ Ⓒ Ⓓ Ⓔ
12. Ⓐ Ⓑ Ⓒ Ⓓ Ⓔ
13. Ⓐ Ⓑ Ⓒ Ⓓ Ⓔ
14. Ⓐ Ⓑ Ⓒ Ⓓ Ⓔ
15. Ⓐ Ⓑ Ⓒ Ⓓ Ⓔ
16. Ⓐ Ⓑ Ⓒ Ⓓ Ⓔ
17. Ⓐ Ⓑ Ⓒ Ⓓ Ⓔ
18. Ⓐ Ⓑ Ⓒ Ⓓ Ⓔ
19. Ⓐ Ⓑ Ⓒ Ⓓ Ⓔ
20. Ⓐ Ⓑ Ⓒ Ⓓ Ⓔ
21. Ⓐ Ⓑ Ⓒ Ⓓ Ⓔ
22. Ⓐ Ⓑ Ⓒ Ⓓ Ⓔ
23. Ⓐ Ⓑ Ⓒ Ⓓ Ⓔ
24. Ⓐ Ⓑ Ⓒ Ⓓ Ⓔ
25. Ⓐ Ⓑ Ⓒ Ⓓ Ⓔ
26. Ⓐ Ⓑ Ⓒ Ⓓ Ⓔ
27. Ⓐ Ⓑ Ⓒ Ⓓ Ⓔ
28. Ⓐ Ⓑ Ⓒ Ⓓ Ⓔ
29. Ⓐ Ⓑ Ⓒ Ⓓ Ⓔ
30. Ⓐ Ⓑ Ⓒ Ⓓ Ⓔ
31. Ⓐ Ⓑ Ⓒ Ⓓ Ⓔ
32. Ⓐ Ⓑ Ⓒ Ⓓ Ⓔ
33. Ⓐ Ⓑ Ⓒ Ⓓ Ⓔ
34. Ⓐ Ⓑ Ⓒ Ⓓ Ⓔ
35. Ⓐ Ⓑ Ⓒ Ⓓ Ⓔ
36. Ⓐ Ⓑ Ⓒ Ⓓ Ⓔ
37. Ⓐ Ⓑ Ⓒ Ⓓ Ⓔ
38. Ⓐ Ⓑ Ⓒ Ⓓ Ⓔ
39. Ⓐ Ⓑ Ⓒ Ⓓ Ⓔ
40. Ⓐ Ⓑ Ⓒ Ⓓ Ⓔ
41. Ⓐ Ⓑ Ⓒ Ⓓ Ⓔ
42. Ⓐ Ⓑ Ⓒ Ⓓ Ⓔ
43. Ⓐ Ⓑ Ⓒ Ⓓ Ⓔ
44. Ⓐ Ⓑ Ⓒ Ⓓ Ⓔ
45. Ⓐ Ⓑ Ⓒ Ⓓ Ⓔ
46. Ⓐ Ⓑ Ⓒ Ⓓ Ⓔ
47. Ⓐ Ⓑ Ⓒ Ⓓ Ⓔ
48. Ⓐ Ⓑ Ⓒ Ⓓ Ⓔ
49. Ⓐ Ⓑ Ⓒ Ⓓ Ⓔ
50. Ⓐ Ⓑ Ⓒ Ⓓ Ⓔ
51. Ⓐ Ⓑ Ⓒ Ⓓ Ⓔ
52. Ⓐ Ⓑ Ⓒ Ⓓ Ⓔ
53. Ⓐ Ⓑ Ⓒ Ⓓ Ⓔ
54. Ⓐ Ⓑ Ⓒ Ⓓ Ⓔ
55. Ⓐ Ⓑ Ⓒ Ⓓ Ⓔ
56. Ⓐ Ⓑ Ⓒ Ⓓ Ⓔ
57. Ⓐ Ⓑ Ⓒ Ⓓ Ⓔ
58. Ⓐ Ⓑ Ⓒ Ⓓ Ⓔ
59. Ⓐ Ⓑ Ⓒ Ⓓ Ⓔ
60. Ⓐ Ⓑ Ⓒ Ⓓ Ⓔ

SKILLS ANALYSIS: READING

1. Ⓐ Ⓑ Ⓒ Ⓓ Ⓔ
2. Ⓐ Ⓑ Ⓒ Ⓓ Ⓔ
3. Ⓐ Ⓑ Ⓒ Ⓓ Ⓔ
4. Ⓐ Ⓑ Ⓒ Ⓓ Ⓔ
5. Ⓐ Ⓑ Ⓒ Ⓓ Ⓔ
6. Ⓐ Ⓑ Ⓒ Ⓓ Ⓔ
7. Ⓐ Ⓑ Ⓒ Ⓓ Ⓔ
8. Ⓐ Ⓑ Ⓒ Ⓓ Ⓔ
9. Ⓐ Ⓑ Ⓒ Ⓓ Ⓔ
10. Ⓐ Ⓑ Ⓒ Ⓓ Ⓔ
11. Ⓐ Ⓑ Ⓒ Ⓓ Ⓔ
12. Ⓐ Ⓑ Ⓒ Ⓓ Ⓔ
13. Ⓐ Ⓑ Ⓒ Ⓓ Ⓔ
14. Ⓐ Ⓑ Ⓒ Ⓓ Ⓔ
15. Ⓐ Ⓑ Ⓒ Ⓓ Ⓔ
16. Ⓐ Ⓑ Ⓒ Ⓓ Ⓔ
17. Ⓐ Ⓑ Ⓒ Ⓓ Ⓔ

18. Ⓐ Ⓑ Ⓒ Ⓓ Ⓔ
19. Ⓐ Ⓑ Ⓒ Ⓓ Ⓔ
20. Ⓐ Ⓑ Ⓒ Ⓓ Ⓔ
21. Ⓐ Ⓑ Ⓒ Ⓓ Ⓔ
22. Ⓐ Ⓑ Ⓒ Ⓓ Ⓔ
23. Ⓐ Ⓑ Ⓒ Ⓓ Ⓔ
24. Ⓐ Ⓑ Ⓒ Ⓓ Ⓔ
25. Ⓐ Ⓑ Ⓒ Ⓓ Ⓔ
26. Ⓐ Ⓑ Ⓒ Ⓓ Ⓔ
27. Ⓐ Ⓑ Ⓒ Ⓓ Ⓔ
28. Ⓐ Ⓑ Ⓒ Ⓓ Ⓔ
29. Ⓐ Ⓑ Ⓒ Ⓓ Ⓔ
30. Ⓐ Ⓑ Ⓒ Ⓓ Ⓔ
31. Ⓐ Ⓑ Ⓒ Ⓓ Ⓔ
32. Ⓐ Ⓑ Ⓒ Ⓓ Ⓔ
33. Ⓐ Ⓑ Ⓒ Ⓓ Ⓔ
34. Ⓐ Ⓑ Ⓒ Ⓓ Ⓔ

35. Ⓐ Ⓑ Ⓒ Ⓓ Ⓔ
36. Ⓐ Ⓑ Ⓒ Ⓓ Ⓔ
37. Ⓐ Ⓑ Ⓒ Ⓓ Ⓔ
38. Ⓐ Ⓑ Ⓒ Ⓓ Ⓔ
39. Ⓐ Ⓑ Ⓒ Ⓓ Ⓔ
40. Ⓐ Ⓑ Ⓒ Ⓓ Ⓔ
41. Ⓐ Ⓑ Ⓒ Ⓓ Ⓔ
42. Ⓐ Ⓑ Ⓒ Ⓓ Ⓔ
43. Ⓐ Ⓑ Ⓒ Ⓓ Ⓔ
44. Ⓐ Ⓑ Ⓒ Ⓓ Ⓔ
45. Ⓐ Ⓑ Ⓒ Ⓓ Ⓔ
46. Ⓐ Ⓑ Ⓒ Ⓓ Ⓔ
47. Ⓐ Ⓑ Ⓒ Ⓓ Ⓔ
48. Ⓐ Ⓑ Ⓒ Ⓓ Ⓔ
49. Ⓐ Ⓑ Ⓒ Ⓓ Ⓔ
50. Ⓐ Ⓑ Ⓒ Ⓓ Ⓔ
51. Ⓐ Ⓑ Ⓒ Ⓓ Ⓔ

52. Ⓐ Ⓑ Ⓒ Ⓓ Ⓔ
53. Ⓐ Ⓑ Ⓒ Ⓓ Ⓔ
54. Ⓐ Ⓑ Ⓒ Ⓓ Ⓔ
55. Ⓐ Ⓑ Ⓒ Ⓓ Ⓔ
56. Ⓐ Ⓑ Ⓒ Ⓓ Ⓔ
57. Ⓐ Ⓑ Ⓒ Ⓓ Ⓔ
58. Ⓐ Ⓑ Ⓒ Ⓓ Ⓔ
59. Ⓐ Ⓑ Ⓒ Ⓓ Ⓔ
60. Ⓐ Ⓑ Ⓒ Ⓓ Ⓔ
61. Ⓐ Ⓑ Ⓒ Ⓓ Ⓔ
62. Ⓐ Ⓑ Ⓒ Ⓓ Ⓔ
63. Ⓐ Ⓑ Ⓒ Ⓓ Ⓔ
64. Ⓐ Ⓑ Ⓒ Ⓓ Ⓔ
65. Ⓐ Ⓑ Ⓒ Ⓓ Ⓔ
66. Ⓐ Ⓑ Ⓒ Ⓓ Ⓔ
67. Ⓐ Ⓑ Ⓒ Ⓓ Ⓔ
68. Ⓐ Ⓑ Ⓒ Ⓓ Ⓔ

SKILLS ANALYSIS: QUANTITATIVE

1. Ⓐ Ⓑ Ⓒ Ⓓ Ⓔ
2. Ⓐ Ⓑ Ⓒ Ⓓ Ⓔ
3. Ⓐ Ⓑ Ⓒ Ⓓ Ⓔ
4. Ⓐ Ⓑ Ⓒ Ⓓ Ⓔ
5. Ⓐ Ⓑ Ⓒ Ⓓ Ⓔ
6. Ⓐ Ⓑ Ⓒ Ⓓ Ⓔ
7. Ⓐ Ⓑ Ⓒ Ⓓ Ⓔ
8. Ⓐ Ⓑ Ⓒ Ⓓ Ⓔ
9. Ⓐ Ⓑ Ⓒ Ⓓ Ⓔ
10. Ⓐ Ⓑ Ⓒ Ⓓ Ⓔ
11. Ⓐ Ⓑ Ⓒ Ⓓ Ⓔ
12. Ⓐ Ⓑ Ⓒ Ⓓ Ⓔ
13. Ⓐ Ⓑ Ⓒ Ⓓ Ⓔ
14. Ⓐ Ⓑ Ⓒ Ⓓ Ⓔ
15. Ⓐ Ⓑ Ⓒ Ⓓ Ⓔ
16. Ⓐ Ⓑ Ⓒ Ⓓ Ⓔ
17. Ⓐ Ⓑ Ⓒ Ⓓ Ⓔ

18. Ⓐ Ⓑ Ⓒ Ⓓ Ⓔ
19. Ⓐ Ⓑ Ⓒ Ⓓ Ⓔ
20. Ⓐ Ⓑ Ⓒ Ⓓ Ⓔ
21. Ⓐ Ⓑ Ⓒ Ⓓ Ⓔ
22. Ⓐ Ⓑ Ⓒ Ⓓ Ⓔ
23. Ⓐ Ⓑ Ⓒ Ⓓ Ⓔ
24. Ⓐ Ⓑ Ⓒ Ⓓ Ⓔ
25. Ⓐ Ⓑ Ⓒ Ⓓ Ⓔ
26. Ⓐ Ⓑ Ⓒ Ⓓ Ⓔ
27. Ⓐ Ⓑ Ⓒ Ⓓ Ⓔ
28. Ⓐ Ⓑ Ⓒ Ⓓ Ⓔ
29. Ⓐ Ⓑ Ⓒ Ⓓ Ⓔ
30. Ⓐ Ⓑ Ⓒ Ⓓ Ⓔ
31. Ⓐ Ⓑ Ⓒ Ⓓ Ⓔ
32. Ⓐ Ⓑ Ⓒ Ⓓ Ⓔ
33. Ⓐ Ⓑ Ⓒ Ⓓ Ⓔ
34. Ⓐ Ⓑ Ⓒ Ⓓ Ⓔ

35. Ⓐ Ⓑ Ⓒ Ⓓ Ⓔ
36. Ⓐ Ⓑ Ⓒ Ⓓ Ⓔ
37. Ⓐ Ⓑ Ⓒ Ⓓ Ⓔ
38. Ⓐ Ⓑ Ⓒ Ⓓ Ⓔ
39. Ⓐ Ⓑ Ⓒ Ⓓ Ⓔ
40. Ⓐ Ⓑ Ⓒ Ⓓ Ⓔ
41. Ⓐ Ⓑ Ⓒ Ⓓ Ⓔ
42. Ⓐ Ⓑ Ⓒ Ⓓ Ⓔ
43. Ⓐ Ⓑ Ⓒ Ⓓ Ⓔ
44. Ⓐ Ⓑ Ⓒ Ⓓ Ⓔ
45. Ⓐ Ⓑ Ⓒ Ⓓ Ⓔ
46. Ⓐ Ⓑ Ⓒ Ⓓ Ⓔ
47. Ⓐ Ⓑ Ⓒ Ⓓ Ⓔ
48. Ⓐ Ⓑ Ⓒ Ⓓ Ⓔ
49. Ⓐ Ⓑ Ⓒ Ⓓ Ⓔ
50. Ⓐ Ⓑ Ⓒ Ⓓ Ⓔ
51. Ⓐ Ⓑ Ⓒ Ⓓ Ⓔ

52. Ⓐ Ⓑ Ⓒ Ⓓ Ⓔ
53. Ⓐ Ⓑ Ⓒ Ⓓ Ⓔ
54. Ⓐ Ⓑ Ⓒ Ⓓ Ⓔ
55. Ⓐ Ⓑ Ⓒ Ⓓ Ⓔ
56. Ⓐ Ⓑ Ⓒ Ⓓ Ⓔ
57. Ⓐ Ⓑ Ⓒ Ⓓ Ⓔ
58. Ⓐ Ⓑ Ⓒ Ⓓ Ⓔ
59. Ⓐ Ⓑ Ⓒ Ⓓ Ⓔ
60. Ⓐ Ⓑ Ⓒ Ⓓ Ⓔ
61. Ⓐ Ⓑ Ⓒ Ⓓ Ⓔ
62. Ⓐ Ⓑ Ⓒ Ⓓ Ⓔ
63. Ⓐ Ⓑ Ⓒ Ⓓ Ⓔ
64. Ⓐ Ⓑ Ⓒ Ⓓ Ⓔ
65. Ⓐ Ⓑ Ⓒ Ⓓ Ⓔ
66. Ⓐ Ⓑ Ⓒ Ⓓ Ⓔ
67. Ⓐ Ⓑ Ⓒ Ⓓ Ⓔ
68. Ⓐ Ⓑ Ⓒ Ⓓ Ⓔ

The MCAT
Model Examination C*

SCIENCE KNOWLEDGE

115 MINUTES
109 QUESTIONS

The following questions are based on your knowledge of science. The questions are varied; therefore, you are advised to pay careful attention to the instructions for each portion.

Biology—38 Questions   Recommended Time—25 minutes

DIRECTIONS: Each of the statements or questions is followed by suggested completions or answers. Choose the one that best completes the statement or answers the question, and mark the letter of your choice on the answer sheet.

1. Which of the following is a major characteristic of mitochondria?
   (A) possess hydrolytic enzymes
   (B) function in protein synthesis
   (C) condense (package) secretory products
   (D) function in energy production

2. Neurotransmitters, such as acetylcholine, are initially detected by which part of a neuron?
   (A) dendrite
   (B) nucleus
   (C) terminal branch
   (D) mitochondrion

3. Which organisms in the food pyramid function as primary consumers?
   (A) bass
   (B) minnows
   (C) copepods
   (D) algae

4. Normally, a complete set of chromosomes (2n) is passed on to each daughter cell as a result of
   (A) reduction division.
   (B) mitotic cell division.
   (C) meiotic cell division.
   (D) nondisjunction.

5. Regulation of the resorption of calcium from bone is controlled by the
   (A) thyroid gland.
   (B) parathyroid glands.
   (C) thymus.
   (D) adrenal glands.
   (E) kidneys.

6. A major function attributed to the adrenal cortex is
   (A) regulation of resorption of calcium from bone.
   (B) regulation of metabolic rate.
   (C) development of a competent immune system.
   (D) production of mineralocorticoids and glucocorticoids.
   (E) production of angiotensins.

---

*Explanations for science answers can be found on p. 391.

7. Oxygen molecules absorbed by moist respiratory surfaces in humans diffuse immediately into
   (A) endocrine glands.
   (B) blood capillaries.
   (C) external tubules.
   (D) skin pores.

8. The energy released from the anaerobic respiration of a glucose molecule is less than that released from the aerobic respiration of a glucose molecule because
   (A) fewer bonds of the glucose molecule are broken in anaerobic respiration than in aerobic respiration.
   (B) more enzymes are required for anaerobic respiration than for aerobic respiration.
   (C) anaerobic respiration occurs 24 hours a day, while aerobic respiration can occur only at night.
   (D) anaerobic respiration requires oxygen but aerobic respiration does not require oxygen.

9. The frequency of traits which presently offer high adaptive value to a population may decrease markedly in future generations if
   (A) conditions remain stable.
   (B) the environment changes.
   (C) all organisms with the trait survive.
   (D) mating remains random.

10. A dominant role in the development of a competent immune system is played by the
    (A) thyroid gland.
    (B) pituitary gland.
    (C) thymus.
    (D) parathyroid glands.
    (E) adrenal glands.

11. Of the following, all are fat-soluble vitamins EXCEPT
    (A) vitamin A.
    (B) vitamin D.
    (C) vitamin E.
    (D) vitamin K.
    (E) vitamin B_1.

12. All of the following affect the affinity of hemoglobin for oxygen EXCEPT
    (A) pH.
    (B) temperature.
    (C) concentration of 2,3-diphosphoglycerate (DPG).
    (D) carbon dioxide concentration.
    (E) ATP concentration in the erythrocyte.

13. All of the following are functions of cholecystokinin EXCEPT
    (A) stimulating pancreatic enzyme secretion.
    (B) increasing the pancreatic bicarbonate response to secretion.
    (C) increasing the distensibility of the stomach.
    (D) inducing gallbladder emptying.
    (E) stimulating pepsinogen secretion.

14. What is the primary pituitary hormone released in response to stress?
    (A) LH
    (B) ACTH
    (C) TSH
    (D) FSH
    (E) Oxytocin

15. Hydra usually reproduce by the process known as budding. This form of reproduction is called as
    (A) cleavage reproduction.
    (B) vegetative reproduction.
    (C) binary fision (mitosis).
    (D) parthenogenesis.
    (E) sexual reproduction.

16. The term "limey," as applied to British individuals, refers to the
    (A) early dietary approach to the prevention of scurvy in the British navy.
    (B) large numbers of lime trees transplanted from Spain to southern Wales in the eighteenth century.
    (C) practice of adding lime slices to the gin drinks ordinarily consumed by British soldiers in India.
    (D) pale green skin seen in many individuals in the British Isles as a result of a combination of diet and insufficient exposure of the skin to sunlight.
    (E) early dietary approach to the prevention of rickets in the British navy.

17. Blood in the pulmonary veins is rich in
    (A) oxyhemoglobin.
    (B) carbaminohemoglobin.
    (C) hemoglobin.
    (D) uric acid.
    (E) carbon dioxide.

18. Fertilization in the human female usually takes place in the upper one-third of the oviduct while implantation occurs in the
    (A) lower one-third of oviduct.
    (B) Mullerian duct.
    (C) vagina.
    (D) peritoneum.
    (E) uterus.

19. A common experiment carried out in the physiology laboratory on the turtle heart involves first destroying the S-A node, observing the heart and then destroying the A-V node and observing and recording the results. After these procedures it is found that the heart now
    (A) beats faster.
    (B) exhibits no change in heart rate.
    (C) beats slower.
    (D) will stop beating.

20. Messenger RNA receives its instructions from
    (A) ribosomes.
    (B) endoplasmic reticulum.
    (C) DNA in the nucleus.
    (D) cytoplasm.
    (E) Golgi zone.

21. Undigested food is eliminated from the body by the process of
    (A) exocytosis.
    (B) excretion.
    (C) egestion.
    (D) catabolism.
    (E) assimilation.

22. The most sensitive tests developed for the accurate detection of very small amounts of hormones to date are
    (A) bio-assays.
    (B) immuno-assays.
    (C) ascorbic acid depletion tests.
    (D) fluorometric assays.
    (E) chromatographic assays.

23. The diagnostic tests for pregnancy utilize the presence of
    (A) progesterone.
    (B) estrogen.
    (C) chorionic gonadotropin.
    (D) oxytocin.
    (E) luteinizing hormone.

24. Photoperiodism is
    (A) the ability to perceive color by the cones of the retina.
    (B) the physiological response of an organism to light and dark periods (cycles).
    (C) the ability to utilize CO_2 to produce O_2.
    (D) not a factor of biological significance.
    (E) the ability to perceive black and white shades by the rods of the retina.

25. The part of the neuron that conducts impulses away from its cell body is called the
  (A) axon.
  (B) dendrite.
  (C) node of Ranvier.
  (D) Schwann sheath.
  (E) nucleus.

26. After fertilization the zygote will develop into a male organism if the
  (A) egg possesses a Y-chromosome.
  (B) sperm possesses an X-chromosome.
  (C) zygote possesses two X-chromosomes.
  (D) zygote possesses two Y-chromosomes.
  (E) sperm possesses a Y-chromosome.

27. Fetal blood is carried to the placenta for oxygenation by the
  (A) umbilical arteries.
  (B) ductus venosus.
  (C) ductus arteriosus.
  (D) foramen ovale.
  (E) umbilical veins.

28. A characteristic of intestinal parasites such as *Ascaris* is a tough protective cuticle which
  (A) protects the parasite from the host's enzymes.
  (B) protects the parasite from other parasites the host carries.
  (C) protects the host from the parasite's enzymes.
  (D) keeps the parasite in a dormant state.

29. Of the following, which is the incorrect pair?
  (A) Robert Hooke—cell wall
  (B) Schleiden and Schwann—cell theory
  (C) Robert Brown—nucleus
  (D) Watson and Crick—DNA model
  (E) Virchow—spontaneous generation of living cells

30. Running to catch the bus to go to work has produced a rapid heart rate, an increase in the respiratory rate, and an increase in blood pressure in an individual. We can attribute these changes to
  (A) the peripheral nervous system.
  (B) the central nervous system.
  (C) the parasympathetic component of the autonomic nervous system.
  (D) increased metabolic rate.
  (E) the sympathetic component of the autonomic nervous system.

31. Homologous structures have
  (A) common embryonic origins.
  (B) similar structures and shapes only in ontogeny.
  (C) different embryonic origins.
  (D) common functions but different shapes.
  (E) different functions but the same shapes.

32. In rabbits, rough coat is dominant over smooth coat. Brown is dominant over gray fur color. A rough, brown male is mated to a couple of smooth, gray females. The offspring present the following ratios: 18 rough, brown; 21 rough, gray; 16 smooth, brown; 24 smooth, gray. If this male had been mated to a female of his own genotype, what proportion of the offspring would have exhibited rough, gray coats?
  (A) 4 out of 16
  (B) 3 out of 32
  (C) 3 out of 16
  (D) 12 out of 16
  (E) 1 out of 16

33. Which of the following is mismatched?
    (A) nervous system—reception, conduction, integration, effect
    (B) skeletal system—posture, protection, locomotion, blood cell production
    (C) epidermis—support, integration, exchange, filtration
    (D) gastrointestinal system—absorption, secretion, digestion, egestion

34. Which of the following muscle types is not under the control of the autonomic (involuntary) nervous system?
    (A) heart (cardiac)   (C) skeletal (striated)
    (B) smooth   (D) arrector pili

35. In animals, cell division takes place throughout the body. In higher plants, regions found at the apices and cambiums of roots and stems are responsible. We speak of these regions as
    (A) young.   (D) meristematic.
    (B) immature.   (E) growth cone.
    (C) differentiated.

36. Mesoderm gives rise to
    (A) the gall bladder.   (C) the lungs.
    (B) the appendix.   (D) muscles.

37. Ectoderm does NOT give rise to
    (A) the skin.
    (B) the lens of the eye.
    (C) the central nervous system.
    (D) the inner lining of the stomach.

38. Endodermal derivation can be ascribed to
    (A) the inner lining of the gut.
    (B) the pituitary.
    (C) the lining of the respiratory system.
    (D) A and C above.

Chemistry—38 Questions   Recommended Time—46 minutes

DIRECTIONS: Each of the statements or questions is followed by suggested completions or answers. Choose the one that best completes the statement or answers the question, and mark the letter of your choice on the answer sheet.

1. $A + B + C \xrightarrow{\text{E (enzyme)}} ABCE \longrightarrow D + F + E$
       (1)   (2)   (3)   (4)

   In the above reaction, the enzyme-substrate complex is represented by
   (A) 1   (C) 3
   (B) 2   (D) 4

2. Which molecule is nonpolar and contains a nonpolar covalent bond?
   (A) F_2 (D) HCl
   (B) CCl_4 (E) H_2O
   (C) HF

3. Which compound reacts with an acid to form a salt and water?
   (A) CH_3Cl
   (B) CH_3COOH
   (C) KCl
   (D) KOH
   (E) CH_4

4. Which bond is formed by the transfer of an electron from one atom to another?
   (A) ionic bond
   (B) covalent bond
   (C) peptide bond
   (D) hydrogen bond
   (E) metallic bond

5. The maximum number of electrons that a single orbital of the $3d$ sublevel may contain is
   (A) 1
   (B) 2
   (C) 3
   (D) 4
   (E) 5

6. Given the following K_{sp} values, which compound will be the least soluble in water?
   (A) $AgBr = 5.0 \times 10^{-13}$
   (B) $AgCl = 1.8 \times 10^{-10}$
   (C) $Ag_2CrO_4 = 1.1 \times 10^{-12}$
   (D) $AgI = 8.3 \times 10^{-17}$

7. Which could act either as an oxidizing agent or a reducing agent?
   (A) Fe^0
   (B) Fe^{2+}
   (C) Fe^{3+}
   (D) Cu^0
   (E) Cu^{2+}

8. The development of our solar system is thought to have proceeded from the condensation of gases composed primarily of
   (A) hydrogen.
   (B) oxygen.
   (C) carbon.
   (D) argon.
   (E) nitrogen.

9. Most enzymes are named to indicate the reaction they catalyze and have the suffix
   (A) -ide.
   (B) -ogen.
   (C) -ase.
   (D) -ose.
   (E) -ade.

Questions 10, 11, 12:

Phenylamine is cooled to 0°C and treated with HCl and $NaNO_2$. After a few minutes of reaction time cuprous bromide is added, and the solution is heated.

10. The solution was cooled because
    (A) the desired reaction proceeds too quickly above 0°, and thus an overreaction may result.
    (B) the intermediate produced at the 0° temperature is unstable at higher temperature.
    (C) HCl and $NaNO_2$ react only at low temperature.
    (D) phenylamine is quite volatile and would evaporate at temperatures above 10°C.

11. What percent nitrogen is contained in the final aromatic product?
    (A) 20
    (B) 15
    (C) 8
    (D) 90
    (E) 0

12. The final product would primarily be a (an)
    (A) azo dye.
    (B) organometallic compound.
    (C) monosubstituted benzene containing no metal.
    (D) disubstituted benzene.
    (E) enzyme.

13. Enzymes are
    (A) proteins that catalyze chemical reactions, but they do not have the usual chemical and physical properties of proteins.
    (B) proteins containing a high concentration of D-amino acids.
    (C) compounds of amino acids, but they cannot be hydrolyzed to form free amino acids.
    (D) proteins and may be considered as such chemically and physically.
    (E) metallic compounds.

14. A covalent bond
    (A) is one in which an orbital electron has been completely transferred from one atom to another.
    (B) is one in which a pair of orbital electrons are shared between two atoms.
    (C) occurs only in inorganic or organometallic compounds.
    (D) occurs only in organic compounds.
    (E) is a very unstable bond.

15. A metabolic process that produces energy to convert ADP^+ phosphate into ATP is the
    (A) production of fructose and glucose from sucrose.
    (B) production of fatty acids and glycerol from triglycerides.
    (C) production of CO_2 and water from fatty acids.
    (D) production of steroids from acetate.
    (E) production of N_2 from fatty acids.

16. If a solution contains equal concentrations of hydroxyl ions and hydrogen ions, its pH is
    (A) around 14.   (D) just very slightly acidic.
    (B) around 0.   (E) just very slightly basic.
    (C) neutral.

17. A molecule possessing NH_2 and COOH groups is classified as a (an)
    (A) glycerol.   (D) carbohydrate.
    (B) protein.   (E) fat.
    (C) amino acid.

18. When CO_2 is dissolved in water, the end product will be
    (A) carbon hydrate.   (D) carbonic acid.
    (B) carbon trioxide.   (E) carbon tetrachloride.
    (C) carbon hydroxide.

19. About twenty of all the elements known are regularly found in protoplasm; this may vary. Which of the items below is present in the smallest quantity (percentage by weight)?
    (A) oxygen   (D) iron
    (B) carbon   (E) nitrogen
    (C) hydrogen

20. Where is messenger RNA synthesized in a cell?
    (A) nucleus   (D) endoplasmic reticulum
    (B) mitochondria   (E) Golgi apparatus
    (C) ribosomes

21. A colloidal solution is influenced greatly by all of the following EXCEPT
    (A) electric charges.   (C) Brownian movement.
    (B) particle size.   (D) gravitational forces.

22. Heating of benzaldehyde with NaOH produces
   (A) no reaction.
   (B) a long chain polymer by aldol condensation.
   (C) benzoic acid and benzyl alcohol.
   (D) benzoic acid and methyl alcohol.
   (E) benzene and sodium carbonate.

23. The Lambert-Beer law
   (A) was developed to explain the nonlinear production of alcohol by yeast in the brewing industry.
   (B) describes the reproduction characteristics of yeast.
   (C) relates the wave length of light to the light absorption of a solution at different wavelengths.
   (D) relates changes in the light absorption at a particular wavelength to changes in thickness and/or concentration of a solution in the light path.
   (E) may be explained in part by all of the statements.

24. Phenol is most soluble in
   (A) aqueous NaOH.
   (B) aqueous $NaHCO_3$.
   (C) aqueous HCl.
   (D) pure water.
   (E) distilled water.

25. The metabolism of which of the following food components produces the greatest energy yield per gram?
   (A) triglyceride
   (B) glucose
   (C) fructose
   (D) protein
   (E) carbohydrate

26. 1,3-Butadiene is a
   (A) cumulative diene.
   (B) conjugated diene.
   (C) isolated diene.
   (D) product of the reaction of calcium carbide with water.

27. An important chemical method for resolution of a racemic mixture utilizes the formation of
   (A) a meso compound.
   (B) geometric isomers.
   (C) diastereomers.
   (D) enantiomers.
   (E) racemers.

28. The four deoxyribonucleotides which make up DNA are
   (A) adenine, guanine, thymine, cytosine.
   (B) adenine, guanine, cytosine, uracil.
   (C) adenine, polyamine, thymine, cytoplasm.
   (D) guanine, adenine, transfer RNA, cytosine.
   (E) adenine, guanine, cytosine, nuclear RNA.

29. The base-catalyzed reaction below produces

$$\begin{matrix} NH_2 & COOH \\ | & | \\ C=O & + & C \\ | & | \\ NH_2 & COOH \end{matrix}$$

   (A) cyclamate.
   (B) nylon.
   (C) barbital.
   (D) saccharin.
   (E) amphetamine.

30. The mechanism of enzymatic action involves
   (A) slow degradation of the enzyme to form an enzyme-substrate complex.
   (B) temporary union of enzyme with substrate.
   (C) no specificity for a given substrate.
   (D) resistance to deactivation by high temperatures.
   (E) rapid degradation of the enzyme to form an enzyme-substrate complex.

31. DNA and RNA are both nucleic acids found in the nucleus; however, DNA differs from RNA in that DNA has
    (A) fewer phosphate components.
    (B) uracil instead of adenine as a nitrogenous base.
    (C) a ribose instead of deoxyribose as a sugar.
    (D) a deoxyribose instead of a ribose as a sugar.
    (E) a shorter chain sugar.

32. The rate with which small molecules enter or leave cells is dependent on several factors; among them is (are)
    (A) the charge they possess.
    (B) their solubility (in lipid, etc.).
    (C) their molecular size.
    (D) all of the above.

33. A compound with the structure $H_2C = \underset{\underset{H}{|}}{C} - CH_2 - \underset{\underset{H}{|}}{C} = O$ is

    (A) an acid.   (C) a ketone.
    (B) an anhydride.   (D) none of the above.

34. An element ordinarily found in monatomic form is
    (A) helium.   (C) neon.
    (B) argon.   (D) all of the above.

35. Hydrolysis of sucrose produces an equimolar mixture of
    (A) fructose and glucose.
    (B) glucose and either ribose or deoxyribose.
    (C) galactose and glucose.
    (D) glucose and maltose.
    (E) none of the above.

36. A compound with the formula C_3H_6 could be
    (A) propane.   (C) cyclopropane.
    (B) propyne.   (D) none of the above.

37. An example of a polyester is
    (A) nylon.   (D) polymixin B.
    (B) Dacron.   (E) achromycin.
    (C) polyethylene.

38. Most home units for softening water
    (A) remove ions such as calcium and replace them with sodium ions.
    (B) remove virtually all ions, producing water of the same chemical purity as distilled water.
    (C) remove primarily anions such as sulfur.
    (D) add small quantities of soap to produce water that feels soft.
    (E) function by osmosis.

Physics—33 Questions   Recommended Time—44 minutes

DIRECTIONS: Each of the statements or questions is followed by suggested completions or answers. Choose the one that best completes the statement or answers the question, and mark the letter of your choice on the answer sheet.

1. A car travels at 30 kilometers/hour for 15 kilometers. It then increases its average speed to 60 km/h for the next 30 kilometers. The overall average speed for the 30 km is:
   (A) 30 km/h.
   (B) 35 km/h.
   (C) 40 km/h.
   (D) 45 km/h.
   (E) 50 km/h.

2. If we neglect friction, the acceleration of a free-falling body near the surface of the earth is about 9.8 m/s^2 This means that the
   (A) velocity at the end of one second will be 19.6 m/s if the body started at rest.
   (B) velocity of a freely falling object increases 9.8 m/s for each second that the object is falling.
   (C) body would drop 9.8 m in the first second.
   (D) velocity does not change as the body falls.
   (E) motion is nonuniform.

3. A gas under 1 atmosphere absolute pressure occupies a 2 cubic meter volume at 293 K. What will the temperature be if the volume is increased to 3 cubic meters and the pressure is 4 atmospheres absolute?
   (A) 0 K
   (B) 273 K
   (C) 373 K
   (D) 1119 K
   (E) 1758 K

4. Which one of the statements below is false?
   (A) An endothermal reaction requires the addition of energy before it can occur.
   (B) An exothermal reaction converts chemical energy to another form.
   (C) The concepts of exothermal and endothermal reactions are relevant in discussing nuclear reactions.
   (D) After an exothermal reaction the final temperature of the components is unchanged.
   (E) During an exothermal reaction heat is released.

5. Isotopes of a given element have the same atomic number but have a different mass number. Which of the statements below is true?
   (A) Isotopes of a given element have a larger number of electrons and protons.
   (B) Isotopes of a given element have a smaller number of electrons and protons.
   (C) Isotopes of a given element have a different number of nucleons in the nucleus.
   (D) All elements have isotopes.
   (E) Isotopes are indistinguishable from one another.

6. The density of a steel block is 7.8 g/cm^3. What is the mass of a steel block whose dimensions are 2 meters by 3 meters by 5 meters?
   (A) 234×10^6 g
   (B) 1234 g
   (C) 7.8×10^6 g
   (D) 178 g
   (E) 30 g

7. What is the kinetic energy possessed by a 100-gram projectile moving with a velocity of 60 m/s?
   (A) 60 joules
   (B) 180 joules
   (C) 360 joules
   (D) 3600 joules
   (E) 6000 joules

8. The basic unit of force in the metric system is a newton which is based on measurement of mass and acceleration in
   (A) g and m/s.
   (B) kg and m/s^2.
   (C) lb. and ft./s^2.
   (D) kg and m/s.
   (E) lb. and m/s.^{2}.

9. In uniform circular motion, the radially inward-directed force to maintain the body in a circular motion is known as
   (A) centrifugal force.
   (B) kinetic friction.
   (C) moment of inertia.
   (D) universal gravitation.
   (E) centripetal force.

10. A 5-kg object is raised 10 meters from the floor. The work done, in joules, was
    (A) 5
    (B) 50
    (C) 98
    (D) 490
    (E) 980

11. A man 2 m tall stands 3 m from an intense source of light at the level of his feet. The man's shadow appears on a wall 15 m from the source of light. How tall is the shadow?
    (A) 6 m
    (B) 10 m
    (C) 12.5 m
    (D) 17.5 m
    (E) 22.5 m

12. When water waves approach the shore at an angle, they will be slowed down in the shallower positions rather than the deeper positions. The portion of the wave in deeper water will consequently swing around until the wave front is almost parallel to shore. This phenomenon of wave action is called
    (A) reflections.
    (B) diffraction.
    (C) dispersion.
    (D) retardation.
    (E) refraction.

13. A car's electric light system is a constant voltage system and not a constant current system. If the resistance in this system is tripled, the resulting power (P) is
    (A) 1/3P.
    (B) 1/2P.
    (C) P (same).
    (D) 2P.
    (E) 3P.

14. A neutral rubber rod is rubbed with fur and acquires a charge of -2×10^{-6} coulomb. The charge on the fur is
    (A) $+1 \times 10^{-6}$ C.
    (B) $+2 \times 10^{-6}$ C.
    (C) -1×10^{-6} C.
    (D) -2×10^{-6} C.

15. In order for standing waves to form in a medium, two waves must
    (A) have the same frequency
    (B) have different amplitudes.
    (C) have different wavelengths.
    (D) travel in the same direction.

16. Only coherent wave sources produce waves that
    (A) are the same in frequency.
    (B) have the same speed.
    (C) are polarized in the same plane.
    (D) have the same wavelength.
    (E) have a constant phase relation.

17. An object is allowed to fall freely near the surface of a planet. The object falls 54 meters in the first 3.0 seconds after it is released. The acceleration due to gravity on the planet is
    (A) 6.0 m/s^2.
    (B) 27 m/s^2.
    (C) 12 m/s^2.
    (D) 108 m/s^2.

18. If the velocity of an automobile is doubled, its kinetic energy
    (A) decreases to one-half.
    (B) doubles.
    (C) decreases to one-fourth.
    (D) quadruples.

19. A ball is at the crest of a hill. The ball moves to a new position after a small amount of displacement. Initially, the ball was in
    (A) stable equilibrium.   (D) unstable equilibrium.
    (B) neutral equilibrium.   (E) productive equilibrium.
    (C) positive equilibrium.

20. A body is submerged in water. The upward force acting upon this body is
    (A) equal to its weight.
    (B) equal to the weight of the displaced fluid.
    (C) the absolute pressure at the surface of the fluid.
    (D) dependent upon its center of gravity.
    (E) directly proportional to its length.

21. The energy of a water wave is directly proportional to the square of its amplitude. If the amplitude is doubled, what occurs to the wave energy?
    (A) It is doubled.   (D) It is halved.
    (B) It is tripled.   (E) It remains the same.
    (C) It is quadrupled.

22. Using the vector diagram below, determine the resultant vector.

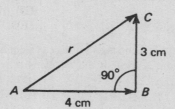

    (A) 5 cm at 37°   (D) 8 cm at 45°
    (B) 0.5 cm   (E) 8 cm at 90°
    (C) 5 cm at 45°

23. In uniformly accelerated motion, the following relationship holds:
$$v = v_0 + at$$
$$x = v_0t + \tfrac{1}{2}at^2$$

    where x = distance moved, t = time, a = acceleration, v_0 = velocity at start, and v = velocity at end. What is the acceleration of a body whose initial velocity of 1340 cm/s increases to 2690 cm/s in 348 m within 15 seconds?
    (A) 15 cm/s²   (D) 60 cm/s²
    (B) 30 cm/s²   (E) 90 cm/s²
    (C) 45 cm/s²

24. What is the radius of a curve if the curve is properly banked for a car traveling at 2500 cm/s and $\tan \theta = v^2/ra$, where r = radius, v = velocity, a = acceleration due to gravity and $\tan \theta = 1$?
    (A) 16 m   (D) 64 m
    (B) 32 m   (E) 80 m
    (C) 48 m

25. The internal energy of water depends on its
    (A) temperature, only
    (B) phase, only
    (C) temperature and mass, only
    (D) temperature and phase, only
    (E) temperature, mass, and phase

26. Under certain conditions, solids will go directly from the solid state to the gaseous state without going through the liquid state. This process is called
    (A) melting.
    (B) freezing.
    (C) vaporization.
    (D) condensing.
    (E) sublimation.

27. The velocity of sound in air is 332 m/s at 0°C. What is the velocity of sound in air at 20°C?
    (A) 344 m/s
    (B) 1268 m/s
    (C) 1420 m/s
    (D) 1484 m/s
    (E) 4975 m/s

28. The velocity of sound in water is 1435 m/s and the velocity of sound in air is 332 m/s. at 0°C. If a tuning fork vibrating at 410 cycles per second is placed in water at 0°C, what is the wavelength of the sound waves that are produced?
    (A) 1.0 m
    (B) 2.5 m
    (C) 3.5 m
    (D) 4.5 m
    (E) 6.0 m

29. A man 2 m tall stands 5 m in front of a plane mirror. How tall is his image?
    (A) 0.5 m
    (B) 1.0 m
    (C) 1.5 m
    (D) 2.0 m
    (E) 2.5 m

30. $$\frac{1}{f} = (n - 1)\left(\frac{1}{R_1} + \frac{1}{R_2}\right)$$

    Which of the following does the equation above represent?

    (A) Bernoulli's equation
    (B) lens-maker's equation—the focal length of a lens is directly related to the index of refraction of the glass and the radius of curvature of each face
    (C) law of universal gravitation—every body in the universe attracts every other body with a force that is directed along a line connecting them and that varies directly with their masses and inversely with the square of the distance between them
    (D) Snell's law
    (E) general gas law—a relationship that relates the pressure, volume, and temperature of a gas

31. A 50-kg crate is being pulled on a horizontal surface against a frictional force of 300 N. It is pulled by a rope, parallel to the ground, which incorporates a scale that reads 400 N. Which of the following statements is correct?
    (A) The crate is in equilibrium with a net force of 100 N.
    (B) The scale must be wrong; it should read 490 N.
    (C) The scale must be wrong; it should read 300 N.
    (D) The crate is accelerated at 8 m/s².
    (E) The crate is accelerated at 2 m/s².

32. A 100-gram rubber ball strikes a wall going 20 m/s and rebounds at 15 m/s. How much impulse does it apply to the wall?

(A) 3.5 N · s

(B) 2.0 N · s

(C) 1.5 N · s

(D) 1.0 N · s

(E) 0.5 N · s

33. The nucleus of a radioactive breakdown product stabilizes by emission of a gamma ray. What change, if any, results in the nucleus?

(A) Its atomic mass number decreases.

(B) No change occurs.

(C) Its mass diminishes slightly.

(D) Its atomic number increases.

(E) Its atomic number decreases.

SCIENCE PROBLEMS

78 MINUTES
60 QUESTIONS: Biology 21; Chemistry 21; Physics 18.

The following questions require you to use your knowledge of science to solve problems.

DIRECTIONS: The following questions and incomplete statements are in groups. Preceding each series of questions or statements is a paragraph or a short explanatory statement, a formula or set of formulas, or a definition. Read the written material and then answer the questions or complete the statements. Eliminate the choices that you think to be incorrect, and mark the letter of your choice on the answer sheet.

For uniformly accelerated angular motion, the following equations hold:

$$w = w_0 + \alpha t$$

$$\theta = w_0 t + \tfrac{1}{2}\alpha t$$

where w = angular velocity, α = angular acceleration, t = time, θ = angular distance, and subscript zero indicates initial condition. A wheel at rest starts rotating with an angular acceleration of 10 radians/sec./sec.

1. What is its angular velocity at the end of 4 seconds?
   (A) 8 radians/sec.
   (B) 16 radians/sec.
   (C) 24 radians/sec.
   (D) 32 radians/sec.
   (E) 40 radians/sec.

2. How many revolutions has the wheel made at the end of 4 seconds?
   (A) 3.2 revolutions
   (B) 6.4 revolutions
   (C) 9.6 revolutions
   (D) 12.7 revolutions
   (E) 15.9 revolutions

3. If the angular velocity of the wheel at the end of the 4 seconds increases to 60 radians/sec. in the next 4 seconds, the magnitude of the angular acceleration changes to
   (A) 5 radians/sec./sec.
   (B) 10 radians/sec./sec.
   (C) 15 radians/sec./sec.
   (D) 20 radians/sec./sec.
   (E) 25 radians/sec./sec.

A protein is least soluble at its isoelectric point since it has an equal number of positive and negative charges. The amino acid residues with their functional groups such as $-NH_3^+$ or $\overset{O}{\overset{\|}{C}}$ $-OH$ or $\overset{O}{\overset{\|}{C}}$ $-O^-$ would, therefore, not have repulsion effects to separate the protein molecules. Increasing turbidity is an indication of insolubility. At a pH below the isoelectric point, more $\overset{O}{\overset{\|}{C}}$ $-O^-$ would be protonated.

4. Given the table below with increasing + indicating increasing turbidity, which is the isoelectric point of the protein?

pH AND SOLUBILITY OF A PROTEIN

pH	5.9	5.6	5.5	5.2	5.0	4.8
Turbidity	0	+	+	++	+	0

   (A) 5.9 or 4.8
   (B) 7
   (C) 5.6
   (D) 5.0
   (E) 5.2

5. What is the net charge on the protein from the previous question?
   (A) 0
   (B) +2
   (C) −2
   (D) +5
   (E) 5.2

6. At pH 4.8 net charge on the protein from above is
   (A) zero.
   (B) positive.
   (C) negative.
   (D) not enough information given.
   (E) equal number of positive and negative charges.

An unknown compound is composed solely of nitrogen, carbon, and hydrogen. An analysis for nitrogen reveals 45.2%. Complete combustion of 0.100 g of the compound produced 0.145 g of water and 0.142 g of carbon dioxide.

7. The empirical formula of the compound is
   (A) CHN.
   (B) CHNO.
   (C) CH_5N.
   (D) C_2H_4N.
   (E) $C_2H_2N_3$.

8. The compound could be a (an)
   (A) olefin.
   (B) organic nitrate.
   (C) substituted pyridine.
   (D) amine.
   (E) nitrile.

9. If it is found that the molecular weight is twice that of the empirical formula, it is possible to write the
   (A) structural formula.
   (B) formula with functional groups indicated.
   (C) molecular formula as $C_2H_{10}N_2$.
   (D) molecular formula as $C_4H_4N_6$.
   (E) none of the above.

The following experiments are designed to illustrate several phenomena. The instructor in a general biology class demonstrates these in the following manner.

Experiment 1:   A piece of spaghetti measuring 3 inches in length is placed in a bowl of warm water and measured after 15 minutes. Its length has increased to 3.7 inches.

10. The increase in length is due to the absorption of water by a (an)
    (A) inert substance.
    (B) semipermeable substance.
    (C) colloidal substance.
    (D) isotonic substance.
    (E) hypertonic substance.

11. The forces observed are substantial and might explain
    (A) the splitting of a concrete driveway by mushrooms.
    (B) the splitting of a sidewalk by the roots of trees.
    (C) the damage (crumbling of rock) observed on a mountainside due to the growth of vegetation.
    (D) all of the above.
    (E) none of the above.

12. The phenomenon demonstrated may best be defined as
   (A) imbibition.
   (B) osmosis.
   (C) concentration.
   (D) turgor.
   (E) plasmolysis.

Experiment 2: Study the illustration below to answer the following three questions.

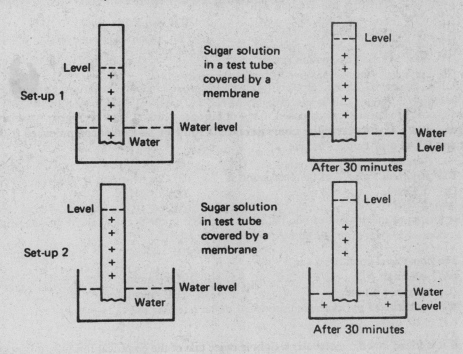

13. From your observation you deduce that the test tubes were placed in a (an)
   (A) hypertonic medium.
   (B) hypotonic medium.
   (C) isotonic medium.
   (D) inert medium.
   (E) saturated medium.

14. Set-up 1 demonstrates the phenomenon of
   (A) imbibition.
   (B) osmosis.
   (C) turgor.
   (D) plasmolysis.
   (E) cyclosis.

15. Set-up 2 demonstrates the phenomenon of
   (A) imbibition.
   (B) osmosis.
   (C) diffusion.
   (D) turgor.
   (E) plasmolysis.

   Avogadro's number may be given as 6.02×10^{23}. Standard temperature and pressure (STP) are 273 K and 760 mm mercury (760 torr).

16. At STP the number of molecules in 1 mole of glucose is
   (A) 22.4×10^{12}.
   (B) 22.4×10^{15}.
   (C) 3.01×10^{20}.
   (D) 6.02×10^{23}.
   (E) 9×10^{23}.

17. Reducing the pressure from 760 to 380 torr would change the number of molecules in one mole of glucose to

(A) 10% of its former value.   (D) 75% of its former value.

(B) 30% of its former value.   (E) none of the above.

(C) 50% of its former value.

18. If a sample contains 3.01×10^{23} molecules of hydrogen in a container at 273 K and a pressure of 760 torr, the volume will be

(A) 6.02 liters.   (D) 44.8 liters.

(B) 11.2 liters.   (E) none of the above.

(C) 22.4 liters.

Sodium metal reacts with anhydrous butyl alcohol to produce sodium butoxide and hydrogen. For the following 3 questions use atomic weights of Na = 23; H = 1; O = 16; and C = 12.

19. How much hydrogen will be produced by the addition of 1 mole of sodium to 10 moles of butyl alcohol?

(A) 1 mole   (D) 22.4 moles

(B) 0.1 mole   (E) none of the above

(C) 0.5 mole

20. Reduction of the amount of butyl alcohol to 1 mole in the problem above would reduce the amount of hydrogen produced by

(A) 10%.   (D) 45%.

(B) 20%.   (E) none of the above.

(C) 40%.

21. The volume (STP) of hydrogen produced in the question above is

(A) 6.02 liters.   (D) 52 liters.

(B) 11.2 liters.   (E) none of the above.

(C) 22.4 liters.

Boyle's law states that the volume of a confined gas varies inversely with the absolute pressure provided that the temperature remains constant. Using this information, apply it to the questions below.

1 liter of oxygen at a pressure of 4 atmospheres is mixed with 5 liters of nitrogen at 2 atmospheres. The mixture is then subjected to 5 atmospheres absolute pressure.

22. What is the pressure of the oxygen in the mixture?

(A) 5.0 atm   (D) 1.67 atm

(B) 4.0 atm   (E) 0.67 atm

(C) 3.33 atm

23. What is the total pressure of the new mixture?

(A) 0.67 atm   (D) 3.00 atm

(B) 1.67 atm   (E) 3.67 atm

(C) 2.34 atm

24. What is the volume of the mixture after it is subjected to 5 atmospheres pressure?

(A) 0.5 liter   (D) 2.8 liters

(B) 1.0 liter   (E) none of the above

(C) 1.8 liters

It has been known for some time that chronic (or in some cases acute) exposure of animals to certain agents results in a fatty degeneration of the liver. Fatty degeneration or fatty liver means an abnormal accumulation of lipid (organic solvent soluble) has occurred. This is a common response of the liver to injury and most often involves an abnormal accumulation of triglyceride (ester of 3 moles of a carboxylic acid and glycerol). Agents capable of producing this effect include such diverse compounds as salts of cerium and other rare earths, carbon tetrachloride, ethyl alcohol, and certain antibiotics. Fatty livers may result from (1) increased liver synthesis of lipid, (2) decreased liver metabolism of lipid, (3) decreased liver secretion of lipid into the blood (as lipoproteins) or combinations of these factors.

25. Long term ingestion of ethyl alcohol can result in liver damage possibly due to
    (A) accumulation of triglycerides.
    (B) increased breakdown of lipids.
    (C) increased secretion of lipid into the blood.
    (D) increased metabolism of lipid.
    (E) all of the above.

26. A person who by profession was a rug cleaner and who still used older methods, such as carbon tetrachloride as a cleaning agent, died under unusual circumstances. On autopsy, organic chemical extract of normal liver showed 1.5% lipid. What might be a reasonable value for an organic chemical extract from the rug cleaner's liver?
    (A) 3.0% lipids
    (B) 1.5% lipids
    (C) 0.5% lipids
    (D) 6% lipids
    (E) 0% lipids

27. For a rat treated with hydrazine and injected with ^{14}C-labeled carboxylic acid after 6 hr., $50\,\mu g/100\,\mu g$ lipoprotein (normal animals injected similarly showed $25\,\mu g/100\,\mu g$) was found. This experiment shows that a fatty liver could NOT be caused by
    (A) increased liver synthesis of lipid
    (B) decreased liver metabolism
    (C) decreased secretion of lipid
    (D) all of the above
    (E) hydrazine

A balloon has been filled with an unknown gas. Having no sophisticated equipment at hand, it is decided to bubble the gas through calcium hydroxide.

28. If a precipitate forms, the gas is identified as
    (A) sulfur dioxide.   (D) butane.
    (B) sulfur trioxide.   (E) none of the above.
    (C) carbon monoxide.

29. Another portion of the unknown gas is passed over a flame. If the gas ignites, this information coupled with the information from the previous question tells us that the gas is
    (A) carbon monoxide.   (D) an ideal gas.
    (B) butane.   (E) a mixture.
    (C) butadiene.

30. A portion of the gas is cooled and then used to fill a beaker. When a lighted splint is inserted into the beaker, the splint is extinguished. This tells us that the gas does not contain a high concentration of
    (A) CO_2.   (D) C_2F_6.
    (B) N_2.   (E) O_2.
    (C) N_2O.

Electrolysis is an important industrial method for the preparation of various chemicals. Electrolysis may be accomplished in aqueous solution or in fused salt depending on the products desired.

31. Which of the following will collect at the anode during electrolysis of aqueous sodium chloride?
    (A) chlorine
    (B) sodium
    (C) hydrogen
    (D) sodium hydroxide
    (E) none of the above

32. Which of the following will collect at the cathode during electrolysis of fused sodium chloride?
    (A) chlorine
    (B) sodium
    (C) hydrogen
    (D) sodium hydroxide
    (E) none of the above

33. Which of the following will collect at the cathode during electrolysis of aqueous sodium chloride?
    (A) sodium
    (B) sodium hydroxide
    (C) hydrogen
    (D) B and C above
    (E) none of the above

Given the circuit diagram below where R_a, R_b, and R_c are respectively the equivalent resistances in series.

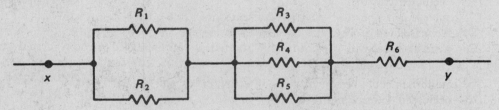

34. The resistance across the parallel resistors R_1 and R_2 can be correctly expressed as
    (A) $R_a = R_1 + R_2$.
    (B) $1/R_a = 1/R_1 + 1/R_2$.
    (C) $R_a = (R_1)(R_2)$.
    (D) $R_a = R_1/R_2$.
    (E) none of the above.

35. If one resistor (R_s) were to replace the entire group of resistors above, its value would be equal to
    (A) $R_s = 1/R_a + 1/R_b + 1/R_c$.
    (B) $R_s = (R_a)(R_b)(R_c)$.
    (C) $R_s = R_a R_b/R_c$.
    (D) $R_s = R_a - R_b/R_c$.
    (E) $R_s = R_a + R_b + R_c$.

36. If total resistance from x to y is 60 ohms and the circuit current of 2 amperes is flowing, what is the potential difference across this resistance?
    (A) 30 volts
    (B) 60 volts
    (C) 120 volts
    (D) 180 volts
    (E) none of the above

Blood, in arteries, exists as a heterogeneous mass which has resistance properties. With this in mind, it is understandable that the greatest rate of flow is experienced in the center of the artery with a concomitant decrease in flow as one approaches the periphery.

37. One can attribute a drop in blood pressure within an artery to
    (A) friction resulting from blood flowing against the wall of an artery.
    (B) the summation of individual shear forces within layers of blood throughout the artery.
    (C) gradual change in the histological construction of the innermost surface of the artery.
    (D) none of the above.
    (E) all of the above.

38. Blood flow is a function of
(A) the amount of elasticity of the arterial wall at a particular point.
(B) the physiological status of the blood.
(C) its compactness as visualized by its radius.
(D) none of the above.

39. Given that the cross-sectional area influences flow by the fourth power of the radius, the flow of a large blood vessel whose diameter is reduced by 50% is in turn reduced to
(A) 1/2.
(B) 1/16.
(C) 1/4.
(D) 1/32.
(E) 1/50.

Reaction equilibria may be affected by temperature or pressure. Consider the reaction
$$X_2 \text{ (gas)} + Y_2 \text{ (gas)} \rightarrow X_2Y_2 \text{ (gas)}$$
which is exothermic in the direction in which it is written.

40. The equilibrium could be shifted in the direction of X_2Y_2 by
(A) increased temperature.
(B) increased pressure.
(C) increased temperature and decreased pressure.
(D) decreased temperature and increased pressure.
(E) none of the above.

41. The equilibrium could be shifted in the direction of X_2 and Y_2 by
(A) decreased temperature.
(B) decreased pressure.
(C) increased temperature and increased pressure.
(D) decreased temperature and decreased pressure.
(E) none of the above.

42. A combination of increased temperature and increased pressure would cause the equilibrium to shift
(A) markedly to the left.
(B) slightly to the left.
(C) markedly to the right.
(D) slightly to the right.
(E) with direction and magnitude unknown or not shift at all.

The half-life of a radioactive element is the time required for one-half of a given amount of an element to disintegrate. The fraction remaining, F, in equation form is $F = \left(\dfrac{1}{2}\right)^{t/T}$ where t = time interval and T = half-life.

43. The half-life of a particular element is 10 seconds. What amount of 10^9 atoms remains after 90 seconds?
(A) 10^9 atoms
(B) 2×10^9 atoms
(C) 2×10^6 atoms
(D) 2×10^3 atoms
(E) 2 atoms

44. What percentage of the original atoms have disintegrated in the 90 seconds?
(A) 99.8%
(B) 50.4%
(C) 41.7%
(D) 49.6%
(E) 0.2%

45. Select the best statement below about elements with a half-life on the order of microseconds.
- (A) Those elements will never totally disintegrate.
- (B) The half-life concept does not apply to them as it does to longer half-life elements.
- (C) Their half-life is adversely influenced by pressure, temperature, and volume.
- (D) They need to be continuously generated through radioactive decay of heavier elements to continue to exist.
- (E) None of the above.

Newton's law of universal gravitation expressed mathematically is $F = G\dfrac{M_1 M_2}{d^2}$ where $G = $ universal physical constant $= 6.67 \times 10^{-11}$ N · m²/kg², M_1 and M_2 are masses of particles attracted, and d is the distance between them.

46. Knowing this law enables us to
- (A) calculate the mass of the earth.
- (B) determine what a person would weigh on the surface of another planet.
- (C) state that the acceleration due to gravity at the surface of planets of equal density is proportional to their radii.
- (D) state that all of the above are true.

47. What is the force of attraction, in newtons, between two bodies separated by 20 m and having masses of 1 kg and 5 kg respectively?
- (A) 7×10^{-11}
- (B) 8×10^{-13}
- (C) 9×10^{-12}
- (D) 2×10^{-9}
- (E) none of the above

48. A deduction from the general gravitation law is an expression for the gravitational force on an object of mass M at the surface of a planet of radius r and density D: $F = \dfrac{4}{3}\pi GMrD$, where G is the universal gravitation constant, 6.67×10^{-11} N·m²/kg². If an object weighs 300 N on earth, how much will it weigh on a planet whose density is the same as the earth's but which has only ¼ of the earth's radius?
- (A) 75 N
- (B) 150 N
- (C) 300 N
- (D) 600 N
- (E) 1200 N

The specific gravity of lead is 11.3.

49. What is the density of lead in g/cm³?
- (A) 1.0
- (B) 2.7
- (C) 7.8
- (D) 11.3
- (E) 13.6

50. What is the volume of a block of lead whose mass is 600 kg?
- (A) 11.3×10^3 cm³
- (B) 53.1×10^3 cm³
- (C) 60×10^3 cm³
- (D) 67.8×10^3 cm³
- (E) none of the above

51. What is the density of lead in lb./ft.³?
- (A) 113.25
- (B) 600.75
- (C) 786.25
- (D) 1678.25
- (E) none of the above

Enzymatic actions are necessary for certain processes to take place. Study the results of the following experiments to answer the questions below.

Experiment 1:
Test tube 1. Compound A + water — after 1 hour no reaction
Test tube 2. Compound B + Compound A — after 1 hour there is a noticeable color change
Test tube 3. Compound B + Water — after 1 hour no reaction

Experiment 2:
Test tube 1. Compound X + Compound Y + Water — no reaction
Test tube 2. Compound X + Acid + Water — no reaction
Test tube 3. Compound X + Compound Y + Acid — reaction product
Test tube 4. Compound X + Compound Y + Solution of bicarbonate — no reaction

Experiment 3:
Test tube 1. Compound Z + Compound W; examined after being left at room temperature for 30 minutes — some reaction product
Test tube 2. Compound Z + Boiled Compound W; examined after being left at room temperature for 30 minutes — no reaction product
Test tube 3. Compound Z + Compound W; examined after being left in an ice bath for 30 minutes — some reaction product

52. In experiment 1, test tube 2 contained the enzyme.
   (A) True
   (B) False

53. The object of experiment 2 was to establish that enzymes are influenced by
   (A) pressure.   (D) all of the above.
   (B) temperature.   (E) none of the above.
   (C) pH.

54. In experiment 3 which of the factors listed below affected the enzymatic reaction?
   (A) pressure   (D) pH
   (B) temperature   (E) all of the above
   (C) boiling

Brown adipose tissue (brown fat) represents only a small percentage of adipose tissue in adult humans. Oxidative metabolism of fat (triacylglycerol) is less efficient in brown adipose tissue, resulting in production of a greater amount of heat and a lesser amount of chemical energy in the form of ATP.

55. A greater proportion of brown fat might be expected in all the following EXCEPT
   (A) lean humans.
   (B) animals being aroused from hibernation.
   (C) newborn animals or humans.
   (D) animals chronically exposed to cold temperatures.
   (E) obese humans.

56. Metabolic oxidation of fatty acids occurs primarily in (on) the subcellular organelles called
   (A) the Golgi apparatus.
   (B) mitochondria.
   (C) smooth endoplasmic reticulum.
   (D) rough endoplasmic reticulum.
   (E) nuclei.

57. The bulk of *de novo* fatty acid synthesis occurs in all animal cells in (on) the
    (A) mitochondria.
    (B) smooth endoplasmic reticulum.
    (C) rough endoplasmic reticulum.
    (D) nonparticulate cytoplasm.
    (E) nuclei.

Three resistors, of 20 Ω, 40 Ω, and 60 Ω, respectively, are connected in series to a 12-volt battery.

58. How is the production of heat distributed in the circuit?
    (A) Rate of heat production is the same for all resistors.
    (B) The 20-Ω resistor produces heat at the fastest rate.
    (C) The 60-Ω resistor produces heat at the fastest rate.
    (D) Total heat produced is the same for all resistors, but rates vary.
    (E) No heat is produced at all.

59. How much is the current in the 20-Ω resistor?
    (A) 0.02 A   (D) 0.60 A
    (B) 0.10 A   (E) 1.1 A
    (C) 0.20 A

60. If the 40-Ω resistor were disconnected and removed from the circuit, with no other change, how much current would there be in the 60-Ω resistor?
    (A) 0.40 A   (D) 0.20 A
    (B) 0.15 A   (E) 0.60 A
    (C) 0 A

SKILLS ANALYSIS: READING

85 MINUTES
68 QUESTIONS

The following questions are to be answered based on your careful reading of selections from scientific writings.

DIRECTIONS: Read each passage carefully, then answer the questions following it. Consider only the material within the passage in answering the questions. Eliminate those choices that you think to be incorrect and mark the letter of your choice on the answer sheet.

It has become obvious in recent years that the decision making power in many school districts is shifting, and is becoming more liberalized as both teachers and parents realize that they are an important facet in the total school operation. They know that without their support and cooperation the system cannot continue to function smoothly.

Consequently, today's educator is no longer content to sit in the background and let decisions be made and programs formulated. New teachers want a voice, they demand a piece of the action, and they are daring enough to question the judgments of the system in their desire to achieve a better educational experience for their students as well as a more economically realistic position for themselves.

Not too many years ago, perhaps as little as a decade in some areas, the decision making power in a school system could have been observed by quickly glancing at an organizational chart which would most probably have looked like this;

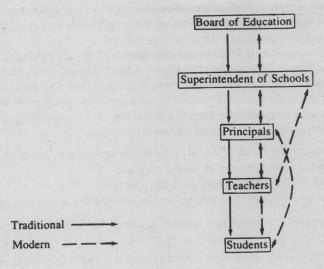

Although much simplified, the chart indicates a flow of power from the school board to the superintendent of schools down to the individual school principals and from there to the teachers and, finally, a minimal involvement of the students themselves.

The board of education was naturally found at the top, for it was assumed that this body represented the taxpaying community. Next in importance was the superintendent, whose word was considered to be law and who would, if so disposed, allow the principal some freedom to make decisions.

By the same token, those principals that prided themselves in being of a democratic nature, would then allow teachers to have a voice in selected matters and would even possibly afford students the opportunity of making minute decisions in appropriate areas.

Within the confines of the individual school, the principal was looked upon as the one person who knew more about educational matters than any other member of the staff. Therefore, he or she was spotlighted not only as the chief administrator, but as the supreme educational leader of the complex. Teachers occupied the place of facilitators, whose main job it was to take the programs that were handed down to them and see that they were carried out satisfactorily. The students were viewed as receptacles for receiving and digesting information. Their major contribution rested in being accepted to an institution of higher learning, thus making the system look good and giving the taxpayers the feeling that the money they spent was, after all, worthwhile.

The entire pattern of decision making, as presented, was based on the very real fact that the board of education controlled the purse strings of a school system. Since money has always been of supreme importance, it was considered the most logical path to follow. Few people thought to question its wisdom or bothered to seek alternatives.

The modern public has slowly come to realize that even though money is still the most crucial factor in operating an efficient school system, there are also other vital and important elements that contribute to its success.

For example, parents are demanding a voice in the operation of local schools. They favor an open door policy which affords them the opportunity to see what is going on in the classrooms and allows many of them to get involved on a parent-volunteer basis. Parents speak out in many cases by manipulating a very vital school input, over which they have strict control, namely their children. Thus we read of such things as parents keeping their offspring out of school to protest situations that they find unsuitable and intolerable. Even though these actions may not in themselves solve the problems, they do cause those in authority to sit up, take notice, and search for possible solutions at a speedy rate.

Every bit as important as the public's realization of its powers, is the teachers' realization that they too have a commodity that is of supreme importance to the system, and that is themselves. When teachers join forces and remove this vital input, school systems are forced to close and the educational machine comes to a halt. Teachers' strikes are now occurring more and more frequently in all areas of the country, and the threat of the entire profession becoming unionized is no longer a laughing matter.

Today's wise school systems have made note of these developments and are attempting to deal with them reasonably. Sharing the decision making power by allowing more realistic and meaningful input from both parents and teachers has become a reality in many districts. While a revised look at the power flow chart today would probably show the players in the same basic positions it would certainly have the arrows of decision coming not only down in a direct line, but also pointing up and out, allowing for a much more liberalized flow of communication and ideas.

The following statements are related to the passage . Based on the information given, select:

(A)   if the statement is *supported by* the information in the passage.
(B)   if the statement is *contradicted by* the information in the passage.
(C)   if the statement is *neither supported nor contradicted by* the information in the passage.

1.   Economics constitutes the prime reason today's teacher clamors for a greater voice in educational decision making.

2.   Parents are becoming increasingly more involved in school situations because they are anxious to determine whether teachers are worth the tax dollars invested in them.

3.   Teachers are more willing than ever to speak out concerning the development of new programs and policies.

4.   Since money is the key factor in operating an efficient school system, and since the board of education holds the purse strings, it stands to reason that the latter should have absolute power over all facets of the educational machine within a district.

5.   The realization that they are of vital importance to the school system has caused teachers to adopt a militant, unionistic attitude.

6.   The National Education Association represents modern educators throughout the United States.

7.   Today's students are radical and demand a share in the decision making process of local school systems.

8. Although a modern organizational chart might resemble one of the past as far as the position of its components is concerned, the flow of power has become more liberalized.

9. Parent-volunteer programs are one avenue of public involvement in local schools.

10. School-systems of the future will probably see an equal division of powers among the board of education, the teachers, and the public.

Performance appraisals— "Who needs them? I'm doing a good job, so why does someone need to sit and put it in writing, then waste my time and theirs talking about it? If I'm doing something that they don't like, let them tell me about it when it happens." This is a typical comment heard from many employees.

The performance appraisal, if completed properly, can be one of the most useful tools a manager can use in developing and training subordinates regardless of what some employees may express. It is a compilation of the employee's strengths and weakness in one concise form. It serves to show the employee the areas in which a good job is being done and also indicates which areas need improvement. The appraisal serves as a permanent record which documents the employee's growth and progress or shows why a promotion is not offered. A performance appraisal forces a manager to discuss an employee's performance on a one-to-one basis and find out more about what the employee's opinions and aspirations might be. This area is often overlooked in the busy day-in and day-out routine of business. It also gives the employee a chance to see what the boss really thinks about his or her work.

An interesting and often very beneficial way of handling a performance appraisal is to give employees a blank evaluation form a few days before the appraisal interview and ask that they rate themselves. When the appraisal takes place, the manager and employee compare their evaluations and work out the areas of disagreement so that each understands the other's position. An unusual result often takes place. Not only do the manager and employee end up with a better knowledge of each other, but they often find that their evaluations are very close to being in agreement. If anything, the employees usually find that they have under-rated themselves. An exception to this result, which the manager must be alert to recognize, is that an unsatisfactory performer may evaluate his or her performance higher than does the manager. The appraisal interview in this situation can often be more valuable than that of the satisfactory performer. It gives the manager an opportunity to counsel an already trained employee and turn around the performance rather than having to seek out and train a replacement. The manager must evaluate the time, expense, and attitude of the present employee against the time and expense of hiring and training a new employee.

Performance appraisals, properly administered, can cut down on turnover and greatly increase the morale of a department. The end result is increased productivity which is really what we are all striving to accomplish.

The following statements are related to the passage above. Based on the information given, select:
(A) if the statement is *supported by* the information in the passage.
(B) if the statement is *contradicted by* the information in the passage.
(C) if the statement is *neither supported nor contradicted by* information in the passage.

11. Managers feel that performance appraisals are a waste of time.

12. A satisfactorily performing employee will rate himself or herself higher than the manager.

13. A performance appraisal only points out the weak areas of performance.

14. The performance appraisal gives the employee and the manager a time to discuss the employee's future in private.

15. Employees and managers can usually work out their differences during the appraisal interview.

16. All performance appraisals are preceded by giving employees blank forms to rate themselves.

17. Performance appraisals often lead to a better understanding between managers and employees and can eventually lead to increased productivity.

18. Most large companies are now using the performance appraisal method because it has been proven a highly effective tool for dismissing unsatisfactory employees.

Time waits for no one. How often we have heard this statement; yet very few of us really pay attention to what it means. We are so busy with all of the things we have to do that we never stop to realize how much we have left undone, or how our priorities have become confused.

It is never too late to learn how to effectively manage our time. The most common response from most people to this suggestion is that they do not have time to learn how to manage their time. These are the people that need time management the most.

Measuring one's time is not as difficult as one might imagine. It merely requires the listing of every activity, regardless of how small, on a piece of paper each day for a week. If there are recurring items, a column can be so headed which will only require a check mark rather than writing out the activity. At the end of the work week, each of the five (5) papers are reviewed to see where time was wasted. These are the main items to be concentrated on during the next week. A side benefit of this analysis may reveal some items which may be delegated to subordinates or eliminated completely.

Another way of managing one's time, is to list all, of the essential activities which must be completed within the next week. Once this list is compiled, go back and organize the activities. Begin with the most important priority and continue it until it is completed, then proceed to the next one and so on. At the end of the week, there may be some items left over which were not completed. Incorporate these in the next week's schedule. They may have moved up in the priority ranking by this time or they may have taken care of themselves and can be eliminated. It is amazing how much can be accomplished with this system. Eventually, the priority items will decrease and there will be available time to be used for other purposes.

You have the essential tools to help you get everything done that you hope to accomplish. Every minute that passes is gone forever.

The following statements are related to the passage above. Based on the information given, select:
(A)   if the statement is *supported by* the information in the passage.
(B)   if the statement is *contradicted by* the information in the passage.
(C)   if the statement is *neither supported nor contradicted by* information in the passage.

19.   Time management is only necessary for experienced managers.

20.   Time management is time consuming if it is done properly.

21.   Time management can be an aid to identify items to be delegated.

22.   With the amount of paper work most people must process, time management is the only way to get things done on time.

23.   Time management helps to identify priorities.

24.   Managing one's time is best learned *before* embarking upon a career.

With the coming of age of the diet generation, amphetamine has taken a place among the most frequently prescribed drugs. It is the chemical structure of amphetamine which gives it resistance to enzymatic destruction and makes it effective after oral ingestion. The compound also exhibits a prolonged ability to activate and stimulate the nervous system. Three forms of the compound exist, with the levorotatory form being the most potent. This is a deviation from usual pharmacodynamic principles since, in most instances, the dextrorotatory form is the most active. Amphetamine is a potent stimulator which mimics many of the actions of the sympathetic nervous system. Adrenalin, the compound released by the sympathetic nervous system, elicits its effect as a result of direct action upon receptors in muscle and glands; amphetamine probably utilizes the same receptor sites as adrenalin. Amphetamine, however, differs from adrenalin in the fact that repeated administration results in a decreasing response of the organism to the drug. If both drugs are administered simultaneously, their action is of an additive nature. The stimulatory response of amphetamine results in an elevated blood pressure, cardiac output, respiratory activity, and basal metabolic rate and hyperirritability. Animals that receive very high doses of the drug become restless, agitated, and sleepless and exhibit tremors but no seizures have been reported. Students during examination week might ingest amphetamine to increase their psychomotor activities. Administration of the drug will result in alertness, and enhancement of initiative, mood, confidence, concentration and expression; however, it has been shown that while the drug allows us to function for longer time periods, it does not enhance the overall performance. Mental ability is not affected by amphetamine.

The following statements are related to the information presented previously. Based on the information given, select:
- (A)   if the statement is *supported by* the information in the passage.
- (B)   if the statement is *contradicted by* the information in the passage.
- (C)   if the statement is *neither supported nor contradicted by* information in the passage.

25.   Repeated administration of adrenalin results in a decreasing response of the organism to the drug.

26.   Amphetamine can be used to treat mental depression.

27.   'Chemically most compounds exhibit increased action if they are present in the levorotatory form.

28.   Amphetamine is a short acting drug.

29.   Adrenalin and amphetamines probably have a similar mechanism of action.

30.   Amphetamine has no effect upon the circulatory system.

31.   Amphetamine may be used in the treatment of certain types of epilepsy.

32.   The overall initiative rather than the ability to do mental tasks is increased by amphetamine.

33.   Considerable danger lies in the promiscuous use of amphetamine.

34.   Psychological and social factors must be considered as components of therapeutic processes.

Tooth development, or odontogenesis, begins at 6½ weeks postconception in the human embryo, and continues for the next 20 years of life. It is initiated as a horseshoe-shaped epithelial thickening in the maxillary and mandibular arches, which sinks into the underlying mesenchyme, and is known as the dental laminae. At 10 discrete regions on this epithelial band of both arches, inductive activity produces lingually oriented outgrowths, known as buds. These buds will then give rise to the enamel organ—the epithelially derived structure that will be responsible for the formation of enamel, as well as for the shape, size, and number of roots the tooth will possess. The mesenchymal tissue of the region surrounding the bud will begin to interact with the epithelially derived bud in several ways. First, a mesenchymal condensation, at the inferior aspect of the bud will direct the future downgrowth of the bud so that a condensation of mesenchymal cells will be surrounded and almost completely enveloped by this epithelial structure. This mesenchymal condensation, the dental papilla, is responsible for the formation of dentin, and will eventually give rise to the pulp of the tooth. The mesenchyme surrounding the rest of the bud will envelop the growing bud and will give rise to the future periodontal ligament and the cementum of the root.

The following statements relate to the passage above. Based on the information given, select: ·
- (A)   if the statement is *supported by* the information in the passage.
- (B)   if the statement is *contradicted by* the information in the passage.
- (C)   if the statement is *neither supported nor contradicted by* information in the passage.

35.   Tooth development is initiated earlier in females than in males.

36.   The bud is the first sign of odontogenesis.

37.   Enamel is mesenchymally derived.

38.   The enamel organ's only function is to determine the shape, size, and number of roots.

39.   The dental papilla is responsible for the formation of dentin and will also give rise to the future pulp of the tooth.

40.   Since enamel is epithelially derived, it is the hardest tissue in the body.

41.   Dentin, pulp, enamel, and periodontal ligament are all derived from the mesenchyme.

42.   Each dental lamina will have 10 buds.

The formation of the palate occurs in several steps. The primary palate, that which contains the five incisors, is formed by the fusion of the globular process of the median nasal process with the right and left lateral palatine shelves of the maxillary process. The secondary palate, or the rest of the hard palate and soft palate, is formed by the fusion of the lateral palatine shelves with each other. Prior to the formation of the palate, the lateral palatine shelves are in the vertical position and the tongue is intervened between them in such a fashion that the tongue occupies both the nasal and oral cavities. At a particular time in development the tongue descends into the prospective oral cavity; and the lateral palatine shelves elevate so that now they are horizontally positioned and in fact act as a dividing plate, separating, almost completely, the oral cavity from the nasal cavity. The two shelves grow medially, contact each other, and fuse. This process is initiated at the middle of the hard palate and spreads both anteriorly and posteriorly, until the secondary palate is completed. If fusion does not occur, cleft palate results. Such clefts may involve the primary palate only, the secondary palate only, a portion of the secondary palate only, or both primary and secondary palates. Additionally, clefts of the primary palate may involve the right side only, the left side only, or both right and left sides, in which case it is referred to as bilateral cleft of the primary palate.

The following statements are related to the passage. Based on the information given, select:
- (A) if the statement is *supported by* the information in the passage.
- (B) if the statement is *contradicted by* the information in the passage.
- (C) if the statement is *neither supported nor contradicted by* information in the passage.

43. Fusion of the secondary palate occurs first in the middle of the soft palate.

44. The primary palate is derived from the lateral palatine shelves and the globular process.

45. Clefts of the secondary palates may be bilateral.

46. The palate separates the nasal and oral cavities from each other.

47. Clefts of the palate are much more common than harelip.

48. The tongue descends into the oral cavity before the palatine shelves elevate.

49. Clefts of the secondary palate are more common than clefts of the primary palate.

50. The lateral palatine processes fuse with each other prior to elevation to the horizontal position.

In long-term care facilities, the medical records department assists the attending physician and the administration of the facility in documenting the course of the patient's illness and medical treatment while an inpatient. It also aids the professional staff in providing good patient care planning. Responsibilities for accurate record keeping and documentation rest with the administration and medical staff, both professional and nonprofessional.

A separate medical record must be maintained for each patient admitted to the facility and kept inviolate and preserved for a statutorily specified period of time after patient's discharge. The medical staff maintains an active clinical record of the resident as documentation of the diagnostic history, medications and treatments provided and their corresponding results, and inpatient care planning. The chart is a tool by which the staff communicates patient care and will serve as documentation to be used in legal proceedings.

For those long-term care facilities participating in federal and state health programs, there are specific requirements relative to the documentation of a resident's plan of care and the skills and training of the personnel executing the documentation and participating in the development of the overall plan of care.

51. From the above passage it can be inferred that
   - (A) medical records are a communication tool.
   - (B) medical records are legal documents recognized in legal proceedings.
   - (C) long term care facilities serve as protectors of patient's rights.
   - (D) A and B.
   - (E) B and C.

52. The phrase that best conveys the central idea of the above passage is
   - (A) clinical records are inviolate.
   - (B) medical records serve as a integral and important function in patient care planning.
   - (C) documentation of total patient care is vital in long-term care facilities.
   - (D) accurate charting makes patient care planning more effective.
   - (E) discharge plans are limited to professional judgments.

53. The writer does NOT state that
    (A) documentation in the clinical records is a responsibility shared by professional and nonprofessional staff.
    (B) discharged medical records are retained for a statutorily specified period of time.
    (C) clinical records are a communication tool.
    (D) release of information from a patient's clinical record is restricted.
    (E) previous diagnoses are to be included in the current clinical record.

54. The clinical record serves all of the following purposes EXCEPT as
    (A) a tool in patient care planning.
    (B) a legal document.
    (C) proof that the best treatment was provided.
    (D) documentation of diagnostic history while an inpatient.
    (E) a means by which a physician orders a treatment plan for a patient.

The limitations of a state's territorial domain are determined by definite boundary lines which mark the extent of the property rights of the state and of its jurisdiction over persons. The existing boundary lines of states have been determined for the most part by definite international conventions. Many of these conventions have materialized as peace treaties following territorial disputes or wars of conquest while still others have been in the form of voluntary agreements between nation states which have brought about an amicable settlement of boundaries.

With respect to constitutional law in the United States, the individual maintains sovereignty not only over the plot of earth that one owns, but, in addition, retains jurisdiction over the acreage in a three-dimensional interpretation. That is, subject to governmental control for aeronautical usage either by the government or by commercial traffic, the sky is the limit. Likewise, retention of mineral rights and subterranean activity is the jurisdiction of the property owner.

It does not necessarily follow, however, that nation states are to follow the same dictum. Unless nation states are participants to binding agreements—made either through international conventions, wars of conquest, or peace treaties—the adjudicatory process lies through international courts of justice or negotiators recognized by and acting on behalf of the parties involved.

55. The subject of this passage is
    (A) determination of boundary lines between nation states.
    (B) individual property rights guaranteed under the Constitution.
    (C) limitations of territorial domain.
    (D) national sovereignty in international boundary disputes.
    (E) origin of property rights.

56. The writer states that
    (A) territorial rights as interpreted from the Constitution are three dimensional.
    (B) international law is derived from participatory judgments of the consenting states.
    (C) periodic international conventions are held to solve boundary disputes between nation states.
    (D) boundary disputes between nation states must be submitted to international courts of justice.
    (E) the best means of determining boundary lines is to fight it out.

57. A method of determining boundary lines not mentioned in the above passage is by
    (A) international convention.
    (B) the Constitution.
    (C) peace treaties.
    (D) voluntary agreements between nation states.
    (E) wars of conquest.

58. Based on the information given in the passage, which of the following is NOT a true statement?
   (A) Boundary lines determine the limitations of a state's territorial domain.
   (B) International boundary lines are generally determined by international conventions.
   (C) Control over the skies is retained by individual nation states.
   (D) Parties to a boundary dispute can take action through international courts of justice to have the dispute resolved.
   (E) All of the above.

With the current emphasis on development of reading skills across the United States (in particular, the standards of quality enacted by the general assembly of the Commonwealth of Virginia and the initiation of the Supplemental Skills Development Program by the Virginia State Department of Education), each school needs to be aware of those areas of reading in which students demonstrated consistent skill weaknesses and, if possible, identify the basic reasons for disparities between ability and achievement in order to develop a supplemental skills program that will improve reading skills.

There are several standardized reading achievement tests and tests measuring educational ability which can be administered that will assist in identifying students who exhibit disparities between levels of ability and of achievement and in what areas of reading weaknesses can be categorized for remediation.

Analysis of information—gleaned from individual student cumulative folders; from interviews with the administrative staff and teachers, former and present, of students identified for remediation and intensification; and by examination of testing materials and testing conditions—may be used as a basis for a quantitative and qualitative study leading to a meaningful intensification program.

59. The central idea conveyed in the above passage is that
   (A) reading skill weaknesses in elementary school children can be attributed to environmental circumstances.
   (B) disparities between achievement and ability levels should be identified before instituting remediation or intensification programs in reading skill development.
   (C) subjective judgments made by educators are prejudicial to identification of a learner's reading weaknesses.
   (D) selection of testing materials will vary disparities in achievement and ability levels.
   (E) enactment of standards of quality will provide the avenue by which reading success may be achieved.

60. The passage specifically states that
   (A) local schools need to identify reading disparities.
   (B) cumulative folders provide valuable information which can be used in a qualitative and quantitative study.
   (C) examination of testing materials and conditions must be used as a basis for quantitative and qualitative study.
   (D) the Supplemental Skills Development Program was enacted by the general assembly.
   (E) student demographic data must be collected to provide a basis for possible study.

61. The writer implies that
   (A) most elementary school age children in Virginia are below the national reading norms.
   (B) Virginia schools are inferior to all other southern school systems.
   (C) standards of quality serve as models for optimum performance by the local school districts in Virginia.
   (D) subjective assessments of a child's home life are valid in determining causative disparities in reading levels.
   (E) remediation programs in reading can be successful if properly developed.

62. The writer mentions each of the following sources of information for qualitative study EXCEPT
    (A) cumulative folders.
    (B) testing materials.
    (C) parental interviews.
    (D) testing conditions.
    (E) teachers and administrative staff.

Just about anyone you talk to nowadays complains about the cost of automobile insurance. It's about time that someone came to the defense of the insurance companies.

We are all familiar with the effects of inflation, but most people forget that the insurance companies are affected, too. An interesting point should be noted. Even though the total costs of producing a policy have been increasing because of increased salaries, paper cost, equipment replacement, etc., the insurance companies' expense ratios have been going down.

If expenses are reduced, then why are premiums going up? Let's look at what makes up the rates that the insurance companies must charge. Automobile repair rates for labor have risen about 20% in the last year and a half. In addition, it has been shown that a new automobile costing $5,000 would cost $20,000 if it were to be repaired with replacement parts (not including the engine). During this same period, a semiprivate hospital room has increased in cost over 22% and physicians' and surgeons' fees have increased 20%. Lawyers continue to ask for larger awards, and the courts are granting them. How can insurance companies continue to pay amounts inflated in this manner without reflecting the increase in their rates?

It is a real shame that the insurance companies don't make these facts known more widely to their customers. A widespread advertising campaign would help to explain their position and make it more tolerable when that next bill comes and has once again increased.

The following statements are related to the passage above. Based on the information given, select:
(A) if the statement is *supported by* the information in the passage.
(B) if the statement is *contradicted by* the information in the passage.
(C) if the statement is *neither supported nor contradicted by* information in the passage.

63. Insurance company expense ratios are continuing to rise with inflation.

64. A car repaired with replacement parts would cost four (4) times as much as a new car.

65. The public is fully aware of why their insurance premiums are increasing.

66. Automobile insurance premiums have risen mainly because of larger awards in law suits.

67. Inflation is affecting the insurance industry and the rates that are charged.

68. Insurance companies are involved in a widespread advertising campaign to make their customers aware of the inflationary problems that have caused rates to rise.

SKILLS ANALYSIS: QUANTITATIVE

85 MINUTES
68 QUESTIONS

The following questions are to be answered based on your knowledge of basic mathematical principles and relationships.

DIRECTIONS: Read each passage carefully, study each table or chart, then answer the questions following it. Consider only the material presented in answering the questions. Eliminate those choices that you think to be incorrect and mark the letter of your choice on the answer sheet.

Using a syringe containing heparin, fifty milliliters of blood were drawn from a healthy male volunteer. Following centrifugation, the "buffy coat" was removed and a lymphocyte rich cell population was obtained by sedimentation through 2% Dextran. After washing in 0.9% saline the lymphocytes were placed in cell culture tubes at a concentration of 5×10^6 cells/ml cell culture medium/tube. To one-half of the tubes was added 5 µg of phytohemagglutinin, a substance which causes lymphocytes to undergo mitosis. The other half of the tubes received no phytohemagglutinin. Radioactive tracers for RNA, DNA, and protein synthesis were then added to all tubes and aliquots removed at selected intervals. The following data were obtained:

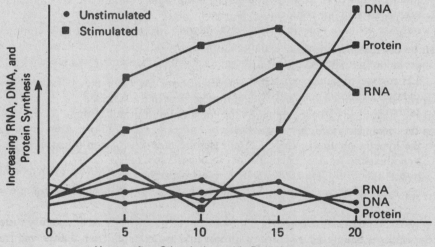

Hours after Stimulation with Phytahemagglutinin

1. The purpose of this experiment was to
   (A) determine the role of heparin in blood clotting.
   (B) determine the sequence of events in cells stimulated to undergo mitosis, and to compare these data to those gathered from unstimulated cells.
   (C) isolate a pure population of lymphocytes.
   (D) determine the life-span of lymphocytes.

2. From these data it can be seen that increased
   (A) RNA synthesis precedes increased protein synthesis.
   (B) DNA synthesis precedes increased protein synthesis.
   (C) protein synthesis precedes increased RNA synthesis.
   (D) DNA synthesis precedes increased RNA synthesis.

3. It may also be assumed that
   (A) DNA synthesis is dependent on previous RNA synthesis.
   (B) protein synthesis is dependent on previous RNA synthesis.
   (C) RNA synthesis is dependent on previous protein synthesis.
   (D) unstimulated lymphocytes synthesize RNA, DNA and protein at a low rate.

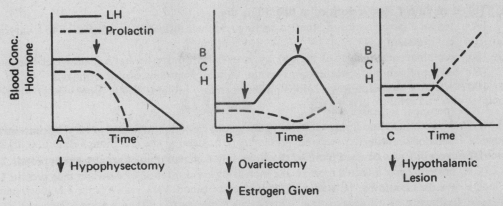

The graphs represent experimental results obtained when the pituitary gland was removed (A), the ovaries were removed (B) and lesions were placed in the hypothalamus (C), that part of the brain most closely related to the pituitary gland. The hormones LH and prolactin were measured in blood by radioimmunoassay.

4. It can be concluded from these results that
    (A) prolactin and LH are removed from the blood at the same rate.
    (B) prolactin and LH are both produced by the pituitary gland.
    (C) both hormones are degraded by the liver.
    (D) only the kidneys remove LH from the blood.

5. It can be concluded from these results that
    (A) prolactin is produced by the ovaries.
    (B) LH release stimulates prolactin release.
    (C) ovarian hormones inhibit LH release, but not prolactin release.
    (D) presence of the ovaries inhibits removal of LH from the blood.

6. It can be concluded from these results that
    (A) the hypothalamus stimulates LH release but inhibits prolactin release.
    (B) hypothalamic lesions are equivalent to hypophysectomy.
    (C) hypothalamic lesions are equivalent to estrogen injections.
    (D) the hypothalamus stimulates LH release, but has no effect on prolactin release.

The urophysis of teleosts secretes a neurohormone directly into the blood circulatory system. This secretory apparatus is believed functional in osmoregulation in fishes from marine and freshwater habitats. Fifteen blueback herring (*Pseudoharengus aestivalis*) were maintained in a marine aquarium at temperatures of 40°-45°. The fish were subjected to increasing salt concentration to a final concentration equal to twice that of seawater. At each concentration four to twelve urophyses were dissected and extracted, and electrophoresis on polyacrylamide gels was performed. Two specific bands of protein were identified as being specific to the urophysis. The amount of protein was determined by microdensitometry. The results are shown in the graph.

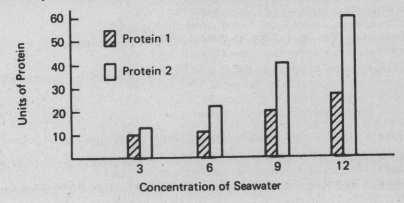

7. This experiment was performed to determine the
   - (A) sexual characteristics of bluefish herring and their influence on adaptation to a varying environment.
   - (B) proteinaceous content of the urophysis in fish from freshwater vs. saltwater habitats.
   - (C) effect of salinity concentrations on the secretory proteins of the urophysis.
   - (D) effect of temperature variations on the secretory proteins of the urophysis.

8. The experiment indicates that
   - (A) the protein material was unaltered in the urophysis of fish subjected to varying concentrations of seawater.
   - (B) protein 1 was affected more by the increasing concentration of seawater than protein 2.
   - (C) protein 2 was affected more by the increasing concentration of seawater than protein 1.
   - (D) the data could not be analyzed.

9. Regarding the functional implications of the urophysis in osmoregulation, which of the following statements is valid?
   - (A) The protein of the urophysis appears to be unaltered by salinity concentration and is not implicated in osmoregulation.
   - (B) The protein secretion is active and directly influences osmoregulation by its action on the gills.
   - (C) Female fish adapt faster to osmotic stress than male fish.
   - (D) None of the above is correct.

An investigator had been studying the interrelationship (cooperation) of various cell types in tissue culture in the immune response to an antigen. The experiments conducted attempted to determine if spleen and mast cells were required for the production of antibody against a pollen. Various donor cells (spleen and mast cells) were injected into recipient rabbits whose immune system had been rendered nonresponsive by whole body X-irradiation. Antibody levels were determined in the serum of the recipients.

Experimental Groups		Antibody Level
A.	Spleen and pollen	0
B.	Spleen	0
C.	Mast cells and pollen	0
D.	Mast cells	0
E.	Spleen and mast cells and pollen	++
F.	Bone marrow and pollen	++
G.	Thymocytes and pollen	++

The following statements are related to the information presented above. Based on the information given, select:
- (A) if the statement is *supported by* the information given.
- (B) if the statement is *contradicted by* the information given.
- (C) if the statement is *neither supported nor contradicted by* information given.

10. In the system under investigation, spleen and mast cells together are required for antibody production.

11. Spleen cells are probably found in the thymus.

12. Spleen cells or mast cells are essential to the antibody production against pollen.

13. In the intact animal, the mast cells would probably be important as a source of antibody.

14. X-irradiation serves as an important tool in immunological experimentation.

Four groups of rats were maintained under identical conditions. Three of the groups received drugs in their drinking water over a period of five weeks. The day before autopsy each rat received one microcurie of ^{131}I. At autopsy the thyroid glands from each group were pooled and weighed. Iodinated intermediates were isolated and their radioactivity determined. Remember iodide is trapped oxidized, proteinated, and stored as part of the thyroid hormone.

^{131}I CONTENT
(counts/min./100 mg Thyroid Tissue)

Groups	Drug	Iodine Ion	Monoiodo-tyrosine	Triiodo-thyronine	Thyroxine	Av. Thyroid Wt. mg/100 g body wt.
1	None	6,120	10,140	7,520	35,990	14
2	A	55	46	13	62	76
3	B	40,976	10	9	14	88
4	C	1,592	2,025	1,970	8,985	4

15. Which group was treated with thyroxine, an inhibitor of the production of thyroid stimulating hormone by the pituitary gland?
    (A) Group 2
    (B) Group 3
    (C) Group 4
    (D) None of the above

16. Which group was treated with thiocyanate, an inhibitor of the iodine pump of the thyroid cells?
    (A) Group 2
    (B) Group 3
    (C) Group 4
    (D) None of the above

17. Which group was treated with propylthiouracil, an inhibitor of iodine oxidation?
    (A) Group 2
    (B) Group 3
    (C) Group 4
    (D) None of the above

18. In which of the above groups is iodine NOT taken up and therefore almost no radioactivity can be measured by the assay?
    (A) Group 1
    (B) Group 2
    (C) Group 3
    (D) Group 4

Many scientists think of the pituitary gland as the master gland responsible for the secretion of many different hormones. A reciprocal relationship operates between the hormones secreted by the pituitary and the hormones produced by the target organs; this delicate control of balance of production of secretory product between the pituitary and the target organs is known as "negative feedback." Among the many hormones produced by the pituitary gland are ACTH, FSH, LH, TSH, and STH. The following experiments were set up to demonstrate the actions of some of the above factors. Twenty-five day-old immature male and female rats were subjected to the following treatment for 10 days: Group 1 was given a 0.5 cc saline injection; Group 2 was given a 0.5 cc FSH injection; and Group 3 was given a 0.5 cc crude pituitary extract injection. The results were recorded in table form.

MALE RATS

Groups	Body Weight grams	Testes mg	Seminal Vesicles mg	Prostate mg	Thyroid mg	Adrenals mg
1	86	3750	18	71	6.0	20
2	82	5310	57	176	6.1	21
3	83	4830	24	163	7.5	27

FEMALE RATS

Groups	Body Weight grams	Ovaries mg	Uterus mg	Thyroid mg	Adrenals mg
1	83	20	25	5.9	22
2	82	43	83	5.7	21
3	84	33	61	7.1	37

The following statements are related to the information presented. Based on the information given, select:

(A)   if the statement is *supported by* the information given.
(B)   if the statement is *contradicted by* the information given.
(C)   if the statement is *neither supported nor contradicted by* information given.

19.   From the table it seems as if the crude pituitary extract had a lesser effect on the sex organs than did FSH.

20.   Pituitary extract affected every organ under investigation.

21.   Hypophysectomy probably would have resulted in a decreased weight of the organs under investigation.

22.   The administration of FSH alone to an immature rat will produce follicular growth, but uterine and vaginal configurations will remain infantile since LH is also needed. The experimental data indicate uterine growth, casting doubt on the purity of the FSH preparation.

23.   Both FSH and LH are necessary for the production of estrogen.

24.   FSH in the male had the greatest effect on the weight of the prostate gland; the tissue is therefore most refractive to it.

25.   The adrenal weight probably would drop if the animals were deprived of ACTH.

26.   In these experiments none of the hormones in the pituitary extract probably were as effective as a purified fraction of them might have been.

27.   FSH has as its target organs the organs of reproduction.

28.   As demonstrated in these experiments ACTH and TSH are produced by the pituitary gland.

After growing turkey red wheat for two years on a dry land farm, John Calendar had accumulated enough capital to move his family to a more fertile area. The first crops he planted on the new 1000-acre farm did well. The bar graphs below indicate his production of wheat and corn over the last five years. Bushels are plotted on the abscissa, and the numbers of acres planted in both crops are shown in parentheses.

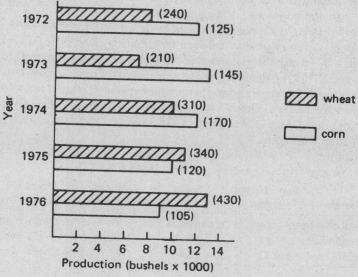

29. What was the average yearly proportion of wheat production to corn production?

(A) 3/2

(B) 7/8

(C) 10/9

(D) 5/7

30. If corn sold for $2.40/bushel in 1973, how many more bushels of wheat at $4.00/bushel would have to be sold to match the income from corn?

(A) 8,800 bushels

(B) 650 bushels

(C) 800 bushels

(D) 1,500 bushels

(E) none of the above

31. How many acres would have to be converted to wheat to obtain a matching output (in bushels) of both crops in 1972?

(A) 94.75 acres

(B) 127.94 acres

(C) 270.25 acres

(D) 30.25 acres

(E) none of the above

32. The average price for wheat and corn in 1976 was $2.90/bushel and $2.40/bushel, respectively. Assuming that the entire farm was planted in these two crops and that an acre of land could grow three times as much corn as wheat, how many acres would be planted in corn to obtain an equal income from both crops?

(A) 327 acres

(B) 287 acres

(C) 204 acres

(D) 275 acres

(E) none of the above

33. Suppose that too great a surplus of wheat was expected in 1977, and the federal government passed a bill to reimburse growers $25 for each acre not planted in that crop, as long as the previous year's income from wheat and corn (in this case, $59,300) was not exceeded. Out of 500 acres, how many could be left unplanted if the remainder were planted in corn which would sell at $2.50/bushel with an average yield of 90 bushels per acre?

(A) 266 acres

(B) 106 acres

(C) 55 acres

(D) 217 acres

(E) none of the above

Three greenhouses were constructed to examine different light cycles and their effects on the growth of several plants.

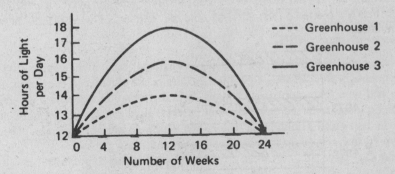

34. Plant X requires 15 hours of light per day for at least three weeks to exhibit a red coloration in its leaves. It may exhibit this highly desired feature in

(A) greenhouse 1.

(B) greenhouse 1 and 2.

(C) greenhouse 2 and 3.

(D) all of the above.

35. Plant Y will only bear fruit when the period of darkness is 8 hours or less. It will not bear fruit in

(A) greenhouse 1.

(B) greenhouse 1 and 2.

(C) greenhouse 2 and 3.

(D) greenhouse 3.

36. Plant Z will only form flowers and seeds when exposed to days of no more than 15 hours in length. It is therefore not native in areas that are simulated by

(A) greenhouse 1.

(B) greenhouse 1 and 2.

(C) greenhouse 2 and 3.

(D) greenhouse 1 and 3.

In order to obtain the results as listed in the table below, golden hamsters were fed 0.05% propylthiouracil (PTU) in their diets. At various times hamsters were sacrificed; the pituitaries were dissected out, fixed in Bouin's solution, dehydrated, embedded in paraffin, and sectioned at a thickness of 6 micra. Sections were stained with a modified Masson trichrome stain. A differential adenohypophyseal cell count was obtained.

PERCENTAGES OF ADENOHYPOPHYSEAL CELLS AFTER ADMINISTRATION OF 0.05% PROPYLTHIOURACIL IN THE DIET

Days of PTU	No. of Animals	Body Wt., grams	Pituitary Wt., mg./100 g B.W.	% Cell Types		
				Acidophils	Basophils	Chromophobes
0	10	129	2.40	29	19	51
3	10	117	3.20[1]	26	36[1]	37[1]
6	10	112	3.40	27	36	37
12	10	120	3.10	27	37	36
15	10	130	4.10	26	36	38

[1]Fisher's "T" significant to .001

37. The objective of the experiment was to

(A) show that propylthiouracil induces thyroidal deficiency which is overcome by the increased production of TSH.

(B) see if propylthiouracil would change the weight of the pituitary gland.

(C) see if propylthiouracil would change the proportion of the various cell types of the pituitary.

(D) prove that chromophobes give rise to basophils which secrete TSH.

38. It was found that

(A) pituitary weight is a good indicator of PTU action.

(B) the mitotic rate of the pituitary increased resulting in an increase of pituitary weight.

(C) there was a percentage increase of basophils with a concomitant decrease in chromophobes.

(D) basophils secrete TSH.

39. The investigator started with the hypothesis that the paucity of mitotic divisions in the adenohypophysis precludes a weight increase as a result of new cell formation. It is believed that one cell type (chromophobe) changes; its transformation to become an active basophil results in an increase in secretory material in it and this increase in metabolic and secretory activity in the gland could bring about this observed weight increase. The differential adenohypophyseal cell count supports such an hypothesis.

(A) True

(B) False

(C) Bad hypothesis

(D) Pure speculation

One hundred ml of blood was drawn from a healthy male donor. Following centrifugation (4°C) and removal of the "buffy coat" by aspiration, hemoglobin was extracted from the pelleted red blood cells. The extracted hemoglobin was then divided into equal aliquots and these were treated as follows:

Aliquot 1: Analyzed on the day of extraction by polyacrylamide gel electrophoresis, followed by densitometer scanning of the stained gel

Aliquot 2: Stored for 30 days at room temperature

Aliquot 3: Stored for 30 days at 4°C

Aliquot 4: Stored for 30 days as a 50% solution (V/V) in glycerol at −20°C

At the end of the 30-day storage period each of the aliquots was analyzed in the same way as aliquot 1. The following densitometer tracings were obtained:

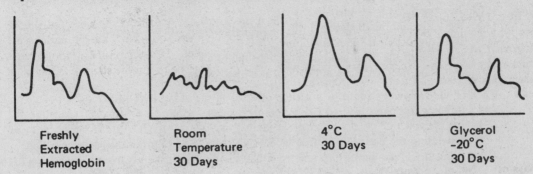

Freshly
Extracted
Hemoglobin

Room
Temperature
30 Days

4°C
30 Days

Glycerol
−20°C
30 Days

40. The purpose of this experiment was to test the effect of
   (A) polyacrylamide gel on hemoglobin concentration.
   (B) removing the buffy coat on red blood cell inability.
   (C) glycerol on hemoglobin concentration.
   (D) different storage conditions on hemoglobin polypeptide composition as revealed by gel electrophoresis.

41. From these data it is clear that
   (A) none of the storage conditions were able to maintain hemoglobin in an unchanged state.
   (B) hemoglobin peptides are strongly affected by heating.
   (C) hemoglobin contains peroxidase activity.
   (D) hemoglobin coupled with oxygen has a longer shelf-life than hemoglobin coupled with CO_2.

42. It may also be seen that
   (A) there are remarkable sex differences in hemoglobin polypeptide patterns.
   (B) centrifugation in the cold may alter oxygen affinity curves for hemoglobin.
   (C) of all the storage methods tried, storage at −20°C in glycerol allowed the least change from the fresh configuration.
   (D) hemoglobin is useful for species identification.

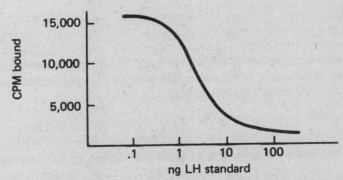

Blood samples from 10 female rats were withdrawn at 5 PM on the day of proestrus, when LH levels in the blood should be high if ovulation were to occur that night. The blood was assayed by double-antibody radioimmunoassay for LH. An antibody specific for LH is allowed to bind with the LH in the sample, then is partially displaced by radio-labeled LH whose binding to the limited amount of anti-LH is inversely proportional to the amount of unlabeled LH present (see standard curve). The antigen-antibody complex is precipitated with an antibody to the anti-LH, and the number of counts per minute bound in the precipitate is determined after the supernatant containing the unbound labeled LH has been poured off. The blood samples from 5 untreated rats (which ovulated) had cpm of 4000, 3000, 5000, 4000 and 3000, whereas those from 5 drug-treated animals had 5000, 13,000, 15,000, 3,000, 13,000.

43. It can be concluded from this study that
    (A) the untreated rats had very little LH in their blood compared to the treated group.
    (B) the drug does not block ovulation.
    (C) the dose of the drug used in this study inhibits LH release in most of the animals.
    (D) ovulation occurred in 3 out of 5 of the treated rats.

44. Each of the following could be a source of error in the assay EXCEPT
    (A) trapping unbound labeled LH in the precipitate.
    (B) the presence of other hormones in the blood.
    (C) separating the bound from free labeled LH before equilibrium had been reached.
    (D) using an LH standard which reacted with the antibody differently from the unknown LH.

45. Which of the following statements is true?
    (A) The antibody cannot be saturated with hormone.
    (B) The antigen-antibody reaction is not reversible.
    (C) Counting error and decay have no effect.
    (D) Only the middle portion of the standard curve is usable.

Selective protein transport from the maternal circulation to the rat fetus is thought to occur via the visceral yolk sac. The maternal proteins are transferred to the yolk sac cavity and then must pass through the visceral endoderm, the visceral basement membrane (VBM), and the vitelline capillary endothelium to reach the fetal blood. Proteins X, Y, and Z were injected into a pregnant rat on day 12 of gestation and then were localized in the layers of the visceral yolk sac at 2 minutes, 6 hours, and 12 hours following injection. The results below demonstrate where each protein was localized at the three postinjection intervals.

Protein	Visceral Endoderm	VBM	Vitelline Endothelium	Fetal Blood
X	2 min.	6 hrs.	12 hrs.	—
Y	2 min., 6 hrs., & 12 hrs.	—	—	—
Z	2 min.	6 hrs.	12 hrs.	12 hrs.

The following statements are related to the information presented above. Based on the information given, select:
    (A) if the statement is *supported by* the information given.
    (B) if the statement is *contradicted by* the information given.
    (C) if the statement is *neither supported nor contradicted by* information given.

46. All three proteins were absorbed at the same rate by the visceral endoderm.

47. The transport of protein X is blocked by the visceral basement membrane.

48. The visceral endoderm appears to block the transport of protein Y.

49. Protein X appears to be transported through the visceral endoderm.

50. Only proteins with a low molecular weight, such as protein Z, pass into the fetal blood.

51. Proteins X and Z are transported at the same rate through the visceral endoderm.

52. The vitelline endothelium appears to block the transport of protein X into the fetal blood.

53. Protein Y is not transported into the fetal circulation because of its large molecular weight.

54. All proteins are transported into the fetal circulation by the visceral yolk sac placenta.

55. Proteins X and Z are absorbed and transported to the vitelline endothelium by the same transport mechanism.

56. Proteins X and Z are transported at the same rate into the vitelline endothelium.

57. Protein transport in the rat occurs only on day 12 of gestation.

The following graph represents an experiment designed to measure the rate of collagen synthesis in developing chondrocytes. Chondrocytes were isolated from developing sterna of chick embryos and incubated in culture media containing proline ^{3}H, a precursor of collagen. Specimens were fixed after various time intervals and prepared for autoradiography. The graph represents number of silver grains counted (μm/square of organelle).

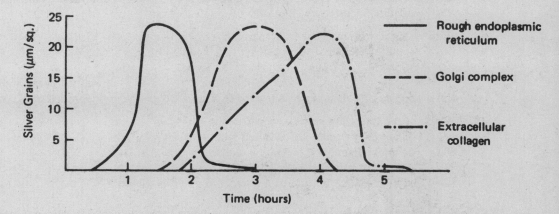

The following statements are related to the information presented. Based on this information, select:
- **(A)** if the statement is *supported by* the information given.
- **(B)** if the statement is *contradicted by* the information given.
- **(C)** if the statement is *neither supported nor contradicted by* information given.

58. The radioactive label found in the rough endoplasmic reticulum is transferred directly into the extracellular collagen without passing through the Golgi complex.

59. Radioactive isotope is incorporated into the extracellular collagen within 2 hours.

60. Collagen is a highly stable molecule and is not degraded.

61. The amount of rough endoplasmic reticulum in the cell increases during collagen synthesis.

EFFECT OF VARIOUS TREATMENTS ON ORGAN WEIGHTS

Treatments	No. of Animals	Body Weight Grams	Organ Weight (mg/100 g Body Weight)		
			Organ 1	Organ 2	Organ 3
Control	8	70	1509 ± 34	223 ± 20	22 ± 0.8
Drug A	8	66	1044 ± 30	87 ± 14	23 ± 1.0
Drug B	8	73	1432 ± 51	224 ± 24	26 ± 0.9
Drug A + B	8	71	1586 ± 68	208 ± 28	25 ± 1.2
Drug C	8	73	1383 ± 80	146 ± 19	31 ± 1.3
Drug B + C	8	65	954 ± 50	61 ± 3	26 ± 2.0

The following statements are related to the table above. Based on the information given, select:
- **(A)** if the statement is *supported by* the information in the table.
- **(B)** if the statement is *contradicted by* the information in the table.
- **(C)** if the statement is *neither supported nor contradicted by* information in the table.

62. Casual evaluation of the results leads one to believe that treatment resulted in significant effects.

63. Drugs B and C seem to have acted in an additive manner.

64. The experimenters should have paid closer attention to body weights.

65. Drug C affected all parameters under investigation.

66. Significant microscopic changes were detected in the organs under investigation.

67. Drugs A and B countered (offset) each other.

68. Organ 3 was least affected by the various treatments.

Model Test C Answers*

SCIENCE KNOWLEDGE

Biology

1.	D	9.	B	17.	A	25.	A	32.	C
2.	A	10.	C	18.	E	26.	E	33.	C
3.	C	11.	E	19.	C	27.	A	34.	C
4.	B	12.	E	20.	C	28.	A	35.	D
5.	B	13.	E	21.	C	29.	E	36.	D
6.	D	14.	B	22.	B	30.	E	37.	D
7.	B	15.	B	23.	C	31.	A	38.	D
8.	A	16.	A	24.	B				

Chemistry

1.	C	9.	C	17.	C	25.	A	32.	D
2.	A	10.	B	18.	D	26.	B	33.	D
3.	D	11.	E	19.	D	27.	C	34.	D
4.	A	12.	C	20.	A	28.	A	35.	A
5.	B	13.	D	21.	D	29.	C	36.	C
6.	D	14.	B	22.	C	30.	B	37.	B
7.	B	15.	C	23.	D	31.	D	38.	A
8.	A	16.	C	24.	A				

Physics

1.	D	8.	B	15.	A	22.	A	28.	C
2.	B	9.	E	16.	E	23.	E	29.	D
3.	E	10.	D	17.	C	24.	D	30.	B
4.	D	11.	B	18.	D	25.	E	31.	E
5.	C	12.	E	19.	D	26.	E	32.	A
6.	A	13.	A	20.	B	27.	A	33.	C
7.	B	14.	B	21.	C				

SCIENCE PROBLEMS

1.	E	13.	B	25.	A	37.	B	49.	D
2.	D	14.	B	26.	D	38.	C	50.	B
3.	A	15.	C	27.	C	39.	B	51.	C
4.	E	16.	D	28.	E	40.	D	52.	A
5.	A	17.	E	29.	E	41.	B	53.	C
6.	B	18.	B	30.	E	42.	E	54.	C
7.	C	19.	C	31.	A	43.	C	55.	E
8.	D	20.	E	32.	B	44.	A	56.	B
9.	C	21.	B	33.	D	45.	D	57.	D
10.	C	22.	E	34.	B	46.	D	58.	C
11.	D	23.	C	35.	E	47.	B	59.	B
12.	A	24.	D	36.	C	48.	A	60.	C

SKILLS ANALYSIS: READING

1.	B	15.	A	29.	A	43.	B	56.	A
2.	C	16.	C	30.	B	44.	A	57.	B
3.	A	17.	A	31.	C	45.	B	58.	C
4.	B	18.	C	32.	A	46.	A	59.	B
5.	C	19.	B	33.	C	47.	C	60.	A
6.	C	20.	B	34.	C	48.	A	61.	E
7.	C	21.	A	35.	C	49.	C	62.	C
8.	A	22.	C	36.	B	50.	B	63.	B
9.	A	23.	A	37.	B	51.	D	64.	A
10.	C	24.	B	38.	B	52.	C	65.	B
11.	C	25.	B	39.	A	53.	D	66.	C
12.	B	26.	C	40.	C	54.	C	67.	A
13.	B	27.	B	41.	B	55.	A	68.	B
14.	A	28.	B	42.	B				

SKILLS ANALYSIS: QUANTITATIVE

1.	B	15.	C	29.	B	43.	C	56.	A
2.	A	16.	A	30.	C	44.	B	57.	C
3.	D	17.	B	31.	D	45.	D	58.	B
4.	B	18.	B	32.	B	46.	A	59.	A
5.	C	19.	A	33.	A	47.	B	60.	B
6.	A	20.	A	34.	C	48.	A	61.	C
7.	C	21.	A	35.	A	49.	A	62.	A
8.	C	22.	A	36.	C	50.	C	63.	A
9.	D	23.	C	37.	C	51.	A	64.	B
10.	A	24.	B	38.	C	52.	A	65.	A
11.	A	25.	C	39.	A	53.	C	66.	C
12.	B	26.	C	40.	D	54.	B	67.	A
13.	C	27.	A	41.	A	55.	C	68.	A
14.	A	28.	B	42.	C				

Explanation of Answers for Science Questions–Model Test C

SCIENCE KNOWLEDGE

Biology

1. **(D)** Mitochondria are the biochemical power-plants of the cell. They recover energy from foodstuff (via Krebs cycle and respiratory chain) and convert it (via phosphorylation) into ATP (adenosine triphosphate). In this manner they produce the energy necessary for the metabolic processes.

2. **(A)** Neutrotransmitters, initially detected by the dendrite of a neuron, are chemicals that carry an impulse from one neuron to another neuron. The dendrites are the short fibers of a neuron which are stimulated by neurotransmitters.

3. **(C)** The copepods function as primary consumers. Primary consumers are herbivores, which feed directly off green plants.

4. **(B)** A complete set of chromosomes ($2n$) is passed on to each daughter cell as a result of mitotic cell division. Cells which are produced mitotically are genetically alike.

5. **(B)** It is believed by some that parathyroid hormone acts upon bone, eliciting changes in calcium and phosphorus. Osteoclasts are the cells stimulated by parathyroid hormone to facilitate the resorption of calcium and phosphorus from bone. Administration of parathyroid hormone to animals without parathyroids results in an increase of phosphorus excretion in the urine, a fall in serum inorganic phosphorus levels, an increase in serum calcium, and an increase of calcium excretion in the urine.

6. **(D)** The function of the adrenal cortex is to secrete (a) sex hormones—androgens, estrogens, and progesterone; (b) corticosteroids—glucocorticoids and mineralocorticoids. These are all steroid hormones. The functional aspects of mineral and carbohydrate control by the adrenal are far more important than the influence it has on the reproductive organs (reproduction).

7. **(B)** Oxygen molecules in humans diffuse immediately into the blood capillaries. The alveoli are thin-walled, moist sacs in the lungs. The blood capillaries surround the alveoli.

8. **(A)** In anaerobic respiration, glucose is converted to two molecules of the 3-carbon compound pyruvic acid. In aerobic respiration glucose is converted to carbon dioxide and water.

9. **(B)** The frequency of traits of adaptive value is maintained by environmental conditions. If these conditions change, the traits no longer have an adaptive value. The organisms with the traits will not survive to reproductive age.

10. **(C)** Lymphocytes, which participate in such immunologic activities as delayed hypersensitivity reactions and graft rejection, are able to do so because of the influence of the thymus. Stem cells for this population are thought to pass through the thymus and, having come under its influence, to seed more peripheral lymphoid organs with their progeny. Removal of the thymus from newborn animals seriously impairs their immunologic system because of the lack of thymic influence.

11. **(E)** Thiamine (Vitamin B_1) is a water-soluble vitamin essential for the proper functioning of the nervous system; it is an acetylcholine antagonist. Deficiency results in beriberi in humans.

12. **(E)** Hemoglobin shows normal affinity for oxygen, even when no ATP is present. A decrease in pH, an increase in temperature, or an increase in DPG will facilitate the release of oxygen in the tissue capillaries. An increase in CO_2 and a decrease in the affinity of hemoglobin for oxygen, with a decrease in pH and an increase in carbamino Hb, is called the Bohr effect.

13. **(E)** Secretin, a polypeptide hormone produced by the small intestines, stimulates pepsinogen secretion. Secretin is released when the pH falls below 4.5.

14. **(B)** Adrenocorticotrophic hormone (ACTH) releases steroids from the adrenal gland in response to stress.

15. **(B)** Budding as in hydra involves the multiplication of cells in one region of the organism and the organization of these cells into a new individual. Binary fission or mitosis is a division of a cell into two equal parts and in this respect two new organisms (cells). Parthenogenesis involves a mechanism in which a single cell is set apart for the purpose of reproduction. This cell has the capability to develop into a new organism.

16. **(A)** The term "limey," as applied to British individuals, refers to the early dietary approach (i.e., providing limes and/or lime juice) of the prevention of scurvy in the British navy while they were on extended absence from access to fresh vegetables and fruits.

17. **(A)** From the right ventricle blood is sent to the lungs via the pulmonary arteries; this blood is rich in carbaminohemoglobin and the CO_2 will be exchanged for O_2. Blood returns from the lungs to the left auricle via the pulmonary veins; this blood has been oxygenated and is rich in oxyhemoglobin. Blood then passes to the left ventricle and then out via the aorta to supply the tissues of the body.

18. **(E)** The uterus is prepared every month via the phases of the menstrual cycle for reception of the fertilized egg. If fertilization does not occur, the endometrium sloughs off (menstruation), is then repaired, and awaits the fertilized egg again. FSH and LH are the gonadotrophins and estrogen and progesterone the hormones responsible for the cyclic changes.

19. **(C)** The heart has its own rhythmicity. The rate of contraction and force of contraction, however, are modified by the sympathetic and parasympathetic influences. The SA node is considered the pacemaker and initiates heart beat; the AV node will take over at a slower rate and its own cardiac rhythmicity will keep the heart beating at a slower rate for some time in this experiment.

20. **(C)** Messenger RNA receives instructions from components which are located in the nucleus.

21. **(C)** Excretion concerns itself with the elimination of water (fluid) while egestion is the process of eliminating undigested food materials. Catabolism is the chemical breakdown of molecules.

22. **(B)** Immuno-assays are the most sensitive of methods available for the detection of many substances.

23. **(C)** Several gonadotropins occur during pregnancy; they are not of pituitary origin. Chorionic gonadotropin (CG) is of placental origin, appears in the urine during pregnancy, resembles LH in some of its actions, and is the basis of most pregnancy tests.

24. **(B)** This is basically a definition. The blooming of plants is influenced by the length of exposure to darkness and is a prime example of photoperiodism.

25. **(A)** Dendrites function in receiving information and conducting it toward the cell body. Axons carry that information away from the cell body and will synapse on dendrites of another neuron.

26. **(E)** A male carries a XY and a female a XX complement of chromosomes. If a male embryo were to result, in our example the sperm that fertilized the egg would have to possess a Y chromosome.

27. **(A)** Umbilical arteries carry deoxygenated blood from the fetus to the placenta for exchange and umbilical veins bring oxygenated blood back to the fetus. Foramen ovale is located between the right and left atria, and in this manner most pulmonary circulation is bypassed. The ductus arteriosus is a communication between the left pulmonary artery and the arch of the aorta through which blood is shunted into the aorta. The ductus venosus is a bypass of the liver in the fetus. All close after birth.

28. **(A)** The cuticle of *Ascaris* protects it from the enzymes that are produced in the intestinal tract of the host.

29. **(E)** Virchow, who was a German physician, is known for his statement that all cells originate from preexisting cells.

30. **(E)** The sympathetic component of the autonomic nervous system mobilizes the body's reserves in case of emergencies.

31. **(A)** Homologous structures exhibit a structural similarity which is attributable to a common genetic and embryologic origin.

32. **(C)** Basic genetic knowledge is applied.

> rough — R (dominant)
> smooth — r (recessive)
> brown — B (dominant)
> gray — b (recessive)

The male is crossed to several smooth gray females; they had to be homozygous recessive genotype. Since all four combinations appeared, we can assume that the male was genotypically heterozygous even though he appeared phenotypically dominant. If first we crossed this heterozygous male RrBb × rrbb, the result would be RrBb; rrBb; rrbb; Rrbb; in other words the four combinations given. Now let us cross the RrBb male × RrBb female; the following combinations would have to be considered in both male and female: RB; Rb; rB; rb. If these are crossed, we find 3 out of 16 possess rough gray coats (namely RRbb; Rrbb and Rrbb).

33. **(C)** Epidermis or, broadly speaking, skin functions in protection against trauma, etc.; it is also important in the regulation of body temperature which it accomplishes by insulation and sweating. Skin possess receptors that make the organism aware of his or her immediate surroundings and it is a depot for glycogen, cholesterol, and water.

34. **(C)** Skeletal (striated) muscle is under voluntary control. The autonomic nervous system innervates cardiac muscle, smooth muscle, and glands. Arrector pili musculature is associated with skin and is smooth musculature.

35. **(D)** Apical meristems are responsible for the extension in length, while cambium meristems are responsible for the increase in thickness. The capacity for division is lost by the main mass of the plant body.

36. **(D)** Mesoderm gives rise to connective tissue, bone, and cartilage; both striated and smooth muscle; blood and lymph cells and the walls of the vascular channels; kidneys; gonads and spleen.

37. **(D)** Ectoderm gives rise to the epidermis, the hypophysis, the central and peripheral nervous system, the epithelium of the sense organs, and the epithelial lining of some other organs.

38. **(D)** Endoderm gives rise to tonsils, thyroid, parathyroids, thymus, liver, and pancreas; epithelial lining of gut, respiratory tract, and urinary bladder.

Chemistry

1. **(C)** Substrate(s) or reactant(s) react(s) with the enzyme to form an enzyme-substrate complex. This complex breaks down into product(s) and frees enzymes ready for formation of a new enzyme-substrate complex.

2. **(A)** Nonpolar covalent bonds are formed between atoms of the same element or atoms with the same electronegativity. The F_2 molecule has one nonpolar covalent bond only and is therefore a nonpolar molecule.

3. **(D)** An acid reacts with a base to form a salt and water. KOH is a base.

4. **(A)** This is a definition of an ionic bond.

5. **(B)** Although different sublevels have different maximum numbers of orbitals, any one orbital can hold a maximum of two electrons.

6. **(D)** The smaller the K_{sp}, the less soluble the salt. Of the four choices, AgI has the smallest K_{sp} (the largest negative exponent).

7. **(B)** A substance can act as both an oxidizing agent and a reducing agent only if the oxidation state of the element can become higher and lower than it is. There are no lower oxidation states for Fe^0 and Cu^0; there are no higher oxidation states for Fe^{3+} and Cu^{2+}.

8. **(A)** The development of our solar system is thought to have proceeded from the condensation of gases composed primarily of hydrogen, the simplest element.

9. **(C)** Most enzymes are named to indicate the reaction they catalyze and have the suffix -ase (e.g., lipase, carboxypeptidase, and amylase).

10. **(B)** We have described conditions for the formation of a diazonium salt and then replacement of the diazonium salt by Br to produce monobromobenzene. (The replacement is known as the Sandmeyer reaction). The intermediate diazonium salt is often unstable at room temperature, so a lower temperature is used.

11. **(E)** See explanation for question 10.

12. **(C)** See explanation for question 10.

13. **(D)** Enzymes and other proteins are primarily composed of L-amino acids, and they may be hydrolyzed to produce free amino acids. Enzymes are proteins and may be considered as such chemically and physically.

14. **(B)** Sharing of a pair of electrons between two atoms results in a covalent bond. This type of bond may occur in organic, inorganic, or organometallic compounds.

15. **(C)** Production of glucose and fructose from sucrose and production of fatty acids and glycerol from triglycerides are both simple hydrolytic reactions in which essentially no energy is gained or lost. Production of steroids from acetate (as is true with most synthetic reactions) requires energy input. Production of CO_2 and water from fatty acids yields large amounts of energy.

16. **(C)** In pure H_2O at 25°C, $[H^+] = [OH^-] = \sqrt{1 \times 10^{-14}} = 1 \times 10^{-7}$ mole/liter. A neutral solution is one in which $[H^+] = [OH^-] = 1 \times 10^{-7}$ mole/liter. In an acid solution $[H^+]$ is greater than 10^{-7} mole/liter, and $[OH^-]$ is less than 10^{-7} mole/liter. In a basic solution $[H^+]$ is less than 10^{-7} mole/liter and $[OH^-]$ is greater than 10^{-7} mole/liter.

17. **(C)** A molecule having NH_2 and COOH groups is an amino acid. Naturally occurring amino acids ordinarily have the NH_2 group on the alpha carbon and are of the L-configuration. Proteins are high molecular weight polymers of amino acids. In proteins one amino acid is attached to the adjacent one

by dehydration to form the peptide bond. In proteins there are very few free amino or carboxyl groups because most are in the peptide bonds.

18. **(D)** $CO_2 + H_2O \rightarrow H_2CO_3$ (i.e., carbonic acid). This reaction occurs nonenzymatically, but it occurs *faster* in the presence of the enzyme, carbonic anhydrase.

19. **(D)** Carbon, oxygen, and hydrogen are the most common elements in protoplasm. These three elements are found in most of the molecules. Only these three plus nitrogen, calcium, and (possibly) phosphorus are in a concentration exceeding 1%.

20. **(A)** The nucleus contains DNA which directs the production of messenger RNA in the nucleus. Messenger RNA leaves the nucleus to influence transfer RNA and eventual production of proteins.

21. **(D)** A colloid is composed of submicroscopic particles which in solution or suspension do not settle out. If such a solution is subjected to spinning in a centrifuge which creates gravitational forces much greater than normally experienced, one can, of course, precipitate colloidal particles.

22. **(C)** Remember that the aldol condensation cannot occur in a compound without alpha-hydrogen. Instead the Cannizarro reaction occurs, resulting in oxidation of one aldehyde molecule and reduction in another. In this case oxidation produces benzoic acid, and reduction produces benzyl alcohol.

23. **(D)** The Lambert-Beer law relates absorption of light (at a particular wavelength) to solution concentration and light path: $\log\left(\frac{I_1}{I_t}\right) - a\,b\,c$ where I_1 = intensity of incident light, I_t = intensity of transmitted light, a = extinction coefficient (a proportionality constant that depends on wavelength and the units of the other variables), b = light path, and c = concentration of the solution.

24. **(A)** Phenol, like many organic compounds, is most soluble in aqueous medium in the ionized form. Phenol will not react with $NaHCO_3$, but it will react with a stronger base (such as $NaOH$) to form the more highly ionized salt, sodium phenolate.

25. **(A)** In general the metabolism of fats (triglycerides) produces about 9 calories per gram as compared with about 4 calories per gram for carbohydrates (e.g., fructose or glucose) or protein.

26. **(B)** A conjugated diene is a compound in which there are double bonds adjacent to a single bond on both sides (e.g., 1,3-butadiene) while a cumulative diene is one in which the double bonds are adjacent to each other (e.g., 1,2-butadiene). An isolated diene is a diene that is neither conjugated nor cumulative (e.g., 1,4-pentadiene).

27. **(C)** Optical isomers that are not mirror images are called diastereomers. In the resolution of racemic lactic acid, we may wish to use L-strychnine to make a salt. The L-strychnine salt of L-lactic acid is a diastereomer of the L-strychnine salt of D-lactic acid. Diastereomers differ somewhat in such physical properties as solubility and may be separated. It is then necessary only that we break down the salt and recover the resolved lactic acid isomers from the L-strychnine.

28. **(A)** DNA is made up of adenine, guanine, thymine, and cytosine; in RNA cytosine is replaced by uracil. These are the nitrogenous bases of the compounds.

29. **(C)** The base-catalyzed reaction of urea with 2,2-diethylmalonic acid (or more likely its diethyl ester) results in a condensation to produce barbital (diethylbarbituric acid).

30. **(B)** See explanation for question 1.

31. **(D)** DNA possesses a deoxyribose while RNA possesses a ribose sugar. For a discussion of their nitrogenous bases see answer to question 28.

32. **(D)** Charge, solubility, and molecular size determine the rate at which molecules enter and leave a cell.

33. **(D)** The compound shown is an unsaturated aldehyde.

34. **(D)** The elements listed are referred to as noble gases. They tend to be unreactive and they are ordinarily found in uncombined monoatomic form.

35. **(A)** Hydrolysis of sucrose produces one molecule each of glucose and fructose for each molecule of sucrose.

36. **(C)** Remember that cycloalkanes and unbranched alkenes have the formula $C_n H_{2_n}$. Thus cyclopropane would be $C_3 H_6$.

37. **(B)** Dacron is a polymer of dicarboxylic acid and a diol; thus it is a polyester. Nylon is a polyamide.

38. **(A)** Most home units for softening water utilize a zeolite with exchangeable sodium ions. The sodium ions exchange for ions such as calcium that are in the untreated water.

Physics

1. **(D)** Average speed is the total distance divided by the total time. First find the times for the two legs:

$$t_1 = \frac{s_1}{v_1} = \frac{15\ \text{km}}{30\ \text{km/h}} = 0.5\ \text{h}$$

$$t_2 = \frac{s_2}{v_2} = \frac{30\ \text{km}}{60\ \text{km/h}} = 0.5\ \text{h}$$

$$v_{\text{average}} = \frac{s_{\text{total}}}{t_{\text{total}}} = \frac{15\ \text{km} + 30\ \text{km}}{0.5\ \text{h} + 0.5\ \text{h}} = 45\ \text{km/h}$$

2. **(B)** This is a statement of uniform acceleration implying that the body will increase its velocity at $9.8\ \text{m/s}^2$ in free-fall.

3. **(E)** The ideal gas law states that $\dfrac{PV}{T} = \dfrac{P_0 V_0}{T_0}$ with temperature and pressure in absolute units. Given: $P_0 = 1$, $V_0 = 2m^3$, $T_0 = 293\ \text{K}$, $P = 4$, $V = 3m^3$, and $T = ?$

$$T = \left(\frac{PV}{P_0 V_0}\right) T_0 = \frac{(4)(3)}{(1)(2)}\ 293$$

$$T = 1758\ \text{K}$$

4. **(D)** During an exothermal reaction, chemical energy is converted to heat energy and therefore the components are heated up.

5. **(C)** Isotopes have different mass numbers, that is, different numbers of nucleons in the nucleus.

6. **(A)** Density (ρ) equals mass (m) per unit volume (V), therefore: $\rho = \dfrac{m}{V}$ where $\rho = 7.8\ \text{g/cm}^3$,

$m = ?$, and $V = 2 \times 3 \times 5 = 30\ \text{m}^3$.

$m = \rho V = (7.8\ \text{g/cm}^3)(30\ \text{m}^3)$

    convert m^3 to cm^3

$m = (7.8)(30)(10^6)\ \text{g}$

$m = 234 \times 10^6\ \text{g}$

7. **(B)** $KE = \dfrac{mv^2}{2}$ where $m = 100$, $g = 0.1\ \text{kg}$ and $v = 60\ \text{m/s}$.
$KE = (0.1)(3600)/2\ \text{kg} \cdot \text{m}^2/\text{s}^2$
$KE = 180\ \text{kg} \cdot \text{m}^2/\text{s}^2 = 180\ \text{joules}$

8. **(B)** One newton is, by definition, the amount of force that will give 1 kg of mass an acceleration of $1\ \text{m/s}^2$.

9. **(E)** The force changing the course of a body from a straight line to a circular motion is known as centripetal force.

10. **(D)** Work = force × distance when force = 5 kg × 9.8 N and distance = 10 m.
Work = $(5)(9.8)(10)$ in joules
Work = 490 joules

11. **(B)** $x_1 = 3\ \text{m}$
$y_1 = 2\ \text{m}$
$x_2 = 15\ \text{m}$
$y_2 = ?$

$\dfrac{x_1}{y_1} = \dfrac{x_2}{y_2}$

$\dfrac{3}{2} = \dfrac{15}{y_2}$

$y_2 = \dfrac{30}{3} = 10\ \text{m}$

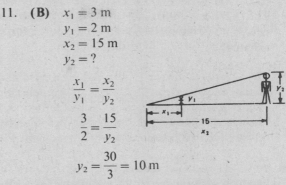

12. **(E)** Refraction can be defined as a change in direction of waves due to a change in their velocity.

13. **(A)** Since $V = IR$, tripling the resistance at constant V reduces the current to 1/3. Then $P = IV$; at constant V, 1/3 I produces 1/3 P.

14. **(B)** When a neutral rubber rod is rubbed with a neutral fur, negative charges are transferred from the fur to the rod, leaving the fur with a positive charge. If the fur loses a charge of -2×10^{-6} coulomb, it is left with a positive charge of $+2 \times 10^{-6}\ \text{C}$.

15. **(A)** Standing waves are produced when two waves having the same frequency and amplitude go through the same medium in opposite directions. Interference takes place, and at certain points, the nodes, no vibration occurs.

16. **(E)** Two sources are defined as coherent sources if their phase relation is constant. They may be in or out of phase, but if there is a difference in phase, the phase difference is kept constant.

17. **(C)** An object falling freely and starting from rest travels a distance equal to one-half the product of the acceleration and the square of the time traveled:

$$s = \tfrac{1}{2}at^2$$

$$54\ \text{m} = \tfrac{1}{2}a(3.0\ \text{s})^2$$

$$a = 12\ \text{m/s}^2$$

18. **(D)** The kinetic energy of an object is proportional to the square of its speed: $E_k = \tfrac{1}{2}mv^2$. When its speed is multiplied by a factor of 2, its kinetic energy is multiplied by a factor 2^2, or 4.

19. **(D)** A body is said to be in unstable equilibrium when it does not return to its original equilibrium position when slightly displaced but moves to another position after displacement.

20. **(B)** A body entirely or partially submerged in a fluid is forced upward in a fluid by a force equal to the weight of the fluid displacement.

21. **(C)** $E = h^2$; when h is doubled
$E = (2h)^2$
$E = 4h^2$, therefore E is quadrupled.

22. **(A)** The magnitude of the vector is found by the law of Pythagoras:

$r = \sqrt{3^2 + 4^2} = 5 \text{ cm}$

The angle with the horizontal is arctan $3/4 = 37°$.

23. **(E)** Use $v = v_0 + at$, where $v = 2690 \text{ cm/s}$, $v_0 = 1340 \text{ cm/s}$, $t = 15 \text{ s}$, and $at = v - v_0$.

$a = \dfrac{v - v_0}{t}$

$a = \dfrac{2690 - 1340}{15} = \dfrac{1350}{15}$

$a = 90 \text{ cm/s}^2$

24. **(D)** $\tan \theta = \dfrac{v^2}{ra}$, where $v = 2500 \text{ cm/s}$, $a = 980 \text{ cm/s}^2$, $r = ?$, and $\tan \theta = 1$.

$r = \dfrac{v^2}{(\tan \theta)a} = \dfrac{v^2}{a}$

$r = \dfrac{(2500 \text{ cm/s})^2}{980 \text{ cm/s}^2}$

$r = 6378 \text{ cm}$

$r = 63.78 \text{ m} = 64 \text{ m}$

25. **(E)** The internal energy of a substance includes the kinetic and internal potential energy of its molecules. The kinetic energy of the molecules depends on the mass of the molecules and their speed ($E_k = \frac{1}{2}mv^2$). The speed of the molecules increases with the temperature of the substance. Additional energy has to be supplied to a substance to change its phase from solid to liquid at constant temperature, as from ice to water. This changes the potential energy of the molecules with respect to each other.

26. **(E)** The process is called sublimation.

27. **(A)** The velocity of sound through an ideal gas is proportional to the square root of the absolute temperature. Therefore, $v/v_0 = (T/T_0)^{1/2}$, where $v_0 = 332 \text{ m/s}$, $T_0 = 273 \text{ K}$, and $T = 293 \text{ K}$.
$v = v_0(T/T_0)^{1/2}$
$v = (332)(293/273)^{1/2}$
$v = 344 \text{ m/s}$

28. **(C)** The velocity (C) of a wave is directly proportional to its wavelength (L) and inversely proportional to its period (T). $C = L/T = fL$ and $C = 1435 \text{ m/s}$ and $f = 410 \text{ cycles/sec}$.
$L = C/f$
$L = 1435/410 = 3.5 \text{ m}$

29. **(D)** Reflection of an object from a plane mirror has an image that is the same size as the object.

30. **(B)** The answer to question 30 is self-explanatory.

31. **(E)** The net force is $400 \text{ N} - 300 \text{ N} = 100 \text{ N}$. Then

$$a = \frac{F}{m} = \frac{100 \text{ N}}{50 \text{ kg}} = 2 \text{ m/s}^2$$

32. **(A)** The impulse is equal to the change in the momentum of the ball. The velocity change is $20 \text{ m/s} - (-20 \text{ m/s}) = 35 \text{ m/s}$, so the change in momentum is $(35 \text{ m/s})(0.10 \text{ kg}) = 3.5 \text{ kg m/s}$.

33. **(C)** The gamma ray has no charge, and its only mass is contained in its energy. The loss of energy by the nucleus diminishes its mass slightly.

SCIENCE PROBLEMS

1. **(E)** Knowing that $\alpha = 10 \text{ radians/sec.}^2$, $w_0 = 0$, $t = 4 \text{ seconds}$, and $w = ?$ Use $w = w_0 + \alpha t$

$w = 0 + (10)(4)$
$w = 40 \text{ radians/sec.}$

2. **(D)** Calculate for the values above by using

$\theta = w_0 t + \dfrac{1}{2}\alpha t^2$

$\theta = 0 + \dfrac{1}{2}(10)(16)(\text{rad/sec.}^2)(\text{sec.}^2)$

$\theta = 80 \text{ radians}$
To convert radians to revolutions, multiply

$80 \text{ radians} \times \dfrac{1 \text{ revolution}}{2 \text{ radians}} = \dfrac{80}{2} \text{ revolutions} =$

12.7 revolutions

3. **(A)** The magnitude of the angular acceleration changes to 5 radians/sec./sec. Use $w = w_0 + \alpha t$, where $w_0 = 40$ radians/sec., $\alpha = ?$, $t = 4$ seconds, $w = 60$ radians/sec., and sec = sec + rad/sec. α.

$60 = 40 + 4\alpha$

$\alpha = 5$ radians/sec.^{2}

(In other words, it slows down.)

4. **(E)** Most insoluble at pH 5.2. The protein is least soluble at the isoelectric point.

5. **(A)** The protein at its isoelectric point has a net zero charge which is why it is least soluble.

6. **(B)** Positive since there will be more $\overset{\displaystyle O}{\overset{\|}{C}} - O^-$ protonated; thus the charge on the protein will be due to $-NH_3^{\oplus}$.

7. **(C)** $4H + O_2 \rightarrow 2H_2O$

$\dfrac{X}{4} = \dfrac{0.145}{36}$ $X = 0.0161$ g H/0.100 g compound

$\dfrac{0.0161}{1} = 0.0161$ g H/0.100 g compound

$C + O_2 \rightarrow CO_2$

$\dfrac{X}{12} = \dfrac{0.142}{44}$ $X = 0.0387$ g C/0.100 g compound

$\dfrac{0.0387}{12} = 0.0032$ g C/0.100 g compound

0.100 g $\times 0.452 = 0.0452$ g N/0.100 g compound

$\dfrac{0.0452}{14} = 0.0032$ g N/0.100 g compound

$\dfrac{0.0161}{0.0032} = 5$ atoms H/atom C

$\dfrac{0.0032}{0.0032} = 1$ atom N/atom C

Empirical formula is CH_5N.

8. **(D)** The compound could only be an amine.

9. **(C)** CH_5N could be written as $C_2H_{10}N_2$.

10-15. **(10-C) (11-D) (12-A) (13-B) (14-B) (15-C)**
The experiments demonstrated basic biological principles. The absorption of water by colloidal substances, such as starch and cellulose, and their subsequent swelling can be defined as inbibition. When the test tubes were placed in the beakers and, as you observed, only solvent or water molecules passed the semipermeable membrane, we speak in terms of osmosis; but when both the solvent and solute pass from a place of higher concentration to one of lower concentration, the principle of diffusion is illustrated. Both processes are related. The test tubes were placed into a hypotonic solution. The following definitions must be considered: (1) isotonic—solutions exhibiting the same osmotic pressure; (2) hypotonic—a solution that possesses a lesser osmotic pressure; and (3) hypertonic—a solution that possesses a greater osmotic pressure.

16. **(D)** The number of molecules in a mole is 6.02×10^{23} (Avogadro's number).

17. **(E)** Pressure has no effect on the number of molecules in a mole.

18. **(B)** One mole contains 6.02×10^{23} molecules. The number given in the question, 3.01×10^{23}, represents 0.5 mole. One mole of gas at STP occupies a volume of 22.4 liters; 0.5 mole occupies a volume of 22.4×0.5 or 11.2 l.

19. **(C)** $Na + Bu—OH \rightarrow Bu—ONa + 0.5\ H_2$
(Remember to balance equations.)

20. **(E)** See answer to previous question. Only one mole of butyl alcohol is required to consume all the sodium.

21. **(B)** Since 1 mole equals 22.4 liters, 0.5 mole equals 11.2 liters.

22. **(E)** 1 liter V_0 and 5 liters V_n are combined to make the total V_m equal to 6 liters. To calculate the pressure of oxygen in the new mixture, use Boyle's law: $P_1V_1 = P_2V_2$ where $P_1 = 4$ atm, $V_1 = 1$ liter, $P_2 = ?$, and $V_2 = 6$ liters.
$(4)(1) = (P)(6)$
$P_2 = 0.67$ atm after mixing

23. **(C)** The total pressure of the new mixture $= P_0 P_n$ after mixing. $P_0 = 0.67$ atm, calculate P_n and add to P_0 for P_t.
original   after mixing
$P_1V_1 = P_2V_2$
$(5)(2) = (P_2)(6)$
$1.67 = P_n$ after mixing
$P_0 + P_n = 0.67 + 1.67 = 2.34$ atm

24. **(D)** What is the volume if the pressure on the container is 5 atm?
$P_1V_1 = P_2V_2$
$(2.34)(6) = (5)(V_2)$
2.8 liters $= V_2$
By subjecting the mixture to 5 atm pressure, the volume is reduced to 2.8 liters.

25. **(A)** Triglycerides, which are esters of glycerol, show a net increase in liver tissue following alcohol ingestion.

26. **(D)** An increase in liver lipids due to net increase in liver triglyceride caused by carbon tetrachloride. Lipids are soluble in organic solvents.

27. **(C)** Note that the lipid has increased from 25 μg to 50 μg in the hydrazine treated liver showing an increased secretion into the blood. Data on A and B is not given and hydrazine is a known factor in fatty liver formation.

28. **(E)** Carbon dioxide is correct but not listed. CO_2 + $Ca(OH)_2 \rightarrow CaCO_3$ + H_2O. The $CaCO_3$ precipitates.

29. **(E)** Carbon dioxide will not ignite; thus the gas must be a mixture.

30. **(E)** If the gas will not support combustion, it does not contain a high concentration of O_2.

31. **(A)** Cations migrate to the cathode, and anions migrate to the anode. Anode 2 $Cl^- \rightarrow Cl_2$ + 2 electrons.

32. **(B)** Electrolysis of the fused salt allows the collection of sodium at the cathode.

33. **(D)** Electrolysis of the aqueous salt does not allow sodium production. Instead, hydrogen gas and sodium hydroxide may be collected at the cathode (provided diffusion of the sodium hydroxide is prevented).

34. **(B)** The parallel resistors in R_a can be expressed as:

$$\frac{1}{R_a} = \frac{1}{R_1} + \frac{1}{R_2}$$

35. **(E)** If one resistor were to replace the entire group of resistors (R_s) it would be equal to the sum of the resistance in each part of the circuit or:

$$R_s = R_a + R_b + R_c$$

36. **(C)** If I = 2 amp and R = 60 ohms the relationship between potential difference, current and resistance can be used and it states that:
$V = IR$
$V = (2)(60)$
$V = 120$ volts

37. **(B)** The cohesiveness of blood by itself causes an increase in viscosity and if there is an increase, a concomitant loss of speed of flow and pressure is observed.

38. **(C)** As the stream becomes more compact, the radius decreases and the layers of blood are brought closer to one another. This results in an increase in viscosity and a decrease in pressure, speed and flow.

39. **(B)** $\frac{1}{2} \times \frac{1}{2} \times \frac{1}{2} \times \frac{1}{2} = \frac{1}{16}$

40. **(D)** An equilibrium shift to the right would be favored by decreased temperature (since it is exothermic) and increased pressure (since the volume is greater on the left side) according to the principle of LeChatelier.

41. **(B)** The equilibrium is favored toward the left by increased temperature and decreased pressure. Decreased pressure is the best choice presented in the question.

42. **(E)** The changes in temperature and pressure would have effects in opposing directions whose total effect could not be predicted from the information given.

43. **(C)** Use $F = \left(\frac{1}{2}\right)^{t/T}$ where T = half-life = 10; t = time = 90

$F = \left(\frac{1}{2}\right)^{90/10} = \left(\frac{1}{2}\right)^{9}$

$F = \frac{1}{512}$

$\left(\frac{1}{512}\right)(10^9)$ = atoms remaining = 2×10^6 atoms

44. **(A)** To calculate the % of disintegration use 100% − % remaining = % disintegrated.

% remaining = $\frac{\text{no. of atoms remaining}}{\text{no. of atoms at start}} \times 100$

$= \frac{2 \times 10^6}{1 \times 10^9} \times 100 = 2 \times 10^{-3} \times 10^2$

$= 2 \times 10^{-1} = 0.2\%$

% disintegrated = 100 − 0.2 = 99.8%

45. **(D)** The answer to the question is self-explanatory.

46. **(D)** All the statements are true.

47. **(B)** $F = GM_1M_2/d^2$:
$F = \frac{(6.67 \times 10^{-11} \text{ N·m}^2/\text{kg}^2)(1 \text{ kg})(5 \text{ kg})}{(20 \text{ m})^2}$
$F = 8.3 \times 10^{-13}$ N

48. **(A)** Since 4/3, π, D and M are constant (the mass of the object does not change) the force on the object (its weight) is proportional only to r:

$$\frac{F_1}{F_2} = \frac{r_1}{r_2} = \frac{4}{1}$$

Therefore, the object will weigh 1/4 as much on the other planet, or 75 N.

49. **(D)** Specific gravity $= \frac{\rho_{\text{substance}}}{\rho_{\text{water}}}$

ρ_{water} in g/cm^3 = 1.0

$$(11.3) \frac{\text{g}}{\text{cm}^3} = \rho_{\text{lead}}$$

50. **(B)** $\rho = \dfrac{M}{\text{Vol.}} = 11.3 \text{ g/cm} = \text{density}, \qquad \text{Vol.} = ?,$

and Mass = 600 kg then Mass = 600×10^3.

$11.3\, V = M$

$V = \dfrac{M}{11.3} = \dfrac{600 \times 10^3 \text{ g}}{11.3 \text{ g/cm}^3}$

$V = 53.1 \times 10^3 \text{ cm}^3$

51. **(C)** $11.3 = \dfrac{\rho_{\text{lead}}}{\rho_{\text{water}}} = \dfrac{\rho_{\text{lead}}}{62.5 \text{ lb./ft.}^3}$

$\rho_{\text{lead}} = (11.3)(62.5) \text{ lb./ft.}^3$

$\rho_{\text{lead}} = 786.25 \text{ lb./ft.}^3$

52-54. **(52-A) (53-C) (54-C)** The answers to these questions are easily deduced from the experimental design.

55. **(E)** Lean humans sometimes have an elevated proportion of brown fat, enabling them to eat more without gaining weight. Many obese humans have little or no brown fat, thus causing weight gain with less food intake. The other three categories represent animals with a greater need for heat production.

56. **(B)** Metabolic oxidation of fatty acids in all tissues occurs primarily in the mitochondria.

57. **(D)** *De novo* fatty acid synthesis occurs primarily in the nonparticulate cytoplasm. Transformation of fatty acids (especially elongation of existing fatty acids) occurs primarily in the mitochondria and the smooth endoplasmic reticulum.

58. **(C)** The rate of heat production is I^2R. In a series circuit, I is the same for all resistors, so the largest resistance generates heat at the fastest rate.

59. **(B)** In a series circuit, resistances add, so the total resistance is 120 Ω. Current is the same in all elements of the circuit and is equal to

$$I = \frac{V}{R} = \frac{12 \text{ V}}{120 \text{ Ω}} = 0.10 \text{ A}$$

60. **(C)** When the resistor is removed, the circuit is broken and there is no current.

Answer Sheet—Model Test D

SCIENCE KNOWLEDGE

Biology

1. Ⓐ Ⓑ Ⓒ Ⓓ Ⓔ   11. Ⓐ Ⓑ Ⓒ Ⓓ Ⓔ   21. Ⓐ Ⓑ Ⓒ Ⓓ Ⓔ   30. Ⓐ Ⓑ Ⓒ Ⓓ Ⓔ
2. Ⓐ Ⓑ Ⓒ Ⓓ Ⓔ   12. Ⓐ Ⓑ Ⓒ Ⓓ Ⓔ   22. Ⓐ Ⓑ Ⓒ Ⓓ Ⓔ   31. Ⓐ Ⓑ Ⓒ Ⓓ Ⓔ
3. Ⓐ Ⓑ Ⓒ Ⓓ Ⓔ   13. Ⓐ Ⓑ Ⓒ Ⓓ Ⓔ   23. Ⓐ Ⓑ Ⓒ Ⓓ Ⓔ   32. Ⓐ Ⓑ Ⓒ Ⓓ Ⓔ
4. Ⓐ Ⓑ Ⓒ Ⓓ Ⓔ   14. Ⓐ Ⓑ Ⓒ Ⓓ Ⓔ   24. Ⓐ Ⓑ Ⓒ Ⓓ Ⓔ   33. Ⓐ Ⓑ Ⓒ Ⓓ Ⓔ
5. Ⓐ Ⓑ Ⓒ Ⓓ Ⓔ   15. Ⓐ Ⓑ Ⓒ Ⓓ Ⓔ   25. Ⓐ Ⓑ Ⓒ Ⓓ Ⓔ   34. Ⓐ Ⓑ Ⓒ Ⓓ Ⓔ
6. Ⓐ Ⓑ Ⓒ Ⓓ Ⓔ   16. Ⓐ Ⓑ Ⓒ Ⓓ Ⓔ   26. Ⓐ Ⓑ Ⓒ Ⓓ Ⓔ   35. Ⓐ Ⓑ Ⓒ Ⓓ Ⓔ
7. Ⓐ Ⓑ Ⓒ Ⓓ Ⓔ   17. Ⓐ Ⓑ Ⓒ Ⓓ Ⓔ   27. Ⓐ Ⓑ Ⓒ Ⓓ Ⓔ   36. Ⓐ Ⓑ Ⓒ Ⓓ Ⓔ
8. Ⓐ Ⓑ Ⓒ Ⓓ Ⓔ   18. Ⓐ Ⓑ Ⓒ Ⓓ Ⓔ   28. Ⓐ Ⓑ Ⓒ Ⓓ Ⓔ   37. Ⓐ Ⓑ Ⓒ Ⓓ Ⓔ
9. Ⓐ Ⓑ Ⓒ Ⓓ Ⓔ   19. Ⓐ Ⓑ Ⓒ Ⓓ Ⓔ   29. Ⓐ Ⓑ Ⓒ Ⓓ Ⓔ   38. Ⓐ Ⓑ Ⓒ Ⓓ Ⓔ
10. Ⓐ Ⓑ Ⓒ Ⓓ Ⓔ   20. Ⓐ Ⓑ Ⓒ Ⓓ Ⓔ

To score add from Science Problems questions: 10–12; 16–18; 22–24; 31–33; 43–48; 55–57.

Chemistry

1. Ⓐ Ⓑ Ⓒ Ⓓ Ⓔ   11. Ⓐ Ⓑ Ⓒ Ⓓ Ⓔ   21. Ⓐ Ⓑ Ⓒ Ⓓ Ⓔ   30. Ⓐ Ⓑ Ⓒ Ⓓ Ⓔ
2. Ⓐ Ⓑ Ⓒ Ⓓ Ⓔ   12. Ⓐ Ⓑ Ⓒ Ⓓ Ⓔ   22. Ⓐ Ⓑ Ⓒ Ⓓ Ⓔ   31. Ⓐ Ⓑ Ⓒ Ⓓ Ⓔ
3. Ⓐ Ⓑ Ⓒ Ⓓ Ⓔ   13. Ⓐ Ⓑ Ⓒ Ⓓ Ⓔ   23. Ⓐ Ⓑ Ⓒ Ⓓ Ⓔ   32. Ⓐ Ⓑ Ⓒ Ⓓ Ⓔ
4. Ⓐ Ⓑ Ⓒ Ⓓ Ⓔ   14. Ⓐ Ⓑ Ⓒ Ⓓ Ⓔ   24. Ⓐ Ⓑ Ⓒ Ⓓ Ⓔ   33. Ⓐ Ⓑ Ⓒ Ⓓ Ⓔ
5. Ⓐ Ⓑ Ⓒ Ⓓ Ⓔ   15. Ⓐ Ⓑ Ⓒ Ⓓ Ⓔ   25. Ⓐ Ⓑ Ⓒ Ⓓ Ⓔ   34. Ⓐ Ⓑ Ⓒ Ⓓ Ⓔ
6. Ⓐ Ⓑ Ⓒ Ⓓ Ⓔ   16. Ⓐ Ⓑ Ⓒ Ⓓ Ⓔ   26. Ⓐ Ⓑ Ⓒ Ⓓ Ⓔ   35. Ⓐ Ⓑ Ⓒ Ⓓ Ⓔ
7. Ⓐ Ⓑ Ⓒ Ⓓ Ⓔ   17. Ⓐ Ⓑ Ⓒ Ⓓ Ⓔ   27. Ⓐ Ⓑ Ⓒ Ⓓ Ⓔ   36. Ⓐ Ⓑ Ⓒ Ⓓ Ⓔ
8. Ⓐ Ⓑ Ⓒ Ⓓ Ⓔ   18. Ⓐ Ⓑ Ⓒ Ⓓ Ⓔ   28. Ⓐ Ⓑ Ⓒ Ⓓ Ⓔ   37. Ⓐ Ⓑ Ⓒ Ⓓ Ⓔ
9. Ⓐ Ⓑ Ⓒ Ⓓ Ⓔ   19. Ⓐ Ⓑ Ⓒ Ⓓ Ⓔ   29. Ⓐ Ⓑ Ⓒ Ⓓ Ⓔ   38. Ⓐ Ⓑ Ⓒ Ⓓ Ⓔ
10. Ⓐ Ⓑ Ⓒ Ⓓ Ⓔ   20. Ⓐ Ⓑ Ⓒ Ⓓ Ⓔ

To score add from Science Problems questions: 4–9; 19–21; 28–30; 37–42; 52–54.

Physics

1. Ⓐ Ⓑ Ⓒ Ⓓ Ⓔ   12. Ⓐ Ⓑ Ⓒ Ⓓ Ⓔ   23. Ⓐ Ⓑ Ⓒ Ⓓ Ⓔ
2. Ⓐ Ⓑ Ⓒ Ⓓ Ⓔ   13. Ⓐ Ⓑ Ⓒ Ⓓ Ⓔ   24. Ⓐ Ⓑ Ⓒ Ⓓ Ⓔ
3. Ⓐ Ⓑ Ⓒ Ⓓ Ⓔ   14. Ⓐ Ⓑ Ⓒ Ⓓ Ⓔ   25. Ⓐ Ⓑ Ⓒ Ⓓ Ⓔ
4. Ⓐ Ⓑ Ⓒ Ⓓ Ⓔ   15. Ⓐ Ⓑ Ⓒ Ⓓ Ⓔ   26. Ⓐ Ⓑ Ⓒ Ⓓ Ⓔ
5. Ⓐ Ⓑ Ⓒ Ⓓ Ⓔ   16. Ⓐ Ⓑ Ⓒ Ⓓ Ⓔ   27. Ⓐ Ⓑ Ⓒ Ⓓ Ⓔ
6. Ⓐ Ⓑ Ⓒ Ⓓ Ⓔ   17. Ⓐ Ⓑ Ⓒ Ⓓ Ⓔ   28. Ⓐ Ⓑ Ⓒ Ⓓ Ⓔ
7. Ⓐ Ⓑ Ⓒ Ⓓ Ⓔ   18. Ⓐ Ⓑ Ⓒ Ⓓ Ⓔ   29. Ⓐ Ⓑ Ⓒ Ⓓ Ⓔ
8. Ⓐ Ⓑ Ⓒ Ⓓ Ⓔ   19. Ⓐ Ⓑ Ⓒ Ⓓ Ⓔ   30. Ⓐ Ⓑ Ⓒ Ⓓ Ⓔ
9. Ⓐ Ⓑ Ⓒ Ⓓ Ⓔ   20. Ⓐ Ⓑ Ⓒ Ⓓ Ⓔ   31. Ⓐ Ⓑ Ⓒ Ⓓ Ⓔ
10. Ⓐ Ⓑ Ⓒ Ⓓ Ⓔ   21. Ⓐ Ⓑ Ⓒ Ⓓ Ⓔ   32. Ⓐ Ⓑ Ⓒ Ⓓ Ⓔ
11. Ⓐ Ⓑ Ⓒ Ⓓ Ⓔ   22. Ⓐ Ⓑ Ⓒ Ⓓ Ⓔ   33. Ⓐ Ⓑ Ⓒ Ⓓ Ⓔ

To score add from Science Problems questions: 1–3; 13–15; 25–27; 34–36; 49–51; 58–60.

SCIENCE PROBLEMS

1. Ⓐ Ⓑ Ⓒ Ⓓ Ⓔ   21. Ⓐ Ⓑ Ⓒ Ⓓ Ⓔ   41. Ⓐ Ⓑ Ⓒ Ⓓ Ⓔ
2. Ⓐ Ⓑ Ⓒ Ⓓ Ⓔ   22. Ⓐ Ⓑ Ⓒ Ⓓ Ⓔ   42. Ⓐ Ⓑ Ⓒ Ⓓ Ⓔ
3. Ⓐ Ⓑ Ⓒ Ⓓ Ⓔ   23. Ⓐ Ⓑ Ⓒ Ⓓ Ⓔ   43. Ⓐ Ⓑ Ⓒ Ⓓ Ⓔ
4. Ⓐ Ⓑ Ⓒ Ⓓ Ⓔ   24. Ⓐ Ⓑ Ⓒ Ⓓ Ⓔ   44. Ⓐ Ⓑ Ⓒ Ⓓ Ⓔ
5. Ⓐ Ⓑ Ⓒ Ⓓ Ⓔ   25. Ⓐ Ⓑ Ⓒ Ⓓ Ⓔ   45. Ⓐ Ⓑ Ⓒ Ⓓ Ⓔ
6. Ⓐ Ⓑ Ⓒ Ⓓ Ⓔ   26. Ⓐ Ⓑ Ⓒ Ⓓ Ⓔ   46. Ⓐ Ⓑ Ⓒ Ⓓ Ⓔ
7. Ⓐ Ⓑ Ⓒ Ⓓ Ⓔ   27. Ⓐ Ⓑ Ⓒ Ⓓ Ⓔ   47. Ⓐ Ⓑ Ⓒ Ⓓ Ⓔ
8. Ⓐ Ⓑ Ⓒ Ⓓ Ⓔ   28. Ⓐ Ⓑ Ⓒ Ⓓ Ⓔ   48. Ⓐ Ⓑ Ⓒ Ⓓ Ⓔ
9. Ⓐ Ⓑ Ⓒ Ⓓ Ⓔ   29. Ⓐ Ⓑ Ⓒ Ⓓ Ⓔ   49. Ⓐ Ⓑ Ⓒ Ⓓ Ⓔ
10. Ⓐ Ⓑ Ⓒ Ⓓ Ⓔ   30. Ⓐ Ⓑ Ⓒ Ⓓ Ⓔ   50. Ⓐ Ⓑ Ⓒ Ⓓ Ⓔ
11. Ⓐ Ⓑ Ⓒ Ⓓ Ⓔ   31. Ⓐ Ⓑ Ⓒ Ⓓ Ⓔ   51. Ⓐ Ⓑ Ⓒ Ⓓ Ⓔ
12. Ⓐ Ⓑ Ⓒ Ⓓ Ⓔ   32. Ⓐ Ⓑ Ⓒ Ⓓ Ⓔ   52. Ⓐ Ⓑ Ⓒ Ⓓ Ⓔ
13. Ⓐ Ⓑ Ⓒ Ⓓ Ⓔ   33. Ⓐ Ⓑ Ⓒ Ⓓ Ⓔ   53. Ⓐ Ⓑ Ⓒ Ⓓ Ⓔ
14. Ⓐ Ⓑ Ⓒ Ⓓ Ⓔ   34. Ⓐ Ⓑ Ⓒ Ⓓ Ⓔ   54. Ⓐ Ⓑ Ⓒ Ⓓ Ⓔ
15. Ⓐ Ⓑ Ⓒ Ⓓ Ⓔ   35. Ⓐ Ⓑ Ⓒ Ⓓ Ⓔ   55. Ⓐ Ⓑ Ⓒ Ⓓ Ⓔ
16. Ⓐ Ⓑ Ⓒ Ⓓ Ⓔ   36. Ⓐ Ⓑ Ⓒ Ⓓ Ⓔ   56. Ⓐ Ⓑ Ⓒ Ⓓ Ⓔ
17. Ⓐ Ⓑ Ⓒ Ⓓ Ⓔ   37. Ⓐ Ⓑ Ⓒ Ⓓ Ⓔ   57. Ⓐ Ⓑ Ⓒ Ⓓ Ⓔ
18. Ⓐ Ⓑ Ⓒ Ⓓ Ⓔ   38. Ⓐ Ⓑ Ⓒ Ⓓ Ⓔ   58. Ⓐ Ⓑ Ⓒ Ⓓ Ⓔ
19. Ⓐ Ⓑ Ⓒ Ⓓ Ⓔ   39. Ⓐ Ⓑ Ⓒ Ⓓ Ⓔ   59. Ⓐ Ⓑ Ⓒ Ⓓ Ⓔ
20. Ⓐ Ⓑ Ⓒ Ⓓ Ⓔ   40. Ⓐ Ⓑ Ⓒ Ⓓ Ⓔ   60. Ⓐ Ⓑ Ⓒ Ⓓ Ⓔ

SKILLS ANALYSIS: READING

1. Ⓐ Ⓑ Ⓒ Ⓓ Ⓔ
2. Ⓐ Ⓑ Ⓒ Ⓓ Ⓔ
3. Ⓐ Ⓑ Ⓒ Ⓓ Ⓔ
4. Ⓐ Ⓑ Ⓒ Ⓓ Ⓔ
5. Ⓐ Ⓑ Ⓒ Ⓓ Ⓔ
6. Ⓐ Ⓑ Ⓒ Ⓓ Ⓔ
7. Ⓐ Ⓑ Ⓒ Ⓓ Ⓔ
8. Ⓐ Ⓑ Ⓒ Ⓓ Ⓔ
9. Ⓐ Ⓑ Ⓒ Ⓓ Ⓔ
10. Ⓐ Ⓑ Ⓒ Ⓓ Ⓔ
11. Ⓐ Ⓑ Ⓒ Ⓓ Ⓔ
12. Ⓐ Ⓑ Ⓒ Ⓓ Ⓔ
13. Ⓐ Ⓑ Ⓒ Ⓓ Ⓔ
14. Ⓐ Ⓑ Ⓒ Ⓓ Ⓔ
15. Ⓐ Ⓑ Ⓒ Ⓓ Ⓔ
16. Ⓐ Ⓑ Ⓒ Ⓓ Ⓔ
17. Ⓐ Ⓑ Ⓒ Ⓓ Ⓔ
18. Ⓐ Ⓑ Ⓒ Ⓓ Ⓔ
19. Ⓐ Ⓑ Ⓒ Ⓓ Ⓔ
20. Ⓐ Ⓑ Ⓒ Ⓓ Ⓔ
21. Ⓐ Ⓑ Ⓒ Ⓓ Ⓔ
22. Ⓐ Ⓑ Ⓒ Ⓓ Ⓔ
23. Ⓐ Ⓑ Ⓒ Ⓓ Ⓔ
24. Ⓐ Ⓑ Ⓒ Ⓓ Ⓔ
25. Ⓐ Ⓑ Ⓒ Ⓓ Ⓔ
26. Ⓐ Ⓑ Ⓒ Ⓓ Ⓔ
27. Ⓐ Ⓑ Ⓒ Ⓓ Ⓔ
28. Ⓐ Ⓑ Ⓒ Ⓓ Ⓔ
29. Ⓐ Ⓑ Ⓒ Ⓓ Ⓔ
30. Ⓐ Ⓑ Ⓒ Ⓓ Ⓔ
31. Ⓐ Ⓑ Ⓒ Ⓓ Ⓔ
32. Ⓐ Ⓑ Ⓒ Ⓓ Ⓔ
33. Ⓐ Ⓑ Ⓒ Ⓓ Ⓔ
34. Ⓐ Ⓑ Ⓒ Ⓓ Ⓔ
35. Ⓐ Ⓑ Ⓒ Ⓓ Ⓔ
36. Ⓐ Ⓑ Ⓒ Ⓓ Ⓔ
37. Ⓐ Ⓑ Ⓒ Ⓓ Ⓔ
38. Ⓐ Ⓑ Ⓒ Ⓓ Ⓔ
39. Ⓐ Ⓑ Ⓒ Ⓓ Ⓔ
40. Ⓐ Ⓑ Ⓒ Ⓓ Ⓔ
41. Ⓐ Ⓑ Ⓒ Ⓓ Ⓔ
42. Ⓐ Ⓑ Ⓒ Ⓓ Ⓔ
43. Ⓐ Ⓑ Ⓒ Ⓓ Ⓔ
44. Ⓐ Ⓑ Ⓒ Ⓓ Ⓔ
45. Ⓐ Ⓑ Ⓒ Ⓓ Ⓔ
46. Ⓐ Ⓑ Ⓒ Ⓓ Ⓔ
47. Ⓐ Ⓑ Ⓒ Ⓓ Ⓔ
48. Ⓐ Ⓑ Ⓒ Ⓓ Ⓔ
49. Ⓐ Ⓑ Ⓒ Ⓓ Ⓔ
50. Ⓐ Ⓑ Ⓒ Ⓓ Ⓔ
51. Ⓐ Ⓑ Ⓒ Ⓓ Ⓔ
52. Ⓐ Ⓑ Ⓒ Ⓓ Ⓔ
53. Ⓐ Ⓑ Ⓒ Ⓓ Ⓔ
54. Ⓐ Ⓑ Ⓒ Ⓓ Ⓔ
55. Ⓐ Ⓑ Ⓒ Ⓓ Ⓔ
56. Ⓐ Ⓑ Ⓒ Ⓓ Ⓔ
57. Ⓐ Ⓑ Ⓒ Ⓓ Ⓔ
58. Ⓐ Ⓑ Ⓒ Ⓓ Ⓔ
59. Ⓐ Ⓑ Ⓒ Ⓓ Ⓔ
60. Ⓐ Ⓑ Ⓒ Ⓓ Ⓔ
61. Ⓐ Ⓑ Ⓒ Ⓓ Ⓔ
62. Ⓐ Ⓑ Ⓒ Ⓓ Ⓔ
63. Ⓐ Ⓑ Ⓒ Ⓓ Ⓔ
64. Ⓐ Ⓑ Ⓒ Ⓓ Ⓔ
65. Ⓐ Ⓑ Ⓒ Ⓓ Ⓔ
66. Ⓐ Ⓑ Ⓒ Ⓓ Ⓔ
67. Ⓐ Ⓑ Ⓒ Ⓓ Ⓔ
68. Ⓐ Ⓑ Ⓒ Ⓓ Ⓔ

SKILLS ANALYSIS: QUANTITATIVE

1. Ⓐ Ⓑ Ⓒ Ⓓ Ⓔ
2. Ⓐ Ⓑ Ⓒ Ⓓ Ⓔ
3. Ⓐ Ⓑ Ⓒ Ⓓ Ⓔ
4. Ⓐ Ⓑ Ⓒ Ⓓ Ⓔ
5. Ⓐ Ⓑ Ⓒ Ⓓ Ⓔ
6. Ⓐ Ⓑ Ⓒ Ⓓ Ⓔ
7. Ⓐ Ⓑ Ⓒ Ⓓ Ⓔ
8. Ⓐ Ⓑ Ⓒ Ⓓ Ⓔ
9. Ⓐ Ⓑ Ⓒ Ⓓ Ⓔ
10. Ⓐ Ⓑ Ⓒ Ⓓ Ⓔ
11. Ⓐ Ⓑ Ⓒ Ⓓ Ⓔ
12. Ⓐ Ⓑ Ⓒ Ⓓ Ⓔ
13. Ⓐ Ⓑ Ⓒ Ⓓ Ⓔ
14. Ⓐ Ⓑ Ⓒ Ⓓ Ⓔ
15. Ⓐ Ⓑ Ⓒ Ⓓ Ⓔ
16. Ⓐ Ⓑ Ⓒ Ⓓ Ⓔ
17. Ⓐ Ⓑ Ⓒ Ⓓ Ⓔ
18. Ⓐ Ⓑ Ⓒ Ⓓ Ⓔ
19. Ⓐ Ⓑ Ⓒ Ⓓ Ⓔ
20. Ⓐ Ⓑ Ⓒ Ⓓ Ⓔ
21. Ⓐ Ⓑ Ⓒ Ⓓ Ⓔ
22. Ⓐ Ⓑ Ⓒ Ⓓ Ⓔ
23. Ⓐ Ⓑ Ⓒ Ⓓ Ⓔ
24. Ⓐ Ⓑ Ⓒ Ⓓ Ⓔ
25. Ⓐ Ⓑ Ⓒ Ⓓ Ⓔ
26. Ⓐ Ⓑ Ⓒ Ⓓ Ⓔ
27. Ⓐ Ⓑ Ⓒ Ⓓ Ⓔ
28. Ⓐ Ⓑ Ⓒ Ⓓ Ⓔ
29. Ⓐ Ⓑ Ⓒ Ⓓ Ⓔ
30. Ⓐ Ⓑ Ⓒ Ⓓ Ⓔ
31. Ⓐ Ⓑ Ⓒ Ⓓ Ⓔ
32. Ⓐ Ⓑ Ⓒ Ⓓ Ⓔ
33. Ⓐ Ⓑ Ⓒ Ⓓ Ⓔ
34. Ⓐ Ⓑ Ⓒ Ⓓ Ⓔ
35. Ⓐ Ⓑ Ⓒ Ⓓ Ⓔ
36. Ⓐ Ⓑ Ⓒ Ⓓ Ⓔ
37. Ⓐ Ⓑ Ⓒ Ⓓ Ⓔ
38. Ⓐ Ⓑ Ⓒ Ⓓ Ⓔ
39. Ⓐ Ⓑ Ⓒ Ⓓ Ⓔ
40. Ⓐ Ⓑ Ⓒ Ⓓ Ⓔ
41. Ⓐ Ⓑ Ⓒ Ⓓ Ⓔ
42. Ⓐ Ⓑ Ⓒ Ⓓ Ⓔ
43. Ⓐ Ⓑ Ⓒ Ⓓ Ⓔ
44. Ⓐ Ⓑ Ⓒ Ⓓ Ⓔ
45. Ⓐ Ⓑ Ⓒ Ⓓ Ⓔ
46. Ⓐ Ⓑ Ⓒ Ⓓ Ⓔ
47. Ⓐ Ⓑ Ⓒ Ⓓ Ⓔ
48. Ⓐ Ⓑ Ⓒ Ⓓ Ⓔ
49. Ⓐ Ⓑ Ⓒ Ⓓ Ⓔ
50. Ⓐ Ⓑ Ⓒ Ⓓ Ⓔ
51. Ⓐ Ⓑ Ⓒ Ⓓ Ⓔ
52. Ⓐ Ⓑ Ⓒ Ⓓ Ⓔ
53. Ⓐ Ⓑ Ⓒ Ⓓ Ⓔ
54. Ⓐ Ⓑ Ⓒ Ⓓ Ⓔ
55. Ⓐ Ⓑ Ⓒ Ⓓ Ⓔ
56. Ⓐ Ⓑ Ⓒ Ⓓ Ⓔ
57. Ⓐ Ⓑ Ⓒ Ⓓ Ⓔ
58. Ⓐ Ⓑ Ⓒ Ⓓ Ⓔ
59. Ⓐ Ⓑ Ⓒ Ⓓ Ⓔ
60. Ⓐ Ⓑ Ⓒ Ⓓ Ⓔ
61. Ⓐ Ⓑ Ⓒ Ⓓ Ⓔ
62. Ⓐ Ⓑ Ⓒ Ⓓ Ⓔ
63. Ⓐ Ⓑ Ⓒ Ⓓ Ⓔ
64. Ⓐ Ⓑ Ⓒ Ⓓ Ⓔ
65. Ⓐ Ⓑ Ⓒ Ⓓ Ⓔ
66. Ⓐ Ⓑ Ⓒ Ⓓ Ⓔ
67. Ⓐ Ⓑ Ⓒ Ⓓ Ⓔ
68. Ⓐ Ⓑ Ⓒ Ⓓ Ⓔ

The MCAT
Model Examination D*

SCIENCE KNOWLEDGE

115 MINUTES
109 QUESTIONS

The following questions are varied; therefore, you are advised to pay careful attention to the instructions for each portion.

Biology—38 Questions   Recommended Time—25 minutes

DIRECTIONS: Each of the statements or questions is followed by suggested completions or answers. Choose the one that best completes the statement or answers the question, and mark the letter of your choice on the answer sheet.

1. To penetrate the corona radiata of the egg in fertilization, sperm utilize
   - (A) spermatase.
   - (B) chondroitin sulfatase.
   - (C) hyaluronidase.
   - (D) deoxyribonuclease.
   - (E) ribonuclease.

2. During gamete production in the human female, how many functional eggs are eventually produced by the cell which undergoes the reduction division (meiosis)?
   - (A) four
   - (B) around three hundred
   - (C) eight
   - (D) one
   - (E) around one hundred

3. A patient has suffered a cerebral hemorrhage that has caused injury and nonfunctioning of the primary motor area of his left cerebral cortex. As a result,
   - (A) he cannot voluntarily move his right arm or hand nor his right leg or foot.
   - (B) he feels no sensation on the left side of his body.
   - (C) reflexes cannot be elicited on the left side of his body.
   - (D) he cannot voluntarily move his right arm nor his left leg.
   - (E) he feels no sensation on the right side of his body.

4. The pituitary (master) gland releases a gonadotrophic hormone which stimulates the production of testosterone by
   - (A) spermatogonia.
   - (B) interstitial cells of Leydig.
   - (C) Sertoli cells.
   - (D) epididymis.
   - (E) ductus deferens.

5. The structure(s) responsible for the production of progesterone is (are)
   - (A) ovarian follicle.
   - (B) corpus albicans.
   - (C) corpus luteum.
   - (D) corpus spongiosum.
   - (E) corpus cavernosum.

---

*Explanations for science answers can be found on p. 446.

6. The sperm count of a normal 25-year-old male would be
   (A) one milion/ml.
   (B) one hundred million/ml.
   (C) one hundred thousand/ml.
   (D) four million/ml.
   (E) ten thousand/ml.

7. Each of the following is under control of the adenohypophysis EXCEPT the
   (A) thyroid.
   (B) adrenal medulla.
   (C) testis.
   (D) adrenal cortex.
   (E) ovary.

8. Mutations
   (A) are changes that take place and will always be passed on to the next generation.
   (B) are influenced by use and disuse of body parts.
   (C) occur spontaneously and cannot be produced experimentally.
   (D) are mainly due to diseases associated with development.
   (E) occur spontaneously and can also be produced by experimental means.

9. The functional unit of a striated muscle is known as the sarcomere. A sarcomere on an electron micrograph is the region between
   (A) two A bands.
   (B) two I bands.
   (C) two H bands.
   (D) two Z bands.

10. Bacteriophages are
    (A) quite dangerous to humans.
    (B) grown by innoculation of sterile broth.
    (C) reproduced only in living cells.
    (D) used as a source of vaccine against many bacterial diseases.
    (E) used in the production of vaccine against specific viral agents.

11. The czarinas of Russia and the queens of England popularized the disease hemophilia. These normal women produced sons suffering from hemophilia, a disease that is caused by a sex-linked recessive gene, h. The more common dominant gene, H, produces normal blood clotting. Genotypically these women must have carried
    (A) HH.
    (B) Hh.
    (C) hh.
    (D) none of the above.

12. Phenotype may be defined as
    (A) genetic makeup of an individual.
    (B) hidden traits of an individual.
    (C) unrelated characteristics.
    (D) visible expression of genotype.
    (E) genetic material carried on the Y chromosome only.

13. Among the defense mechanisms available to humans to ward off their destruction by the environment is (are)
    (A) skin.
    (B) white blood corpuscles.
    (C) antibodies.
    (D) sebaceous secretions.
    (E) all of the above.

14. Alleles are genes which
    (A) arise during the cross-over process.
    (B) are linked to one chromosome only.
    (C) are always sex-linked and are transmitted from mothers to their sons.
    (D) occupy corresponding positions on homologous chromosomes.
    (E) are sex-linked and are transmitted from fathers to their daughters.

15. The neurotransmitter acetylcholine is released by
    (A) axon terminals.
    (B) dendrite terminals.
    (C) Golgi apparatus of neuron cell bodies.
    (D) Schwann cells.
    (E) node of Ranvier.

16. Two people are planning to have a family. The woman has blood type A/A and the man B/B. Their children might have the following
    (A) A and B.
    (B) B only.
    (C) A/B only.
    (D) A and B and A/B.

17. A man with blood cell genotype B/O marries a woman with type A/B. Their offspring could have any of the following
    (A) A/B, B/B, A/O, B/O.
    (B) A/B and B/O only.
    (C) A/O and B/B only.
    (D) none of the combinations above.

18. Of the pairs below which one is mismatched?
    (A) lymphatics: contain amino acids, salt, water, but no blood corpuscles
    (B) hepatic portal vein: drains the intestinal tract and carries nutrients
    (C) inferior vena cava: carries oxygenated blood and has a low blood pressure
    (D) hypothalamus: secretes releasing factors that influence pituitary-target organ relationships
    (E) pulmonary veins: carry oxygenated blood

19. A lack of iodine in the diet usually is associated with which disorder?
    (A) acromegaly
    (B) goiter
    (C) rickets
    (D) skin rash
    (E) tetanus

20. One enzyme that is important in protein digestion is
    (A) ptyalin.
    (B) trypsin.
    (C) maltose.
    (D) pancreatic lipase.
    (E) rennin.

21. If we examine the three types of muscles in respect to their characteristics, which of the series below is false?

	Characteristic	Cardiac	Skeletal	Smooth
(A)	No. of Nuclei	Several	Several	One
(B)	Position of Nuclei	Central	Central	Central
(C)	Striations	Present	Present	Absent
(D)	Control	Autonomic	Voluntary	Autonomic

22. Twinning is an interesting biological phenomenon. Identical twins usually result from fertilization of
    (A) two eggs by one sperm.
    (B) one egg by two sperms.
    (C) one egg by one sperm and separation of cells during the early cleavage division.
    (D) one egg and one polar body.
    (E) two eggs by two sperms.

23. The basic scientific finding that finally led to the development of the oral contraceptive (pill) used by many females in our society was that the preovulatory surge of LH can be prevented by the administration of
    (A) FSH.
    (B) estrogen.
    (C) progesterone.
    (D) ICSH.
    (E) androgen.

24. Dialysis (as is used for the treatment of chronic kidney ailments) differs from the process of osmosis in the respect that
    (A) both solvent and solute pass through the membrane.
    (B) solute selectively passes through the membrane only.
    (C) solvent selectively passes through the membrane only.
    (D) gases are the only substances that pass the membrane and blood is cleansed.

25. A foreign protein, when introduced into the body, is recognized and elicits an immunologic response; this substance is known as a (an)
    (A) antigen.
    (B) antibody.
    (C) complement.
    (D) vitamin.
    (E) enzyme.

26. In vasectomy, which of the following is (are) cut, with a portion removed, and the two ends sutured?
    (A) epididymis
    (B) spermatic cords
    (C) oviducts
    (D) urethra
    (E) seminal vesicles

27. Sweating is a mechanism of temperature regulation by the body. This mechanism is usually far less effective in cooling the organism if the person is in an environment where the
    (A) wind is of hurricane proportion.
    (B) humidity is at least 0°.
    (C) humidity is almost 0°.
    (D) all of the above.
    (E) none of the above.

28. Hypersecretion of which hormone will result in acromegaly (giantism)?
    (A) TSH—thyroid stimulating hormone
    (B) STH—somatotropin (growth hormone)
    (C) ACTH—adrenocorticotrophic hormone
    (D) thyroxin
    (E) adrenalin

29. Conservation of body heat is aided by
    (A) constriction of the capillaries of the skin.
    (B) decreased respiratory activity.
    (C) decreased heart rate.
    (D) decreased sweating.
    (E) all of the above.

30. Testosterone is produced by
    (A) spermatogonia of the testes.
    (B) interstitial cells of the testes (Leydig cells).
    (C) the glans penis.
    (D) the prostate gland.
    (E) Sertoli cells.

31. Glucagon, which is produced by the pancreas, and epinephrine, which is produced by the adrenal glands, are hormones which
    (A) raise blood sugar level.
    (B) lower blood sugar level.
    (C) do not affect blood sugar markedly.
    (D) markedly increase liver glycogen.

32. Abnormal blood clots (thrombi) occur more frequently in people with
    (A) prothrombin deficiency.
    (B) impeded venous blood flow.
    (C) vitamin K deficiency.
    (D) platelet deficiency.
    (E) none of the above.

33. Growth hormone releasing factor is
    (A) a precursor of growth hormone.
    (B) the same as growth hormone (somatotropin).
    (C) a hypothalamic releasing factor.
    (D) a dietary stimulant regulating positive nitrogen balance.
    (E) an enzyme.

34. The large intestine functions mainly in
    (A) absorption of water.
    (B) excretion of water.
    (C) absorption of sodium and potassium.
    (D) finishing the digestive process.
    (E) excretion of digestive enzymes.

35. Blood pH is influenced by respiration; experimental hyperventilation in a physiology laboratory will result in the student's blood pH being
    (A) lowered.
    (B) raised.
    (C) unaffected.
    (D) raised to pH6.

36. Heart beat is initiated by the
    (A) vagus nerve.
    (B) sympathetic nervous system.
    (C) A-V (atrio-ventricular) node.
    (D) Purkinje system.
    (E) S-A (sino-atrial) node.

37. Which of the following is a grossly incorrect dimension?
    (A) diameter of an animal cell: 10 micrometers
    (B) distance between two covalently bonded atoms: 0.1 nanometer
    (C) length of a human embryo at 1 month development: 5 millimeters
    (D) thickness of a cell membrane: 10 nanometers
    (E) thickness of human epidermal layer: 25 micrometers

38. A patient is awaiting surgery and routine blood tests are conducted. It is found that problems may arise due to the patient's abnormally long clotting time. This patient may be deficient in
    (A) vitamin K.
    (B) platelets.
    (C) prothrombin.
    (D) any or all of the above.

Chemistry—38 Questions   Recommended Time—46 minutes

DIRECTIONS: Each of the statements or questions is followed by suggested completions or answers. Choose the one that best completes the statement or answers the question, and mark the letter of your choice on the answer sheet.

1. The basic building block of proteins is (are)
   (A) nitrogenous bases.
   (B) amino acids.
   (C) ammonia.
   (D) transfer RNA.
   (E) messenger RNA.

2. Catalytic hydrogenation of phenyl diazonium bromide produces
   (A) bromobenzene.
   (B) phenylhydrazine.
   (C) benzene.
   (D) phenylamine.

3. In transcription of RNA from DNA, thymine will form a base pair only with
   (A) adenine.
   (B) guanine.
   (C) cytosine.
   (D) uracil.
   (E) thymine.

4. Calcium carbide reacts with water to produce
   (A) carbon dioxide.
   (B) methane.
   (C) carbohydrate.
   (D) acetylene.
   (E) ethylene.

5. Addition of water to metallic sodium produces
   (A) oxygen and sodium hydride.
   (B) hydrogen and sodium hydroxide.
   (C) sodium hydrate.
   (D) nitrogen and sodium hydride.
   (E) no reaction.

6. The common lead storage battery produces electricity by two hall cell reactions, one of which is (written in the direction of production of electricity)
   (A) $PbSO_2 + 2H_2O \rightarrow PbO_2 + 4H^+ + SO_4^{2-} + 2e^-$
   (B) $PbSO_4 + 2e^- \rightarrow Pb + SO_4^{2-}$
   (C) $Pb + SO_4^{2-} \rightarrow PbSO_4 + 2e^-$
   (D) none of the above

7. If one wished to remove substantially all of the chloride ions from an aqueous solution, this could be done by the addition of an aqueous solution of
   (A) KNO_3.
   (B) Na_2SO_4.
   (C) $AgNO_3$.
   (D) starch.
   (E) gelatin.

8. How many organic products are produced when methyl iodide and *n*-propyl iodide are reacted with sodium metal?
   (A) 2
   (B) 3
   (C) 4
   (D) 6
   (E) 8

9. In question 8 the compound listed below that would be produced in greatest yield is
   (A) *n*-hexane.
   (B) sodium propane.
   (C) hexyl iodide.
   (D) *n*-butane.
   (E) none of the above.

10. If it is known that H_2S is a weak acid that ionizes to form $2H^+$ and S^{2-}, lowering the pH of a solution of H_2S by adding HCl should
    (A) raise the S^{2-} concentration.
    (B) lower the S^{2-} concentration.
    (C) have no effect on S^{2-} concentration.
    (D) not be possible.

11. Which of the following aqueous solutions will have the lowest freezing point?
    (A) 1 M NaCl
    (B) 0.3 M Na_2SO_4
    (C) 1.5 M glucose
    (D) 0.5 M $BaSO_4$
    (E) H_2O

12. Consider this reaction: $Fe^{2+} \rightleftarrows Fe^{3+} + e^-$. Which of the following is correct?
    (A) The reaction toward the right is an oxidation.
    (B) The reaction toward the right is a reduction.
    (C) The reaction toward the left is a reduction.
    (D) A and C are correct.
    (E) None of the above is correct.

13. A negative iodoform test (i.e., no yellow precipitate) will be the result when NaOH + I₂ is reacted with

    (A) $CH_3 - CH - CH_3$
          $\quad\quad\quad |$
          $\quad\quad\quad OH$

    (B) $CH_3 - C - CH_2 - CH_3$
          $\quad\quad\quad \|$
          $\quad\quad\quad O$

    (C) $\phi - \overset{\overset{\textstyle O}{\|}}{C} - CH_3$

    (D) $CH_3 - CH_2 - CH_2 - \overset{\overset{\textstyle H}{|}}{C} = O$

14. The hydronium ion is
    (A) a protonated water molecule.
    (B) formed by removal of H^- from a water molecule.
    (C) really a free radial rather than an ion.
    (D) an ion with the formula of H_2O^+.
    (E) an uranium byproduct.

15. The alpha helix in a protein is classified as the
    (A) primary structure.
    (B) secondary structure.
    (C) tertiary structure.
    (D) quaternary structure.
    (E) permanent structure.

16. How many milliliters of 0.50N NaOH are required to neutralize 50 ml of 0.25N HCl?
    (A) 25
    (B) 50
    (C) 0.25
    (D) 2.5
    (E) none of the above

17. How many carbon atoms are present in the smallest organic ring compound that may be synthesized?
    (A) 3
    (B) 4
    (C) 5
    (D) 6
    (E) 7

18. Factor(s) that influence(s) enzymatic activity is (are)
    (A) temperature.
    (B) pH.
    (C) concentration, substrate, cofactors
    (D) enzyme poisons.
    (E) all of the above.

19. A zwitterion is a molecule containing
    (A) both cationic and anionic functions.
    (B) more than one cationic or anionic function.
    (C) polar and nonpolar groups.
    (D) a Z^+ charge.
    (E) none of the above.

20. Prolonged boiling of animal fat with lye is called
   (A) hydrolysis.
   (B) stain removal.
   (C) saponification.
   (D) alchemy of glyceridization.
   (E) conjugation.

21. Without considering stereoisomers the number of possible dibromobutane isomers is
   (A) 3.
   (B) 4.
   (C) 5.
   (D) 6.
   (E) 8.

22. The reaction of HBr with 1-propene in the presence of peroxides will produce primarily
   (A) 1-bromopropane.
   (B) 2-bromopropane.
   (C) 1,2-dibromopropane.
   (D) 2-bromopropene.
   (E) 1,3-dibromopropane.

23. Theoretically, how many isomers could be produced from the ring monobromination of 4-bromo-1,2-dimethylbenzene?
   (A) 1
   (B) 2
   (C) 3
   (D) 4
   (E) 5

24. In a titration of iodine with sodium thiosulfate, the formation of a blue color on the addition of colorless starch solution indicates that
   (A) all of the iodine has not been oxidized.
   (B) the glassware has not been washed sufficiently.
   (C) all of the iodine has not been reduced.
   (D) a blue complex of starch, iodine, and sodium thiosulfate has been produced.
   (E) the temperature is above 50°C.

25. Of the compounds listed below which has the greatest affinity for combining with hemoglobin?
   (A) nitrogen, N_2
   (B) carbon dioxide, CO_2
   (C) oxygen, O_2
   (D) helium
   (E) carbon monoxide, CO

26. Use of helium is preferred over use of hydrogen in airships (e.g., blimps) because
   (A) helium has a lower density.
   (B) helium is chemically less reactive.
   (C) both of the above.
   (D) none of the above.

27. Of what two types of sugars are nucleotides composed?
   (A) glucose and maltose.
   (B) glucose and ribose.
   (C) maltose and deoxyribose.
   (D) ribose and deoxyribose.
   (E) none of the above.

28. The process of fermentation can be considered to be
   (A) oxidation.
   (B) dehydration.
   (C) aerobic respiration.
   (D) anaerobic respiration.
   (E) hydrolytic.

29. Low molecular weight mercaptans are often added to natural gas to
   (A) increase the flammability.
   (B) slightly retard the burning.
   (C) produce a pleasant deodorant during burning.
   (D) provide a stench which is helpful in the detection of gas leaks.
   (E) prevent corrosion of the pipelines.

30. In the reaction sequence used in breakdown of glycogen in the liver or muscle—glycogen → glucose-1-phosphate → glucose-6-phosphate → glucose—the first step is
    (A) catalyzed by phosphorylase.
    (B) catalyzed by pepsin.
    (C) catalyzed by pancreatic amylase.
    (D) nonenzymatic.
    (E) catalyzed by trypsin.

31. An inorganic cation has been precipitated from water by the addition of NaOH. When we find that the precipitate may be redissolved upon the addition of NaOH or dilute HNO_3, we may conclude that the precipitate was
    (A) colloidal.   (D) amorphous.
    (B) amphoteric.   (E) crystalline.
    (C) anthromorphic.

32. The inorganic cation in the question above could be
    (A) silver.   (D) nickel.
    (B) ferric.   (E) barium.
    (C) aluminum.

33. Transuranium elements are
    (A) found on earth as a result of bombardment by particles from the planet Uranus.
    (B) found naturally in abundance greater than that of uranium isotopes.
    (C) man-made elements with more than 92 protons in the nucleus.
    (D) elements that have been postulated but not found naturally or produced artificially.

34. The particles which spin around the nucleus of an atom and are negatively charged are the
    (A) neutrons.   (D) electrons.
    (B) positrons.   (E) ions.
    (C) protons.

35. Given an atom with electron configuration $1s^2 2s^2 2p^3$, how many orbitals are completely filled?
    (A) 1   (C) 3
    (B) 2   (D) 4

36. The heat of fusion of a substance is the energy measured during a
    (A) phase change.   (C) chemical change.
    (B) temperature change.   (D) pressure change.

37. How many moles of water are contained in 0.250 mole of $CuSO_4 \cdot 5H_2O$?
    (A) 1.25   (C) 40.0
    (B) 4.50   (D) 62.5

38. Which of the following reactions is a decomposition reaction?
    (A) $CO_2 + H_2O \rightarrow H_2CO_3$ (D) $HCl + NaOH \rightarrow NaCl + H_2O$

    (B) $2HgO \overset{\Delta}{\rightarrow} 2Hg + O_2$ (E) $2H_2 + O_2 \rightarrow 2H_2O$

    (C) $Zn + CuSO_4 \rightarrow ZnSO_4 + Cu$

Physics—33 Questions   Recommended Time—44 minutes

DIRECTIONS: Each of the statements or questions is followed by suggested completions or answers. Choose the one that best completes the statement or answers the question, and mark the letter of your choice on the answer sheet.

1. If the uniform acceleration near the surface of the earth is about 9.8 m/s² for a free-fall, **what is the velocity at the end of 2 seconds of fall (neglect friction)?**
   (A)   19.6 m/s
   (B)   17.0 m/s
   (C)   14.6 m/s
   (D)   12.2 m/s
   (E)   9.8 m/s

2. The amount of heat measured in calories needed to raise the temperature of 1 gram of substance by 1 degree Celsius is known as
   (A)   coefficient of expansion.
   (B)   specific heat.
   (C)   heat of fusion.
   (D)   mechanical equivalent of heat.
   (E)   latent heat.

3. If a force of 300 N acts on a 60 kg mass, calculate the resulting acceleration.
   (A)   0.5 m/s²
   (B)   2 m/s²
   (C)   5 m/s²
   (D)   6 m/s²
   (E)   9.8 m/s²

4. If an object is moving with a constant acceleration, the net force acting on that body is
   (A)   constant.
   (B)   increasing.
   (C)   decreasing.
   (D)   zero.
   (E)   none of the above.

5. What is the potential energy of a 10 kg steel ball which has been raised vertically 9 m above the floor?
   (A)   90 joules
   (B)   98 joules
   (C)   441 joules
   (D)   882 joules
   (E)   1938 joules

6. If the mass of a moving projectile is tripled and its velocity is doubled, the kinetic energy will be multiplied by
   (A)   2.
   (B)   6.
   (C)   8.
   (D)   12.
   (E)   16.

7. The direction of the force exerted on a surface by a liquid at rest is
   (A)   tangential to the surface.
   (B)   parallel to the surface.
   (C)   normal to the surface.
   (D)   45° to the surface.
   (E)   30° to the surface.

8. The volume of a confined gas varies inversely with the absolute pressure provided that the temperature remains unchanged. This statement is known as
   (A)   Avogadro's law.
   (B)   Bernoulli's law.
   (C)   the gas law.
   (D)   Dalton's law.
   (E)   Boyle's law.

9. Which ratio below best defines the efficiency of simple machines?
   (A) $\dfrac{\text{useful work output}}{\text{work input}} \times 100\%$
   (B) $\dfrac{\text{work input}}{\text{work output}} \times 100\%$
   (C) $\dfrac{\text{theoretical mechanical advantage}}{\text{actual mechanical advantage}} \times 100\%$
   (D) $\dfrac{\text{centrifugal force}}{\text{centripetal force}} \times 100\%$
   (E) $\dfrac{\text{useful work input}}{\text{useful work output}} \times 100\%$

10. You are standing 1000 m from the point where a steel block strikes the sidewalk. How long will it take the sound to reach your ears if the speed of sound in air at 0°C is about 333 m/s?
    (A) 1 second
    (B) 2 seconds
    (C) 3 seconds
    (D) 4 seconds
    (E) 5 seconds

11. In simplest terms, the energy of a wave is directly proportional to the square of its
    (A) period.
    (B) length.
    (C) reflection.
    (D) refraction.
    (E) amplitude.

12. Shadows consist of two portions, the umbra and the penumbra. Which statement below applies ONLY to the umbra?
    (A) It is circular in shape.
    (B) It is always the longest portion.
    (C) It is a partial shadow.
    (D) It receives no light from any part of the source.
    (E) It receives light from part of the source.

13. What is the work done in joules if a 100-kg ball is raised to 3 m above the floor in 1 second?
    (A) 300 joules
    (B) 980 joules
    (C) 1960 joules
    (D) 2940 joules
    (E) 3240 joules

14. Virtual images can be formed by
    (A) converging lenses, only.
    (B) diverging lenses, only.
    (C) neither converging nor diverging lenses.
    (D) either converging or diverging lenses.

15. Three resistances of 2 ohms, 4 ohms, and 6 ohms are connected in parallel. The equivalent resistance of the three resistors is
    (A) less than 2 ohms.
    (B) between 2 ohms and 4 ohms.
    (C) between 4 ohms and 6 ohms.
    (D) greater than 6 ohms.

16. An object starts from rest and falls freely. What is the velocity of the object at the end of 3.00 seconds?
    (A) 9.81 m/s
    (B) 19.6 m/s
    (C) 29.4 m/s
    (D) 88.2 m/s
    (E) 176.4 m/s

17. The driver of a car hears the siren of an ambulance which is moving away from her. If the actual frequency of the siren is 2,000 hertz, the frequency heard by the driver may be
    (A) 1,900 Hz
    (B) 2,000 Hz
    (C) 2,100 Hz
    (D) 4,000 Hz
    (E) 6,000 Hz

18. A resultant force of 10. newtons is made up of two component forces acting at right angles to each other. If the magnitude of one of the components is 6.0 newtons, the magnitude of the other component must be
    (A) 16 N
    (B) 8.0 N
    (C) 6.0 N
    (D) 4 N
    (E) 2 N

19. Which of the statements below is correct?
    (A) If a road is properly banked for the speed of the vehicle, the resultant force on the vehicle is a horizontal centripetal force.
    (B) The resultant force action on a vehicle will be that which maintains it in a circular path.
    (C) There is no tendency for the vehicle to skid if a road is banked for the speed at which the vehicle is moving.
    (D) The angle of bank for a road is obtained from a consideration of the centripetal force required.
    (E) All of the above statements are correct.

20. How far will a body free-fall in 1 second if released from rest?
    (A) 0.0 m   (D) 14.7 m
    (B) 4.9 m   (E) 19.6 m
    (C) 9.8 m

21. A resultant force of 440 N is acting on a body whose acceleration is 10 m/s^2. Calculate the mass of the body.
    (A) 4.5 kg   (D) 980 kg
    (B) 44.1 kg   (E) 1960 kg
    (C) 450 kg

22. $F = Gm_1m_2/d_2$ is the equation representing Newton's law of universal gravitation. Which of the statements below is true?
    (A) G is called the gravitation constant.
    (B) The law can be used to calculate the mass of an object on another planet if the mass and radius of that planet are known.
    (C) Knowing the value of G, one can easily calculate the mass of the earth.
    (D) The force of attraction of the earth for a body is equal to the force of attraction of the body for the earth.
    (E) All of the above are true.

23. Two forces of 45 N and 40 N act on a body in opposite directions. What is the resultant force?
    (A) 5 N   (D) 85 N
    (B) 40 N   (E) 90 N
    (C) 45 N

24. A good floor lamp has a wide heavy base to increase its stability through
    (A) raising the center of gravity.   (D) neutral equilibrium.
    (B) lowering the center of gravity.   (E) none of the above.
    (C) banking.

25. When analyzed, most complicated machines are found to consist of a combination of various simple machines. Which machine below is NOT a simple machine?
    (A) wheel-and-axle   (D) electric motor
    (B) pulley   (E) inclined plane
    (C) lever

26. The velocity of a test sled propelled from rest by a device that has 2500 joules of available energy to propel a sled of 50-kg mass is
    (A) 50 m/s.   (D) 5 m/s.
    (B) 25 m/s.   (E) 1 m/s.
    (C) 10 m/s.

27. The figure below represents a pipe in which a fluid flows into another pipe that has a smaller cross section. If v_1 and v_2 are velocities and P_1 and P_2 are pressures, which of the following is correct?
    (A) $v_1 > v_2$
    (B) $P_1 > P_2$
    (C) $v_1 = v_2$
    (D) $P_1 = P_2$
    (E) $P_2 > P_1$

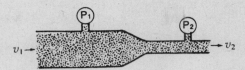

28. If the density of a given body is 10 g/cm³, what is its specific gravity?
    (A) 0.01 g/cm³
    (B) 1.0 g
    (C) 0.01
    (D) 10.0
    (E) 1.0

29. The amount of a liquid's cohesive force per unit of length is called
    (A) apparent weight.
    (B) adhesion.
    (C) depression.
    (D) surface tension.
    (E) capillary rise.

30. When light is reflected from a surface it can be either regular reflection or diffuse reflection. The essential difference between regularly and diffusely reflecting surfaces is that
    (A) the regularly reflecting surface is coarser than the diffusely reflecting surface.
    (B) only mirrors reflect in a regular manner, every other surface reflects diffusely.
    (C) regularly reflecting surfaces are smoother than diffusely reglecting surfaces.
    (D) light can not be reflected from a diffusely reflecting surface.
    (E) all of the above are essential differences between regularly and diffusely reflecting surfaces.

31. A crate is being slid up an inclined plane. What happens as the angle of the plane is made steeper?
    (A) Friction increases; coefficient of friction remains constant.
    (B) Friction and coefficient of friction decrease.
    (C) Friction and coefficient of friction increase.
    (D) Friction decreases; coefficient of friction remains constant.
    (E) Friction remains constant; coefficient of friction decreases.

32. Two points in an electric circuit are at potentials 20 V and 80 V. Two resistors, one of 20 Ω and the other of 40 Ω, are connected in parallel between the points. How much is the current in the 20-Ω resistor?
    (A) 5 A
    (B) 4.5 A
    (C) 4 A
    (D) 3 A
    (E) 1 A

33. How does the sound produced by a piano playing high C compare with that from middle C, an octave lower?
    (A) Wavelength is half as much; velocity is the same.
    (B) Wavelength is twice as much; velocity is the same.
    (C) Frequency and velocity are twice as much.
    (D) Frequency is twice as much; wavelength is the same.
    (E) Wavelength and frequency are twice as much.

SCIENCE PROBLEMS

78 MINUTES
60 QUESTIONS: Biology 21; Chemistry 21; Physics 18.

The following questions require you to use your knowledge of science to solve problems.

DIRECTIONS: The following questions or incomplete statements are in groups. Preceding each series of questions or statements is a paragraph or short explanatory statement, a formula or set of formulas, or a definition. Read the written material and then answer the questions or complete the statements. Eliminate the choices that you think to be incorrect and mark the letter of your choice on the answer sheet.

In uniformly accelerated motion the following equations hold:

$$v = v_0 + at$$

$$x = v_0 t + \frac{1}{2}at^2$$

when x = displacement, v = velocity at time t, v_0 = initial velocity, t = time, and a = acceleration. A ball is projected directly upward at a velocity of 15 m/s.

1. What is the distance above the ground after 3 seconds?
   (A) 0 m
   (B) 0.9 m
   (C) 1.8 m
   (D) 2.7 m
   (E) 3.6 m

2. What is its velocity at that point?
   (A) 14.4 m/s upward
   (B) 14.4 m/s downward
   (C) 29.4 m/s upward
   (D) 29.4 m/s downward

3. What is the highest point this ball will reach?
   (A) 9.80 m
   (B) 11.48 m
   (C) 38.66 m
   (D) 22.95 m
   (E) 1.53 m

In the dark, bromine adds to double bonds to produce dibromo additional compounds. The addition of bromine to conjugated dienes can produce 1,2-dibromo-3-alkenes or 1,4-dibromo-2-alkenes.

4. The reaction of 1 mole of 1,3-butadiene with 1 mole of bromine would be expected to result in production of
   (A) 1,4-dibromo-3-butene.
   (B) 1,4-dibromobutane.
   (C) 1,2-dibromo-2-butene.
   (D) 1,3-dibromo-2-butene.
   (E) none of the above.

5. Another example of the reaction of bromine with conjugated dienes is that in which bromine reacts with
   (A) acetylene.
   (B) allene (propadiene).
   (C) 1,4-pentadiene.
   (D) B and C.
   (E) none of the above.

6. The formation of 1,4-addition products with conjugated dienes is evidence of
   (A) ionic mechanism.
   (B) free radical mechanism.
   (C) radiant energy.
   (D) A and B.
   (E) none of the above.

The solubility of compound R in water is 5 g/100 ml. The distribution coefficient between water and ether, $K_{H_2O/ether}$, is 2 at room temperature.

7. How many grams of compound R will be in the ether phase when 50 ml of water containing 1.0 g of compound R is extracted with 50 ml of ether?
   (A) 1.0 g
   (B) 0.5 g
   (C) 0.33 g
   (D) 0.1 g
   (E) 0.05 g

8. A second extraction of the remaining aqueous solution by another 50 ml of ether would result in the extraction of an additional
   (A) 0.1 g.
   (B) 0.2 g.
   (C) 0.3 g.
   (D) 0.5 g.
   (E) 0.55 g.

9. How many milliliters of ether must be used to remove 0.8 g in the first extraction?
   (A) less than 150 ml
   (B) 200 ml
   (C) 300 ml
   (D) 400 ml
   (E) more than 475 ml

Assume that the membrane of a neuron is unimolecular, and that an impulse travelling along the nerve involves the same type of ions regardless of location along the fiber. While examining with the oscilloscope the nature of an impulse traveling along the sciatic nerve of a test animal, an unusually large spike is visualized and seems out of phase.

10. One can assume that the unusually large spike height visualized is
    (A) typical of a repeated nerve impulse.
    (B) an artifact.
    (C) not typical of a nerve impulse but definitely a result of the nerve's physiology.
    (D) all of the above.
    (E) none of the above.

11. The usual wave function seen while studying neural impulses is an example of
    (A) an all or none response.
    (B) a gradient response.
    (C) subthreshold transmission.
    (D) all of the above.
    (E) none of the above.

12. The spike height of the wave can be altered by
    (A) external application of a saline solution to the nerve.
    (B) injecting a saline solution into the nerve fiber.
    (C) increasing the voltage of the applied stimulus.
    (D) all of the above.
    (E) none of the above.

A block with a mass of 1 kg = 1000 grams is totally submerged in a liquid whose specific gravity is 1.25. It is attached to a spring scale that reads 800 grams.

13. What is the mass equivalent of the buoyant force?
    (A) 125 g
    (B) 200 g
    (C) 800 g
    (D) 1000 g
    (E) 1800 g

14. What is the volume of the body or that of the displaced liquid?
    (A) 50 cm^3
    (B) 160 cm^3
    (C) 250 cm^3
    (D) 350 cm^3
    (E) 450 cm^3

15. What is the density of the body?
    (A) 1 g/cm³
    (B) 2 g/cm³
    (C) 3 g/cm³
    (D) 6.25 g/cm³
    (E) 5 g/cm³

Use the following graph to answer questions 16-18:

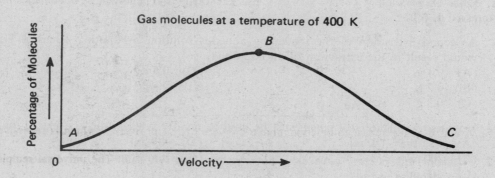

16. In the graph above, point B is
    (A) the escape velocity.
    (B) the average velocity.
    (C) the most probable velocity.
    (D) the maximum velocity.
    (E) B and C

17. Point C indicates
    (A) cessation of motion.
    (B) escape velocity.
    (C) maximum velocity.
    (D) an improbable velocity under these conditions.
    (E) an impossible velocity under these conditions.

18. If the above velocity plot were changed to 500 K, the peak of the curve would
    (A) be displaced to the right.
    (B) remain unchanged.
    (C) be displaced to the left.
    (D) have three maxima.
    (E) be flattened to such an extent that no maximum could be observed.

The equilibrium constant for the reaction $C + D \rightleftharpoons E + 2F$ may be represented by the equation:

$$K_{eq} = \frac{[E]\,[F]^2}{[C]\,[D]}$$

19. Doubling the concentration of C will
    (A) double the equilibrium constant.
    (B) halve the equilibrium constant.
    (C) increase the equilibrium constant by a factor of 3.
    (D) increase the equilibrium constant by a factor of 4.
    (E) do none of the above.

20. Doubling the concentration of D would result in
    (A) an increase in the concentration of E.
    (B) an increase in the concentration of F.
    (C) a decrease in the concentration of C.
    (D) all of the above.
    (E) none of the above.

21. The greatest change in the equilibrium constant would be noted upon
    (A) doubling the concentration of A.
    (B) doubling the concentration of B.
    (C) doubling the concentration of C.
    (D) doubling the concentration of D.
    (E) none of the above.

The A B O blood grouping system is explained on the basis of a single triallelic system with genes A, B, and O operating at a single genetic locus. Phenotypic and genotypic characteristics may be expressed as follows:

Phenotype	Genotype
A	A/A; A/O
B	B/B; B/O
O	O/O
AB	A/B

The A and B genes appear to be codominant; they are dominant over O, which is recessive.

22. Utilizing this system, transfusions have become relatively safe. The universal recipient is considered to be type
    (A) A.
    (B) B.
    (C) O.
    (D) AB.
    (E) Rh.

23. Which of the following agglutinogens do these individuals carry on their red blood cells?
    (A) A.
    (B) B.
    (C) O.
    (D) A,B.
    (E) None.

24. A person of blood type A can receive blood of type(s)
    (A) A.
    (B) B; A.
    (C) O.
    (D) A; O.
    (E) A; AB.

The equation of Snell's law is $\dfrac{\sin \theta_i}{\sin \theta_r} = \dfrac{N_r}{N_i}$ where θ_i = angle of incidence, θ_r = angle of refraction, N_r = index of refraction of pass through medium, and N_i = index of refraction of incident medium.

A beam of light is traveling through air and strikes a medium whose index of refraction is 1.414 at 45° with a normal to the glass.

25. The ray of light as it enters will
    (A) bend toward the normal.
    (B) bend away from the normal.
    (C) be totally reflected.
    (D) travel along the normal.
    (E) do none of the above.

26. The index of refraction can be defined as the velocity of light in a vacuum divided by the velocity in the medium ($N = \dfrac{C}{S}$). Then if a beam enters a medium from a vacuum, Snell's law states that
    (A) $\dfrac{S_i}{S_r} = \dfrac{N_r}{N_i}$
    (B) $\dfrac{\sin \theta_i}{\sin \theta_r} = \dfrac{C_i}{S_i}$
    (C) $\dfrac{\sin \theta_i}{\sin \theta_r} = \dfrac{C_r}{S_r}$
    (D) $\dfrac{\sin \theta_i}{\sin \theta_r} = \dfrac{S_i}{S_r}$
    (E) $\dfrac{\sin \theta_i}{\sin \theta_r} = \dfrac{S_r}{S_i}$

27. What is the velocity of the light entering a medium from a vacuum if $Sin\ \theta_i = 0.707$, $Sin\ \theta_r = 0.500$, and the velocity of light in a vacuum is 3.0×10^8 m/s?
    (A) 1.4×10^8 m/s   (D) 3.5×10^8 m/s
    (B) 2.1×10^8 m/s   (E) 4.2×10^8 m/s
    (C) 2.8×10^8 m/s

Two containers of equal volume are filled with helium gas at different temperatures and pressures.

28. If container X is at 760 torr and 0°C while container Y is at 137°C and 1140 torr, then container X (compared to container Y) has
    (A) fewer atoms of gas and a higher average velocity.
    (B) more atoms of gas and a lower average velocity.
    (C) an equal number of atoms of gas and an equal average velocity.
    (D) fewer atoms of gas and a lower average velocity.
    (E) none of the above.

29. Increasing the number of atoms in container X while retaining the volume constant would result in
    (A) increased pressure.   (D) decreased temperature.
    (B) decreased pressure.   (E) Choices A and C.
    (C) increased temperature.

30. If containers X and Y (above) had been at the temperatures and pressures given but container Y had contained argon rather than helium, then container X (compared to container Y) would be observed to have
    (A) fewer atoms of gas and a higher average velocity.
    (B) more atoms of gas and lower average velocity.
    (C) an equal number of atoms of gas with an equal average velocity.
    (D) an equal number of atoms of gas with an unknown average velocity.
    (E) none of the above.

A muscle fiber is a single muscle cell. Each fiber is composed of numerous cylindrical fibrils running the entire length of the fiber. The fibril exhibits light and dark bands—the I and A bands respectively. The I band is bisected by the M line. There is a somewhat lighter band within the A band that is called the H band. These striations are produced by the arrangement within the fibril of myofilaments; myosin is the thick myofilament while actin is considered the thin myofilament.

31. A sarcomere is the area between
    (A) two A bands.   (D) two Z bands.
    (B) two H bands.   (E) two M bands.
    (C) two I bands.

32. During contraction the lengths of the thick and thin myofilaments
    (A) increase.   (C) remain the same.
    (B) decrease.

33. If we could imagine observing a muscle contraction under a light microscope we would see the narrowing of the
    (A) H and I bands.   (D) H bands only.
    (B) A bands.   (E) I bands only.
    (C) Z bands.

Given the circuit diagram below:

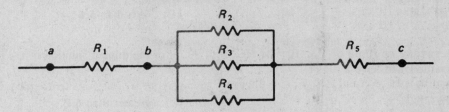

with the resistors $R_1 = 5$ ohms, $R_2 = 2$ ohms, $R_3 = 4$ ohms, $R_4 = 12$ ohms and $R_5 = 5$ ohms. The current through the circuit is 10 amperes.

34. What is the potential difference across R_1?
    (A) 10 volts
    (B) 20 volts
    (C) 30 volts
    (D) 40 volts
    (E) 50 volts

35. What is the resistance in the parallel resistors?
    (A) 1.2 ohms
    (B) 5.6 ohms
    (C) 6.0 ohms
    (D) 18 ohms
    (E) 28 ohms

36. What is the potential difference across the parallel resistors?
    (A) 12 volts
    (B) 60 volts
    (C) 120 volts
    (D) 180 volts
    (E) none of the above

An unknown organic compound is observed to react with phenylhydrazine to form a crystalline derivative. Mild oxidation produces one or more acidic compounds.

37. The compound could be
    (A) acetone.
    (B) 1,3-butadiene.
    (C) ethylene glycol.
    (D) butanal.
    (E) all of the above.

38. Another compound fulfilling the requirements would be
    (A) glycerol.
    (B) ethanol.
    (C) acetic acid.
    (D) aniline.
    (E) none of the above.

39. If oxidation with permanganate and then oxidation with periodic acid are performed before the reactions with phenylhydrazine and the mild oxidation (treatment and results mentioned above), the compound could be
    (A) 2-butene.
    (B) acetone.
    (C) 2-butanone.
    (D) butane.
    (E) 2-butanol.

Strong acids such as HCl are considered to be completely ionized unless they are at very high concentrations.

40. A 1×10^{-4} M solution of HCl in water will have a pH of
    (A) 11.
    (B) 7.
    (C) 9.
    (D) 4
    (E) less than 3.

41. A 1:10,000 dilution of the above solution with water will have a pH of
    (A) greater than 8.5.   (D) 6.
    (B) 8.   (E) less than 5.6.
    (C) 7.

42. A mixture of 10 ml of 1×10^{-4} M HCl with 90 ml of the diluted solution of the previous question will have a pH of
    (A) 0.4.   (D) 5.
    (B) 3.1.   (E) greater than 6.2.
    (C) 4.

The diagram illustrates a typical single neuron; the basic unit of the nervous system. Neurons connect with each other and in that manner an impulse is conducted and transmitted throughout the body. Two types of cell processes are indicated.

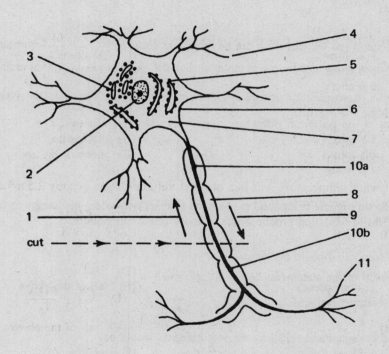

43. An impulse on the skin will be picked up by
    (A) 4.   (D) 10.
    (B) 6.   (E) 11.
    (C) 7.

44. The genetic material of the cell is located in
    (A) 2.   (D) 7.
    (B) 3.   (E) 9.
    (C) 5.

45. Protein synthesis is carried out under the direction of
    (A) 3 in 5.   (D) 2 in 7.
    (B) 2 in 3.   (E) 5 in 2.
    (C) 2 in 5.

A person has been in an accident and the physician is conducting a neurological examination. Sensation is lost over several fingers and the examiner fears that a nerve has been cut. Note the cut indication on the diagram preceding question 43.

46. Which process would completely degenerate?

    (A) 4   (D) 10b

    (B) 8   (E) 11

    (C) 10a

47. Retrograde degeneration would be visible in

    (A) 2.   (D) 10b.

    (B) 3.   (E) 11.

    (C) 6.

48. The impulse in the neuron is normally conducted in which direction?

    (A) 9

    (B) 1

The general gas law equation can be written as follows: $\frac{PV}{T} = \frac{P_0 V_0}{T_0}$ with the temperature and pressure in absolute units. A gas is maintained at 0°C in a volume of 5 m³ at atmospheric pressure.

49. If the atmospheric pressure is maintained, but the temperature is raised to 20°C, what will be the volume?

    (A) 2.50 m³   (D) 5.36 m³

    (B) 3.75 m³   (E) 6.65 m³

    (C) 4.65 m³

50. At what temperature will this original volume of gas occupy 2.5 m³ at 4 atmospheres absolute pressure?

    (A) 273 K   (D) 546 K

    (B) 373 K   (E) 679 K

    (C) 456 K

51. Which of the statements below is (are) true?

    (A) $\dfrac{P}{P_0} = \dfrac{T}{T_0}$ (D) $\dfrac{PV}{T} = \dfrac{P_0 V_0}{T_0}$

    (B) $\dfrac{V}{V_0} = \dfrac{T}{T_0}$ (E) all of the above

    (C) $PV = P_0 V_0$

A newly synthesized, weakly ionized acid is being studied. It is found to have an ionization constant of 1×10^{-7}.

52. A 0.1 N solution of the acid will have a pH of

    (A) 4.   (D) 6.9.

    (B) 5.5.   (E) none of the above.

    (C) 6.1.

53. A tenfold dilution of the above solution with water will have a pH between

    (A) 3.5 and 4.5.   (D) 6.75 and 7.1.

    (B) 4.6 and 5.5.   (E) none of the above.

    (C) 5.6 and 6.7.

54. Assuming the acid is highly soluble in water, prediction of pH at very high concentrations might be in error because of
  (A) higher temperatures in the solution.
  (B) errors in that area of logarithm tables.
  (C) decreased ionization at higher concentrations.
  (D) all of the above.
  (E) none of the above.

  Serum cholesterol levels are seen as a risk factor in the development of atherosclerotic plaques in the circulatory systems. The risk is modified, however, by the relative amounts of cholesterol that are carried by two lipoproteins: low-density lipoproteins (LDL) and high-density lipoproteins (HDL).

55. Which best describes the cholesterol in blood serum?
  (A) not present
  (B) free, unattached to lipoproteins
  (C) attached to only one lipoprotein
  (D) attached to only two lipoproteins
  (E) attached to more than two lipoproteins

56. An elevated numerical value of serum LDL cholesterol/HDL cholesterol is indicative of
  (A) reduced risk of atherosclerosis.
  (B) elevated risk of atherosclerosis.
  (C) inability to synthesize proteins.
  (D) inability to synthesize cholesterol.
  (E) reduced total serum cholesterol.

57. Cholesterol may be described as
  (A) totally without benefit in the human body, serving only in the development of atherosclerosis.
  (B) a required precursor of prostaglandins.
  (C) a required precursor of bile acids.
  (D) a required precursor of bile pigments.
  (E) a required precursor of certain polyunsaturated fatty acids.

  A 10-kg sled on a horizontal surface is pushed from rest with a force of 40 N, causing it to accelerate at 3 m/s^2 for 6 seconds.

58. How far did the sled go?
  (A) 54 m
  (B) 108 m
  (C) 18 m
  (D) 36 m
  (E) 9 m

59. How much was the force of friction?
  (A) 10 N
  (B) 30 N
  (C) 40 N
  (D) 60 N
  (E) 120 N

60. How much work was done in moving the sled the first 5 m?
  (A) 200 N
  (B) 150 N
  (C) 490 N
  (D) 50 N
  (E) 120 N

SKILLS ANALYSIS: READING

85 MINUTES
68 QUESTIONS

The following questions are to be answered based on your careful reading of selections from scientific writings.

DIRECTIONS: Read each passage carefully, then answer the questions following it. Consider only the material within the passage in answering the questions. Eliminate those choices that you think to be incorrect and mark the letter of your choice on the answer sheet.

The origin of the ovarian follicle has long been a subject of confusion. It is generally recognized that germ cells arise extragonadally during fetal development and migrate to the prospective gonadal region. There is still confusion, however, concerning the manner by which these germ cells enter the gonad and become enveloped by the follicular epithelium.

In their study of ovarian development in mice, Doctors Odor and Blandau suggested that stromal cells within the ovary surround the germ cells which have migrated into this region. The stromal cells thus become the follicular epithelium. Observations of previous investigators, however, suggest that the situation in the primate may be different. Witschi in 1948 described the migration of germ cells in humans. He stated that these cells were present in the endoderm (the epithelium of the presumptive gut), the mesothelium (an epithelium lining the body cavity) adjacent to the gut, and the mesenchymal tissue (which lies between these two epithelia). According to Dr. Witschi, the cells within the endoderm leave this epithelium and migrate through the mesenchymal tissue to the presumptive gonadal region which is a thickening of the mesenchyme of the body wall covered by a continuation of the same mesothelium found in proximity to the gut. In another investigation, Dr. Gillman described the presence of cords of cells within the fetal ovary. These cords were continuous with the mesothelium of the ovary. Initially these cords were devoid of germ cells; however, in the later stage of development the germ cells which had been seen in the stroma were incorporated into the cords. These cords subsequently split up into follicles. More recently, Dr. Merchant has reexamined ovarian development in the rat. By injecting a mitotic poison into a pregnant female at the time of germ cell migration, he has produced offspring which are lacking germ cells. In these animals follicles are absent but epithelial cell cords which are continuous with the ovarian mesothelium are present. Other investigators have also noted the presence of cords in the ovaries of normal laboratory animals.

Studies of human ovaries during the early stages of development are difficult because of technical as well as legal and medical problems. Nevertheless, observations by this investigator of ovaries from human and monkey fetuses after germ cell migration, confirm Gillman's observation that germ cells are present in the epithelial cords and that from these cords follicles are produced. However, this investigator is not in agreement with the proposed method by which the germ cells become incorporated into the cords. We have observed germ cells in the ovarian mesothelium which is in continuity with the epithelial cords. At the points of continuity, dividing cells within the mesothelium are oriented so that their mitotic spindles are perpendicular to the plane of the mesothelium. One daughter cell from such a division would be retained in the mesothelium, while the other would become part of the underlying cord. These observations suggest that the germ cell-containing cords arise from inward growth of a germ cell containing mesothelium. An extension of this conclusion would be that it is the germ cells which are found in the mesothelium in the region of the gut rather than those in the gut itself which are the cells that populate the gonad; and that this region of the mesothelium because of differential growth is, at a later time, positioned over the stroma of the presumptive gonad where the inward growth takes place.

The following statements are related to the passage above. Based on the information given, select:
  (A) if the statement is *supported by* the information in the passage.
  (B) if the statement is *contradicted by* the information in the passage.
  (C) if the statement is *neither supported nor contradicted by* information in the passage.

1. The manner by which the germ cells are enveloped by follicle cells is generally agreed on.

2. Germ cells arise within the ovary by differentiation of ovarian stromal cells.

3. In primates follicles arise by splitting off of ovarian cords.

4. Ovarian cords grow from the ovarian mesothelium.

5. Germ cells are moved by ciliary action.

6. The author believes that germ cells move independently of surrounding cells.

7. Due to less rigid abortion laws, studies on humans will increase and allow for the solution of the problem.

Does the order of a child's birth in a family have a bearing on his or her personality and on the type of adult he or she will grow up to be, or is the entire theory of ordinal position simply a bag of tricks that makes for interesting cocktail party conversation but little else?

While it has been the highlight of numerous debates and most certainly the subject of various studies, ordinal position remains a little-understood personality variable.

Consider the oldest child in a family of three children. Parents often claim that their first-born has a solid head on his or her shoulders, behaves in a mature manner, and is capable of getting along with adults. This important family member often exhibits a quiet front, yet is able to take the lead, care for his or her siblings and act like a miniature adult. Parents view the first-born as an intelligent individual who will grow up to be a pillar of the community.

What on earth happened to the second-born (again in a family of three children) to make him or her so different from the eldest? This child is much more lively, less willing to take orders, does not show the same interest in adults, and often has difficulty communicating with them. He or she may even become a "problem" child in school. Teachers have been heard to complain that "B— is not in the least like A— was. . . ." Could it be that the second-born is striking out in an attempt to find his or her own place? The problems of the second child in a family seem to intensify even more when the "baby" comes along and moves him or her into the "middle-child" position. Now he or she has to contend not only with a successful older brother or sister, but also with the youngest who seems to be the favorite. The youngest, on the other hand appears not to feel the need to measure up to anyone and goes along his or her own way to develop into an often exuberant, well-rounded individual. Because he or she is the baby, the mother doesn't expect this third sibling to function like a miniature adult, and she considers "cute" a great number of the actions that were viewed as unsatisfactory in the case of the other children.

Surely the questions related to ordinal position will provide research material for years to come. The problem is much like that of the chicken and the egg in that it is difficult to tell whether the numerical place a child occupies in a family *or* the attitudes which parents have developed in connection to child-rearing through years of trial and error, have the greatest effect on his or her personality.

The following statements are related to the information presented above. Based on the information given, select:

    (A) if the statement is *supported by* the information in the passage.
    (B) if the statement is *contradicted by* the information in the passage.
    (C) if the statement is *neither supported nor contradicted by* information in the passage.

8. It is a proven fact that the first-born always grows up to be a responsible citizen.

9. Ordinal position has been the topic of research for many years.

10. Parents often claim that first-born children behave in a more mature manner than later-born.

11. To date, ordinal position is a little-understood personality variable.

12. Second-born children who later move into the "middle-child" position achieve on a higher plane in school than do second-born who remain in the same position.

13. Comparison to older siblings, by teachers and other adults is the best method for stimulating the middle child to work harder.

14. By the time the third child comes along, mothers no longer seem to put the same emphasis on certain aspects of behavior that they did when raising their first-born.

15. The best place to discuss ordinal position is at a cocktail party, because it is such an interesting topic of conversation.

16. The youngest child is most adversely affected by his or her family position because he or she has more than one sibling to live up to.

17. The "baby" of the family is often a child with an outgoing personality.

Two systems modulate, integrate, and control the activities of the body; they are the nervous and endocrine systems. The response in nervous control is rapid while control via the endocrine system is fairly slow and longer lasting. The endocrine glands are ductless glands and secrete their products called hormones into the capillaries (bloodstream). Hormones are substances that are secreted into the bloodstream and travel to their target organs to elicit their effects. The product of the target organ may also feed back upon the organ that stimulated its activity and production; and manipulate in this respect its cycle of function. It may shut off the supply of stimulating hormone; this activity is called a negative feedback. The controlling mechanism can be though of as a neuro-endocrine-somatic tissue relationship, or the brain affecting the pituitary gland, which in turn affects the target organs, which then elicit their effect upon the body tissues and cells. Hormones cannot be classified into one chemical class; they are, however, all organic substances and may be proteins, peptides, amino acids (or amino acid derivatives), and steroids, or prostaglandins (derivatives of essential fatty acids). Generally the glands which produce protein hormones embryologically originate from the alimentary tract; they are the anterior pituitary, thyroid, parathyroids, and pancreas. Glands which produce steroid products are derived from the celomic mesothelium and are the testes, ovaries, and adrenal cortex. Glands whose products are small molecular weight amines arise from cells of nervous tissue derivation and are the neurohypophysis and the adrenal medulla.

The following statements are related to the information presented above. Based on the information given, select:
   (A)   if the statement is *supported by* the information in the passage.
   (B)   if the statement is *contradicted by* the information in the passage.
   (C)   if the statement is *neither supported nor contradicted by* information in the passage.

18. Nervous impulses are conducted quickly and produce long-acting effects.

19. The endocrine system achieves its functions via the bloodstream.

20. Releasing factors produced by the hypothalamus affect the pituitary gland.

21. Hormones are similar in nature.

22. The pancreas produces hormones that are proteins.

23. Steroids are produced by the reproductive organs.

24. The cells of the adrenal medulla may be thought of as postganglionic sympathetic cells.

Contraction in a skeletal muscle is triggered by the generation of an action potential in the muscle membrane. Each motor neuron upon entering a skeletal muscle loses its myelin sheath and divides into branches with each branch innervating a single muscle fiber, forming a neuromuscular junction. Each fiber normally has one neuromuscular junction which is located near the center of the fiber. A motor unit consists of a single motor neuron and all the muscle fibers innervated by it. The motor end plate is the specialized part of the muscle fiber's membrane lying under the nerve.

The impulse arriving at the end of the motor neuron causes liberation of acetylcholine from vesicles in the nerve terminal. The acetylcholine acts at specific sites normally found only on the motor end plate section of the fiber membrane and increases the permeability of the motor end plate. The resulting $Na+$ influx produces a depolarizing potential called the end plate potential. This in turn depolarizes adjacent areas of the fiber membrane, triggering an action potential which is propagated in both directions from the central neuromuscular junction toward the fiber ends. Normally the magnitude of the end plate potential is sufficient to discharge the muscle membrane, so that each impulse in the nerve ending produces a response in the muscle. The acetylcholine is rapidly destroyed by the enzyme acetylcholinesterase which is found in high concentrations at the neuromuscular junction.

The following statements are related to the information presented. Based on the information given, select:

(A)   if the statement is *supported by* in the passage.
(B)   if the statement is *contradicted by* the information in the passage.
(C)   if the statement is *neither supported nor contradicted by* information in the passage.

25.   The contraction of skeletal muscle is quicker and of shorter duration than the activation of smooth muscle.

26.   Acetylcholinesterase is released at the motor end plate.

27.   Motor neurons are myelinated.

28.   Acetylcholine is produced by muscle.

29.   While there is a sodium ion influx, potassium ions leave the cell.

30.   Sodium ion influx plays a role in the conduction of a nerve impulse.

31.   Magnitude of the end plate potential is of critical importance.

Primogeniture was the custom of allowing the oldest member of a family, in most situations this meant the oldest male member, to inherit all lands and possessions of his parents, to the exclusion of his siblings.

The ordinal position of being the first-born male therefore carried much power, as the first-born was considered to be intelligent, level-headed, and capable of taking over as family protector and landlord once the father died. Theoretically the oldest would be unselfish and see to the care of the younger family members, but in actuality this was often not the case.

The custom of primogeniture was particularly popular during the feudal period and was practiced in many countries of Europe, especially in France and England, where, for example, a fief descended intact to the oldest son. One European country where this custom was not in force during the Middle Ages was Germany.

Outlawed in the United States and no longer the mode of inheritance in Europe for today's population as a whole, primogeniture was in evidence as late as the 1920s and can still be seen in degree with some of Europe's royal families.

The following statements are related to the information presented above. Based on the information given, select:

(A)   if the statement is *supported by* the information in the passage.
(B)   if the statement is *contradicted by* the information in the passage.
(C)   if the statement is *neither supported nor contradicted by* information in the passage.

32.   Countries in Europe that have royal families still practice the custom of primogeniture

33.   Ordinal position was of utmost importance in medieval Europe

34.   In Germany during the feudal period the oldest son could be certain of inheriting his father's fief intact.

35.   In the United States each sibling receives the same amount of inheritance.

36.   Modern society often calls upon the first-born male to be the executor of his parents' will.

37.   The first-born male was thought to be the most intelligent level-headed sibling and therefore considered the proper landlord of his parents' holdings.

38.   Under the primogeniture custom, younger brothers and sisters were granted their fair share.

39.   France and England were two of the countries where primogeniture was practiced during the federal period.

40.   Today the royal family of England carries on this custom.

41.   The oldest child—whether male or female—*always* inherited everything.

A term that has been very much in vogue over the past five years or so is that of behavior modification or the changing of a subject's behavior from an unacceptable to an acceptable pattern.

While it may be argued that behavior is continually being altered and modified, the term as used here refers to a very structured approach by which the undesirable behavior is identified and specific monitored steps are undertaken to modify and move it into the path of becoming acceptable. A token system is included so that progress in the correct direction can be rewarded immediately.

This type of management system has been widely used by educators, especially at the elementary level, so that when children come home on any given afternoon with scores of M&M's in their pockets, mothers realize that teachers are busily modifying some aspect of behavior and that the candy is the reward system. Education does not, however, have a monopoly on behavior modification techniques. They have proven to be successful in certain scientific areas as well as many other fields.

Consider the person who has a weight problem yet claims to consume very little at meal time. Often this frustrated soul will eat next to nothing morning, noon, and evening, thus convinced that he or she is starving, but will forget to account for the 20 sidetrips to the refrigerator.

Such a person would be wise to use behavior modification techniques. Two charts are called for in this case. The first to cover every waking hour for one week with a check to indicate the times when something was eaten. The second could be identical except that the subject would now make a conscious effort to reduce the checks and give a token each time this happens. Thus, for instance, for each check missing a dime could be thrown in a kitty and saved for a nonfood splurge later on. Hopefully the subject would eventually alter his or her previous habit without the need for charting.

The following statements are related to the information presented above. Based on the information given, select:

(A) if the statement is *supported by* the information in the passage.
(B) if the statement is *contradicted by* the information in the passage.
(C) if the statement is *neither supported nor contradicted by* information in the passage.

42. The only way behavior can be altered is through use of a token system.

43. Doctors should suggest behavior modification to their overweight patients.

44. One area where this technique is used frequently is in elementary education.

45. Overweight people often eat too many carbohydrates and too little proteins.

46. Behavior modification can be classified as a type of management system.

47. In order to be successful, a person using behavior modification must first identify the undesirable behavior and then plan specific structured steps to change it.

48. Problem identification is an important facet of the behavior modification process.

49. Just because they are in vogue does not mean that behavior modification techniques are reliable.

50. Charting a specific behavior is often one way of pinpointing the undesirable action.

51. Once the problem has been spotted behavior modification will always eliminate it.

The major structural and functional cellular unit of nervous tissue is the neuron. The neuronal cell body or soma, like all cells, contains a distinct nucleus and nucleolus and a cytoplasm rich in organelles.

Prominent among these organelles are mitochondria, the Golgi apparatus, and profiles of rough-surfaced endoplasmic reticulum. Extending from the neuronal cell bodies are numerous appendages which are characterized as either axons or dendrites. The dendrites are generally multiple in number and from their primary shafts secondary, tertiary, and higher order branches arise.

Frequently, extending from the dendritic surfaces are numerous spines or gemmules which are reminiscent of thorns extending along the branches of a rose bush. The dendrites and their associated spines provide a greatly increased neuronal surface area which ultimately allows for increased interaction with other neuronal elements. Unlike their dendritic counterparts, the axons are usually singular and generally are quite long and thin. Many axons are encompassed by a lipoprotein sheath known as myelin and this myelin sheath displays periodic discontinuities referred to as the Nodes of Ranvier At terminal points these axons transmit impulses to the dendrites of other neurons and such sites of contacts between individual neurons are called synapses. In the human nervous system there are approximately 8 billion neurons, all of which display great variability in both size and form. Also, in addition to these 8 billion neurons, there exist 80 billion supportive elements known as glial cells. In view of both the number and complexity of the neurons and their supportive elements, it is readily apparent as to why our present understanding of nervous tissue interaction and function is quite limited.

The following statements are related to the passage. Based on the information given, select:
(A) if the statement is *supported by* the information in the passage.
(B) if the statement is *contradicted by* information in the passage.
(C) if the statement is *neither supported nor contradicted by* information in the passage.

52. Axons and dendrites are appendages of neuronal cell bodies and as such are structurally and functionally the same.

53. Dendrites greatly increase the neuronal surface area.

54. The neurons and glial cells are structurally and functionally comparable.

55. The site of functional contact between two individual neurons constitutes a synapse.

56. It is clear from the preceding passage that the precise nature of nervous tissue interaction has been completely elucidated.

Local anesthetics are frequently used and because of this widespread clinical use, knowledge concerning the effects of these drugs at the cellular level is desirable. Most local anesthetics produce a cytotoxic effect; tissues that are affected usually degenerate, and the fragments are phagocytized. This process is followed by a phase of regeneration. There is evidence that the severity of the effect—recognized by the size of the lesion produced—varied with the potency of the anesthetic, the concentration of the anesthetic, the route of administration, and the sequence of injections. The significance of potency—that is, the variability of effect produced by different local anesthetics at the same concentration—was clearly demonstrated when tetracaine produced more severe lesions than lidocaine which in turn produced more severe lesions than procaine. The severity of the lesion increased as the concentration increased. Differences in route of injection were apparent as more severe lesions were produced following intramuscular injection of the anesthetic when compared with subcutaneous injection. Muscle degeneration and subsequent regeneration is found irrespective of the sequence of injection (as for example, one large dose or two smaller doses). No muscular damage has been found following an injection when the same volume of physiologic saline, instead of the anesthetic, is administered. Limited information is available concerning the effect of local anesthetics on enzyme activity in the highly ordered metabolic machinery of the cell.

The following statements are related to the passage above. Based on the information given, select:
(A) if the statement is *supported by* the information in the passage.
(B) if the statement is *contradicted by* the information in the passage.
(C) if the statement is *neither supported nor contradicted by* information in the passage.

57. All local anesthetics are alike.

58. Local anesthetics are used more often by dentists than physicians.

59. Potency and concentration may be considered one and the same.

60. Severity of lesion and concentration show a direct relationship.

61. Physiologic saline can provide the same effects as an anesthetic.

62. General anesthesia does not result in any damage.

63. Tissues are sensitive to local anesthetics.

Because protons and neutrons are found in the nucleus of an atom, they are referred to collectively as nucleons. The number of protons of an atom determines its atomic number. All atoms of the same element have the same number of protons and, therefore, the same atomic number. Atoms of different elements have different atomic numbers. Thus, the atomic number identifies the element. The English scientist Henry Moseley first determined the atomic numbers of the elements.

Since the actual mass of a proton or a neutron is a very small number when expressed in grams, scientists use atomic mass units instead. An atomic mass unit (amu) is defined as 1/12 the mass of a carbon atom with 6 protons and 6 neutrons. Thus, the mass of each proton or neutron is 1 amu, and the mass of any atom is expressed relative to the mass of the carbon atom.

The sum of the number of protons and neutrons is called the mass number. Since only protons and neutrons are used to find the mass of the atom, the mass number also represents the mass of an atom in atomic mass units.

64. The atomic number of an element is determined by its
  (A) number of nucleons.
  (B) number of neutrons.
  (C) number of protons.
  (D) number of neutrons minus the number of protons.
  (E) number of protons minus the number of neutrons.

65. An atomic mass unit is equal in mass to
  (A) 1 hydrogen atom.
  (B) 1/12 of a carbon atom.
  (C) 1 carbon atom.
  (D) 1/5 of a hydrogen atom.
  (E) 1/2 of an oxygen atom.

66. The scientist who first determined the atomic numbers of the elements came from
  (A) England.
  (B) Russia.
  (C) France.
  (D) the United States.
  (E) Sweden.

67. The sum of the protons and neutrons is called the
  (A) atomic number.
  (B) atomic charge.
  (C) mass unit.
  (D) mass number.
  (E) atomic weight.

68. If atomic number is subtracted from mass number, the result is the number of
  (A) neutrons.
  (B) protons.
  (C) electrons.
  (D) nucleons.
  (E) amus.

SKILLS ANALYSIS: QUANTITATIVE

85 MINUTES
68 QUESTIONS

The following questions are to be answered based on your knowledge of basic mathematical principles and relationships.

DIRECTIONS: Read each passage carefully, study each table or chart, then answer the questions following it. Consider only the material presented in answering the questions. Eliminate those choices that you think to be incorrect and mark the letter of your choice on the answer sheet.

Diet	Losing Weight	Mortality
Balanced Diet	4%	2%
Diet A	90%	74%
Diet A + Vitamin C	84%	72%
Diet A + Vitamin B	4%	2%
Diet A + Vitamin A	88%	76%

Groups of 50 mice were fed the diets listed in the table, and the percentage losing more than 10% of their initial body weight and the percentage mortality after 30 days were recorded.

1. The study was designed to determine
   (A) what vitamins are missing from a balanced diet.
   (B) what vitamins aid in losing weight.
   (C) what vitamins were missing from diet A.
   (D) what mice need that humans do not.

2. The best conclusion to be drawn from this study is that
   (A) diet A is a good reducing diet.
   (B) diet A lacks B vitamins.
   (C) vitamin C is not necessary for life.
   (D) vitamin A is necessary for life.

3. The difference between percentage losing weight and percentage mortality within each group is best explained by
   (A) individual variation among mice within each group.
   (B) variations in importance of the different vitamins.
   (C) the fact that the effectiveness of vitamins is reduced by purification and later addition to food.
   (D) the fact that some mice were overweight and therefore were not resistant.

The epiphyseal cartilage plate is very sensitive to somatotrophin (growth hormone) and, therefore, can be used as an assay for this compound. Species variations exist and other hormones such as estrogen, thyroxine, and several antibiotics also have an effect upon cartilage growth. The assay must be carried out on hypophysectomized animals.

The following experiments were conducted as can be seen from the table:

Test Groups	No. of Animals	Cartilage Growth in μ	
		1 Injection Daily	2 Injections/Day (½ amount each time)
Control (normal) (saline)	20 (10/injecting group)	100	100
Hypophysectomized (saline)	20	60	60
Hypox + 100 mg STH	20	150	160
Hypox + 300 mg STH	20	180	195
Stressed normal animals (saline)	20	175	190
Hypox & stressed (saline)	20	50	50
Stressed normal + 100 mg STH	20	200	210
Hypox, stressed + 100 mg STH	20	110	120

4. The reason the assay must be carried out on hypophysectomized rats is
   (A) just to add another sophisticated method to the experiment.
   (B) because the pituitary produces its own growth hormone and it might interfere with the assay.
   (C) to study the pituitary composition of growth hormone.
   (D) to obtain the animals' own growth hormone.

5. These experiments show
   (A) the route of administration was critical.
   (B) the route of administration made no difference.
   (C) the route should be adjusted from procedure to procedure.
   (D) none of the above.

6. Twice daily administration proved to be
   (A) less effective in eliciting a response.
   (B) more effective in eliciting a response.
   (C) of no great consequence in the experiment.
   (D) none of the above.

7. Stressed animals
   (A) do not need growth hormone.
   (B) produce substances that act like growth hormone.
   (C) produce growth hormone that has an additive affect upon stress factors.
   (D) both B and C.

The following experimental protocol was carried out. Bean seeds were picked for their uniformity and 20 were planted/pot. One hundred percent germination was observed; and when the seedlings were 9 days old, the seedlings of uniform growth were selected for treatment with X-rays. Four hundred r units/minute were applied at a distance of 30 cm from the object. Seedlings were exposed up to 60 minutes with up to 24,000 r. After exposure, seedlings were placed in a greenhouse and kept at uniform light, temperature, and moisture conditions. Seedlings were measured as indicated in the table.

CODE

I	II
1 From ground to cotyledon (a mark was made on the seedling near the ground with india ink)	A 0 minutes — control
	B 7.5 minutes — 3,000 r
2 Cotyledon to 1st node	C 15 minutes — 6,000 r
3 Petiole length of 1st leaf	D 30 minutes — 12,000 r
4 Midrib of 1st leaf	E 60 minutes — 24,000 r
5 From 1st node to tip of the plant (when included).	

EXPERIMENTAL RESULTS

	10 Days					17 Days					33 Days				
	A	B	C	D	E	A	B	C	D	E	A	B	C	D	E
1	6.20	6.58	7.30	5.45	4.43	7.08	6.73	8.00	6.99	5.82	7.21	6.73	8.00	7.00	6.05
2	2.17	2.16	2.30	1.15	.76	8.06	7.11	5.36	2.50	1.63	8.07	7.11	5.48	2.65	1.65
3	.87	1.11	1.10	0.65	.53	4.12	4.50	4.15	2.13	1.70	4.33	4.61	4.86	2.30	1.90
4	3.00	3.23	3.02	2.03	1.86	5.44	5.27	5.68	5.33	4.97	5.50	5.50	6.13	5.91	5.25
5											12.56	11.38	5.27		

8. The purpose of this experiment was
   (A) to observe the germination rate.
   (B) to check for uniform growth rate.
   (C) test output and scatter of the X-ray machine.
   (D) observe X-ray effect on growth.

9. At the termination of the experiment the plants that had received 3000 r units were only 2.66 cm shorter than the controls. What was the height of the control plants?
   (A) 25.11
   (B) 27.84
   (C) 37.67
   (D) 18.06

10. When 12,000 r units were employed, plant growth did not go beyond the first node and these plants were 18.19 cm shorter than the controls. Growth from the mark on the stem to the cotyledon was comparable to that in control plants, but growth beyond the cotyledon was greatly diminished. Which of the following is true?
    (A) This cannot be determined from the data given.
    (B) These statements are absolutely correct.
    (C) Too many assumptions are made.
    (D) All of the above are confusing statements.

11. As seen from the table, the plants exposed to 24,000 r units show a marked effect. Growth from the cotyledon to the first node is greatly decreased. This was the part most affected; the midrib lengths were not affected. Which of the following is true?
    (A) The statements are unfounded.
    (B) The statements are partly correct.
    (C) The statements are correct.
    (D) Too many assumptions are made.

Both sexes carry a complete complement of sex-linked genes. A female, however, with the XX arrangement will only exhibit a recessive gene if she has received it from both parents (a rare event if we are dealing with an uncommon gene of the population); while in the male with the XY arrangement the recessive gene cannot be masked since there is no partner X chromosome and, therefore, a larger number of recessive genes are expressed (examples are hemophilia and color blindness). A man receives his X chromosome from his mother and passes it on to his daughters not his sons. His daughters in this respect are the carriers of his sex-linked traits and their sons will be the affected ones. Let us illustrate with an example. The normal czarinas of Russia produced sons suffering from hemophilia, a disease that is caused by a sex-linked recessive gene, h. The more dominant gene, H, produces normal blood clotting. Genotypically, these women must have carried Hh (X_H and X_h). A daughter, depending on the father (X_HY or X_hY), could have carried X_HX_h or X_HX_H while a son could have been born either with an X_HY or a X_hY (hemophilic) chromosomal complement.

The following statements are related to the information presented above. Based on the information given, select:
   (A) if the statement is *supported by* the information given.
   (B) if the statement is *contradicted by* the information given.
   (C) if the statement is *neither supported nor contradicted by* information given.

12. A cattle breeder has in a herd a Y-linked trait. A male calf sired by a bull carrying this trait is born. The chances of the inheritance of the trait are 50%.

13. A female calf was born; the chances of exhibiting the trait are zero.

14. If the sex in the above cross is known, there is no doubt about whether a calf has the trait.

15. All males would exhibit the trait.

16. Females in this case would not be the carriers of this trait.

Melanoma tumors were implanted into three strains of mice. Experiments were then performed to determine the types and amounts of host serum antibodies produced against the lipid components of the virus contained in the melanoma cells. The results are summarized in the table below.

Host	Ag A Phenotype	Mg Equivalent Day 40 Post Implant	Antilipid Antibody Day 60 Post Implant
Strain 1	3/3	4.5 ± 0.3	6.3 ± 1.7
Strain 2	1/3	3.4 ± 0.4	5.5 ± 1.3
Strain 3	1/1	1.3 ± 0.1	1.3 ± 0.3

The following statements are related to the information presented above. Based on the information given, select:

   (A) if the statement is *supported by* the information given.

   (B) if the statement is *contradicted by* the information given.

   (C) if the statement is *neither supported nor contradicted by* information given.

17. Strain 1 produced less antilipid antibody at both time periods measured than the other two hosts.

18. On the basis of this information, Strain 1 animals are less resistant to melanoma-type cancers than either Strain 2 or 3 animals.

19. All three hosts produced more antibody at 60 days than they did at 40 days.

20. An Ag A phenotype containing three seems to be related to higher antibody production.

21. If it has a 1/3 Ag A phenotype, a mouse resulting from a cross of Strain 2 with one of Strain 3 would probably be a better antibody producer than a sibling having a 1/1 Ag A phenotype.

During wound healing, proliferation of cells in epithelial tissues, connective tissues, and vascular tissues occurs in order to fill in and resurface the defect caused by necrotic (dead) tissue. In experimental studies of the cellular kinetics of wound healing, it is often necessary to assess the amount of proliferation in various cell populations. Because cells replicate DNA within 8 to 12 hours before dividing, determination of the frequency of DNA synthesis at a particular time among cells in a population is a good index of the rate of cell division. DNA synthesis can be determined by tagging replicating DNA with radioactive thymidine. By the procedure of autoradiography, the nuclei of cells which have incorporated radioactive thymidine can be identified on histological sections. The percentage of cells labeled with radioactive thymidine is called the labeling index.

The following table includes data on the labeling index of endothelial cells which form the lining of blood vessels.

[3]H-THYMIDINE INDEX IN WOUND HEALING

Wound Age	Amount of Epidermal Resurfacing	Endothelial Labeling Index
1 day	0%	3.5%
2 days	0%	13.3%
3 days	0-5%	10.5%
6 days	60-70%	5.6%
10 days	90-100%	2.5%

The following statements are related to the information presented. Based on the information given, select:

    (A)   if the statement is *supported by* the information given.
    (B)   if the statement is *contradicted by* the information given.
    (C)   if the statement is *neither supported nor contradicted by* information given.

22. The ³H-thymidine labeling index, and hence the amount of endothelial proliferation, increased before epidermal resurfacing had become evident.

23. The endothelial labeling index, after day two, decreased both with advancing wound age and with advancing surface coverage.

24. The increased endothelial proliferation at two and three days led to the formation of new blood vessels, which then induced epidermal resurfacing.

25. Endothelial proliferation ceases when the wounds are 90-100% resurfaced with epidermis.

26. Synthesis of DNA may not lead to cell division, but rather may lead to an increase in the ploidy of the cell.

Androgen compounds are responsible for maintaining the secondary sex organs and characteristics of organisms. An endocrinology class was divided into 4 groups to conduct a blind experiment and at the end was asked to compare results. Each group received a compound and injected a similar amount. The experimental protocol in male animals was: 1) Unoperated control animals; 2) Unoperated control animals receiving vehicle only; 3) Bilaterally castrated (testes) animals; and 4) Bilaterally castrated animals receiving unknown. The results were summarized in table form.

Experimental Groups	Prostate Weight-mg Student Groups				Seminal Vesicle Weight-mg Student Groups			
	1	2	3	4	1	2	3	4
Unoperated Control	33	31	29	34	68	65	63	67
Unoperated Control and Vehicle	31	32	30	31	69	70	65	64
Bilaterally Castrated	10	9	7	8	12	14	10	15
Bilaterally Castrated and Unknown	37	33	28	31	70	64	61	59

The following statements are related to the information presented above. Based on the information given, select:

    (A)   if the statement is *supported by* the information given.
    (B)   if the statement is *contradicted by* the information given.
    (C)   if the statement is *neither supported nor contradicted by* information given.

27. Different compounds were used by the different groups.

28. The compounds used were in the androgen group.

29. The parameters used were not the proper ones.

30. The prostate gland is most sensitive to a lack of androgens.

31. These experiments were not properly controlled.

32. The results obtained are probably not statistically significant.

33. When these data are plotted on graph paper, it is found that the percentage of increase in organ weight corresponds to a dose relationship.

34. Bilateral castration removes a major source of sex hormones.

35. In the absence of the testes, the hypophysis exhibits an increased production of gonad stimulating hormones.

36. The absence of androgens affects the behavior of the animal.

In the laboratory experiment, red blood cells were placed into 0.5M solutions and the appearance of the solutions was observed two hours later with the naked eye.

Solution	Cells
0.5M glucose	no change
0.5M sucrose	no change
0.5M urea	hemolysis of RBCs
0.5M glycerol	hemolysis of RBCs

37. How can the solutions of urea and glycerol be described with respect to the red blood cells?

(A) isotonic   (C) hypertonic

(B) hypotonic   (D) none of the above

38. The reason for these results is that:

1. the number of particles in the urea and glycerol solutions is greater than that in the glucose and sucrose solutions.
2. glucose and sucrose form coatings around the red blood cells which prevent their breaking.
3. glucose and sucrose enter the cells but are immediately metabolized, therefore water does not enter the cells.
4. urea and glycerol can enter the cell, water follows them into the cell because it is then in greater concentration outside.

(A) 1 and 2   (C) 3 and 4

(B) 1 and 3   (D) 4

39. The property of the cell membrane that allows for this phenomenon to be demonstrated is called

(A) diffusion.   (C) impermeability.

(B) osmosis.   (D) semipermeability.

A 75-kg person and a 1-kg steel ball fall simultaneously from an airplane 5000 feet above ground level. The following graph and table summarize the kinetic data for the first few seconds of the fall.

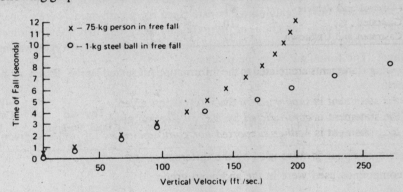

Time of Fall (sec.)	Vertical Velocity (ft./sec.)		Distance of Fall (feet)	
	Person	**Steel Ball**	**Person**	**Steel Ball**
1	32	32	32	
2	64	64	96	
3	96	96	192	
4	115	128	307	
5	126	160	433	
6	141	192	574	
7	152	224	726	
8	159	256	895	
9	163		1058	
10	166		1224	
11	169		1393	
12	170		1563	

40. The greatest increase in downward velocity for the person occurs
   (A) during the first 5 seconds of the fall.
   (B) between 3 and 6 seconds of the fall.
   (C) between 6 and 9 seconds of the fall.
   (D) between 8 and 12 seconds of the fall.

41. Comparing the first 5 seconds with seconds 8-12 of the person's fall, the later velocity changes can be explained by
   (A) the force of gravity being greater than atmospheric resistance.
   (B) the force of gravity being less than atmospheric resistance.
   (C) atmospheric resistance approaching the acceleratory force of gravity.
   (D) none of the above.

42. After 7 seconds of the fall, how far is the steel ball from the person (vertical distance)?
   (A) 96 feet   (C) 144 feet
   (B) 108 feet   (D) 170 feet

43. Assuming the person's velocity does not change after 12 seconds (170 ft./sec.), the person will hit the ground
   (A) 20 seconds after start of the fall.
   (B) 24 seconds after start of the fall.
   (C) 32 seconds after start of the fall.
   (D) Cannot be calculated from data provided.

44. The person will hit the ground how many seconds after the steel ball? (Assume ball's velocity remains constant after 8 seconds of fall).
   (A) 6 seconds   (C) 9 seconds
   (B) 8 seconds   (D) 11 seconds

Gerbils were used for this experiment. One group served as a control; one group was thyroidectomized and maintained on 1% calcium gluconate since the parathyroids were probably removed also; one group received daily injections of thyroxin; and one group that was thyroidectomized and maintained as described above also received daily injections of thyroxin. Oxygen was measured in a standard manner. The following were the results.

Groups	Initial Body Weight gm	Final Body Weight gm	Thyroid Gland Weight mg	Liter of O_2 Consumed hour/ meter^2
Normal	143	150	5.0	1.54
Hypothyroid	160	174	0.0	0.16
Hyperthyroid	123	120	8.0	7.33
Hypothyroid + thyroxin	164	158	4.9	1.23

The following statements are stated on the information presented above. Based on the information given, select:
   (A) if the statement is *supported by* the information given.
   (B) if the statement is *contradicted by* the information given.
   (C) if the statement is *neither supported nor contradicted by* information given.

45. The quantity of heat liberated by an organism as calculated on the basis of respiratory exchange is decreased by deficiencies and elevated by excesses of the active thyroid principle.

46. After total thyroidectomy the basal metabolic rate falls to 10% of its normal value.

47. Hypothyroid animals probably exhibited sluggishness.

48. Hypothyroidism is accompanied by a depression of the oxidative processes in the tissues and slight obesity probably due to the relatively slow burning of the consumed food.

49. Thyroxin probably is the active thyroid principle.

50. Animals can be made hyperthyroid if given thyroxin.

51. In thyroidectomized animals, glucose absorption is slower in the intestinal tract.

A manufacturer is testing a newly designed line of autoclaves that will be marketed. Calibration of timers and temperature controls is critical to insure destruction of bacteria.

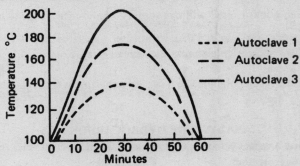

52. Bacteria X requires a minimum of 140°C for at least 20 minutes to be destroyed. Which is (are) the only autoclave(s) that can accomplish that task?

(A) autoclave 1
(B) autoclave 1 and 2
(C) autoclave 2 and 3
(D) autoclave 3

53. Virus Y requires 180°C or more. The technician would not place material in

(A) autoclave 1.
(B) autoclave 1 and 2.
(C) autoclave 2 and 3.
(D) autoclave 3.

54. Bacteria Z will only grow when the temperature is below 160°C. Therefore to be destroyed it can not be put into

(A) autoclave 1.
(B) autoclave 1 and 2.
(C) autoclave 2 and 3.
(D) autoclave 3.

The pineal complex is implicated in the modulation of reproductive functions of the golden hamster. Surgical removal of the eyes produced atrophy of the testes and seminal vesicles within four to six weeks, and simultaneous pinealectomy prevented the atrophy. In the following experiment the drug MTPH was injected subcutaneously daily for 30 days to learn if there was an enhancement of atrophy. The results are summarized below.

Treatment	Number of Hamsters Treated	Organ Weight (mg/100 g body weight)	
		Testes	Seminal Vesicles
Untreated Control	6	2884	722
Blinding	6	1695[a]	396[a]
Pinealectomy	6	2600	544
Blinding, Pinealectomy	6	2580	577
MTPH, No Surgery	6	3069	699
MTPH, Blinding	6	1419[a]	398[a]
MTPH, Pinealectomy	6	2875	591
MTPH, Blinding, Pinealecomy	6	2635	577

[a]($p < 0.05$)

The following statements are related to the information presented above. Based on the information given, select:

(A) if the statement is *supported by* the information given.
(B) if the statement is *contradicted by* the information given.
(C) if the statement is *neither supported nor contradicted by* information given.

55. Drug MTPH increased the testicular atrophy in blinded hamsters when compared with blinded hamsters not receiving MTPH.

56. Drug MTPH increased the seminal vesicle atrophy in blinded hamsters when compared with blinded hamsters not receiving MTPH.

57. Drug MTPH had no effect on atrophy, either testicular or seminal vesicles.

58. Drug MTPH had no effect on the weights of testes or seminal vesicles.

59. Drug MTPH when administered without surgery would affect reproductive organ weight.

The table represents the results obtained in a certain experiment analyzing hydrocarbon A with a new fluorometric procedure.

ANALYSIS OF HYDROCARBON A

Sample	Hydrocarbon A Concentration, mole/ml	Fluorescence in delta units	Determinations
Blank	0.00	0.00	40
1	2.95×6^{-14}	1.26 ± 0.24	40
2	4.12×6^{-14}	2.21 ± 0.35	40
3	7.36×6^{-14}	3.48 ± 0.48	40
4	10.63×6^{-14}	4.84 ± 0.60	40
5	14.79×6^{-14}	6.67 ± 0.67	40
6	22.21×6^{-14}	10.14 ± 0.54	40
7	29.50×6^{-14}	13.42 ± 0.61	40

The following statements are related to the information presented above. Based on the information given, select:

(A) if the statement is *supported by* the information given.
(B) if the statement is *contradicted by* the information given.
(C) if the statement is *neither supported nor contradicted by* information given.

60. The table represents data for multiple analyses of hydrocarbon A exhibiting a range of 3×6^{-14} to 30×6^{-14} mole/ml.

61. Average deviations varied from 20% for the lowest concentration to 5% for the highest.

62. The variations in the blank obviously affected the reliability of the analysis more at the higher concentrations.

63. A fluorescence of 53.68 units corresponds to a hydrocarbon A concentration of 118×10^{-14} mole/ml.

The graph represents the vapor pressure curves of three substances. The boiling point of each of these liquids is defined as the temperature at which its vapor pressure equals atmospheric pressure. The *normal* boiling point is the temperature at which the vapor pressure equals *standard* atmospheric pressure.

Vapor Pressure Curves

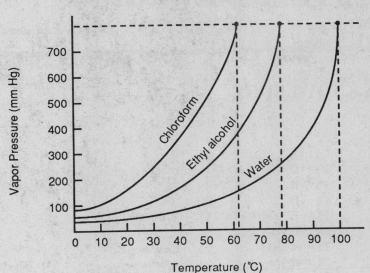

64. Compared to the vapor pressures of chloroform and water, the vapor pressure of ethyl alcohol is
    (A) constant.
    (B) greater than either.
    (C) greater than that of chloroform, but less than that of water.
    (D) less than either.
    (E) less than that of chloroform, but greater than that of water.

65. In degrees Celsius, the normal boiling point of chloroform is approximately
    (A) 50.   (D) 100.
    (B) 61.   (E) 760.
    (C) 78.

66. The graph indicates that standard atmospheric pressure, in millimeters of mercury (Hg), is
    (A) between 0 and 100.
    (B) less than 760.
    (C) 100.
    (D) 760.
    (E) greater than 100, but less than 760.

67. At the top of a mountain where atmospheric pressure is less than standard atmospheric pressure, the boiling point of water is
    (A) less than its normal boiling point.
    (B) more than its normal boiling point.
    (C) the same as that of chloroform and that of ethyl alcohol.
    (D) the same as that of chloroform.
    (E) the same as that of ethyl alcohol.

68. At what atmospheric pressure would the boiling point of water equal the normal boiling point of ethyl alcohol?
    (A) 100   (D) 700
    (B) 300   (E) 760
    (C) 500

Model Test D Answers*

SCIENCE KNOWLEDGE

Biology

1.	C	9.	D	17.	A	25.	A	33.	C
2.	D	10.	C	18.	C	26.	B	34.	A
3.	A	11.	B	19.	B	27.	B	35.	B
4.	B	12.	D	20.	B	28.	B	36.	E
5.	C	13.	E	21.	B	29.	E	37.	E
6.	B	14.	D	22.	C	30.	B	38.	D
7.	B	15.	A	23.	C	31.	A		
8.	E	16.	C	24.	A	32.	B		

Chemistry

1.	B	9.	D	17.	A	25.	E	33.	C
2.	B	10.	B	18.	E	26.	B	34.	D
3.	A	11.	A	19.	A	27.	D	35.	B
4.	D	12.	D	20.	C	28.	D	36.	A
5.	B	13.	D	21.	D	29.	D	37.	A
6.	C	14.	A	22.	A	30.	A	38.	B
7.	C	15.	B	23.	C	31.	B		
8.	B	16.	A	24.	C	32.	C		

Physics

1.	A	8.	E	15.	A	22.	E	28.	D
2.	B	9.	A	16.	C	23.	A	29.	D
3.	C	10.	C	17.	A	24.	B	30.	C
4.	A	11.	E	18.	B	25.	D	31.	D
5.	D	12.	D	19.	E	26.	A	32.	D
6.	D	13.	D	20.	B	27.	B	33.	A
7.	C	14.	D	21.	B				

SCIENCE PROBLEMS

1.	B	13.	B	25.	A	37.	D	49.	D
2.	B	14.	B	26.	D	38.	E	50.	D
3.	B	15.	D	27.	B	39.	A	51.	E
4.	E	16.	E	28.	E	40.	D	52.	A
5.	E	17.	D	29.	E	41.	C	53.	B
6.	A	18.	A	30.	D	42.	D	54.	C
7.	C	19.	E	31.	D	43.	A	55.	E
8.	B	20.	D	32.	C	44.	A	56.	B
9.	D	21.	E	33.	A	45.	C	57.	C
10.	B	22.	D	34.	E	46.	D	58.	A
11.	A	23.	D	35.	A	47.	A	59.	A
12.	C	24.	D	36.	A	48.	A	60.	A

SKILLS ANALYSIS: READING

1.	B	15.	C	29.	C	43.	C	56.	B
2.	B	16.	B	30.	A	44.	A	57.	B
3.	A	17.	A	31.	B	45.	C	58.	C
4.	A	18.	B	32.	B	46.	A	59.	B
5.	C	19.	A	33.	A	47.	A	60.	A
6.	B	20.	A	34.	B	48.	A	61.	C
7.	C	21.	B	35.	C	49.	C	62.	C
8.	C	22.	A	36.	C	50.	A	63.	A
9.	A	23.	A	37.	A	51.	B	64.	C
10.	A	24.	C	38.	B	52.	B	65.	B
11.	A	25.	C	39.	A	53.	A	66.	A
12.	C	26.	C	40.	C	54.	C	67.	D
13.	B	27.	A	41.	B	55.	A	68.	A
14.	A	28.	B	42.	B				

SKILLS ANALYSIS: QUANTITATIVE

1.	C	15.	A	29.	B	43.	C	56.	B
2.	B	16.	A	30.	B	44.	C	57.	A
3.	A	17.	B	31.	B	45.	A	58.	A
4.	B	18.	C	32.	B	46.	A	59.	B
5.	D	19.	B	33.	B	47.	A	60.	A
6.	B	20.	A	34.	A	48.	A	61.	A
7.	B	21.	A	35.	C	49.	A	62.	C
8.	D	22.	A	36.	C	50.	A	63.	C
9.	B	23.	A	37.	B	51.	C	64.	E
10.	C	24.	C	38.	D	52.	C	65.	B
11.	C	25.	B	39.	D	53.	B	66.	D
12.	A	26.	C	40.	A	54.	A	67.	A
13.	A	27.	B	41.	C	55.	B	68.	B
14.	A	28.	A	42.	D				

Explanation of Answers for Science Questions-Model Test D

SCIENCE KNOWLEDGE

Biology

1. **(C)** Hyaluronidase is an enzyme carried by sperm, capable of hydrolysis of hyaluronic acid, promoting fertilization (penetration of sperm). Hyaluronidase is medically used to promote the diffusion and absorption of many injected medications.

2. **(D)** During meiosis in the female one functional gamete (egg) and three polar bodies are produced.

3. **(A)** Control of these functions is due to crossing of the fibers, and control of the right side is by the left cerebral hemispheres.

4. **(B)** The interstitial cells are stimulated be ICSH (interstitial cell stimulating hormone) a gonadotrophin of the pituitary to produce androgens. Testosterone is an androgen.

5. **(C)** Progesterone is produced by the corpus luteum.

6. **(B)** Between 3 to 4 ml of semen comprise one ejaculate which contains between 300-400 million sperm cells.

7. **(B)** The adrenal medulla can be considered to house the post ganglionic neurons for part of the sympathetic portion of the autonomic nervous system and is responsible for epi- and norepinephrine production.

8. **(E)** A mutation may be thought of as a sudden change in the genetic make up of the organism. It may be beneficial or harmful. It may occur spontaneously or may be experimentally produced with chemicals, X-rays, cosmic rays, etc. It may not be passed on to the next generation because, or example, it may be lethal or otherwise preclude reproduction.

9. **(D)** A sarcomere is the region between two Z bands. In simple terms we are dealing with this unit: ZIAHAIZ. Contraction of the sarcomeres due to the fine filaments (actin) sliding between the thick filaments (myosin) pulling the Z bands which

they are attached with them. This pulls the Z bands closer together, and so the sarcomeres are shortened.

10. **(C)** A bacteriophage is a virus that is a parasite of bacteria; sometimes lysis of the bacterial cell is a result.

11. **(B)** Hemophilia, a frequent disease of the royal houses of Europe, is a bleeding disorder transmitted through a sex-linked recessive gene. It results in abnormal coagulation; hemophilia A is the classical true hemophilia resulting from a deficiency of factor VIII.

12. **(D)** Genotype refers to the genetic makeup of the organism. The genotype is expressed via phenotypic characteristics that are visible and observable under normal circumstances.

13. **(E)** Humans are very well protected against the dangers of their surroundings. The external layer of skin is practically impermeable; it protects against trauma, bacteria, drying, water penetration, ultraviolet light, noxious agents, etc. White blood cells are influential in the mobilization of the immunological machinery of the body and also have the capability to engulf bacteria, etc., and destroy them. After an antigen enters the organism the immune system counters by producing antibodies to neutralize the effect and in many cases to protect the organism against susceptibility to the same agent in the future (the basis of immunization).

14. **(D)** An allele is one of a pair of genes that occupies the same locus on homologous chromosomes.

15. **(A)** The chemical mediator of cholinergic nerve impulses is acetylcholine and is released by the axon terminals.

16. **(C)** The ABO blood grouping system is explained on the basis of a single triallelic system with genes A, B, and O operating at a single genetic locus. Phenotypic and genotypic characteristics may be expressed as follows:

Phenotype	Genotype
A	A/A; A/O
B	B/B; B/O
O	O/O
AB	A/B

The A and B genes appear to be codominant; they are dominant over O, which is recessive.

17. **(A)** See explanation for question 16.

18. **(C)** The inferior vena cava empties into the right atrium, carries deoxygenated blood, and blood pressure is low at that point.

19. **(B)** Acromegaly is a result of pituitary oversecretion of growth hormone. Lack of iodine will result in goiter development of the thyroid gland. Rickets is due to a vitamin D deficiency. A skin rash is not a specific lesion that can be associated with only one specified cause as the others listed.

20. **(B)** Trypsin is the enzyme that is functional in protein digestion. Ptyalin (salivary amylase) acts on starches while pancreatic lipase (steapsin) acts on fats. Maltose is not an enzyme but a sugar.

21. **(B)** In skeletal muscle the nuclei are found peripherally. To complete the chart the speed of contraction should also be mentioned. Skeletal muscle is the fastest working, smooth the slowest, and cardiac muscle occupies an intermediate position.

22. **(C)** Identical twins arise from the same egg. One egg is fertilized by one sperm and a splitting (separation) occurs during the early cleavage divisions. Fraternal twins arise from the fertilization of two eggs, each by one sperm. Identical twins always are the same sex. Fraternal twins may be of either sex (50-50 proposition).

23. **(C)** While on the pill no new eggs are produced; the female is kept in the progestational phase (second half) of the menstrual cycle.

24. **(A)** Osmosis is a process in which solvent passes from an area of lower solute concentration to an area of higher solute concentration. In dialysis solvent and solute both pass through the membrane.

25. **(A)** Any substance that has the capability to elicit an immunological response, such as the production of antibody that is specific to that substance is considered an antigen.

26. **(B)** Vasectomy involves an interruption of the spermatic cords (vas deferens) in the male.

27. **(B)** After the secretion of sweat, evaporation of this product is the key to the cooling of the organism. In an environment of high humidity the effectiveness of this mechanism is decreased.

28. **(B)** Acromegaly and (or) giantism is due to overactivity of the alpha cells of the pituitary which secrete growth hormone. If a person is affected before puberty, he or she will develop into a fairly well proportioned giant. After maturity, an increase in the size of the hands and feet and massive development of the bones comprising the face are consequences. In the adult strictly speaking the term acromegaly must be applied to this condition.

29. **(E)** The question lists the most important features.

30. **(B)** Most researchers feel that the interstitial cells of Leydig of the seminiferous tubules are the source of androgen and possibly testicular estrogen. The most potent androgen is testosterone.

31. **(A)** Glucagon is released into the bloodstream in response to diminishing blood sugar levels. The main action of glucagon is to promote liver glycogenolysis; as a consequence glycogen stores of the liver diminish. Epinephrine secreted by the adrenal medulla has the same general effect. Epinephrine is an important factor in the normal organism for counteracting the hypoglycemic action of insulin.

32. **(B)** Impeded or sluggish venous blood flow, especially of the veins of the lower extremity, can lead to the formation of blood clots. The disease, thrombophlebitis, is characterized by an inflammation of veins with thrombosis.

33. **(C)** The releasing factors that have been isolated and identified to date are produced in hypothalamic areas.

34. **(A)** One of the main functions of the large intestine is the reabsorption of water.

35. **(B)** Hyperventilation is abnormally rapid, deep breathing resulting in a loss of CO_2 and an increase in blood pH. A person would be in the state of respiratory alkalosis since a decreased blood concentration of hydrogen ion is the result of pulmonary CO_2 elimination.

36. **(E)** Heart beat is initiated by the S-A (sino-atrial) node.

37. **(E)** The epidermal layer of skin is typically about 20 to 30 cells thick, or about 250 micrometers.

38. **(D)** Prothrombin is a plasma precursor to the clotting fibrin; platelets provide a phospholipid needed as a cofactor for clotting reactions; vitamin K is necessary for the synthesis of prothrombin and other clotting factors.

Chemistry

1. **(B)** Amino acids represent the basic structure of proteins.

2. **(B)** $\emptyset N_2{}^+Br^- + H_2 \xrightarrow{\text{catalyst}} \emptyset\text{-NH-NH}_2$

3. **(A)** In DNA there are principally 4 nitrogen bases: adenine, thymine, guanine, and cytosine. In RNA uracil is present instead of thymine. During transcription of RNA from DNA, the DNA bases of adenine, thymine, guanine, and cytosine will pair with the RNA bases of uracil, adenine, cytosine, and guanine, respectively.

4. **(D)** $CaC_2 + 2H_2O \rightarrow C_2H_2 + Ca(OH)_2$

5. **(B)** $H_2O + Na \rightarrow H_2 + NaOH$

6. **(C)** During the production of electricity the two half-cell reactions of the storage battery are
$Pb + SO_4{}^{2-} \rightarrow PbSO_4 + 2e^-$
$PbO_2 + 4H^+ + SO_4{}^{2-} + 2e^- \rightarrow PbSO_4 + 2H_2O$
During recharging of the battery the two half-cell reactions are reversed.

7. **(C)** Silver ions will react with chloride ions and precipitate as AgCl.

8. **(B)** The three organic products of this Wurtz reaction and n-hexane, n-butane, and ethane. On the basis of probability only, the butane should represent 50% of the product on a molar basis.

9. **(D)** See explanation for question 8.

10. **(B)** $H_2S \rightleftarrows 2H^+ + S^{2-}$. By the common ion effect, lowering the pH (increasing the H^+ concentration) will lower the S^{2-} concentration by displacing the reaction to the left. $K_i = \dfrac{[H^+]^2[S^{2-}]}{[H_2S]}$. If $[H^+]$ increases, $[S^{2-}]$ must decrease.

11. **(A)** Freezing point depression in water depends only on the number of solute particles per unit volume
$1\,M$ NaCl $= 2 \times 1 \times 6.02 \times 10^{23}$ particles per liter
0.3 $Na_2SO_4 = 3 \times .03 \times 6.02 \times 10^{23}$ particles per liter
1.5 M glucose $= 1 \times 1.5 \times 6.02 \times 10^{23}$ particles per liter
$0.5\,M$ $BaSO_4 = 2 \times 0.5 \times 6.02 \times 10^{23}$ particles per liter
Dividing by 6.02×10^{23} we can see that the comparative figures are NaCl, 2; Na_2SO_4, 0.9; glucose, 1.5; and $BaSO_4$, 1.0. Thus, the NaCl solution has the greatest number of particles per unit volume (considering the ionization of NaCl, Na_2SO_4 and $BaSO_4$), and it will have the lowest freezing point.

12. **(D)** A reaction in which electrons (e^-) are removed is termed an oxidation reaction; the adding of electrons to an atom or molecule is termed a reduction reaction.

13. **(D)** A yellow precipitate of iodoform is produced in this reaction with methyl ketones, alcohols that may be oxidized to methyl ketones, or acetaldehyde.

14. **(A)** The hydronium ion, H_3O^+, is a protonated water molecule. $2H_2O \rightleftarrows H_3O^+ + OH^-$

15. **(B)** The alpha helix contributes to the secondary structure of proteins, but not all proteins (nor all regions of proteins) contain the alpha helix secondary structure.

16. **(A)** As long as the volume units are the same, $N_1V_1 = N_2V_2$
$$V_2 = \frac{N_1V_1}{N_2} = \frac{(50)(0.25)}{0.50} = 25 \text{ ml}$$

17. **(A)** Cyclopropane, containing 3 carbon atoms, is the smallest organic ring compound.

18. **(E)** Enzymes are influenced by:
temperature
1. inactivated usually above 60°C
2. rate of reaction is controlled as in any chemical reaction; the rate is approximately doubled by each 10°C increase
3. low temperatures slow the reaction
pH
there is an optimum pH for every reaction

concentration
the rate of a reaction is directly proportional to the amount of enzyme present in relation to substrate. If a coenzyme or specific activator is required, that substance may control the overall rate of the reaction also

poisons
some enzymes themselves can be harmful to the organism but they are also susceptible to compounds like cyanide, etc., which inactivate them

19. **(A)** This is a definition of the zwitterion; an example is the amino acid, glycine.

20. **(C)** Lye soap was produced in earlier days by boiling animal fat with lye. This process of forming the salt of fatty acids by treating a fat with alkali is called saponification.

21. **(D)** The different isomers are 1,1; 1,2; 1,3; 2,2; 1,4; and 2,3. There might appear to be other possibilities; but 2,4 is more properly 1,3 and 3,4 is more properly 1,2.

22. **(A)** Markovnikov's rule predicts that in the absence of peroxides the addition of hydrogen halide across a double bond will occur with hydrogen being added to the carbon, which already contains the most hydrogen. In the presence of peroxides, however, a free radical mechanism results in hydrogen bromide being added in the opposite orientation.

23. **(C)** The starting compound may be pictured as

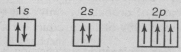

Monobromination in the 3, 5, or 6 position will produce different compounds. The identity of the alkyl groups is not important since ring monobromination was specified.

24. **(C)** $I_2 + 2S_2O_3^{2-} \rightarrow 2I^- + S_4O_6^{2-}$. Iodine is being reduced. Iodine (i.e., I_2) but not iodide (i.e., I^-) reacts with starch to form a blue complex.

25. **(E)** Hemoglobin is the oxygen carrier in red blood cells of all vertebrates. With carbon monoxide hemoglobin forms carboxyhemoglobin. The binding capacity (affinity) of hemoglobin for carbon monoxide is over 100 times that of the binding capacity for oxygen.

26. **(B)** Helium has a higher density and cost than hydrogen, but it is much safer. Hydrogen readily escapes through tiny holes, and if ignited, it reacts quite readily with oxygen. Helium is essentially inert chemically.

27. **(D)** This information should be learned.

28. **(D)** Anaerobic oxidation is far less efficient than aerobic oxidation. Pasteur showed that fermentation can take place in the absence of air. The common equations are written in the following manner:
Aerobic respiration:
$C_6H_{12}O_6 + 6O_2 \rightarrow 6H_2O + 6CO_2$ + Energy (673 calories)
Anaerobic respiration (Alcoholic Fermentation):
$C_6H_{12}O_6 \rightarrow 2C_2H_5OH + 2CO_2$ + Energy (25 calories)

29. **(D)** Low molecular weight mercaptans have a very unpleasant odor even in low concentration. They are added to give an odor to the odorless natural gas. This is quite helpful in detecting leaks and thus avoiding explosions.

30. **(A)** Conversion of glycogen to glucose-1-phosphate is catalyzed by the enzyme, phosphorylase. Pancreatic amylase is usually not in contact with glycogen (except dietary glycogen); in any case it would not catalyze the formation of glucose-1-phosphate.

31. **(B)** This precipitate reacts with acid or base and, therefore, is amphoteric. It could be aluminum hydroxide.
$Al(OH)_3 + 3H^+ \rightarrow Al^{3+} + 3H_2O$
$Al(OH)_3 + OH^- \rightarrow Al(OH)_4$

32. **(C)** See explanation for question 31.

33. **(C)** Transuranium elements are those having more than the 92 protons of uranium. Several may be produced by neutron bombardment of lighter elements such as uranium.

34. **(D)** The electron is the negatively charged particle that forms part of an atom outside the nucleus.

35. **(B)** Electrons fill orbitals in order of increasing energy level. In a given sublevel, a second electron will not enter any orbital until all orbitals in that sublevel have one electron. In this atom, the electrons will fill the orbitals as follows:

1s	2s	2p
↑↓	↑↓	↑ ↑ ↑

36. **(A)** The heat of fusion is defined as the number of calories needed to change one gram of a substance from the solid to the liquid phase at its melting point. During phase change, the temperature and pressure remain constant. Phase change is a physical change.

37. **(A)** In 1 mole of $CuSO_4 \cdot 5H_2O$ there are 5 moles of H_2O. Therefore, in 0.250 mole of the hydrate there are 1.25 moles of water.

38. **(B)** The first reaction $CO_2 + H_2O \rightarrow H_2CO_3$ is a synthesis reaction.
The second reaction $2HgO \xrightarrow{\Delta} 2H_g + O_2\uparrow$ is a decomposition reaction.
The third reaction $Zn + CuSO_4 \rightarrow ZnSO_4 + Cu$ is a single replacement reaction.
The fourth reaction $HCl + NaOH \rightarrow NaCl + H_2O$ is a double replacement reaction (as well as a neutralization reaction).

Physics

1. **(A)** At a uniform acceleration of 9.8 m/s^2 the body goes from 0 to 9.8 m/s in the first second and from 9.8 to 19.6 m/s at the end of the 2nd second of fall.

2. **(B)** The amount of heat needed to raise the temperature by 1 degree Celsius of 1 gram of substance is known as specific heat.

3. **(C)** Use $f = ma$, where $m = 60$ kg and $f = 300$ N.
$a = f/m = 300$ N$/60$ kg
$a = 5$ m/s^2

4. **(A)** $F = ma$ if $m =$ mass of body and $a =$ constant. Since both m and a are constant, F must be constant.

5. **(D)** $PE = mgh = (10$ kg$)(9.8$ m/s$^2)(9$ m$) = 882$ J.

6. **(D)** $KE = \frac{1}{2}mv^2$
$KE_0 = \frac{1}{2}m_0v_0^2$
Increase m_0 to $3m_0$, increase v_0 to $3v_0$, then:
$KE = \frac{1}{2}(3m_0)(2v_0)^2$
$KE = \frac{1}{2}(12)(m_0v_0^2)$
Therefore KE will be multiplied by 12.

7. **(C)** The direction of the force exerted against a surface by a fluid at rest is normal or perpendicular to the surface.

8. **(E)** The statement is known as Boyle's law.

9. **(A)** Efficiency $= \dfrac{\text{useful work output}}{\text{work input}} \times 100\%$, by definition, or,
Efficiency $= \dfrac{\text{actual mechanical advantage}}{\text{theoretical mechanical advantage}} \times 100\%$

10. **(C)** Speed of sound $(v) = \dfrac{\text{distance } (x)}{\text{time } (t)}$ where $x = 1000$ m and $s = 333$ m/s.
$v = x/t$, therefore
$t = x/v$
$t = \dfrac{1000 \text{ m}}{333 \text{ m/s}} = 3$ seconds

11. **(E)** Energy of a wave is proportional to the square of its amplitude.

12. **(D)** The umbra is that portion of a shadow which does not receive light from any part of the light source.

13. **(D)** Work = force × distance; the force is the weight of the object = $(100$ kg$)(9.8$ m/s$^2) = 980$ N. Then the work is $(980$ N$)(3$ m$) = 2940$ J.

14. **(D)** Diverging (or concave) lenses produce virtual images for all distances of the object from the lens. The convex (or converging) lens produces a virtual image only when the object distance from the lens is less than one focal length.

15. **(A)** When resistors are connected in parallel, their combined resistance is less than the smallest resistance. Since the smallest resistance here is 2 ohms, the equivalent resistance of all three must be less than 2 ohms.

16. **(C)** For an object starting from rest the velocity at any time is equal to the product of the acceleration due to gravity and the elapsed time:
$v = gt$
$= (9.8$ m/s$)(3.0$ s$)$
$= 29.$ m/s

17. **(A)** This is an example of the Doppler effect. As the distance between the listener and the source of the constant-frequency sound increases, the frequency heard by the listener decreases. This is so because fewer cycles reach the listener per second as a result of the increasing distance; each part of the cycle has to travel a greater distance than the preceding part.

18. **(B)** If you think in terms of a right triangle, you may recognize this as an application of the 3–4–5 right triangle, with the sides being 6–8–10. If not, sketch a right triangle in which the hypotenuse is the resultant force of 10. N and one of the other sides is 6.0 N. In a right triangle the square of the hypotenuse is equal to the sum of the squares of the other two sides:
$(10. \text{ N})^2 = (6.0 \text{ N})^2 + F^2$
$F = 8.0$ N

19. **(E)** All of the above are true statements regarding the banking of a roadbed.

20. **(B)** Use $x = v_0 + \frac{1}{2}at^2$ where $x =$ distance of fall, $v_0 =$ initial velocity $= 0$, $a =$ acceleration, 9.8 m/s^2, and $t = 1$ second.
$x = 0 + \frac{1}{2}at^2$
$x = (\frac{1}{2})(9.8)(1)^2$
$x = 4.9$ m

21. **(B)** $F = ma$ where $F = 440$ N, $m = ?$, and $a = 10$ m/s^2
$m = F/a = \dfrac{440 \text{ kg} \cdot \text{m/s}^2}{10 \text{ m/s}^2}$
$m = 44$ kg

22. **(E)** All the statements are correct concerning the application and characteristics of Newton's law of universal gravitation.

23. **(A)** $\sum F_x = 45 - 40 = 5$ N

(40 subtracted from 45 because the forces are in direct opposition to one another).

24. **(B)** Lowering the center of gravity increases the stability of the table lamp.

25. **(D)** The six devices known as simple machines are: inclined plane, lever, pulley, screw, wedge, and wheel-and-axle.

26. **(A)** $KE = \dfrac{mv^2}{2}$, where $KE = 2500$ joules, $m = 50$ kg, and $v = ?$

$$2500 = \frac{50}{2}(v^2)$$
$$100 = v^2$$
$$v = 10 \text{ m/s}$$

27. **(B)** The fluid must speed up on entering the narrow pipe. Bernoulli's theorem states that pressure goes down when velocity goes up.

28. **(D)** Specific gravity is numerically equal to density, so long as density is measured in g/cm^3.

29. **(D)** Definition of surface tension.

30. **(C)** The smoother the surface, the more regularly reflecting the surface is. Mirrors are smooth enough that they reflect in a regular fashion.

31. **(D)** The coefficient of friction depends only on the nature of the two surfaces. As the angle increases, the normal force decreases and the friction gets smaller.

32. **(D)** The potential difference is $80 - 20 = 60$ V, and the current in the 20-Ω resistor is

$$I = \frac{V}{R} = \frac{60 \text{ V}}{20\Omega} = 3\text{A}$$

In a parallel circuit, the other resistor has no effect.

33. **(A)** Velocity depends only on the temperature of the air. Since $v = \lambda v$, doubling the frequency (up an octave) reduces the wavelength to half.

SCIENCE PROBLEMS

1. **(B)** Choose the upward direction as negative and downward as positive. Then $v_0 = 15$ m/s and

$a = 9.8$ m/s^2 at $t = 3$ seconds, $x = ?$
$x = v_0 t + \frac{1}{2}at^2$
$x = (-15)(3) + (\frac{1}{2})(9.8)(3)^2$
$x = -45 + 44.1$
$x = -0.9$ m above ground

2. **(B)** What is v?
$v = v_0 + at$
$v = -15 + (9.8)(3)$
$v = -15 + 29.4$
$v = 14.4$ m/s downward

3. **(B)** At highest point $v = 0$, $v_0 = -15$ m/s, $a = 9.8$ m/s^2, and $t = ?$

$v = v_0 + at$
$0 = -15 + 9.8t$
$15 = 9.8t$
$1.53 = t$
$x = (-15)(1.53) + \frac{1}{2}(9.8)(1.53)^2$
$x = -22.95 + (4.9)(2.34)$
$x = -22.95 + 11.47$
$x = 11.48$ m above the ground

4. **(E)** 1,4-dibromo-2-butene and 1,2-dibromo-3-butene would be the products.

5. **(E)** None of these are conjugated dienes.

6. **(A)** The diene removes Br$^+$ from the bromine molecule to form a 1-bromocarbonium ion. The double bond shifts to the 2 position and the positive charge primarily to the 4-position prior to reaction of the carbonium ion with Br$^-$ to form the final product.

7. **(C)** $K = \dfrac{(1.0 - X)/50}{X/50}$

$2 = \dfrac{1.0 - X}{X}$
$2X = 1.0 - X$
$3X = 1.0$
$X = 0.33$ g

8. **(B)** $K = \dfrac{(0.67 - X)/50}{X/50}$

$2 = \dfrac{0.67 - X}{X}$
$2X = 0.67 - X$
$3X = 0.67$
$X = 0.22$ g

9. **(D)** $K = \dfrac{(1.0 - 0.8)/50}{0.8/X} = 2$

$2 = \dfrac{0.2X}{(0.8)(5)}$
$X = \dfrac{(2)(0.8)(50)}{0.2} = 400$ ml

10-12. **(10-B) (11-A) (12-C)** The large spike encountered was probably due to an artifact since if the membrane is unimolecular and the same type of ions are present on the surface of the membrane, the same membrane potential should be existing and the spike should have the same height at all times. The normal impulse is due to an all or none response; there is no gradual (gradient) increase or decrease with respect to neural impulses. External increase in voltage will alter the height of the spike.

13. **(B)** A force diagram of this body would show the following, where F_u = apparent weight, B = buoyant force, and F_d = weight.

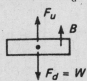

Since there is equilibrium $F_{up} = \Sigma F_{down}$ therefore $F_u + B = F_d$. Knowing F_u and F_d, B is easily established as $F_d - F_u$
$B = 100 \text{ g} - 800 \text{ g}$
$B = 200 \text{ g}$

14. **(B)** In the metric system specific gravity is numerically equal to density. Here the B force = weight of the displaced fluid by definition

$V = \dfrac{B}{d}$

$V = \dfrac{200}{1.25}_{cm^3}$

$V = 160 \text{ cm}^3$ = volume of the body and the displaced liquid.

15. **(D)** To calculate density of body
$\rho = \dfrac{m}{V} = \dfrac{1000}{160} = 6.25 \text{ g/cm}^3$

16. **(E)** By inspection of the graph, the largest number of molecules of a single velocity is at point C. The graph appears symmetrical and thus this would be also the average velocity.

17. **(D)** Both points A and C are improbable according to the graph. Very few molecules would achieve the high velocity represented by point C.

18. **(A)** The peak of the curve (i.e., the most probable velocity) would be shifted to the right, indicating a higher velocity.

19. **(E)** A change in concentration of any of the components of the equilibrium will not change the equilibrium constant for that temperature.

20. **(D)** As stated above, the equilibrium does not change. Thus the concentrations of the other components of the equilibrium must change in the stated directions.

21. **(E)** The equilibrium constant does not change unless temperature changes.

22-24. **(22-D) (23-D) (24-D)** As can be seen from the table, there are four major blood types and the explanation as to universal donor and recipient is based on the following:

Type	Agglutinogens on Cells	Agglutinins in Serum and Plasma
AB — can receive A, B, AB, or O (universal recipient)	A, B	none
A — can receive A, O	A	anti b
B — can receive B, O	B	anti a
O — can receive only O, but can give to all; therefore, O is the universal donor	O	anti ab

25. **(A)** The answer is simple in that we know that $N_r = 1.5$ and $N_l = 1.0$, $\therefore \dfrac{N_r}{N_l} > 1.0$; therefore, the ray of light slows down and bends towards the normal.

26. **(D)** $N = \dfrac{C}{S}$; $\therefore N_r = \dfrac{C}{S_r}$ and $N_l = \dfrac{C}{S_l}$. Substituting in the Snell's law given $\dfrac{\operatorname{Sin} \theta_i}{\operatorname{Sin} \theta_r} = \dfrac{\frac{C}{S_r}}{\frac{C}{S_l}}$

where C = speed of light in vacuum and S_l and S_r are speeds of light in medium. Then $\dfrac{\operatorname{Sin} \theta_i}{\operatorname{Sin} \theta_r} = \dfrac{S_i}{S_r}$

27. **(B)** Using $\dfrac{\operatorname{Sin} \theta_i}{\operatorname{Sin} \theta_r} = \dfrac{S_i}{S_r}$ and knowing that

$S_i = 3 \times 10^8 \text{ m/s}$

$S_r = S_i \left(\dfrac{\operatorname{Sin} \theta_r}{\operatorname{Sin} \theta_i} \right) = (3 \times 10^8) \left(\dfrac{0.500}{0.70} \right)$

$S_r = (3)(.7)(10^8)$
$S_r = 2.1 \times 10^8 \text{ m/s}$

28. **(E)** $PV = nRT$ where P = pressure, V = volume, n = molecules (in the case of helium, atoms) of gas, R = universal gas constant, and T = temperature, K. Since the volumes are equal, $\dfrac{P}{T}$ is proportional to the number of atoms.

$$\dfrac{P_X}{T_X} = \dfrac{760 \text{ torr}}{273 \text{ K}} = 2.78$$

$$\dfrac{P_Y}{T_Y} = \dfrac{1140 \text{ torr}}{410 \text{ K}} = 2.78$$

Without calculating the numbers of atoms, we can see that the numbers are equal. The average velocity will be higher in the container of the higher temperature.

29. **(E)** $\dfrac{PV}{T} = nR$. If n increases, both P and T will increase unless an attempt is made to control one or the other.

30. **(D)** $\dfrac{P_X}{T_X}$ still equals $\dfrac{P_Y}{T_Y}$ so the number of atoms is equal. There is sufficient information to allow a comparison of average velocities of the two gases.

31-33. **(31-D) (32-C) (33-A)** These questions essentially detail the activities carried out during a muscular contraction and are self-explanatory.

34. **(E)** To calculate the potential difference recall that V = potential difference, and $V = IR$ where I = current and R = resistance. In our case
$V = (10)(5)$
$V = 50$ volts

35. **(A)** To calculate the parallel resistance we can use the fact that $\dfrac{1}{R} = \dfrac{1}{R_2} + \dfrac{1}{R_3} + \dfrac{1}{R_4}$

Therefore, $\dfrac{1}{R} = \dfrac{1}{2} + \dfrac{1}{4} + \dfrac{1}{12} = \dfrac{6 + 3 + 1}{12}$
$10R = 12$
$R = 1.2$ ohms

36. **(A)** Again, $V = IR$ as above when $R = 1.2$ ohms and $I = 10$ amps.
$V = (10)(1.2)$
$V = 12$ volts

37. **(D)** The compound must be an aldehyde or ketone based on the first information. It must not be a ketone based on the second test.

38. **(E)** See explanation for question 37.

39. **(A)** Permanganate oxidation would oxidize the unsaturated 2-butene to a glycol. Periodic acid would oxidize the glycol to 2 molecules of acetaldehyde.

40. **(D)** pH $= -\log [H^+] = -\log (1 \times 10^{-4}) = 4$

41. **(C)** $1/10{,}000 = 1 \times 10^{-4}$
$1 \times 10^{-4} \times 1 \times 10^{-4} = 1 \times 10^{-8}$
$(1 \times 10^{-8}) + 1 \times 10^{-7}$ (from water ionization) $= 1.1 \times 10^{-7}$
$-\log (1.1 \times 10^{-7}) = -(-6.96) = 6.96$
Although you could not make this complete calculation without logarithm tables, you should be aware that this small amount of acid would have a small effect on the pH of 7 in water.

42. **(D)** This is essentially a 1:10 dilution with water since the diluted solution (above) is essentially water and the volume of the second dilution is 10 ml to 90 + 10 ml.
$\dfrac{1 \times 10^{-4}}{10} = 1 \times 10^{-5}$
pH $= -\log [H^+] = -\log (1 \times 10^{-5}) = 5$

43-48. **(43-A) (44-A) (45-C) (46-D) (47-A) (48-A)** Let us identify the components of the neuron numbered: (2) nucleus with nucleolus, containing the genetic material of the cell and directing the synthetic activity of the cell; (3) Golgi apparatus (zone), the packaging and concentrating area of the cell's secretory activity; (4) dendrites; dendrites are the processes that pick up an impulse and carry it towards the cell body; (5) endoplasmic reticulum (rough in this case—ribosomes are attached), the synthetic machinery of the cell (proteins etc.,); (6) cell membrane, semipermeable and the protector of the cell from its environment; (7) cytoplasm (specifically the area here is called the axon hillock); (8) myelin sheath (Schwann cell covered by its neurilemma, the insulator of the axon; (9) direction of conduction of an impulse; axons (10a) conduct impulses away from the cell body to the function with the dendrites of another neuron. The junction point is known as the synaptic area; the impulse can cross the synapse only from the axon to the dendrite and no backflow is permitted; (11) terminal branches of the axon. In a lesion (cut) the process distal from the cell body would completely degenerate; retrograde degeneration would be detected in the proximal portion and the cell body, however, the proximal portion has the capacity and will regenerate.

49. **(D)** Using the general gas law $\dfrac{PV}{T} = \dfrac{P_0 V_0}{T_0}$, where $0°C = 273 \text{ K} = T_0$, $5 \text{ m}^3 = V_0$, $1 \text{ atm} = P_0$, $T_r = 293 \text{ K}$, $V = ?$, and $P_r = 1$ atm.

$\dfrac{V}{T} = \dfrac{V_0}{T_0}$

$\dfrac{V}{293} = \dfrac{5}{273}$

$273 V = 1465$

$V = 5.36 \text{ m}^3$

50. **(D)** Again using $\dfrac{PV}{T} = \dfrac{P_0 V_0}{T_0}$, where $V_0 = 5 \text{ m}^3$,

$P_0 = 1$ atm, $T_0 = 273$ K, $V = 2.5 \text{ m}^3$, $P = 4$ atm, and $T = ?$ Solving for T one gets

$$T = \frac{PVT_0}{P_0 V_0} = \frac{(4)(2.5)(273)}{(1)(5)}$$

$$T = \frac{2730}{5} = 546 \text{ K}$$

51. **(E)** All are correct statements and, combined, express Charles' law, Boyle's law, and the general gas law.

52. **(A)** $K_i = \dfrac{[H^+][X^-]}{[HX]} = 1 \times 10^{-7}$

$\dfrac{[H^+][X^-]}{0.1} = 1 \times 10^{-7}$

Since $[H^+] = [X^-]$ in the ionization,
$[H^+][X^-] = [H^+]^2 = 0.1 \times 1 \times 10^{-7} = 1 \times 10^{-8}$
$[H^+] = \sqrt{1 \times 10^{-8}} = 1 \times 10^{-4}$
$\text{pH} = 4$

53. **(B)** $1 \times 10^{-4} \times 0.1 = 1 \times 10^{-5}$
$\text{pH} = 5$

54. **(C)** Ionization constants are useful only at reasonably low concentrations.

55. **(E)** Cholesterol is attached to (or a part of) a number of serum lipoproteins, particularly high-density lipoproteins (HDL), low-density lipoproteins (LDL), very-low-density lipoproteins (VLDL), and chylomicrons.

56. **(B)** LDL cholesterol is considered to be cholesterol on its way to the tissues (from the liver in particular). This cholesterol may be deposited in the circulatory system as part of the development of atherosclerosis. HDL cholesterol is considered to be cholesterol on the way from tissues to the liver. In the liver this cholesterol may be converted to bile acids and released into the bile.

57. **(C)** Cholesterol is required in the body as a precursor of the bile acids (see above), the adrenal steroids, the estrogens, the androgens, and progesterone.

58. **(A)** $s = \frac{1}{2}at^2 = \frac{1}{2}(3 \text{ m/s}^2)(6 \text{ s})^2 = 54$ m

59. **(A)** The unbalanced force is $ma = (10 \text{ kg})(3 \text{ m/s}^2) = 30$ N. The rest of the force, another 10 N, was accounted for by friction.

60. **(A)** $W = Fs = (40 \text{ N})(5 \text{ m}) = 200$ J.

Appendix

LOGARITHMS AND EXPONENTS

Logarithms

The logarithm of any number is the exponent of the power to which 10 must be raised to produce the number. The logarithm X of the number N to the base 10 is the exponent of the power to which 10 must be raised to give N (for example, $\log_{10} N = X$). Logarithms consist of two parts. First, there is the "characteristic," which is determined by the position of the first significant figure of the number in relation to the decimal point. If we count leftwards from the decimal point as positive and rightwards as negative, the characteristic is equal to the count ending at the right of the first significant figure. Thus, the characteristic of the logarithm of 2340 is 3, and of 0.00234 is -3. Second, there is the "mantissa." It is always positive, is found in logarithm tables, and depends only on the sequence of significant figures. Thus, the mantissa for the two numbers is the same, namely 0.3692. The logarithm of a number is the sum of the characteristic and the mantissa. Thus, $\log 2340 = 3.3692$ while $\log 0.00234 = -3 + 0.3692 = -2.6308$.

The logarithms of the whole integers 1 to 10 are given below.

$$\log 1.0 = 0.000 \qquad \log 6.0 = 0.778$$
$$\log 2.0 = 0.301 \qquad \log 7.0 = 0.845$$
$$\log 3.0 = 0.477 \qquad \log 8.0 = 0.903$$
$$\log 4.0 = 0.602 \qquad \log 9.0 = 0.954$$
$$\log 5.0 = 0.699 \qquad \log 10.0 = 1.000$$

Useful Rules in Handling Logarithms

1. The logarithm of a product is equal to the sum of the logarithms of the factors:

$$\log ab = \log a + \log b$$

(Check this out by solving for log 6, using log 2 + log 3.)

2. The logarithm of a fraction is equal to the logarithm of the numerator minus the logarithm of the denominator:

$$\log \frac{a}{b} = \log a - \log b$$

Example:

$$\log \frac{10}{2} = \log 10 - \log 2 = \log 5$$

How about log 2.5? The answer from the log tables is 0.398.

3. The logarithm of the reciprocal of a number is the negative logarithm of the number:

$$\log \frac{1}{a} = \log 1 - \log a$$

Since $\log 1 = 0$, then

$$\log \frac{1}{a} = -\log a$$

Equally,

$$\log \frac{1}{2} = -\log 2 = -0.301$$

4. The logarithm of a number raised to a power is the logarithm of the number multiplied by the power:

$$\log a^b = b \log a$$
$$\log 2^2 = 0.603$$

Exponents

It is convenient to express large numbers as 10^x, where x represents the number of places that the decimal must be moved to place it after the first significant figure. This also represents $10 \cdot 10$ for x times. For example, $1,000,000$ may be expressed as 1×10^6; 3663 as 3.663×10^3; and so on. To multiply, the exponents are added, but coefficients are multiplied. To divide, the exponents are subtracted, but coefficients are divided.

Multiplying: $\quad (1 \times 10^x) \cdot (1 \times 10^y) = 1 \times 10^{x+y}$

$\qquad\qquad\quad (4 \times 10^2) \cdot (2 \times 10^3) = 8 \times 10^5$

Dividing: $\quad (1 \times 10^x) \div (1 \times 10^y) = 1 \times 10^{x-y}$

$\qquad\qquad\quad (4 \times 10^2) \div (2 \times 10^3) = 2 \times 10^{-1}$

Numbers less than 1 are 10^{-x}. For example, 0.000001 is 1×10^{-6}.

Multiplying: $\quad (1 \times 10^{-x}) \cdot (1 \times 10^{-y}) = 1 \times 10^{-(x+y)}$

$\qquad\qquad\quad (4 \times 10^{-2}) \cdot (2 \times 10^{-3}) = 8 \times 10^{-5}$

A large number multiplied by a small number:

$$(4 \times 10^{-2})(2 \times 10^3) = 8 \times 10^1$$

(Logarithms and Exponents are reproduced through the courtesy of Dr. Richard B. Brandt, Dept. of Biochemistry, MCV, VCU, Richmond, Virginia, 23298).

Table of Common Logarithms

Numbers	0	1	2	3	4	5	6	7	8	9
10	0000	0043	0086	0128	0170	0212	0253	0294	0334	0374
11	0414	0453	0492	0531	0569	0607	0645	0682	0719	0755
12	0792	0828	0864	0899	0934	0969	1004	1038	1072	1106
13	1139	1173	1206	1239	1271	1303	1335	1367	1399	1430
14	1461	1492	1523	1553	1584	1614	1644	1673	1703	1732
15	1761	1790	1818	1847	1875	1903	1931	1959	1987	2014
16	2041	2068	2095	2122	2148	2175	2201	2227	2253	2279
17	2304	2330	2355	2380	2405	2430	2455	2480	2504	2529
18	2553	2577	2601	2625	2648	2672	2695	2718	2742	2765
19	2788	2810	2833	2856	2878	2900	2923	2945	2967	2989
20	3010	3032	3054	3075	3096	3118	3139	3160	3181	3201
21	3222	3243	3263	3284	3304	3324	3345	3365	3385	3404
22	3424	3444	3464	3483	3502	3522	3541	3560	3579	3598
23	3617	3636	3655	3674	3692	3711	3729	3747	3766	3784
24	3802	3820	3838	3856	3874	3892	3909	3927	3945	3962
25	3979	3997	4014	4031	4048	4065	4082	4099	4116	4133
26	4150	4166	4183	4200	4216	4232	4249	4265	4281	4298
27	4314	4330	4346	4362	4378	4393	4409	4425	4440	4456
28	4472	4487	4502	4518	4533	4548	4564	4579	4594	4609
29	4624	4639	4654	4669	4683	4698	4713	4728	4742	4757
30	4771	4786	4800	4814	4829	4843	4857	4871	4886	4900
31	4914	4928	4942	4955	4969	4983	4997	5011	5024	5038
32	5051	5065	5079	5092	5105	5119	5132	5145	5159	5172
33	5185	5198	5211	5224	5237	5250	5263	5276	5289	5302
34	5315	5328	5340	5353	5366	5378	5391	5403	5416	5428
35	5441	5453	5465	5478	5490	5502	5514	5527	5539	5551
36	5563	5575	5587	5599	5611	5623	5635	5647	5658	5670
37	5682	5694	5705	5717	5729	5740	5752	5763	5775	5786
38	5798	5809	5821	5832	5843	5855	5866	5877	5888	5899
39	5911	5922	5933	5944	5955	5966	5977	5988	5999	6010
40	6021	6031	6042	6053	6064	6075	6085	6096	6107	6117
41	6128	6138	6149	6160	6170	6180	6191	6201	6212	6222
42	6232	6243	6253	6263	6274	6284	6294	6304	6314	6325
43	6335	6345	6355	6365	6375	6385	6395	6405	6415	6425
44	6435	6444	6454	6464	6474	6484	6493	6503	6513	6522
45	6532	6542	6551	6561	6571	6580	6590	6599	6609	6618
46	6628	6637	6646	6656	6665	6675	6684	6693	6702	6712
47	6721	6730	6739	6749	6758	6767	6776	6785	6794	6803
48	6812	6821	6830	6839	6848	6857	6866	6875	6884	6893
49	6902	6911	6920	6928	6937	6946	6955	6964	6972	6981
50	6990	6998	7007	7016	7024	7033	7042	7050	7059	7067
51	7076	7084	7093	7101	7110	7118	7126	7135	7143	7152
52	7160	7168	7177	7185	7193	7202	7210	7218	7226	7235

53	7243	7251	7259	7267	7275	7284	7292	7300	7308	7316
54	7324	7332	7340	7348	7356	7364	7372	7380	7388	7396
55	7404	7412	7419	7427	7435	7443	7451	7459	7466	7474
56	7482	7490	7497	7505	7513	7520	7528	7536	7543	7551
57	7559	7566	7574	7582	7589	7597	7604	7612	7619	7627
58	7634	7642	7649	7657	7664	7672	7679	7686	7694	7701
59	7709	7716	7723	7731	7738	7745	7752	7760	7767	7774
60	7782	7789	7796	7803	7810	7818	7825	7832	7839	7846
61	7853	7860	7868	7875	7882	7889	7896	7903	7910	7917
62	7924	7931	7938	7945	7952	7959	7966	7937	7980	7987
63	7993	8000	8007	8014	8021	8028	8035	8041	8048	8055
64	8062	8069	8075	8082	8089	8096	8102	8109	8116	8122
65	8129	8136	8142	8149	8156	8162	8169	8176	8182	8189
66	8195	8202	8209	8215	8222	8228	8235	8241	8248	8254
67	8261	8267	8274	8280	8287	8293	8299	8306	8312	8319
68	8325	8331	8338	8344	8351	8357	8363	8370	8376	8382
69	8388	8395	8401	8407	8414	8420	8426	8432	8439	8445
70	8451	8457	8463	8470	8476	8482	8488	8494	8500	8506
71	8513	8519	8525	8531	8537	8543	8549	8555	8561	8567
72	8573	8579	8585	8591	8597	8603	8609	8615	8621	8627
73	8633	8639	8645	8651	8657	8663	8669	8675	8681	8686
74	8692	8698	8704	8710	8716	8722	8727	8733	8739	8745
75	8751	8756	8762	8768	8774	8779	8785	8791	8797	8802
76	8808	8814	8820	8825	8831	8837	8842	8848	8854	8859
77	8865	8871	8876	8882	8887	8893	8899	8904	8910	8915
78	8921	8927	8932	8938	8943	8949	8954	8960	8965	8971
79	8976	8982	8987	8993	8998	9004	9009	9015	9020	9025
80	9031	9036	9042	9047	9053	9058	9063	9069	9074	9079
81	9085	9090	9096	9101	9106	9112	9117	9122	9128	9133
82	9138	9143	9149	9154	9159	9165	9170	9175	9180	9186
83	9191	9196	9201	9206	9212	9217	9222	9227	9232	9238
84	9243	9248	9253	9258	9263	9269	9274	9279	9284	9289
85	9294	9299	9304	9309	9315	9320	9325	9330	9335	9340
86	9345	9350	9355	9360	9365	9370	9375	9380	9385	9390
87	9395	9400	9405	9410	9415	9420	9425	9430	9435	9440
88	9445	9450	9455	9460	9465	9469	9474	9479	9484	9489
89	9494	9499	9504	9509	9513	9518	9523	9528	9533	9538
90	9542	9547	9552	9557	9562	9566	9571	9576	9581	9586
91	9590	9595	9600	9605	9609	9614	9619	9624	9628	9633
92	9638	9643	9647	9652	9657	9661	9666	9671	9675	9680
93	9685	9689	9694	9699	9703	9708	9713	9717	9722	9727
94	9731	9736	9741	9745	9750	9754	9759	9763	9768	9773
95	9777	9782	9786	9791	9795	9800	9805	9809	9814	9818
96	9823	9827	9832	9836	9841	9845	9850	9854	9859	9863
97	9868	9872	9877	9881	9886	9890	9894	9899	9903	9908
98	9912	9917	9921	9926	9930	9934	9939	9943	9948	9952
99	9956	9961	9965	9969	9974	9978	9983	9987	9991	9996

Periodic Table of the Elements

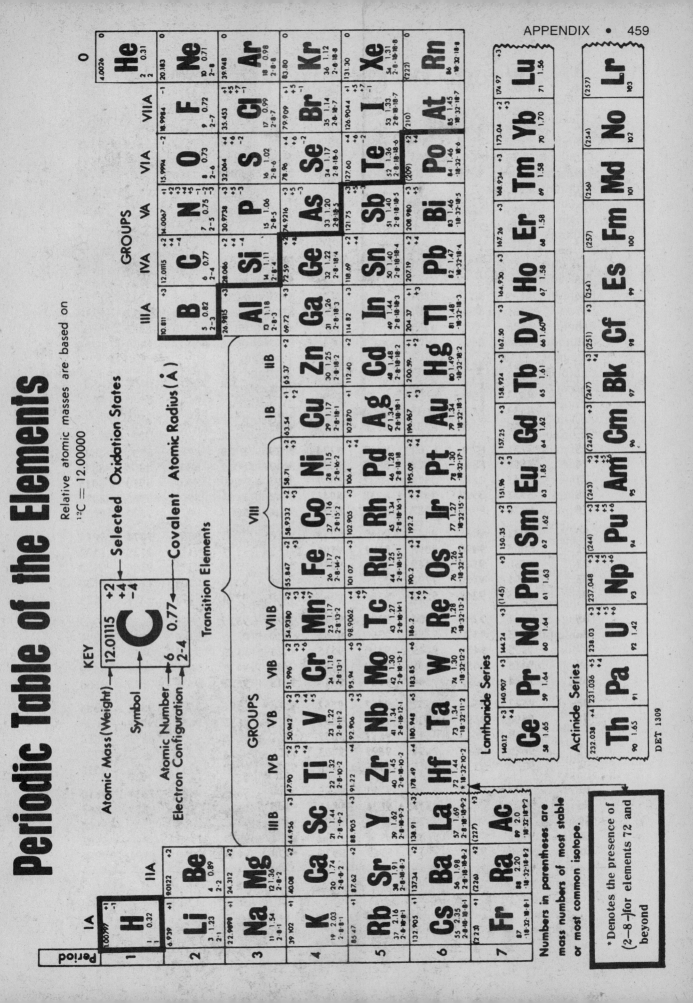

LIST OF ELEMENTS WITH THEIR SYMBOLS

Element	Symbol	Element	Symbol
Actinium	Ac	Mendelevium	Md
Aluminum	Al	Mercury	Hg
Americium	Am	Molybdenum	Mo
Antimony	Sb	Neodymium	Nd
Argon	Ar	Neon	Ne
Arsenic	As	Neptunium	Np
Astatine	At	Nickel	Ni
Barium	Ba	Niobium	Nb
Berkelium	Bk	Nitrogen	N
Beryllium	Be	Nobelium	No
Bismuth	Bi	Osmium	Os
Boron	B	Oxygen	O
Bromine	Br	Palladium	Pd
Cadmium	Cd	Phosphorus	P
Calcium	Ca	Platinum	Pt
Californium	Cf.	Plutonium	Pu
Carbon	C	Polonium	Po
Cerium	Ce	Potassium	K
Cesium	Cs	Praseodymium	Pr
Chlorine	Cl	Promethium	Pm
Chromium	Cr	Protactinium	Pa
Cobalt	Co	Radium	Ra
Copper	Cu	Radon	Rn
Curium	Cm	Rhenium	Re
Dysprosium	Dy	Rhodium	Rh
Einsteinium	Es	Rubidium	Rb
Element 106		Ruthenium	Ru
Erbium	Er	Samarium	Sm
Europium	Eu	Scandium	Sc
Fermium	Fm	Selenium	Se
Fluorine	F	Silicon	Si
Francium	Fr	Silver	Ag
Gadolinium	Gd	Sodium	Na
Gallium	Ga	Strontium	Sr
Germanium	Ge	Sulfur	S
Gold	Au	Tantalum	Ta
Hafnium	Hf	Technetium	Tc
Helium	He	Tellurium	Te
Holmium	Ho	Terbium	Tb
Hydrogen	H	Thallium	Tl
Indium	In	Thorium	Th
Iodine	I	Thulium	Tm
Iridium	Ir	Tin	Sn
Iron	Fe	Titanium	Ti
Krypton	Kr	Tungsten	W
Lanthanum	La	Uranium	U
Lawrencium	Lr	Vanadium	V
Lead	Pb	Xenon	Xe
Lithium	Li	Ytterbium	Yb
Lutetium	Lu	Yttrium	Y
Magnesium	Mg	Zinc	Zn
Manganese	Mn	Zirconium	Zr

Reference Tables for Chemistry

PHYSICAL CONSTANTS AND CONVERSION FACTORS

Name	Symbol	Value(s)	Units
Angstrom unit	Å	1×10^{-10} m	meter
Avogadro number	N_A	6.02×10^{23} per mol	
Charge of electron	e	1.60×10^{-19} C	coulomb
Electron volt	eV	1.60×10^{-19} J	joule
Speed of light	c	3.00×10^8 m/s	meters/second
Planck's constant	h	6.63×10^{-34} J·s	joule-second
		1.58×10^{-37} kcal·s	kilocalorie-second
Universal gas constant	R	0.0821 L·atm/mol·K	liter-atmosphere/mole-kelvin
		1.98 cal/mol·K	calories/mole-kelvin
		8.31 J/mol·K	joules/mole-kelvin
Atomic mass unit	μ(amu)	1.66×10^{-24} g	gram
Volume standard, liter	L	1×10^3 cm^3 = 1 dm^3	cubic centimeters, cubic decimeter
Standard pressure, atmosphere	atm	101.3 kPa	kilopascals
		760 mmHg	millimeters of mercury
		760 torr	torr
Heat equivalent, kilocalorie	kcal	4.18×10^3 J	joules

Physical Constants for H$_2$O

Molal freezing point depression	1.86°C
Molal boiling point elevation	0.52°C
Heat of fusion	79.72 cal/g
Heat of vaporization	539.4 cal/g

STANDARD UNITS

Symbol	Name	Quantity
m	meter	length
kg	kilogram	mass
Pa	pascal	pressure
K	kelvin	thermodynamic temperature
mol	mole	amount of substance
J	joule	energy, work, quantity of heat
s	second	time
C	coulomb	quantity of electricity
V	volt	electric potential, potential difference
L	liter	volume

Selected Prefixes

Factor	Prefix	Symbol
10^6	mega	M
10^3	kilo	k
10^{-1}	deci	d
10^{-2}	centi	c
10^{-3}	milli	m
10^{-6}	micro	μ
10^{-9}	nano	n

RELATIVE STRENGTHS OF ACIDS IN AQUEOUS SOLUTION AT 1 atm AND 298 K	
Conjugate Pairs *ACID* *BASE*	K_a
$HI = H^+ + I^-$	very large
$HBr = H^+ + Br^-$	very large
$HCl = H^+ + Cl^-$	very large
$HNO_3 = H^+ + NO_3^-$	very large
$H_2SO_4 = H^+ + HSO_4^-$	large
$H_2O + SO_2 = H^+ + HSO_3^-$	1.5×10^{-2}
$HSO_4^- = H^+ + SO_4^{2-}$	1.2×10^{-2}
$H_3PO_4 = H^+ + H_2PO_4^-$	7.5×10^{-3}
$Fe(H_2O)_6^{3+} = H^+ + Fe(H_2O)_5(OH)^{2+}$	8.9×10^{-4}
$HNO_2 = H^+ + NO_2^-$	4.6×10^{-4}
$HF = H^+ + F^-$	3.5×10^{-4}
$Cr(H_2O)_6^{3+} = H^+ + Cr(H_2O)_5(OH)^{2+}$	1.0×10^{-4}
$CH_3COOH = H^+ + CH_3COO^-$	1.8×10^{-5}
$Al(H_2O)_6^{3+} = H^+ + Al(H_2O)_5(OH)^{2+}$	1.1×10^{-5}
$H_2O + CO_2 = H^+ + HCO_3^-$	4.3×10^{-7}
$HSO_3^- = H^+ + SO_3^{2-}$	1.1×10^{-7}
$H_2S = H^+ + HS^-$	9.5×10^{-8}
$H_2PO_4^- = H^+ + HPO_4^{2-}$	6.2×10^{-8}
$NH_4^+ = H^+ + NH_3$	5.7×10^{-10}
$HCO_3^- = H^+ + CO_3^{2-}$	5.6×10^{-11}
$HPO_4^{2-} = H^+ + PO_4^{3-}$	2.2×10^{-13}
$HS^- = H^+ + S^{2-}$	1.3×10^{-14}
$H_2O = H^+ + OH^-$	1.0×10^{-14}

Note: $H^+(aq) = H_3O^+$

Sample equation: $HI + H_2O = H_3O^+ + I^-$

CONSTANTS FOR VARIOUS EQUILIBRIA
AT 1 atm AND 298 K

$$H_2O(\ell) = H^+(aq) + OH^-(aq) \qquad K_w = 1.0 \times 10^{-14}$$

$$H_2O(\ell) + H_2O(\ell) = H_3O^+(aq) + OH^-(aq) \qquad K_w = 1.0 \times 10^{-14}$$

$$CH_3COO^-(aq) + H_2O(\ell) = CH_3COOH(aq) + OH^-(aq) \qquad K_b = 5.6 \times 10^{-10}$$

$$Na^+F^-(aq) + H_2O(\ell) = Na^+(OH)^- + HF(aq) \qquad K_b = 1.5 \times 10^{-11}$$

$$NH_3(aq) + H_2O(\ell) = NH_4^+(aq) + OH^-(aq) \qquad K_b = 1.8 \times 10^{-5}$$

$$CO_3^{2-}(aq) + H_2O(\ell) = HCO_3^-(aq) + OH^-(aq) \qquad K_b = 1.8 \times 10^{-4}$$

$$Ag(NH_3)_2^+(aq) = Ag^+(aq) + 2NH_3(aq) \qquad K_{eq} = 8.9 \times 10^{-8}$$

$$N_2(g) + 3H_2(g) = 2NH_3(g) \qquad K_{eq} = 6.7 \times 10^5$$

$$H_2(g) + I_2(g) = 2HI(g) \qquad K_{eq} = 3.5 \times 10^{-1}$$

Compound	K_{sp}	Compound	K_{sp}
AgBr	5.0×10^{-13}	Li_2CO_3	2.5×10^{-2}
AgCl	1.8×10^{-10}	$PbCl_2$	1.6×10^{-5}
Ag_2CrO_4	1.1×10^{-12}	$PbCO_3$	7.4×10^{-14}
AgI	8.3×10^{-17}	$PbCrO_4$	2.8×10^{-13}
$BaSO_4$	1.1×10^{-10}	PbI_2	7.1×10^{-9}
$CaSO_4$	9.1×10^{-6}	$ZnCO_3$	1.4×10^{-11}

STANDARD ENERGIES OF FORMATION OF COMPOUNDS AT 1 atm AND 298 K

Compound	Heat (Enthalpy) of Formation* kcal/mol ($\triangle H_f^o$)	Free Energy of Formation* kcal/mol ($\triangle G_f^o$)
Aluminum oxide $Al_2O_3(s)$	−400.5	−378.2
Ammonia $NH_3(g)$	−11.0	−3.9
Barium sulfate $BaSO_4(s)$	−352.1	−325.6
Calcium hydroxide $Ca(OH)_2(s)$	−235.7	−214.8
Carbon dioxide $CO_2(g)$	−94.1	−94.3
Carbon monoxide $CO(g)$	−26.4	−32.8
Copper (II) sulfate $CuSO_4(s)$	−184.4	−158.2
Ethane $C_2H_6(g)$	−20.2	−7.9
Ethene (ethylene) $C_2H_4(g)$	12.5	16.3
Ethyne (acetylene) $C_2H_2(g)$	54.2	50.0
Hydrogen fluoride $HF(g)$	−64.8	−65.3
Hydrogen iodide $HI(g)$	6.3	0.4
Iodine chloride $ICl(g)$	4.3	−1.3
Lead (II) oxide $PbO(s)$	−51.5	−45.0
Magnesium oxide $MgO(s)$	−143.8	−136.1
Nitrogen (II) oxide $NO(g)$	21.6	20.7
Nitrogen (IV) oxide $NO_2(g)$	7.9	12.3
Potassium chloride $KCl(s)$	−104.4	−97.8
Sodium chloride $NaCl(s)$	−98.3	−91.8
Sulfur dioxide $SO_2(g)$	−70.9	−71.7
Water $H_2O(g)$	−57.8	−54.6
Water $H_2O(\ell)$	−68.3	−56.7

* Minus sign indicates an exothermic reaction.

Sample equations:

$$2Al(s) + \frac{3}{2}O_2(g) \rightarrow Al_2O_3(s) + 400.5 \text{ kcal}$$

$$2Al(s) + \frac{3}{2}O_2(g) \rightarrow Al_2O_3(s) \quad \triangle H = -400.5 \text{ kcal/mol}$$